Treatment Resource Manual

FOR SPEECH-LANGUAGE PATHOLOGY

5th Edition

Froma P. Roth, Ph.D.

Colleen K. Worthington, M.S.

University of Maryland
College Park
Department of Hearing
and Speech Sciences

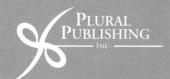

PLURAL
PUBLISHING
INC.

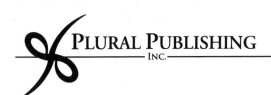

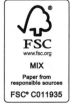

5521 Ruffin Road
San Diego, CA 92123

e-mail: info@pluralpublishing.com
website: http://www.pluralpublishing.com

This book was previously published by: Cengage Learning. Original printing 2015.

Printed in the United States of America by McNaughton & Gunn

Library of Congress Cataloging-in-Publication Data

Names: Roth, Froma P., author. | Worthington, Colleen K., author.
Title: Treatment resource manual for speech-language pathology / Froma P. Roth and Colleen K. Worthington.
Description: 5th edition. | San Diego, CA : Plural Publishing, [2018] | Reprint. Originally published: Clifton Park, NY : Cengage Learning, [2016]. | Includes bibliographical references and index.
Identifiers: LCCN 2018018241| ISBN 9781635501346 (alk. paper) | ISBN 1635501342 (alk. paper)
Subjects: | MESH: Speech Therapy—methods | Language Therapy—methods | Communication Disorders—therapy
Classification: LCC RC424.7 | NLM WL 340.3 | DDC 616.85/5—dc23
LC record available at https://lccn.loc.gov/2018018241

DEDICATION

For **Ilana** and **Eli**, each unique and extraordinary, who continue to
fill my life with light and infinite delight; and to **Graydn Robert ("G")**,
our newest and brightest light.
FPR

For **Leigh-Anne**, the small miracle who remains the heart of my heart.
CKW

Contents

PART ONE   PREPARING FOR EFFECTIVE INTERVENTION

CHAPTER 2

Information Reporting Systems and Techniques 67

PART TWO   PROVIDING TREATMENT FOR COMMUNICATION DISORDERS

CHAPTER 3   Intervention for Articulation and Phonology in Children.......107

List of Tables

Case Examples by Disorder

Disorder	Example Profile	Selection of Therapy Targets	Sample Activities	Helpful Hints
Alaryngeal Speech [Chapter 10]	429	429	429	432
Autism Spectrum [Chapter 6]	289	289	NA	NA
	289	290	NA	NA
	290	290	NA	291
Aphasia [Chapter 7]	316	317	317	NA
	318	319	319	NA
	321	322	322	324
Apraxia of Speech [Chapter 8]	361	361	361	NA
	362	363	363	364
Articulation [Chapter 3]				
Cleft Palate [Chapter 3]	132	133	133	134
Childhood Apraxia of Speech [Chapter 3]	143	144	144	145
Functional [Chapter 3]	119	120	120	NA
	121	121	121	NA
	123	123	124	125
Hearing Impairment [Chapter 3]	137	138	138	140
Phonological [Chapter 3]	125	126	127	NA
	128	129	129	130

TABLE *(Continued)*

Disorder	Example Profile	Selection of Therapy Targets	Sample Activities	Helpful Hints
Dysarthria [Chapter 8]	349	349	349	NA
	350	350	351	NA
	352	352	352	354
Fluency [Chapter 9]	385	385	NA	386
	388	388, 389	388, 389	NA
	390	390, 391	390, 391	NA
	392	392, 393	392, 394	395
Language				
Birth–3 years old [Chapter 4]	174	174	174	175
3–5 years old [Chapter 4]	184	184	185	NA
	187	187	187	189
5–10 years old [Chapter 5]	236	236	237	NA
	242	242	242	NA
10–18 years old [Chapter 5]	246	246	247	NA
	253	253	254	260
Voice [Chapter 10]	417	417	417	NA
	420	420	420	NA
	421	422	422	423

List of Forms and Figures

LIST OF FORMS

LIST OF FIGURES

Preface

The original purpose of this manual was to provide beginning speech-language pathology graduate students with a practical introductory guide to intervention. It also provided practicing clinicians with a single resource for specific therapy techniques and materials for a wide variety of communication disorders. This new edition continues to fulfill these aims and also reflects the changing information and recent advances in the field of speech-language pathology that are essential to address in a text of this kind. The revisions made in the fifth edition constitute substantial changes in content compared to previous editions. Selected examples include: (a) new, comprehensive chapter on autism spectrum disorder (ASD), which includes coverage of a wide variety of treatment approaches; (b) two separate and expanded chapters on adult neurogenic communication disorders; (c) greatly expanded section on treatment for dysphagia; and (d) new section on the Common Core State Standards (CCSS), including the central role of speech-language pathologists (SLPs) and implementation of the CCSS within a Response to Intervention (RTI) instructional model. We have carefully updated each chapter in the areas of treatment efficacy and evidence-based practice to ensure that the book reflects the most current thinking in the research and clinical spheres. Two main factors created the need for a resource of this kind for students. First, speech-language pathology programs across the country are rapidly adopting a pre-professional model of education that minimizes clinical practicum experience at the undergraduate level. Thus, even students with undergraduate degrees in communication disorders are entering graduate school with very little direct knowledge of basic therapy approaches, techniques, and materials. Second, master's programs in speech-language pathology are attracting an increasing number of students with bachelor's degrees in areas other than the hearing and speech sciences. These students enter clinical training without any supporting background. As a result, a genuine need exists for a user-friendly and comprehensive source of effective, practical suggestions to guide beginning clinicians through their first therapy experiences.

Another primary use of this book is as a text for undergraduate- and graduate-level courses in clinical methods. Traditional textbooks for such courses tend to be largely theoretical in nature and lack useful information on how to do therapy. Thus, instructors are often faced with the task of assembling their own clinical materials to complement the text. One of the aims of this text is to provide such supplementary information in a single source. In response to requests from readers, this new edition is accompanied by a premium website containing the forms and appendices in the book for easy download and use.

This manual also was written with the practicing clinician in mind. Speech-language pathologists are handling caseloads/workloads with a broader spectrum of communication disorders than ever before. This trend is occurring in all clinical settings, from hospitals to public schools to early childhood centers. Moreover, there has been a dramatic increase in private practice as a service-delivery model in the field of speech-language pathology. Many practitioners work independently and may not be able to consult readily with colleagues about the management of communication disorders that are outside of their main areas of expertise. This manual can serve as an accessible and reliable source of basic treatment information and techniques for a wide range of speech and language disorders.

The information in this book is based on existing knowledge about communication disorders and available research data, as well as the combined clinical experiences of the authors. It is not intended as a cookbook approach to intervention. The complexities of communication disorders preclude such a parochial approach. The therapy targets and activities we have included are meant to serve as illustrations of basic intervention practice, and only as starting points in the therapeutic process. By their very nature, therapy programs for communication disorders should be designed to accommodate each client's unique strengths and weaknesses as well as individual learning styles.

TEXT ORGANIZATION

The manual is organized into two main sections. The first section (Chapters 1 and 2) covers basic principles of speech-language intervention and information reporting systems. The second section includes eight chapters (Chapters 3–10) devoted to therapy strategies for specific communication disorders. Each of these chapters includes a brief description of the disorder, example case profiles, specific suggestions for the selection of therapy targets, and sample therapy activities. These have been designed to illustrate the most common characteristics of a given disorder, as well as typical approaches to treatment. Each chapter concludes with a set of helpful hints on intervention and a selected list of commercially available therapy materials.

The second section also includes Chapter 11, which offers practical suggestions for beginning clinicians regarding effective client and family counseling skills. Finally, the book concludes with Chapter 12, which presents discussion and guidelines regarding multicultural issues in speech-language interventions. Reference tables, charts, and reproducible forms are included throughout the manual.

The focus of this manual is on the most common characteristics and treatment approaches for a given disorder. Unusual or atypical populations are beyond the scope of this book. This book is written from the perspective of Standard American English. The information, procedures, and activities contained in each chapter should be adapted in a culturally appropriate manner.

NEW TO THIS EDITION

This fifth edition of our book features many changes that serve two main purposes: (a) update material from the previous edition to reflect current knowledge and practices in the field and (b) respond to feedback and suggestions received from instructors, practitioners, and students. Highlights of the new material contained in this edition include the following:

- New, comprehensive chapter on autism spectrum disorder (ASD) includes discussion of DSM-5 criteria, detailed information on characteristics/severity levels of ASD, and substantial coverage of a wide variety of treatment approaches.

- Information on adult neurogenic communication disorders is expanded and now comprises two separate chapters: Chapter 7, Intervention for Adult Aphasia with Introduction Traumatic Brain Injury (TBI); and Chapter 8, Intervention for Motor-Speech Disorders: The Dysarthrias, Apraxia of Speech, and Dysphagia.

- Greatly expanded information on treatment strategies for aphasia/TBI, including script training, noninvasive electrical brain stimulation, and response elaboration training, as well as a discussion of the principle of neuroplasticity.

- Greatly expanded section on treatment for dysphagia, including postural techniques, oral-motor maneuvers/exercises, sensory stimuli, and dietary modifications.

- New section on the Common Core State Standards (CCSS), including the central role of SLPs, implementation of the CCSS within an RTI instructional model, and the importance of collaborative practices to optimize student achievement.

- Expanded discussion of treatment strategies for young children with language disorders, including a section, with examples, on a new scientifically validated phonological awareness instructional program (*Promoting Awareness of Sounds in Speech, PASS*) for preschool children, including those with communication impairments and English language learners.

- New discussion of theoretical models of human learning as it relates to language development and disorders.

- New or expanded sections on professional issues such as telepractice, coding/reimbursement, and the Health Insurance Portability and Accountability Act (HIPAA).

- Expanded discussion of clinical considerations in multilingual populations with language disorders.

- Updated/expanded information on specific approaches to intervention for articulation and phonology.

- Expanded discussion of characteristics of older students with language-learning disabilities (LLD), including a new section on "transition documentation" for adolescents at the postsecondary level.

- New tables on (1) the stages of cognitive development and (2) gross and fine motor development.

PluralPlus Companion Website

Purchase of Treatment Resource Manual for Speech-Language Pathology, Fifth Edition comes with complimentary access to printable clinical forms on a PluralPlus companion website.

The companion website is located at:

http://www.pluralpublishing.com/publication/trmslp5e
To access the materials, you must register on the companion website and log in using the passcode on the inside front cover of the book.

Acknowledgments

We thank the many people who have contributed their time, efforts, and talents to the preparation of this revised edition. Enormous appreciation is extended to our colleagues who generously shared with us their insights, expertise, and libraries: Vivian Sisskin and Yasmeen Faroqui Shah.

In the previous edition, we acknowledged the invaluable technical support of our colleague, Emily Mineweaser. In this fifth edition, we express our deep gratitude and respect for her extended contribution as co-author of the new section on traumatic brain injury. Emily's content knowledge, her enthusiasm for clinical practice, and her ability to consistently produce excellent work under tight timelines served as a genuine source of inspiration to both of us.

REVIEWERS

Lynette Austin, M.A., Ph.D., CCC-SLP
Licensed Speech Language Pathologist
Associate Professor
Department of Communication Sciences
and Disorders
Abilene Christian University
Abilene, TX

Nancy Carlino, M.A., CCC-SLP
Assistant Professor
Department of Communication Disorders
California University of Pennsylvania
California, PA

Ellen Cohn, Ph.D., CCC-SLP
ASHA Fellow
Professor and Associate Dean for
Instructional Development
School of Health and Rehabilitation
Sciences
University of Pittsburgh
Pittsburgh, PA

Liz DeVelder, M.A., CCC-SLP
SLP Clinic Coordinator
University of South Dakota
Vermillion, SD

Martine Elie, Ph.D., CCC-SLP
Clinic Director
Howard University/Howard University
Speech and Hearing Clinic
Washington, D.C.

Amy J Hadley, Ed. D., CCC-SLP
Associate Professor of Communication
Disorders
Director, Communication Disorders
Program
School of Health Sciences
The Richard Stockton College of New
Jersey
Galloway, NJ

Melanie L. Houk, M.A., CCC-SLP
Assistant Professor
Ball State University
Muncie, IN

Carol Kaminski, M.A., CCC-SLP
Assistant Professor
Department of Communication Disorders
California University of Pennsylvania
California, PA

Janet A Lovet, M.S., CCC-SLP/L
Director of Practice
Saint Mary's College
Notre Dame, IN

Claudia J. Mornout, M.S., CCC-SLP
Clinical Professor
Director of Clinical Education-SLP
Purdue University
W. Lafayette, IN

Hope C. Reed, SLP D, CCC-SLP, C.O.M.
Associate Professor
Communicative Sciences & Disorders
Program
Alabama A & M University
Huntsville, AL

Marla S. Staab, M.S., CCC-SLP
ASHA Fellow
Faculty Emerita
Department of Communication Disorders
Fort Hays State University
Hays, KS

About the Authors

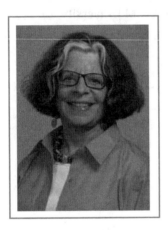

Froma P. Roth

is a Professor Emeritus at the University of Maryland, College Park, Maryland, in the Department of Hearing and Speech Sciences. She currently serves as the Associate Director of Academic Affairs and Research Education at the American Speech-Language-Hearing Association in Rockville, Maryland. Professor Roth received her bachelor's degree from Hunter College, her master's degree from Queens College, and her doctoral degree from the Graduate Center of the City University of New York. Dr. Roth's current research and clinical interests focus on language/literacy and learning disabilities.

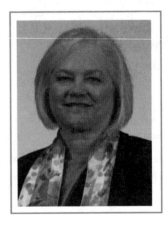

Colleen K. Worthington

is a Clinical Professor and the Director of Clinical Education in Speech-Language Pathology within the Department of Hearing and Speech Sciences at the University of Maryland, College Park. She received her bachelor's degree from the University of Maryland and her master's degree from Loyola College, Baltimore. Ms. Worthington's primary professional interests include articulation/phonology and the supervisory process.

PART ONE

Preparing for

Effective Intervention

CHAPTER 1

PHILOSOPHY

In the field of communication disorders, the domains of research and clinical practice are frequently regarded as distinctly separate entities. It is true that the aims of the two activities are very different. The main purpose of research is to add to the existing knowledge base in a given area, whereas the ultimate goal of clinical work is to change behavior. However, the two activities also share many common characteristics, and these similarities outweigh the differences. The most fundamental similarity is that both research and clinical practice are scientific processes based on the highest quality of evidence available (often referred to as evidence-based practice). Therefore, it is our view that intervention, like research, should be based on the principles of the scientific method. Both research and intervention involve the following:

- Identification of a problem
- Review of existing knowledge regarding the problem area
- Formulation of hypotheses about how to solve the problem
- Manipulation of the independent variable(s)
- Collection and analysis of data
- Formulation of conclusions about the validity of the original hypotheses

Speech and language intervention is a dynamic process that follows a systematic progression. It begins with the diagnosis of a communication disorder and is followed by the selection of appropriate therapy targets. Training procedures are then implemented to facilitate the acquisition of the target behaviors. The intervention process is complete when mastery of these behaviors is achieved. Periodic follow-up is performed to monitor retention and stability of the newly acquired behaviors. Throughout all stages of therapy, advocacy is an important role for the speech-language pathologist (SLP). All clinicians should be aware of the Americans with Disabilities Act (1990). This federal legislation (Public Law 101-336) and its amendments (Public Law 110-325) prohibit discrimination and ensure equal opportunity in public accommodations, employment, transportation, government services, and telecommunications (see www.ada .gov for more specific information). Speech-language pathology is a dynamic profession that is continually evolving. The **scope of practice** in speech-language pathology is delineated by the American Speech-Language-Hearing Association, or ASHA (ASHA, 2007b). SLPs are responsible for fully understanding the areas of communication and swallowing that they are qualified to address (e.g., voice, language, fluency) as well as the range of services that they are eligible to deliver (e.g., screening, consultation, treatment). A related document of major importance to all SLPs is the 2010 **ASHA Code of Ethics** (see Appendix A at the end of this book). This document outlines standards for professional behavior with regard to several areas (e.g., client welfare, SLP competence level, public understanding of the profession).

UNIVERSAL DESIGN PRINCIPLES FOR LEARNING: AN OVERARCHING FRAMEWORK

In 2000, Rose and Meyer put forth a framework based on the premise that every individual, regardless of physical, cognitive, sensory, learning, or other type of disability, is entitled to universal access to information and to learning. Their model is characterized by three universal design principles for learning (UDL): multiple means of representation, multiple means of expression, and multiple means of engagement. As applied to educational and clinical settings, it is meant to be a theoretical framework for providing the most appropriate supports for children and adults and includes:

- *Multiple Means of Representation:* There must be multiple methods available by which individuals can access and learn important information and skills (e.g., traditional textbook supplemented by CD-ROM, speech-to-text media).
- *Multiple Means of Expression:* Various methods and modalities must be available for individuals to demonstrate their mastery of information and skills.
- *Multiple Means of Engagement:* Individuals must be provided with enough successful learning opportunities and meaningful interactions to maintain adequate motivation for learning.

The crux of UDL is instructional flexibility to provide the most suitable options for different learners. For individuals with disabilities, UDL includes accommodations, modifications, and assistive technology. **Accommodations** are changes that help clients overcome or compensate for their disability, such as preferential seating or allowing written rather than spoken communication. **Modifications** are changes in informational content or expectations of an individual's performance. Examples include decreased amount of classwork/homework or reduced goals for productivity or learning.

Also inherent in UDL is the use of **assistive technology (AT)** as supports for students and adults with disabilities (Dalton, Pisha, Eagleton, Coyne, & Deysher, 2002; Hall, Meyer, & Rose, 2012; Ralabate, 2011; Strangman, 2003). AT may include speech-to-text software that converts speech into text documents, translation software for English language learners, and Internet access as a means of information gathering. In all cases, adequate training must be provided so that individuals can use the AT successfully and reliably. We must emphasize that these technologies are supportive and do not replace direct instruction.

General Principles of Intervention

The basic principles of effective intervention are consistent with a UDL framework and apply to clients of all ages and disorders. These include:

- Intervention is a dynamic rather than static process in which the clinician continuously assesses a client's progress toward established goals and modifies them as necessary.
- Intervention programs should be designed with careful consideration of a client's verbal and nonverbal cognitive abilities. Knowledge of a client's level of cognitive functioning is critical to making decisions about eligibility for treatment and selecting appropriate therapy objectives.
- The ultimate goal of intervention is to teach strategies for facilitating the communication process rather than teaching isolated skills or behaviors (to the extent possible). Whereas skills are required to achieve specific outcomes in given situations, strategies enable the individual to know when and how to use these skills in new and varied learning contexts.
- Speech and language abilities are acquired and used primarily for the purpose of communication and therefore should be taught in a communicative context. To the

extent possible, therapy should occur in realistic situations and provide a client with opportunities to engage in meaningful communicative interactions.

■ Intervention should be individually oriented, based on the nature of a client's specific deficits and individual learning style.

■ Intervention should be designed to ensure that a client experiences consistent success throughout all stages of the therapy program.

■ Intervention is most effective when therapy goals are tailored to promote a client's knowledge one step beyond the current level.

■ Intervention should be terminated once goals are achieved or the client is no longer making demonstrable progress.

■ Intervention practices must be based on the best scientific evidence available.

■ Intervention should be sensitive to a client's values and beliefs as well as cultural and linguistic background.

To provide effective intervention for any type of communication disorder, speech-language pathologists must acquire certain essential clinical skills. These skills are based on fundamental principles of human behavior and learning theory. The following categories of clinical skills are the building blocks of therapy and serve as the foundation for all disorder-specific treatment approaches:

■ *Programming:* Selection, sequencing, and generalization of therapy targets

■ *Behavior modification:* Systematic use of specific stimulus-response-consequence procedures

■ *Key teaching strategies:* Use of basic training techniques to facilitate learning

■ *Session design:* Organization and implementation of therapy sessions, including interpersonal dynamics

■ *Data collection:* Systematic measurement of client performance and treatment efficacy

Successful intervention requires the ability to effectively integrate these five parameters into a treatment program. Appendix 1-A at the end of this chapter provides a checklist of clinician behaviors that correspond to each of the parameters. This checklist can be used by students as a guide for observing therapy sessions or by supervisors for evaluating student clinician performance. The remainder of this chapter is devoted to a detailed discussion of each basic skill area.

PROGRAMMING

Programming involves the selection and sequencing of specific communicative behaviors. New behaviors are introduced and taught in highly structured situations with multiple prompts and maximal support provided by the clinician. Subsequent activities progress through a hierarchy of difficulty and complexity, with decreasing support from the clinician. The client demonstrates generalization of each newly learned behavior by using it in novel situations or contexts. The programming process culminates with a client's habitual and spontaneous use of a behavior in everyday speaking and listening situations.

Selection of Therapy Targets

The first step in programming is identification of the communication behaviors to be acquired over the course of the treatment program. These therapy targets are often referred to as **long-term goals.** Initial information about potential therapy targets should be obtained by reviewing the results of previous diagnostic findings. Frequently, assessment data are based, in part, on the administration of standardized tests. These tests typically are designed to sample only one or two exemplars of a given communication behavior. However, a single incorrect response does not constitute a sufficient basis for the inclusion of a behavior as a target in a treatment program. It indicates only a potential area of weakness, which then must be sampled more extensively to determine whether a genuine deficit exists. In addition, it is essential that a clinician consider the client's cultural and linguistic background when identifying potential therapy targets. Speech and language differences arising from dialect usage or a non-English native language do not constitute a communicative disorder. Refer to Chapter 12 for common characteristics of African American English, Spanish-influenced English, and Asian-influenced English.

This sampling is accomplished through the administration of **pretreatment baselines.** Baselines are clinician-designed measures that provide multiple opportunities for a client to demonstrate a given communicative behavior. A good rule of thumb is to include a minimum of 20 stimuli on each pretreatment baseline. The ratio of correct versus incorrect responses is calculated; the resulting percentage is used to determine whether the behavior should be selected as a therapy target. Many clinicians view a performance level of 75% accuracy or higher as an indication that the communication skill in question is not in need of remediation. Baseline measures that fall below the 75% accuracy level represent potential intervention targets. Ultimately, however, the selection of appropriate therapy targets relies heavily on clinical judgment. Some clinicians believe that behaviors that occur with at least 50% accuracy represent targets with the best potential for improvement. Other clinicians argue strongly that behaviors with much lower baseline rates of accuracy may be the most appropriate choices based on individual client characteristics (e.g., intelligibility level, age, and so on).

Often, clients present with several behaviors that qualify as candidates for remediation. For individuals who demonstrate a large number of errors, clinicians may choose a *broad* programming strategy that attacks as many targets as possible in a given time frame. Alternatively, clinicians may select a *deep* programming strategy for clients who demonstrate either relatively few or highly atypical errors. In addition, clinicians typically employ one of two basic approaches for choosing among potential targets: developmental/normative or client-specific.

The Developmental/Normative Strategy. This strategy is based on known normative sequences of communicative behaviors in typically achieving individuals. Therapy targets are taught in the same general order as they emerge developmentally. When two or more potential targets are identified from baseline procedures, the earliest emerging behaviors are selected as the first therapy objectives. Following are two examples that illustrate use of the **developmental** strategy.

A 5-year-old child with an articulation disorder produces the following speech sound errors on baseline procedures:

1. /p/ for /f/ as in *p*inger for *f*inger
2. /t/ for /ʃ/ as in *t*ip for *sh*ip
3. /d/ for /dʒ/ as in *d*uice for *j*uice
4. /d/ for /b/ as in *d*oat for *b*oat

Use of the developmental strategy guides the clinician to select /b/ as the initial therapy target because typically developing children demonstrate mastery of this sound earlier than the others. According to a developmental progression, /f/ is the next logical target, followed by /ʃ/ and /dʒ/.

A 4-year-old child with a language disorder exhibits the following grammatical errors on baseline procedures:

1. Omission of present progressive tense, as in "The boy *play*" for "The boy *is* play*ing*"
2. Omission of the plural marker on regular nouns, as in "I see two *bike*" for "I see two *bikes*"
3. Overgeneralization of regular past tense, as in "He *runned* down the street" for "He *ran* down the street"

Use of the developmental strategy dictates that the first target for therapy is the present progressive form (*is* + *verb* + *-ing*), because it is the earliest of the three structures to emerge. The plural marker is the next behavior to be targeted, followed by the regular past-tense form.

Note: With clients from different cultural/linguistic backgrounds, these grammatical forms may reflect a language difference rather than a language disorder. Therefore, intervention may not be warranted.

The developmental strategy tends to be most effective for articulation and language intervention with children. This strategy has less application for adults and disorders of voice and fluency.

A developmental strategy for target selection should be implemented with careful consideration of at least two factors. The sample population from which the norms were derived may have been too small to permit valid generalization of the findings to other populations. Moreover, the characteristics of the standardization sample (e.g., ethnicity, gender, socioeconomic status) may differ significantly from those of an individual client. Consequently, it may be difficult to draw direct comparisons between the client's performance and the group norms.

The Client-Specific Strategy. Using the **client-specific** strategy, therapy targets are chosen based on an individual's specific needs rather than according to developmental norms. Relevant factors in the selection of treatment objectives include: (1) the frequency with which a specific communicative behavior occurs in a client's daily activities; (2) the relative importance of a specific communicative behavior to the client, regardless of how often it occurs; and (3) the client's potential for mastery of a given communication skill. This last factor addresses the notion of *stimulability*, which is typically defined as the degree to which a client can approximate the correct production of an error pattern on imitation. Following are two examples that illustrate the use of the client-specific strategy.

Mr. Max Asquith, a 52-year-old computer programmer, demonstrates the following speech and language characteristics on pretreatment baseline procedures:

1. Omission of final consonants such as /s/, /k/, and /θ/
2. Distortion of vowels in all word positions
3. Misarticulation of consonant blends such as /br/, /pl/, /fl/, /ks/, and /skw/
4. Omission of the copula forms (*is* and *are*) as in "He sad" for "He is sad"
5. Difficulty with the accurate use of spatial, temporal, and numerical vocabulary
6. Difficulty with subject-verb agreement, especially third-person singular constructions, as in "He *drink* milk" for "He *drinks* milk"

From the client-specific perspective, initial speech intervention targets could consist of /ks/ and /skw/ because these blends occur in the client's name and therefore constitute a high priority for him. An appropriate initial language target for this client would be vocabulary words that convey number concepts because his position as a computer programmer relies heavily on the use of this terminology.

A 6-year-old child with an articulation disorder exhibits the following speech sound errors on baseline procedures:

1. /θ/ for /s/ as in *th*un for *s*un
2. /g/ for /d/ as in *g*uck for *d*uck
3. /w/ for /l/ as in *w*ight for *l*ight
4. /ʃ/ for /tʃ/ as in *sh*ew for *ch*ew

Using the client-specific strategy, the initial therapy target would be /s/, regardless of developmental considerations. The results of stimulability testing conducted during the diagnostic test indicated that this child's ability to imitate /s/ was superior to performance on the other error sounds. In addition, /s/ occurs far more frequently in English than /l/, /w/, and /tʃ/.

Unlike the developmental approach, a client-specific strategy can be implemented across a wide range of communication disorders with both pediatric and adult populations. In addition, a combination of the two strategies is often an effective way to approach therapy target selection for children with speech and language impairments.

Sequencing of Therapy Targets

Following therapy target selection and prioritization, programming involves the development of a logical sequence of steps that will be implemented to accomplish each objective. Three major factors determine the progression of the therapy sequence: *stimulus type*, *task mode*, and *response level*. The following outline presents a hierarchy of complexity for each of these factors.

Stimulus Type (nature of input used to elicit target responses)

1. Direct physical manipulation
2. Concrete symbols
   - Objects
   - Photographs/color pictures
   - Black-and-white line drawings
3. Abstract symbols
   - Oral language
   - Written language

Task Mode (type of clinician support/scaffolding provided to obtain desired responses)

1. Imitation
2. Cue/prompt
3. Spontaneous

Response Level (degree of difficulty of target responses)[1]

1. Increase length and complexity of desired response
   - Isolation
   - Syllable
   - Word
   - Carrier phrase (e.g., "I see a ___.")
   - Phrase
   - Sentence
   - Text (conversation, narration)
2. Decrease latency (actual time) between stimulus presentation and client response

The sequencing process starts with a decision regarding the most appropriate level to begin training on each target behavior. Pretreatment baseline data for a given target are analyzed to determine the entry training level. One rule of thumb that can be used is the following:

- If a client obtained a baseline score lower than 50% accuracy, training on that behavior should begin just below the level of difficulty of the baseline stimulus items.

---

[1]This response level hierarchy pertains to oral responses only. Other response types such as gesture, sign, and writing may require alternative hierarchies of difficulty.

■ If the score was between 50% and 75% accuracy, training can begin at the same difficulty level as the baseline stimuli.

For example, a 5-year-old client scored the following on baseline measures for initial /s/: word level = 65%; carrier phrase level = 40%; and sentence level = 30%. In this example, therapy would begin at the word level of difficulty.

Adherence to these procedures generally will result in a progression of targets at the appropriate levels of difficulty. However, there may be occasions when a client does not perform as predicted; a chosen task turns out to be too difficult or too easy for the individual at this time. The clinician must recognize this situation when it occurs and immediately modify the task rather than persisting with the original plan. This modification is known as **branching** and is achieved by increasing or decreasing the difficulty level by one step according to the therapy sequence hierarchies listed previously.

As the client's performance improves and initial training objectives are mastered, the stimulus type, task mode, and response level should be manipulated systematically to gradually increase the difficulty of therapy tasks until the final criterion is met for a given target. This criterion level is generally set at 90% accuracy or higher in everyday conversational interactions.

The following sample behavioral objectives illustrate the manipulation of each of the three factors.

Behavioral objective: The client will imitatively produce /s/ in the initial position of single words with 90% accuracy while naming 20 photographs.

Modified stimulus type: The client will imitatively produce /s/ in the initial position of single words with 90% accuracy while naming 20 *written* words.

Modified task mode: The client will *spontaneously* produce /s/ in the initial position of single words with 90% accuracy while naming 20 photographs.

Modified response level: The client will imitatively produce /s/ in the initial position of *words in carrier phrases* with 90% accuracy in response to 20 photographs.

Generalization/Carryover

A crucial consideration in programming involves a client's ability to transfer newly mastered communicative behaviors from the clinical setting to the everyday environment. Generalization is enhanced when intervention is provided in the most authentic, realistic contexts possible. Generalization should not be viewed as a distinct event that occurs only in the final phase of the therapy process. Rather, it is an integral part of programming that requires attention from the very beginning. Three main factors can influence the degree to which successful generalization occurs. A variety of **stimuli** (objects, pictures, questions) should be used during therapy activities to avoid tying learning to only a small set of specific stimulus items. Similarly, the clinician should vary the **physical environment** (location in room, location in building, real-world locations) in which therapy occurs as soon as a new target behavior has been established. This will minimize a client's natural tendency to associate target behaviors with a particular setting. Finally, clinicians should bear in mind that target behaviors frequently become attached to the individual who consistently reinforces them (i.e., the clinician). Therefore, it is important to vary the **audience** (familiar adult, sibling, unfamiliar adult) with whom therapy targets are practiced, to maximize the likelihood of successful generalization.

Termination of Therapy

It is difficult to definitively state the point at which intervention services are no longer warranted. At the current time, there are no valid empirical data that can be used to determine appropriate dismissal criteria for any particular communicative disorder. Therefore, it is beyond the scope of this book to indicate realistic time frames for the duration of intervention. General discharge guidelines used by many clinicians include: (1) attainment of communication skills that are commensurate with a client's chronological/developmental age or premorbid status, (2) attainment of functional communication skills that permit a client to operate in the daily environment without significant handicap, and (3) lack of discernible progress persisting beyond a predetermined time period. The authors strongly believe that the establishment of reliable treatment outcome measures is critical in the current climate of professional accountability in both the public and private sectors. Within the past few years, the availability of efficacy data has increased significantly for a variety of communication disorders. This information will be presented throughout the book in pertinent chapters.

Formulation of Behavioral Objectives

Once long-term goals and initial treatment levels have been identified, the clinician develops short-term objectives designed to culminate in the achievement of the selected long-term goals. (In education settings, student progress is measured through *benchmarks*, which are sets of skills required to achieve specific learning standards.) These objectives must be clearly delineated to ensure appropriate and effective intervention programming. A widely used approach to task design is the formulation of **behavioral objectives**. A behavioral objective is a statement that describes a specific target behavior in observable and measurable terms. There are three main components of a behavioral objective:

1. "Do" (action) statement
2. Condition
3. Criterion

The **"do" statement** identifies the specific action the client is expected to perform. Thus, behavioral objectives should contain verbs that denote observable activity; nonaction verbs should be avoided. List 1 contains examples of verbs that are appropriate for inclusion in behavioral objectives; list 2 is made up of verbs that are unacceptable because they refer to behaviors that cannot be observed.

List 1		List 2	
point	say	understand	know
label	write	think	appreciate
repeat	count	learn	remember
match	vocalize	believe	apply
name	ask	improve	comprehend
tell	elevate	discover	feel

An easy way to check the appropriateness of a verb is to ask yourself, "Will I be able to count (tally) how many times this behavior occurs?" (Mowrer, 1988). For example, consider the following pair of statements: (1) "to repeat single syllable words" and (2) "to learn single syllable words." Only the first is an appropriate "do" statement. Number of repetitions can be easily counted, whereas "learning" is a behavior that cannot be directly observed.

The **condition** portion of a behavioral objective identifies the situation in which the target behavior is to be performed. It specifies one or more of the following: when the behavior will occur, where it will be performed, in whose presence, or what materials and cues will be used to elicit the target. Following are common examples of condition statements:

Given the clinician's model

In response to a question from the teacher

In the presence of three classmates

During book report presentation

Given a list of written words

In the home environment

During a job interview

Using pictures

During free play

In the presence of other group therapy members

During storybook reading time

Condition statements are critical parts of behavioral objectives because clients may demonstrate adequate mastery of a communicative behavior in one situation and yet be completely unable to perform the same behavior under different conditions. For example, a client's ability to perform a "do" statement, such as "Produce 1 minute of connected speech without disfluency," is likely to be quite different if the condition statement specifies "while talking to a familiar clinician" versus "while talking to a potential date."

The **criterion** specifies how well the target behavior must be performed for the objective to be achieved. It can be expressed in several ways, including percent correct, within a given time period, minimum number of correct responses, or maximum number of error responses. A list of criterion measures typically used in speech-language therapy follows:

90% accuracy

8 correct out of 10 trials

Less than four errors over three consecutive sessions

80% accuracy over two consecutive sessions

90% agreement between clinician and client judgments

Continuously over a 2-minute period

A well-formulated behavioral objective allows the client, as well as the clinician, to know exactly what the therapy target is, how it is to be accomplished, and what constitutes successful performance. The following examples illustrate how to formulate behavioral objectives.

Example A

1. "Do" statement: Verbally segment words into syllables.
2. Condition: Given a written list of 100 multisyllabic words
3. Criterion: With no more than four errors

Behavioral objective: The client will verbally segment 100 written multisyllabic words into their component syllables with no more than four errors.

Example B

1. "Do" statement: Use a slow rate of speech (four syllables per second).
2. Condition: Reading single sentences
3. Criterion: With 85% accuracy or better over two consecutive sessions

Behavioral objective: The client will use a slow rate of speech (four syllables per second) with 85% accuracy or higher while reading single sentences over two consecutive sessions.

Example C

1. "Do" statement: Say /s/ in the initial position of single words.
2. Conditions: Given the clinician's model
                Name pictures of animals
3. Criterion: With 90% accuracy

Behavioral objective: Given the clinician's model, the client will say /s/-initial single words with 90% accuracy while naming animal pictures.

Additional examples of behavioral objectives and worksheets are provided in Appendixes 1-B and 1-C at the end of this chapter. Appendix 1-D contains a sample Daily Therapy Plan that illustrates the following components of a single session: behavioral objectives, client data, and clinician comments. (A reproducible copy of the Daily Therapy Plan form is provided in Appendix 1-E and on the CD-ROM that accompanies this book, along with a sample form for documenting observation hours in Appendix 1-F.)

THEORIES OF LEARNING

Different philosophies regarding the nature of human learning have led to the development of a variety of theories of how we learn information and skills. Different theories result in different intervention approaches and strategies. No single theory is applicable to all clients. To evaluate how well a model fits a specific client, clinicians may find it helpful to ask themselves the following questions:

Has this approach been evaluated experimentally?

Have the results been favorable?

Has the approach been replicated across settings, clinicians, and clients?

Is the model appropriate for my client? (e.g., cognitive issues, cultural issues)

Can the environment be manipulated to implement procedures that are required for this approach? (e.g., hospital versus school versus clinic)

Is my client improving?

Three of the major theoretical approaches to learning are the innateness/biological model, the behavioral model, and the constructivism model. An overview of each model is presented in the following sections. The behavioral model will be discussed at length in this chapter, and the other models will be incorporated into later chapters as they relate to specific communication disorders.

Innateness Theory/Biological Model (Chomsky, 1965; Fodor, 1975; Piaget, 1973)

The hypothesis is that human beings have an innate predisposition to acquire knowledge. Children use these innate capacities to develop concepts, ideas, and linguistic rules. Exposure to the environment serves as an "on-off" switch that activates the linguistic system.

When applied to clinical intervention:

- Clinical programming follows patterns of typical developmental sequences in areas such as cognition, language, and motor skills.
- Variations of the biological approach stress different facets of development. For example, a cognitive model emphasizes the experiences necessary to activate cognitive capacities, whereas a linguistic model stresses teaching semantic-syntactic relationships.

Behavioral Model (Skinner, 1957)

- The hypothesis is that children learn because their behaviors are selectively rewarded by significant others in their environment. This is the "tabula rasa" view and claims that human minds begin as blank slates and that the environment is the major determinant of learning. In this manner, children's responses to their environmental experiences are gradually shaped through feedback; desirable behaviors are reinforced and unwanted behaviors are faded.

When applied to clinical intervention:

- Clinical programming emphasizes development of functional behaviors without the assumption of a stage-wise progression or prerequisite behaviors.
- There is a heavy reliance on systematic application of behavior-modification techniques such as reinforcement, punishment, and extinction.

Constructivism/Interactionist/Integrative Model (Bruner, 1960; Piaget, 1973; Vygotsky, 1978)

The main hypothesis is that children are biologically predisposed to learn, and their experiences help them to construct knowledge (an integration of the two previous models). Learning is an active process in which children construct ideas and concepts through experience. Learners continuously test and refine knowledge through interactions with others, as well as their environment. This allows the learner to extract unique meaning from information and experiences.

When applied to clinical intervention:

- This model fosters client-centered learning in which learners play an active role.
- Clinical programming is designed as a reciprocal process between clients and clinicians and emphasizes intervention tailored to an individual's specific needs and abilities.
- Because learning is a combination of inborn capacity and extrinsic environmental factors, it can be affected by certain constraints (e.g., attention/memory deficits; severe disabilities). Some individuals with severe disabilities may learn primarily through behavioral principles that emphasize repetition and practice.

Another way of capturing the variation among theoretical approaches is through the lens of a "continuum of naturalness." According to Fey (1985), the continuum represents the degree to which intervention contexts reflect everyday communication situations and interactions (see Figure 1-1). According to this view, intervention approaches fall along a continuum into one of three groups: *clinician-directed, hybrid,* and *client-centered.* In directive strategies, the clinician takes charge of all aspects of therapy, including the selection of goals, therapy materials, procedures, and the order of tasks and target responses to be elicited. Imitation and indirect modeling (response is not expected from the client) are two examples of clinician-directed techniques. Directive approaches are not considered naturalistic because of the degree of clinician control and the absence of natural reciprocal communication.

Client-centered approaches emphasize the use of authentic communication in natural communication situations. In contrast to directive strategies, these approaches involve following the client's lead (waiting for the client to initiate a behavior), treating the client's verbal and nonverbal initiations as intentional communications, and providing natural responses. These approaches are based on the premise that individuals will attain therapy goals more quickly and transfer newly learned behaviors more spontaneously when they are taught in natural contexts using familiar activities. Examples of responsive strategies used with children are expansions, extensions, and recasts (see p. 22 for definitions). For adult clients, two examples of client-centered techniques are functional communication (practicing communication activities of daily living such

FIGURE 1–1
Continuum of naturalness.

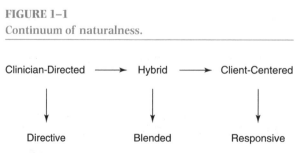

SOURCES: Adapted from Fey, M. (1985); Language intervention with young children. Baltimore, MD: Allyn & Bacon; and the American Speech-Language-Hearing Association (2005).

as making a doctor's appointment) and conversational group therapy with other clients and the clinician. Both of these strategies permit clients to receive natural feedback on the relevance, intelligibility, and appropriateness of their turns from others in the group and the clinician.

Hybrid approaches represent a blending of clinician-directed and client-centered approaches. Hybrid approaches promote generalization by teaching new behaviors in natural environments using behavioral strategies. An example of a hybrid approach that is used with both children and adults is focused stimulation (concentrated exposure to a target form in a natural context, such as reading a book or restaurant menu).

The continuum of naturalness also applies to clients who use assistive technology (AT) to augment their speech production capabilities and those who rely completely on alternative modes of communication (AC) because speech is not a realistic communication mode. These accommodations are known collectively as AAC.

BEHAVIOR MODIFICATION

The fundamental purpose of intervention is to either increase desired behavior or decrease unwanted behavior. (The term *behavior* refers to communication targets as well as a patient's degree of cooperation and attentiveness.) This is accomplished through application of the principles of behavior modification. **Behavior modification** is based on the theory of operant conditioning and involves the relationship among a stimulus, a response, and a consequent event (Skinner, 1957). A **stimulus** (or antecedent event) is an event that precedes and elicits a response. A **response** is the behavior exhibited by an individual on presentation of the stimulus. A **consequence** is an event that is contingent on and immediately follows the response. There are different types of consequent events. Consequences that increase the probability that a particular behavior will recur are known as **reinforcement.** Those that are designed to decrease the frequency of a behavior are termed **punishment.**

Types of Reinforcement

There are two basic types of reinforcement: **positive reinforcement** and **negative reinforcement.** Both types are used to increase the frequency of a target response.

Positive Reinforcement. Positive reinforcement is a rewarding event or condition that is presented contingent on the performance of a desired behavior.

Primary. These are contingent events to which a client reacts favorably due to the biological makeup or physiologic predisposition of the individual. Food is the most common example of a primary reinforcer. This type of reinforcer is very powerful and is used most effectively to establish new communicative behaviors (i.e., behaviors not previously present in the client's repertoire). Low-functioning clients often respond well to the basic nature of primary reinforcers. There are known disadvantages of primary reinforcement. First, it can be difficult to present the reinforcement immediately after every occurrence of the target behavior. In addition, this type of reinforcement is susceptible to **satiation;** that is, it loses its appeal as a reward if presented too often. Finally, skills that are taught using these contingent events are often difficult to generalize outside the therapy setting, because primary reinforcers do not occur naturally in the real world.

Secondary. These are contingent events that a client must be taught to perceive as rewarding. This category includes the following subtypes of reinforcers:

- **Social:** This group of reinforcers consists of events such as smiling, eye contact, and verbal praise. It is the most commonly used type of reinforcement in speech-language remediation programs. Social reinforcers are extremely easy to administer after each target response and generally do not disrupt the flow of a therapy session. In addition, this type of contingent response is not very susceptible to satiation (although it is not totally immune) and does occur in a client's natural daily environment.

- **Token:** This group of reinforcers consists of symbols or objects that are not perceived as valuable in and of themselves. However, the accrual of a specified number of these tokens will permit a client to obtain a previously agreed-on reward. Examples include stickers, checkmarks, chips, and point scores. These reinforcers are generally regarded as very powerful because they are easy to administer contingent on each occurrence of a target behavior and are relatively resistant to satiation.

- **Performance feedback:** This category of reinforcers involves information that is given to a client regarding therapy performance and progress. Many individuals find it rewarding to receive information about the quality of their performance. It is not intended to function as praise and need not be presented verbally. Feedback regarding client performance can be delivered in various formats, including percentage data, frequency of occurrence graphs, numerical ratings, and biofeedback devices. Provision of this type of contingent event decreases a client's reliance on external sources of reinforcement by encouraging the development of intrinsic rewards (i.e., internal satisfaction and motivation) for mastering and maintaining a target behavior.

Negative Reinforcement. An unpleasant event/condition is removed contingent on the performance of a desired behavior.

Escape. This type of reinforcer requires the presence of a condition that the client perceives as aversive. Each performance of the target behavior relieves or terminates this aversive condition, thus increasing the probability that the specified behavior will recur. For example, a clinician might place her hands firmly over a child's hands and remove them only when the child exhibits the target behavior of imitatively producing /s/.

Avoidance. With this type of negative reinforcer, each performance of a target behavior prevents the occurrence of an *anticipated* aversive condition. This contingent event results in increased rates of performance of the desired response on subsequent occasions. For example, a clinician might inform a child that each imitative production of the target /s/ will prevent the imposition of hand restraint.

Use of negative reinforcement is relatively uncommon in the treatment of communication disorders because it repeatedly exposes clients to unpleasant or aversive situations. Use of positive reinforcement is the preferred method for increasing the frequency of desired responses. Positive reinforcement also can improve a client's motivational level and foster an effective interpersonal relationship between clinician and client.

Punishment. An event is presented contingent on the performance of an undesired behavior, to decrease the likelihood that the behavior will recur.

Type I. This involves the prompt presentation of an aversive consequence after each demonstration of an unwanted behavior. Examples of this consequence type that might be used in speech-language remediation programming include verbal utterances such as "No!", frowning, or the presentation of bursts of white noise.

Type II. This type of punishment requires withdrawal of a pleasant condition contingent on the demonstration of an unwanted behavior. Time-out and response cost are the two most common forms used in speech-language intervention. **Time-out** procedures involve the temporary isolation or removal of a client to an environment with limited or no opportunity to receive positive reinforcement. A modified version can be accomplished by turning the client's chair toward a blank wall in the therapy room or simply withholding direct eye contact from the client for short periods of time. **Response-cost** contingencies occur when previously earned positive reinforcers are deducted or taken back each time the undesirable behavior is demonstrated. This type of punishment can take various forms, including removal of stickers earned for previous correct responses or the partial subtraction of points already accrued by the client earlier in a therapy session. Sometimes, the clinician may choose to give a client several unearned tokens at the beginning of a session or task to institute response cost procedures.

Several factors influence the effectiveness of punishment procedures (adapted from Hegde & Davis, 2010):

- Punishment should be delivered after *every* instance of the unwanted behavior.
- Punishment should be presented *immediately* following the undesirable behavior.
- Punishment should occur at the *earliest* signs of the unwanted behavior rather than waiting until the behavior is full-blown.
- Punishment should not be programmed in graduated levels of intensity; this creates the potential for client habituation to the punishing stimulus, thus reducing its effectiveness.
- Punishment duration should be as brief as possible; lengthy periods of punishment call into question the strength of the chosen punishing stimulus.

Punishment procedures should be employed with caution in the therapy setting because there are undesirable effects associated with their use. These may include client anger, aggression, a reluctance to engage in any communicative behavior with the therapist, and the avoidance or actual termination of treatment.

If no contingent consequences occur following a targeted behavior, the frequency of that behavior will gradually decrease and ultimately disappear from a client's repertoire. This phenomenon is known as **extinction** and is used in therapy to eliminate behaviors that interfere with effective communication. Extinction does not occur immediately. In fact, a temporary increase in emission rate may be observed when the behavior is initially ignored. Behaviors that receive reinforcement on a continuous basis are most vulnerable to extinction, whereas those that are only periodically reinforced over a long period of time are least susceptible to this procedure. It is recommended that extinction procedures that are implemented for an undesired behavior (e.g., ignoring crying behavior) be combined with positive reinforcement for the converse behavior (e.g., rewarding noncrying behavior).

Positive Behavioral Supports

Application of all the principles just discussed does not guarantee that a therapy session will run smoothly. The clinician should anticipate the possibility that a patient may not pay attention or cooperate with the session plan. This may occur due to a patient's developmental level of attention, boredom, frustration, lack of self-motivation, or a neurological behavior disorder. The clinician must now focus on **behavior management** in addition to behavior modification.

Currently, a system of **positive behavioral supports (PBS)** is recommended for dealing with challenging behaviors. PBS is a proactive approach that uses interpersonal and environmental strategies to minimize opportunities for problematic behavior and encourages more socially useful behaviors. Thus, PBS shifts the emphasis of behavior management from a reactive, aversive approach to one that is more preventative and positive in nature. Helpful information on this topic can be found at several Web sites, including the Center for Effective Collaboration and Practice (cecp.air.org/) and the Center on Positive Behavior Interventions and Supports (www.pbis.org/). A PBS plan can be developed for individuals, classrooms, school districts, or state-wide systems. A positive behavior support plan (see Appendix 1-H) generally identifies the following information:

- A description of the problematic behavior(s), an explanation of why it impedes learning, and an estimate of its severity (frequency, intensity, duration)
- Antecedent events that appear to trigger the behavior(s)
- The desired or alternative behavior(s)
- The supports (teaching strategies or environmental modifications) that will help the client achieve the desired behavior(s)

From the SLP's perspective, most behavior problems can be prevented if the therapy materials are creative, the activities are interesting, and the session is well paced.

Schedules of Reinforcement

Once the appropriate type of reinforcer has been selected for a given client, the clinician must decide how often the reinforcer will be delivered. The two main schedules of reinforcement are *continuous* and *intermittent*.

Continuous Reinforcement. A reinforcer is presented after *every* correct performance of a target behavior. This schedule, sometimes characterized as "dense," tends to generate a very high rate of response. It is most commonly used to shape and establish new communication behaviors. It also can be used when transitioning an already established skill from one level of difficulty to the next (e.g., from word to sentence level). Use of a **continuous** schedule reduces the risk that a client's production of a target behavior will "drift" from the intended response. The primary disadvantage of this schedule is that behaviors reinforced at such a high density level are very susceptible to extinction. It also may interfere with a client's production of a steady flow of responses.

Intermittent Reinforcement. With this schedule, only some occurrences of a correct response are followed by a reinforcer. **Intermittent** reinforcement, often termed *lower density*, is most effective in strengthening responses that have been previously established.

This reinforcement schedule reduces the probability of satiation during treatment and results in behaviors that are extremely resistant to extinction. The four types of intermittent schedules are as follows.

Fixed Ratio. A specific number of correct responses must be exhibited before a reinforcer is delivered (e.g., every two responses, every 10 responses, every 35 responses). The required number is determined by the clinician and remains unchanged throughout a therapy task. This reinforcement schedule generally elicits a high rate of response.

Fixed Interval. Reinforcement is delivered for the first correct response made after a predetermined time period has elapsed (e.g., every 3 minutes, every 50 seconds). The main disadvantage of this schedule is that response rate tends to decline dramatically immediately following presentation of the reinforcer, and therefore a fixed interval schedule may be an inefficient use of therapy time.

Variable Ratio (VR). The number of correct responses required for the delivery of a reinforcer varies from trial to trial according to a predetermined pattern set by the clinician. For example, the pattern might be as follows: after the third response; then after the tenth response; then after the fourth response; then after the seventh response. This ratio, represented as VR: 3, 10, 4, 7, would be repeated throughout a therapy task. This schedule tends to be more effective than a fixed ratio schedule because the client cannot predict the seemingly random pattern of delivery and anticipates that every response has an equal chance of being reinforced.

Variable Interval (VI). This schedule is similar to a variable ratio except that the clinician varies the time period required for reinforcement delivery rather than the number of responses. For example, one interval pattern might be as follows: after 3 minutes; then after 10 minutes; then after 1 minute; then after 4 minutes. This pattern, represented as VI: 3, 10, 1, 4, would be repeated throughout a therapy task.

In general practice, continuous reinforcement is used to establish a new target behavior. Intermittent schedules are introduced in subsequent stages of therapy to promote maintenance and generalization. One rule of thumb is to switch to lower-density intermittent schedules when the target response rate increases 30% to 50% over the original baseline measures.

KEY TEACHING/SCAFFOLDING STRATEGIES

Several basic training techniques are commonly used in intervention programs to facilitate the acquisition of communication behaviors. The following strategies are used for a variety of purposes and are implemented at different points throughout the remediation process:

- *Direct modeling:* Clinician demonstrates a specific behavior to provide an exemplar for the client to imitate.
- *Indirect modeling:* Clinician demonstrates a specific behavior frequently to expose a client to numerous well-formed examples of the target behavior.
- *Shaping by successive approximation:* A target behavior is broken down into small components and taught in an ascending sequence of difficulty.

- *Prompts:* Clinician provides additional verbal or nonverbal cues to facilitate a client's production of a correct response.

- *Fading:* Stimulus or consequence manipulations (e.g., modeling, prompting, reinforcement) are reduced in gradual steps while maintaining the target response.

- *Expansion:* Clinician reformulates a client's utterance into a more mature or complete version.

- *Recast:* Clinician reformulates a client's utterance into a different sentence type.

- *Negative practice:* The client is required to intentionally produce a target behavior using a habitual error pattern. This procedure is generally employed to facilitate learning by highlighting the contrast between the error pattern and the desired response.

- *Target-specific feedback:* The clinician provides information regarding the accuracy or inaccuracy of a client's response relative to the specific target behavior. This type of feedback contrasts with generalized feedback or consequences.

Direct modeling is the teaching technique most frequently used in the early stages of therapy. It is also employed whenever a target behavior is shifted to a higher level of response difficulty because this type of modeling provides the maximum amount of clinician support. Typically, clinicians augment direct models with a variety of visual and verbal cues to establish correct responses at the level of imitation. Direct modeling also minimizes the likelihood that a client will produce his or her customary error response. Initially, a direct model is provided before each client response.

Once a target behavior is established, continuous modeling should be eliminated because it does not facilitate strengthening or maintaining a target response. Direct modeling can be terminated abruptly or faded gradually. Gradual **fading** can be accomplished in at least two ways. One requires a client to produce multiple imitations for each model demonstrated by the clinician (e.g., three imitative responses are required after each direct model). The second method involves the progressive reduction of the length of the behavior modeled by the clinician. For example, the direct model of "The boy is running" is shortened first to "The boy is . . . ," and then to "The boy . . . ," while the client's imitative response in all three cases is the production of the complete target sentence, "The boy is running." In general, fading procedures can be initiated once a client is able to produce at least five consecutive correct imitative responses.

In some cases, the stimulus alone is not sufficient to elicit the desired response. **Prompts** are extra verbal and nonverbal cues designed to help a client produce the target behavior. Prompts can be categorized as attentional or instructional. **Attentional** cues improve performance by focusing a client's concentration on the task at hand. Examples include "Look at me," "Watch my mouth," "Remember to pay attention," and "Are you ready?" Clinicians also can draw attention to a target by modeling the behavior with exaggerated loudness and duration. **Instructional** cues provide information that is directly related to the specific target behavior being attempted. This may include verbal prompts such as "Remember to elevate your tongue tip at the beginning of each word," "Don't forget to segment your words into syllables if you get stuck," or "Be sure that your answer has at least three words in it." Instructional cues also can be nonverbal, such as an index card with the name of the targeted fluency technique written on it, a gesture to indicate that voice loudness should be increased, or drawings that represent the grammatical categories of subject, verb, and object.

Some target behaviors are too complex for a client to perform successfully and even the provision of a direct model accompanied by prompts may not elicit a correct imitative response. In such instances, procedures for **shaping by successive approximation** are usually instituted. The simplification of a difficult target into a series of more manageable tasks fosters client success at each step. Each successive step moves progressively closer to the final form of the desired response.

Target-specific feedback is a technique that is useful throughout all phases of the therapy process. It serves three main functions. First, clients benefit from feedback that consists of more than simple accuracy judgments regarding their responses. Target-specific feedback provides precise information about why responses are correct or incorrect (e.g., "Good, I didn't see your tongue peeking out when you said, 'Soup'," rather than simply "Good job!"). Second, use of this strategy tends to maintain a client's awareness of the exact response being targeted without the need for continuous reinstruction during a therapy activity. Finally, this type of feedback assists clinicians in maintaining client focus on the communication behavior being targeted by a given therapy activity. It is a particularly helpful strategy for beginning clinicians who may get too involved in the details or rules of an activity and lose sight of the true purpose of the therapy task.

Negative practice is a strategy intended to enhance a client's awareness of the salient characteristics of his or her error pattern. It is used primarily to illustrate the differences between an "old" response and the intended target. This procedure generally is implemented only after a client demonstrates the ability to produce a given target consistently at the level of imitation. Negative practice is a powerful technique that is best used on a short-term basis. Devoting a significant amount of therapy to client practice on incorrect responses is of questionable value.

In addition to the specific training techniques just discussed, clinicians frequently use the general stimulation procedures of **indirect modeling, expansion, and recasting.** These strategies can be employed at any stage in the therapy process. They provide a client with increased exposure to instances of desirable speech, language, or communication behaviors but are not intended to elicit immediate specific responses. For example, a clinician working with a client on the production of /s/ may implement indirect modeling by including a significant number of /s/-initial words in her off-task comments throughout a session. Expansions are used almost exclusively in language therapy programs and may involve the clinician's interpretation of the client's intended meaning (e.g., Client: "Daddy cookie"; Clinician: "Yes, Daddy is eating the cookie."). An example of recasting is changing the client's declarative statement to an interrogative form (e.g., Client: "Doggie is barking"; Clinician: "Is the doggie barking?").

Homework

Once a target communication behavior has been established in therapy using the teaching strategies specified in the previous section, **homework assignments** can be given to strengthen the response and facilitate its generalization outside the clinical setting. Certain guidelines for the design and implementation of homework can increase its effectiveness as an intervention strategy:

- The purpose of homework is to provide the client with practice on an *existing* skill rather than teaching something new. Therefore, it should focus only on targets that have been solidly established in therapy.

- Homework should be instituted only after a client has demonstrated a basic ability to accurately evaluate his or her performance on a given target.

- To increase the likelihood that homework will be completed, it should be assigned in amounts that are perceived as manageable by a client or family. For example, activities that involve a daily commitment of 5 to 10 minutes may be more effective than those that require 30 to 45 minutes once a week.

- Homework should be assigned on a regular basis throughout the course of therapy.

- Homework assignments should always be accompanied by simple written instructions that specify exactly what the client is expected to do.

- Review and check homework during the initial portion of the next therapy session.

- Homework activities can be supervised by a variety of individuals (e.g., teacher, spouse, babysitter).

SESSION DESIGN

Once therapy targets have been appropriately programmed, the clinician must determine the organizational flow of each therapy session. The first decision to be made is whether treatment will be delivered in an individual or group setting. **Session design** for both of these formats requires consideration of the basic factors discussed in the sections that follow. Elements that are specific to design for a group session will be addressed later in this chapter.

Basic Training Protocol

Regardless of disorder type or severity level, speech, language, and communication therapy is carried out using the same basic training protocol. This protocol is the distillation of the therapy process and consists of the following five steps (see Table 1-1 for guidelines on giving instructions):

1. Clinician presents stimulus.
2. Clinician waits for the client to respond.
3. Clinician presents appropriate consequent event.
4. Clinician records response.
5. Clinician removes stimulus (as appropriate).

   This sequence represents a single trial for a given target and is repeated continuously throughout a therapy session. The acceptable latency period between stimulus presentation and client response may vary according to disorder type as well as individual client characteristics. It is critical that the consequent event (reinforcement/punishment) follow the response immediately, so that the contingent relationship between the two is obvious to the client. For this reason, data recording should not delay the delivery of the consequence.

Task Order

Another important component of session design is the order in which tasks are conducted. Appropriate task order enhances the overall effectiveness of treatment. An ideal progression follows an "easy-hard-easy" pattern. A session should begin with therapy tasks with

TABLE 1–1
Guidelines for Effective Instructions

- Instructions should be worded as clearly and concisely as possible. Long, complicated explanations can be counterproductive to a client's understanding of the intended task. (Beginning clinicians may benefit from writing an actual script of instructions prior to a session.)

- State instructions in the declarative form. Directions that are presented indirectly in the form of requests (e.g., "Would you say /s/ for me?") are pragmatically confusing and understandably may elicit negative replies (e.g., "No" or "I don't want to.").

- Be sure to allow clients sufficient time to respond before repeating the instructions. Resist the temptation to repeat instructions or stimuli too quickly, because individuals with communication impairments often require increased processing time. Waiting is a strategy that may facilitate correct responses more consistently than repetition of instructions.

- If it becomes necessary to re-administer instructions, try to avoid significant reformulation of the original wording. This is particularly important with clients who have language disorders, because rewording tends to become a source of confusion rather than clarification.

- The main emphasis of instructions should always be on the targeted behavior rather than on the details of the activity or game being used to elicit the behavior. (This aspect poses particular difficulty for beginning clinicians, who must learn to create the appropriate balance between the amount of time spent explaining elaborate therapy activities versus working on target behaviors.)

which a client can be relatively successful without excessive expenditure of effort. This could entail a review of completed homework assignments or nearly mastered targets from a previous session. The central portion of the session should consist of behavioral objectives that are most challenging to the client. The final segment should return to tasks that elicit fairly accurate performance with minimal effort. This task order increases the likelihood that a given therapy session will begin and end on a positive note. This success-oriented session design promotes high levels of client motivation even during difficult stages of the therapy process.

Dynamics of Therapy

Thus far, this chapter has focused on the technical aspects of intervention. However, the therapy process involves another critical dimension: the dynamics of therapy. Therapy dynamics contribute significantly to session design and include factors such as the clinician-client relationship, work efficiency/pace, materials, and proxemics.

The Clinician-Client Relationship. The nature of the clinician-client relationship influences the success of a therapy program as powerfully as the technical design. One of the most important aspects of the therapeutic relationship is the professional personality of the clinician. Clearly, personal attributes among clinicians vary tremendously. In general, a calm, positive, and firm demeanor is most effective in enhancing clinician-client interaction.

Further, clinicians need to maintain a conscious awareness of their body language, intonation patterns, and social speaking style to prevent client confusion. Body language and voice intonation patterns must be monitored to ensure that they do not conflict with accompanying verbal messages. For example, the message, "You're doing a great job!" may not be perceived by a client as a positive remark if it is delivered without eye contact and in an apathetic tone of voice. Further, the use of overly diplomatic forms of speech should be minimized because they may contradict the message that a clinician intends to convey. For example, beginning clinicians who are reluctant to risk hurting a client's feelings may react to an incorrect response with a big smile, while saying, "Good! Let's try that again!" rather than clearly stating that the attempt was inaccurate.

In any interpersonal interaction, there may be a mismatch between an intended message and the perceived message. A persistent mismatch can have a negative influence on the therapeutic alliance. It is the responsibility of clinicians to adapt their interactive styles (comprising energy level, humor, talkativeness, and vocabulary) to accommodate the comfort level of each client rather than the other way around. It is also important to remember that clients can be easily overwhelmed and intimidated by the excessive use of unfamiliar technical jargon. To maintain a professional yet warm atmosphere, clinicians need to determine on a case-by-case basis the appropriate balance between their use of technical versus more colloquial language forms.

Moreover, clinicians must establish the parameters of the therapeutic relationship from the very first session. This entails an explicit definition of the roles and responsibilities of each partner. This will clearly differentiate the nature of a professional relationship from a personal one. At the beginning of a therapeutic relationship, clients do not always feel comfortable volunteering information about their goals for therapy. Clinicians should make a point of asking clients about their expectations. Whenever possible, clients (and their families) should be active participants in the target selection phase of therapy, by identifying the communication behaviors that are the highest priorities in their daily lives.

Clinicians can minimize client anxiety and confusion by providing a clear rationale regarding the purpose of each activity implemented in a therapy session. Intervention tends to be less effective if clients do not understand why they are being asked to perform particular tasks. Further, difficult client questions should be addressed in a manner that allows the clinician to maintain credibility. For instance, instead of responding with "I haven't had that course yet," it is more effective to simply say, "I don't know. I'll do some research on the topic and give you the information at our next session."

Clinicians need to create a balance between responding to and ignoring off-task comments made by clients. Sometimes clients genuinely need to talk about topics that are not part of the clinician's original lesson plan but are important to address (e.g., questions regarding lack of progress, comments concerning family reactions to new communicative behaviors). At other times, off-task comments are meant simply to distract the clinician from a therapy task that a client perceives as difficult or boring.

Ultimately, the success of any therapeutic relationship will be influenced by the clinician's recognition that it is the client, and not merely the disorder, that is the main focus of treatment.

Work Efficiency/Pace. This aspect of session dynamics entails consideration of two main issues. First, every session should be efficiently designed to provide a client with the maximum number of opportunities to practice target behaviors. Second, the pace of each session must be geared to the learning rates and styles of individual clients. A pace that is either too fast or too slow may cause frustration for a client and interfere with successful performance.

Materials. The materials selected for therapy must be appropriate for a client's age, developmental status, language level, gender, cultural background, and linguistic needs. In addition to these criteria, it is important to consider the interest value of therapy materials based on individual client preferences. For example, when selecting materials for a 12-year-old boy with a learning disability who reads at a second-grade level, the clinician must ensure that any stories used in therapy are sufficiently interesting for a preteen, yet written at a manageable difficulty level. Finally, clinicians should avoid the use of time-consuming and complicated materials or activities. Materials that require lengthy physical manipulation (e.g., cutting, gluing, intricate board games) may negatively affect the efficiency of a session by reducing the amount of time available for client responses.

Proxemics. For the purposes of the present discussion, **proxemics** involves the spatial arrangement or relationships between the clinician and client(s) within the therapy setting. Proxemics should take into account the spatial factors that affect any social interaction. One of the most important considerations for SLPs is to determine a socially acceptable (and, in some cases, culturally acceptable) physical proximity between the clinician and the client. Seating arrangements that are extremely far apart may be perceived by the client as an indication of aloofness or lack of interest on the part of the clinician. In contrast, clients may be very uncomfortable with clinicians who sit too close and invade their personal space. Clinicians may deliberately use proxemics as a strategy to influence client behavior (e.g., reducing impulsive or distractible behavior by sitting very close to a child).

In addition to having social implications, proxemics also influence the effective implementation of certain therapy procedures. For example, monitoring the degree of tongue protrusion for an interdental lisp (i.e., /θ/ for /s/) will be difficult if the clinician cannot see the client's face. On the other hand, a face-to-face seating arrangement may interfere with an activity that requires the clinician and client to read from the same stimulus sheet. Seating arrangements should always be selected based on the goal of a given therapy objective. The three most common sitting arrangements (chair or floor) for conducting individualized therapy are face to face, side by side, and side by side in front of a mirror.

Group Therapy

The use of a group therapy model requires attention to several unique aspects of session design that are not pertinent to individual treatment. Unfortunately, there is a paucity of information on group intervention and even less empirical study of this process in the field of speech-language pathology. However, group therapy is critical to any discussion of session design, because it is a frequently used service delivery mode—in fact, it is becoming the dominant model in many therapeutic settings (such as the public schools). Therefore, group therapy is treated as a separate topic in this chapter to provide clinicians with fundamental information on the effective design and execution of these programs.

Clinicians implement a group intervention model for a variety of purposes. Some groups are intended to teach new communication skills at introductory levels. Others are designed primarily to provide clients with practice on skills previously established in individual sessions. Still others have socialization, self-help, or counseling as their main purpose.

The stage of therapy at which group intervention is initiated also varies. Some clinicians employ a group model from the very beginning of the therapy process; others use it mainly in the final stages to facilitate carryover. In many cases, a combination of individual and group formats is used throughout all stages of the therapy process.

Group Size. The size of a group will vary depending on its purpose, the setting, and client age. Groups whose primary purpose is to teach new skills tend to be smaller than those geared for the generalization of previously mastered skills. Group size is also determined by the availability of clients in different service delivery settings. Institutions such as metropolitan hospitals and public schools lend themselves more readily to the formation of larger therapy groups than do private practices or small clinics.

Based on the available literature, the recommended group size for children is approximately two to six members (Blosser & Neidecker, 2002; Weiss, Gordon, & Lillywhite, 1987). Guidelines for adults differ. For example, E. Cooper and C. Cooper (2003) recommend 7 to 12 members for adult stuttering groups. They also caution that groups of fewer than five clients are undesirable for several reasons: (1) personality characteristics of individual group members are more prominent, (2) the absence of a single member can interfere with the group's ability to function, and (3) small groups are more susceptible to domination by a single member.

Group Composition. The primary client characteristics to be considered in the formation of a group are age, gender, disorder type, and disorder severity. Other factors that may be relevant to some groups include intelligence, socioeconomic status, education level, and personality type. As a general rule, the two most important factors are client age and disorder type. Effective groups tend to be relatively homogeneous with respect to one or both of these variables. Clinicians may choose to organize groups in either a closed or open format. *Closed groups* frequently operate for predetermined time periods and maintain the same membership throughout. In contrast, *open groups* have revolving membership and accept new individuals whenever space becomes available. One rule of thumb for pediatric groups is that the age or developmental level of the members should be within two or three years of one another, because cognitive abilities and social maturity can significantly influence group interaction.

Clinician's Role. The role of the clinician is to function as group leader. Leadership style can be directive or nondirective. A *directive* style is typically used with groups composed of young children. In addition, it is more common in the early stages of therapy when a group model is being used to teach new communication behaviors. In this role, the clinician sets the agenda, chooses the materials and activities, provides specific instruction, and gives corrective feedback. A *nondirective* approach is more commonly used in the carryover stages of therapy and with self-help groups. In this style, the clinician does not perform a primary teaching function. Instead, group members take charge of session activities, while the clinician serves as a facilitator who oversees rather than directs group interactions. Regardless of style, a group leader is responsible for establishing and maintaining group cohesion, mediating conflicts between members, and ensuring that each member of the group is progressing adequately toward established therapy goals.

Procedures. Several procedures can be used in group settings to maintain the active participation of all members throughout the entire session. In one method, the clinician presents a stimulus and pauses before choosing a particular group member to respond. This strategy increases the likelihood that all members will pay attention and prepare answers to every stimulus in anticipation of being called on. In another strategy, clients can take turns modeling target behaviors for other group members to repeat in unison. Finally, clients can be required to listen, watch, and evaluate the performance of a target behavior by fellow group members.

Clinicians can use a variety of techniques to facilitate group interaction. The following examples are applicable to any type of communicative disorder:

- Reinforce client behaviors and comments that are consistent with treatment goals.
- Model the target behaviors or techniques group members are attempting to develop.
- Focus attention and group time on members who are making progress toward established goals.
- Encourage interaction within the group by asking one member to demonstrate a target behavior for the other members.
- Ask open-ended questions that require longer than one- or two-word responses.
- Cue a group member to focus on a particular therapy target before she or he begins speaking.
- Restructure comments or topics so they have appeal for all members of the group.
- Use behaviors of individual members to form generalizations that are applicable to the group as a whole.

Advantages and Disadvantages. The delivery of therapy services through a group model has both advantages and disadvantages. The main advantages are as follows:

- Carryover is facilitated.
- Clients stimulate and motivate each other.
- More opportunities exist for natural-speaking situations.
- Clients recognize that others have problems similar to their own.
- More occasions exist for clients to engage in critical listening.
- A broader variety of activities and materials can be used.
- The setting provides for socialization and peer interaction.
- Increased opportunities exist to learn by observing others.
- Self-monitoring is encouraged by reducing the client's dependence on the clinician as the sole evaluator of communication behavior.

The primary disadvantages of group intervention include the following:

- Each group member receives less direct attention from the clinician than is given in individual sessions.
- Fewer opportunities exist to address the specific weaknesses of each client, especially when the group is not homogeneous with respect to disorder.
- Clients who are shy, reticent, or of different cultural backgrounds may be reluctant to participate.
- One or two members may become dominant and monopolize the group.
- The group's rate of progress may be too fast for the slowest members and too slow for the most advanced members.

Perhaps the heart of successful group therapy is a clinician's ability to establish and maintain a true group dynamic; otherwise, the sessions merely consist of multiple clients receiving individualized treatment in a group room.

DATA COLLECTION

Speech-language pathologists are accountable for the efficiency as well as the effectiveness of the intervention services they provide. Clients and their families invest valuable time, resources, and effort in the therapy process. The primary mechanism for ensuring clinician accountability is data collection. Information obtained from the data collection process serves two important functions. It allows the clinician to monitor a client's progress from one session to the next. Data collection systems also can be designed to permit documentation of the efficacy of a given treatment strategy. Clinicians need to recognize that best practices in service delivery are data driven.

Recording Session Data

Data recording is greatly facilitated by behavioral objectives that are written properly (i.e., in specific and measurable terms). In most cases, data collection difficulties occur because objectives are written in a vague and unclear manner. Following are guidelines for a comprehensive approach to data collection:

1. Appropriate data recording sheets should be designed or selected prior to the onset of a therapy session. (Samples of reproducible data forms and instructions for their use are included in Appendix 1-G at the end of this chapter.)

2. The notation system should provide the type of information that is most relevant to a specific client or disorder. A binary system of "correct" versus "incorrect" is not the only option. Interval scales can be developed to rate responses on a continuum (e.g., degree of correctness or latency of response).

3. The data collection system must allow the clinician to clearly distinguish among imitative, cued/prompted, self-corrected, and spontaneous responses.

4. Once therapy tasks reach the conversational level of complexity, it is often more efficient to use a data recording system that is based on time rather than on total number of responses. For example, it may be easier to document the number of errors per minute rather than to identify all occurrences of a target behavior to calculate the percentage correct.

5. Reinforcement tokens or stimulus items can be used as an alternative to paper-and-pencil or online recording of client responses. One useful approach is to organize the items or tokens in groups of 10 or 20. The number and percentage of correct responses can be calculated easily by (a) counting the number of unearned reinforcement tokens remaining at the end of an activity or (b) checking the number of stimulus items (e.g., picture cards) that the clinician has placed in a "correct response" pile.

6. Record *every* stimulus-response event. Even the absence of a response to a particular stimulus should be recorded.

Data collection systems are used to maximize a clinician's effectiveness. It is important to recognize that data yield information regarding a client's status on a particular objective. However, data alone do not identify specific programming changes that may need to be made or how to implement them. These clinical decisions can be made only through a clinician's careful analysis and interpretation of the recorded data.

Probes

Probes are instruments administered periodically throughout treatment to measure a client's progress. They are designed to assess generalization of a trained target behavior (Hegde, 1998). Probes consist of a set of novel stimuli that are equivalent to, but different from, those used for treatment. For example, after teaching the production of initial /s/ with a set of picture cards, the clinician may probe a client's generalization by presenting a new set of unfamiliar pictures to elicit this phoneme (good rule of thumb: 20 stimulus items for each probe).

Probes are similar to baselines in that client responses are elicited without target-specific instruction and do not receive any reinforcement. However, lengthy periods of nonreinforcement may be undesirable for some clients, particularly in the early stages of therapy. Therefore, a **mixed probe** may be instituted, whereby both trained and untrained stimulus items are presented in an alternating sequence. In this procedure, the client continues to receive reinforcement for responses to the trained stimuli.

The findings obtained from probe procedures are used by the clinician to determine the next step in the therapy program. If the predetermined criterion from the behavioral objective has not been achieved, training should continue at the current level. If the criterion has been met, the clinician may choose to shift to a higher level of response complexity in the same target area or move on to a new communicative behavior. Periodic administration of probes is especially important, because it minimizes the risk of continuing therapy that is no longer effective or necessary.

SERVICE-DELIVERY MODELS

The traditional approach to providing speech-language intervention has been the individual model, where clients receive therapy in a one-to-one setting. However, there has been a growing trend toward the provision of therapy in a variety of different service-delivery models. The hallmark characteristic of this trend is collaborative partnership.

Collaborative Partnership

Collaboration is critical to promoting better communication among different professionals, all of whom possess specialized knowledge and skills. For example, SLPs have a deep understanding of the linguistic underpinnings of literacy in both typically developing children and children with learning problems. On the other hand, teachers and special educators have expertise in strategies, materials, and standards for teaching literacy. In medical and educational settings, health professionals from different disciplines regularly team with one another to problem-solve and provide interprofessional patient care.

Often, professionals do not have an appreciation for the knowledge and skills possessed by one another. Partnerships offer an opportunity for professionals to engage in focused and frequent exchanges about effective intervention and instruction. They are able to leverage their combined knowledge and skills to implement best practices and improve outcomes for diverse groups of clients (Roth & Troia, 2006).

Collaboration is highly valued by SLPs and other professionals, and although research findings suggest that it is a service-delivery model of choice, collaboration often does not occur because it requires a substantial degree of coordination and planning (Beck & Dennis, 1997). One means of making collaboration more manageable is to strategically select a client(s) for whom the potential benefits of co-treatment are most evident. Once success is experienced in this initial venture, collaborative efforts can be extended more broadly across a clinician's workload.

Eight guiding principles for effective collaborations (Paul, Blosser, & Jakubowitz, 2006) that promote effective communication and build good relationships among professionals and families follow:

1. Engage in mutual problem solving and shared responsibility for positive client outcomes.
2. Establish communication goals and priorities for clients on the basis of their strengths and needs.
3. Form partnerships that are nonhierarchical and based on co-equal participation.
4. Recognize that collaboration is a dynamic process: the size, composition, goals, and function of teams change as client needs change.
5. Respect different professional perspectives.
6. Make partnerships a priority.
7. Establish realistic expectations for the partnership.
8. Celebrate success.

Effective implementation of these principles across a wide variety of service delivery settings can be maximized with the following strategies:

- Maintain ongoing communication with collaborative partners to promote clear understanding of roles and responsibilities of different partners.
- Use technology to maintain communication and exchange of information.
- Involve people who have significant relationships with the student (e.g., teachers, families, spouses, and peers).
- Engage in pre-professional training and professional development opportunities to learn and implement partnership models.

Many collaborative partnership models are easily adapted to the educational setting and can be used instead of or in combination with the traditional pull-out model, in which a student leaves the classroom and receives therapy in either individual or group sessions. Some of the most commonly used collaborative models are as follows:

Consultative: The clinician acts as a resource for professionals who work directly with a child and parents to help solve problems related to the child's communicative deficit. In this model, the agent of intervention is someone other than the SLP.

Team teaching: The clinician and the teacher share the responsibility for classroom instruction on a regular basis. In this model, a comprehensive program with strong language and academic components can be provided within the context of the classroom.

Self-contained: The clinician alone serves as the classroom teacher and is responsible for developing and implementing all aspects of the curriculum. Classroom activities in all topic areas are specifically designed to promote the development of language skills.

Many states and localities now use an inclusion model of education in which students with disabilities receive all needed services and supports in the general education classroom. In addition, there has been a growing trend toward the provision of therapy in a wider variety of service-delivery models.

An increasingly well-regarded collaborative model is interprofessional practice (IPP) where different health and social care professionals regularly work together to improve patient/client outcomes. Along with the IPP model, current health care and education reforms are prompting some rethinking about the academic and clinical preparation of future professionals in health-related professions (including speech-language pathology and audiology). One iteration of this rethinking is **interprofessional education** (IPE). The core feature of IPE is interactive student learning, where students from different disciplines (e.g., speech-language pathology, physical therapy, occupational therapy, nursing, social work, and nutrition) learn and work side by side, both academically and clinically. Simulation activities are frequently used in clinical practica in which learners from different disciplines are given a "real-life" clinical situation and, together, they must reflect on and solve the problem. **Telepractice** (and its educational counterpart, telesupervision) is a relatively recent clinical model that is used for the provision of services to clients and as a clinical educational model. It involves the use of telecommunications technology to deliver clinical services at a distance. SLPs use telepractice to treat clients who cannot participate in face-to-face therapy because of distance, mobility issues, or unavailability of SLPs in underserved regions, or to provide access to SLPs in specialized areas of expertise (ASHA, 2013 practice portal). From the perspective of clinical education, telesupervision, or e-supervision, refers to the use of video/audio conferencing technologies or electronic messaging (such as email) to provide clinical supervision to students at a distant site.

Two common descriptors of these service/education models are synchronous and asynchronous. Synchronous telepractices occur between a client and clinician in real time using video- or audio-conferencing and simulate traditional face-to-face therapy sessions. In synchronous telesupervision, the student and supervisor communicate in real time using web-conferencing technologies. This provides live supervision of student clinicians in off-campus clinical placements. In asynchronous models of telepractice and telesupervision (also called "store and forward"), images or data are captured and transmitted for later viewing, reviewing, or interpretation by a professional (e.g., voice clips, session segments). Sometimes, these two models are used in combination with one another and are referred to as hybrid applications. Telepractice/telesupervision can be implemented in any setting as long as the services comply with national, state, institutional, and professional regulations or policies. These settings include schools, medical centers, rehabilitation hospitals, community health centers, outpatient clinics, universities, homes, residential health care facilities, and childcare centers. Patient privacy concerns should be considered carefully when telepractice is chosen as a service-delivery mechanism. Many current video-conferencing systems (e.g., Skype, Facetime, etc.) are not compliant with the Health Insurance Portability and Accountability Act (HIPAA). More information about confidentiality in telepractice can be found in Cohn and Watzlaf (2011) and on.asha.org/privacy-telepractice. When used appropriately, these "long-distance" models may help address the following:

- persistent and growing shortages of SLPs by increasing the number of qualified SLPs from Communication Science Disorders (CSD) programs
- issues of limited clinical capacity while ensuring a high-quality supervisory experience
- the persistent issue of available extern practicum sites by increasing the number and variety of potential clinical practicum placements and experiences for students
- the needs of some students whose geographic locations require long-distance clinical supervision

Ultimately, the selection of a particular service-delivery model is determined by (1) the needs of a child, (2) the size and composition of a clinician's workload, and (3) scheduling constraints.

RESPONSE TO INTERVENTION

In the reauthorization of the **Individuals with Disabilities Education Act** (2004), **Response to Intervention (RTI)** was sanctioned as an approach for identifying students with learning disabilities and determining their eligibility for services. It was developed as an alternative to the traditional discrepancy criterion approach. With the *discrepancy criterion*, students need to demonstrate a significant gap (usually defined as 1.5 standard deviations) between cognitive ability and academic achievement. Researchers and educators have long viewed this approach as a "wait-to-fail" model because most children do not demonstrate the needed discrepancy until third or fourth grade. RTI focuses on earlier identification and intervention when students first experience academic difficulties. Its goal is to improve the achievement of all students, including those with language-learning disabilities.

RTI models involve a collaborative, problem-solving process with the following components (Fuchs & Fuchs, 2006; Roth & Troia, 2009):

- Universal screening/assessment
- High-quality classroom-wide instruction
- Progress monitoring
- Multi-tiered instruction/intervention
- Family engagement

The most widely used RTI model includes the three tiers described in Table 1-2 along with suggested roles for SLPs within each tier. The intensity and duration of services (i.e., progression through the tiers) is determined by a student's responsiveness to intervention.

In RTI, the identification of a learning disability (LD) is based on a "dual discrepancy" (Fuchs, 2003). That is, despite *high-quality instruction* AND *remedial instruction*, a student does not progress at the expected rate. Although originally conceived as a model for primary grades, there is growing support for applying developmentally appropriate RTI approaches in preschool settings as a means of prevention, earlier identification, and early intervention for children at risk for educational failure (Coleman, Roth, & West, 2009; Justice, 2006).

TABLE 1–2
Response to Intervention Tiers

Tier	Description	Suggested Roles of SLPs
1	All students receive high-quality, scientifically based core classroom curriculum in the general education setting. Teachers monitor student learning on an ongoing basis (compared to age, grade, classmates' performance) to track child progress and guide differentiated instruction for children according to their needs.	■ SLPs can use their extensive knowledge of the structures and functions of language (e.g., phonological awareness, vocabulary, morphology/syntax) to educate school staff about the fundamental relationships between oral language, literacy, and academic learning. ■ Help teachers make appropriate adaptations in academic language (e.g., reducing linguistic complexity, marking important information, providing concrete and relevant examples for abstract concepts). ■ Contribute to the creation of literacy-rich classroom learning environments. ■ Help teachers systematically implement screening and progress monitoring measures and interpret the results. ■ Provide in-class modeling or co-teaching of language-based emergent literacy activities (e.g., phonological awareness, shared book-reading).
2	Students whose performance and rate of progress lag those of behind peers receive more specialized instruction within the general education curriculum.	■ Adapt their training in "diagnostic" observation and analysis to assist in the delivery of targeted interventions for struggling learners (e.g., provide specifically tailored instruction retrieval strategies for students who read slowly). ■ Continue professional education efforts to help school staff with progress monitoring and identification of students with learning disabilities. ■ Consult with school staff to ensure consistency and continuity among the multiple individuals who provide instruction to the same struggling learners (e.g., reading specialists, English as a second language/bilingual education teachers, paraeducators, community volunteers).
3	Students who show continued need for support are considered for more intensive, individualized instruction and/or are referred for comprehensive evaluation to determine eligibility for special education services.	■ Implement direct treatment for students with language or learning deficits who have not benefited from Tier 1 or Tier 2 services. ■ Confer with special educators to focus resources on students who need the greatest amount of support to succeed in the classroom. ■ Provide services in the quickest possible time frame to minimize the gap between struggling students and their classroom peers.

Source: Adapted from Roth, F. P., & Troia, G.A. (2009). Applications of responsiveness to intervention and the speech-language pathologist in elementary school settings. Seminars in Speech & Language, 30, 75-89.

An emerging body of evidence shows that tier-based early intervention approaches can improve the academic performance of at-risk students (e.g., Murray, Woodruff & Vaughn, 2010; Orosco & Klingnen, 2010). Results of a state-wide survey of RTI implementation (Hoover, Baca, Wexler-Love, & Saenz, 2008) indicated that tier-based models are currently in use or are in development in almost every state. Survey findings also revealed that (1) state-wide RTI professional development training efforts are under way in 90% of the states; and that (2) most states are using or plan to use a combined problem-solving assessment and treatment model for making tier-based educational decisions (Hoover & Patton, 2009). A systematic review of 16 well-designed studies indicated that five factors were constant across effective programs. Of these five, at least three involved collaborative efforts (i.e., involvement of all school personnel, administrative support at the building and system level, adequate meeting time for teaming and coordination) (Hughes & Dexter, 2011).

Current Challenges of RTI

Information about the effectiveness of RTI models is still evolving. Clinicians should be aware of several issues that require further study:

- RTI models have focused on early identification and intervention. No studies are available that report the long-term effects of Tier 1 and Tier 2 services on later academic achievement and learning outcomes. RTI may miss identifying and addressing the needs of students with late-emerging reading or writing disabilities (Badian, 1999; Catts, Hogan, & Adlof, 2005; Leach, Scarborough, & Rescorla, 2003; Nation, 2005).

- Application of RTI has largely been limited to the domain of reading; consequently, its applicability to other domains (e.g., oral language, writing) is unknown.

- It is unclear how long a student should remain in a particular tier of service and what specific criteria should be met to judge responsiveness as adequate or inadequate (e.g., Duhon, Mesmer, Atkins, Greguson, & Olinger, 2009; Speece & Hines, 2008).

- RTI models evaluate risk and disability status in the classroom setting (Fuchs, 2002, 2003). This context is relative because demands vary not only across grades, but across teachers, schools, districts, and states. When discrepancy is based on comparisons between performance of the struggling student and his or her peers at the local level, identification of LDs becomes much more relative (Kavale, Holdnack, Mostert, & Schmied, 2003).

Treatment Efficacy/Evidence-Based Practice

Treatment efficacy is a general term that encompasses three basic factors: effectiveness (Does treatment work?), efficiency (Does one treatment work better or faster than another?), and effects (In what ways does treatment alter behavior?). For certain communicative disorders, such as those involving voice and fluency, the definition of successful treatment should account for subjective variables (e.g., client feelings, willingness to communicate) as well as objective variables (e.g., number of stuttered words, maintenance of specified optimal pitch).

In the context of clinical intervention, the most typical approach to data collection is the following single subject design: pretreatment baseline of a target → treatment → post-treatment baseline of the same behavior (in which the baseline measures are identical to one another and different from the treatment items). The information obtained from this data collection method is useful in documenting the amount of change or progress for a specific client. However, it does not address treatment efficacy in that this design does not permit the clinician to determine whether the intervention itself was responsible for the observed change.

To more adequately document the efficacy of treatment, a **multiple-baseline** design can be implemented. A simple multiple-baseline procedure involves the selection of at least three target behaviors of similar complexity that are in need of remediation. It is important to choose a set of targets for which direct transfer of learning is not expected to occur from one behavior to the others. For example, it is inappropriate to include phonemes that differ from each other by only one feature (e.g., voicing). Baseline measures are used to ascertain pretreatment status of the targets and treatment procedures are then implemented for one of them. After the criterion has been reached on the trained behavior, the clinician repeats the baseline measures on the untrained targets. If the results show no significant change from the original baseline scores, the clinician can be confident that the treatment, and no other factor, was responsible for the client's improvement on the trained target. One of the remaining targets is then selected for training and the treatment/posttreatment baseline sequence is repeated. This procedure is continued until all therapy targets have been trained.

An **evidence-based practice (EBP)** approach to intervention is best conceptualized as the integration of three main components: (1) current best scientific evidence; (2) clinician expertise; and (3) client values, beliefs, and preferences, including cultural/linguistic factors. Information in the professional literature can be categorized according to levels of scientific design and quality. Table 1-3 provides an evidence rating hierarchy that ranges from most to least scientifically robust. ASHA provides a valuable compendium of systematic literature reviews that clinicians can consult to guide their "best practices." This resource, the National Center for Evidence-Based Practice in Communication Disorders (N-CEP), can be accessed at www.asha.org/members/ebp/EBSRs/ and facilitates clinicians' ability to incorporate evidence into their clinical decision making in a variety of disorder areas.

From a practical perspective, clinicians should realize that "gold-standard" evidence (levels I and II) is frequently unavailable in the research literature for our profession. Clinicians should evaluate existing information from the other levels of the hierarchy to guide

TABLE 1–3

Evidence Rating Hierarchy

IA	Well-designed meta-analysis of more than one randomized, controlled study
IB	One well-designed, randomized, controlled study
IIA	One well-designed, controlled study without randomization
IIB	One well-designed, quasi-experimental study
III	Well-designed, nonexperimental studies (i.e., correlational and case studies, including multiple-baseline designs)
VI	Expert committee report, consensus conference, clinical experience of respected authorities

SOURCE: Adapted from Robey, R. (2004, April 13). Levels of evidence. The ASHA Leader. Retrieved from http://www.asha.org/Publications/leader/2004/040413/f040413a2.htm.

their decision making, to the extent possible. Implementation of an EBP approach may take many forms. Key steps in the process generally include the following:

1. Ask an answerable and intelligent clinical question.
2. Search for the best available evidence.
3. Critically evaluate the evidence.
4. Consider individual client characteristics and needs.
5. Make a clinical decision with client input.
6. Implement treatment plan and document progress/outcome(s).

Treatment Intensity and Dosage

In 2007, Warren, Fey, and Yoder (2007) presented a formal definition of treatment intensity: ". . . the product of rate [teaching episodes] per minute or hour, the number of hours of intervention per specified time period (e.g., a day or a week), and the full length of the interventions in weeks, months, or years . . ." (p. 71). This definition has been interpreted many different ways by both researchers and clinicians, resulting in considerable variability in treatment intensity. From the clinical practice perspective, the heart of the issue is "How much therapy, of what frequency and overall duration, and in which forms, is necessary to attain treatment goals?" Because little scientific evidence exists, clinicians must base their decisions on the individual characteristics and circumstances of each client.

Following is a list of the most common terminology used to describe treatment intensity: dose, dose form, dose frequency, total intervention duration, and cumulative intervention intensity (adapted from Breit-Smith, Justice, McGinty, & Kaderavek, 2009; Warren et al., 2007). An explanation of each of these terms follows:

- Dose: The number of times a strategy or technique is presented within a session
  - Example: 10 wh- questions produced in one session
- Dose Form: The delivery form for presenting the stimuli
  - Example: Semantic maps
- Dose Frequency: How often the intervention is provided
  - Example: 3 times per week
- Total Intervention Duration: The entire length of time the intervention is provided
  - Example: 14 weeks
- Cumulative intervention intensity: The numerical result of multiplying the values from dose, dose frequency, and total duration time
  - Example: 100 treatment sessions

SETTING-SPECIFIC PROFESSIONAL TERMINOLOGY

In the field of speech-language pathology, clinicians work in a variety of settings. Much of the information in the profession is considered "core" and applicable across settings. However, some jargon or terminology is specific to certain populations or work environments. Clinicians need to adapt the information contained in this book to their settings. To illustrate this point, Table 1-4 provides key examples of terminology used in two different settings: medical/hospital and educational/school.

TABLE 1–4
Examples of Terminology

Medical/Hospital Setting	Educational/School Setting
Modified barium swallow study: X-ray images are analyzed by a radiologist and SLP to evaluate the structure and function of swallowing mechanism. This is also known as VFSS (videofluoroscopic swallow study).	**Decodable texts:** A type of text used in beginning reading instruction in which words are restricted to spelling patterns that students can already decode given their existing knowledge of letter-sound correspondence.
Fiber-optic endoscopic evaluation of swallowing (FEES): SLP uses a flexible tube with a light attached to evaluate an individual's ability to swallow food/liquid safely and comfortably.	**Differentiated instruction:** Adapting teaching strategies to the needs of individual students or groups of children within a classroom to ensure that all students can learn effectively regardless of ability differences.
Skilled nursing facility (SNF): A facility that primarily provides inpatient care and rehabilitative services but does not provide the level of care or treatment available in a hospital.	**Embedded phonics:** An approach to classroom reading instruction in which letter-sound correspondence training is woven into authentic reading experiences.
Tracheostomy tube: A small plastic tube placed in a surgically created airway opening in the trachea to facilitate breathing.	**Guided reading:** Small-group reading instruction strategy in which teachers use a variety of prompts/scaffolds (e.g., context cues, definitions, word pronunciations) to improve the reading ability of students.
Ventilator: A machine designed to mechanically move breathable air in and out of the lungs.	**Language Experience Approach:** A reading instruction strategy that utilizes the personal experiences of students or a shared class experience to increase young readers' abilities to decode and understand written text.
Passy-Muir speaking valve (PMSV): A one-way valve that attaches to the outside opening of a tracheostomy tube. It allows air to pass into the tracheostomy but not out through it. The valve opens when the client breathes in, but stays closed during exhalation. This directs airflow around the tube and up through the vocal folds, permitting speech production.	**Leveled texts:** A system for organizing texts/books at different difficulty levels. Books are generally categorized by grade level using alphabetic lettering (A to Z) or by stages of difficulty (e.g., Stage 1, Stage 2, etc.).
NG (naso-gastric) tube: A long, flexible tube is placed through the nose into the stomach to allow liquid nutrition to be provided to individuals unable to eat by mouth.	**Locus of control:** Refers to a person's beliefs about the causes of good and bad predicaments in one's life. There are two main forces: external (fate, luck) and internal (one's own decisions and efforts). Belief in internal forces is associated with high levels of motivation.
G (gastrostomy) tube: A tube is placed in a surgically created opening to the stomach to allow nutrition to be provided to individuals unable to eat by mouth.	
Acute rehab: Rehabilitation services provided in a medical setting for patients whose health status requires continued hospitalization.	

(continues)

TABLE 1–4 *(Continued)*

Medical/Hospital Setting	Educational/School Setting
Subacute rehab: Programs/facilities that provide comprehensive inpatient rehabilitation services to clients after their discharge from the hospital.	**Readability:** An estimate of the relative difficulty or ease of a reading passage, based on counting the number of syllables, words, or sentences in a passage. There are three levels:
NPO: An abbreviation for a Latin term meaning "nothing by mouth."	■ Independent: Level at which student can read without adult support
Arteriovenus malformation (AVM): An abnormal collection of blood vessels that block the flow of blood to brain tissue.	■ Instructional: Level at which student can read with adult guidance ■ Frustration: Level at which student cannot read even with adult assistance
RUE/LUE: An acronym for right and left upper extremity (i.e., arms).	**Structural analysis:** A teaching strategy to help students understand the meaning of new words. It involves dividing words into
Functional independence measure (FIM): A seven-level scale sensitive to client changes over the course of a comprehensive inpatient rehabilitation program.	their parts (i.e., roots, prefixes, suffixes) and figuring out the meaning of the word parts.
Functional assessment measure (FAM): An adjunct set of items to the FIM that specifically address cognitive, behavioral, and communicative skill areas.	**Think-alouds:** An instructional strategy in which students are asked to say out loud what they are thinking about before, during, and after reading, solving math problems, or responding to questions posed by the teacher or other students. The think-aloud process is first modeled by the teacher to demonstrate practical ways of approaching difficult/new tasks or materials.
Cerebrovascular accident (CVA): Damage to brain cells due to the lack of oxygen that occurs when blood flow is impaired by blockage or rupture of an artery. This is also referred to as a *stroke*.	
ICD codes: Alphanumeric codes that are used to uniformly describe every medical diagnosis, description of symptoms, and cause of death.	**Thinking map:** A type of visual graphic organizer that shows the structure of different text genres (e.g., description, cause-effect, compare-contrast).
CPT codes: Numbers assigned to every task and service a practitioner may provide to a client, including medical, surgical, and rehabilitation diagnostic services.	

REIMBURSEMENT AND CODING

Reimbursement is an important and complex issue in health care. New developments in this area occur frequently and rapidly. Therefore, a comprehensive discussion of reimbursement issues is beyond the scope of this book. However, a brief introduction to several important concepts will be provided in this paragraph. Clinicians should be aware that insurers require the use of sets of alphanumeric codes to identify important information about patients. Descriptions of a client's diagnosis or condition must be assigned an appropriate code from the International Classification of Diseases–Tenth Revision (ICD-10), whereas descriptions of services provided/procedures performed need to be identified with codes from the Current Procedural Terminology (CPT). Several Web sites provide detailed information about appropriate use of these code sets. Clinicians can refer to the Centers for Medicare and Medicaid (www.cms.gov/Medicare/Coding/ICD10/index .html?redirect=/ICD10/), the American Medical Association (www.ama-assn.org/ama/ pub/physician-resources/solutions-managing-your-practice/coding-billing-insurance .page?), and the American Speech-Language-Hearing Association (www.asha.org/ practice/reimbursement/coding/default/) for more information.

TROUBLESHOOTING TIPS FOR THERAPY SESSIONS

If your client is not making adequate progress or seems bored and inattentive, ask yourself the following questions:

1. Are the reinforcers that I am using during therapy activities really motivating for this client?
2. Am I delivering the reinforcers fast enough for the client to connect them with the target behavior?
3. Did I shift from a continuous reinforcement schedule to an intermittent schedule too soon?
4. Am I teaching the target behavior in small enough steps?
5. Am I presenting the stimuli when the client is not paying attention or not making eye contact?
6. Is the patient bored because the same therapy materials are being used too often?
7. Is the client confused because I tend to phrase instructions in the form of requests rather than directions?
8. Am I programming a sufficient variety of target behaviors during each session to maintain the client's interest and motivation level?
9. Am I providing enough prompts/scaffolding during difficult therapy tasks to ensure that the client is relatively successful?
10. Am I allowing the client to make too many errors in a row without modifying the task?
11. Am I telling the patient what he or she does well or giving feedback only about incorrect responses?
12. Am I giving the client enough time to respond before repeating or rephrasing the stimuli?
13. Did I anticipate the unexpected and prepare 50% more material than I thought I needed?

CONCLUSION

This chapter has presented basic information, protocols, and procedures for intervention for communicative disorders at an *introductory* level. This information is intended only as a starting point in the reader's clinical education and training. For in-depth coverage of this area, the following readings are recommended:

Edwards, M., Stedler-Brown, A., & Houston, K. T. (2012). Expanding use of telepractice in speech-language pathology and audiology. *The Volta Review, 112*(3), 227–242.

Efficacy information on the Internet in speech-language pathology and audiology. Retrieved from http://www.mnsu.edu/comdis/efficacy/efficacy.html

Evidence-based practice. Retrieved from http://www.asha.org/members/ebp/

Hegde, M. N., & Davis, D. (2010). *Clinical methods and practicum in speech-language pathology.* (5th ed.) Clifton Park, NY: Delmar, Cengage Learning.

Paul, R., & Casella, P. (2013). *Introduction to clinical methods on communication disorders.* (3rd ed.) Baltimore, MD: Paul H. Brookes.

Speech and Language Forum: Evidence-Based Practice (EBP) Briefs. Retrieved from http://www.speechandlanguage.com/ebp-briefs

ADDITIONAL RESOURCES

Therasimplicity Inc.
228 Paperjack Drive, Suite 4
New Richmond, WI 54017
Phone: 800-906-8302
Fax: 715-246-3565
Web site: http://www.therasimplicity.com

Therasimplicity

A series of "books" that allow clinicians to access and print therapy materials such as cards, sequences, photographs, and pictures for a wide range of communication disorders. Also includes a medical encyclopedia and graphics for creating cards, templates, and certificates. Provides information on products in 23 areas (e.g., feeding, motor development).

Tactus Therapy Solutions
E-mail address: info@tactustherapy.com
Web site: http://tactustherapy.com/

Professional Apps for Speech Therapy

A series of apps designed to target the adult rehabilitation population. A variety of strategies and programs are provided to target skills such as language comprehension, naming, conversation skills, and memory/recall. Programs can be altered to allow clients to receive varying amounts of prompting and supports throughout the treatment process. The programs also enable clients to continue working on therapy targets at home.

APPENDIX 1-A

FORM 1–1 THERAPY OBSERVATION CHECKLIST

Date: _____

Clinician: _____

Supervisor: _____

Client: _____

KEY:

4 = Outstanding   1 = Weak

3 = Above average   0 = Unsatisfactory

2 = Average   N/A = Not applicable

PROGRAMMING

_____ Clear rationale for behavioral objectives/activities

_____ Appropriate written formulation of objectives ("do" statement, condition, criterion)

_____ Data from previous session used to determine behavioral goals

_____ Skill in revising goals/procedures as necessary during session (branching)

BEHAVIOR MODIFICATION

_____ Appropriate type of reinforcement

_____ Appropriate schedule of reinforcement

_____ Client behavior managed consistently in a firm yet nonthreatening manner

KEY TEACHING STRATEGIES

_____ Target behaviors modeled accurately

_____ Target-specific feedback provided consistently

_____ Brief summary of performance given after each activity

_____ Therapy techniques appropriate for client's age/developmental level and disorder

_____ Appropriate home assignments given with written instruction and demonstration

SESSION DESIGN

_____ Clear preinstruction given for each target behavior

_____ Communication style adapted to needs of the client (vocabulary, language level, nonverbal communication)

_____ Appropriate interpersonal skills; establishing rapport, motivating client

_____ Poised, confident demeanor

_____ Appropriate pace and amount of target productions

_____ Creative and appropriate therapy materials

_____ Appropriate proxemics

_____ Objectives for each client integrated into group sessions

DATA COLLECTION

_____ Ability to judge responses accurately

_____ Consistent, accurate data collection

APPENDIX 1-B

FORM 1–2 WORKSHEET FOR IDENTIFYING BEHAVIORAL OBJECTIVES

INSTRUCTIONS: The objectives listed below are stated incorrectly. Identify the errors in each objective by placing a check mark in the appropriate column(s). Answer key is on the next page.

Objective	"Do"	Condition	Criterion
1. Client will understand the concept of "red" with 90% accuracy when shown 30 cards.			
2. Client will produce /f/ several times given the clinician's model.			
3. Client will produce a complete sentence in four out of five trials.			
4. Client will use the regular past tense with no errors.			
5. Client will improve voice quality while reciting nursery rhymes with less than one parameter break per minute.			
6. To elicit /s/ and /z/ in single words by presenting familiar objects.			
7. Client will produce "is + verb + -ing" with 80% accuracy.			
8. Client will comprehend two-stage directions 100% of the time.			
9. Client will use the stuttering modification technique of "pull-out" frequently during a 1-minute monologue.			
10. Student will write 10 behavioral objectives that meet the criteria as discussed in this chapter.			

(continues)

ANSWER KEY: WORKSHEET FOR IDENTIFYING BEHAVIORAL OBJECTIVES

INSTRUCTIONS: The objectives listed below are stated incorrectly. Identify the errors in each objective by placing a check mark in the appropriate column(s).

Objective	"Do"	Condition	Criterion
1. Client will understand the concept of "red" with 90% accuracy when shown 30 cards.	X		
2. Client will produce /f/ several times given the clinician's model.			X
3. Client will produce a complete sentence in four out of five trials.		X	
4. Client will use the regular past tense with no errors.		X	
5. Client will improve voice quality while reciting nursery rhymes with less than one parameter break per minute.	X		
6. To elicit /s/ and /z/ in single words by presenting familiar objects.	X		
7. Client will produce "is + verb + -ing" with 80% accuracy.		X	
8. Client will comprehend two-stage directions 100% of the time.	X	X	
9. Client will use the stuttering modification technique of "pull-out" frequently during a 1-minute monologue.			X
10. Student will write 10 behavioral objectives that meet the criteria as discussed in this chapter.		X	X

APPENDIX 1-C

FORM 1–3 WORKSHEET FOR FORMULATING AND WRITING BEHAVIORAL OBJECTIVES

1. "Do" statement: Maintain phonation of a vowel for an average of 1.8 seconds
   Conditions: Using the inhalation method
   Criterion: 9 correct of 10 trials

   BEHAVIORAL OBJECTIVE: _____

   _____

   _____

2. "Do" statement: Manipulate objects
   Conditions: Given oral directions containing the concepts up-down, in-out, on-under
   Criterion: With no errors

   BEHAVIORAL OBJECTIVE: _____

   _____

   _____

3. "Do" statement: Imitate nonspeech vocalizations
   Conditions: Given the clinician's model
                     Given no more than two verbal prompts
   Criterion: 90% accuracy

   BEHAVIORAL OBJECTIVE: _____

   _____

   _____

4. "Do" statement: Tally instances of disfluency
   Conditions: While watching a videotape of himself speaking
   Criterion: 95% agreement with the clinician's tally

   BEHAVIORAL OBJECTIVE: _____

   _____

   _____

(continues)

5. "Do" statement: Produce fricatives /f/, /v/, /s/ in CV syllables

   Conditions: In imitation of the clinician

   In response to pictures

   Criterion: With 90% accuracy over two consecutive sessions

   BEHAVIORAL OBJECTIVE: _____

   _____

   _____

6. "Do" statement: Use easy onset of phonation

   Conditions: On the telephone

   While reading a written script

   Criterion: With less than two errors

   BEHAVIORAL OBJECTIVE: _____

   _____

   _____

7. "Do" statement: Sort 20 pictures of common objects

   Conditions: According to categories named by clinician

   Criterion: 18 correct of 20 trials

   BEHAVIORAL OBJECTIVE: _____

   _____

   _____

8. "Do" statement: Say words with /sw/ in the initial position

   Conditions: While looking in a mirror

   Criterion: 100% accuracy

   BEHAVIORAL OBJECTIVE: _____

   _____

   _____

9. "Do" statement: Maintain correct production of all forms of the verb "to be"

   Conditions: In spontaneous conversation with the clinician

   Criterion: No more than one error per 3-minute segment

   BEHAVIORAL OBJECTIVE: _____

   _____

   _____

APPENDIX 1-D

FORM 1–4 SAMPLE DAILY THERAPY PLAN

Client: __John Adams__   Clinician: __Marie Landers__

Date: __March 8, 2010__   Disorder: __Articulation/Language__

Behavioral Objectives	Data/Results
1. Given 10 pictures for each position and asked to create a sentence for each word, John will produce /f/ in the initial, medial, and final positions (IMF) with 90% accuracy.	/f/ I = 100% /f/ M = 90% /f/ F = 60% He was heard to use /f/ initial correctly in off-task comments. 5/6 errors in final position were θ/f.
2. John will correctly label the position of a block in relation to another object as "on" or "under" with 90% accuracy.	30/40 = 75%. Was only required to say "on" or "under," but on the last six responses client used a phrase as the answer (i.e., "on the chair").
3. John will follow two-step commands with four linguistic elements in response to clinician's verbal directions for 9 out of 10 trials.	5/10—had to be reminded to refrain from responding until entire command was presented.
4. John will imitatively produce CVC words maintaining final consonant with 90% accuracy.	28/50 = 56%

Reinforcement = 1:1 token + verbal praise
20 tokens = 1 puzzle piece

(continues)

OBSERVATION AND COMMENTS

CLIENT: John has met the criterion for /f/ I and M. Next session we will work only on F position. His spontaneous use of phrases during the preposition activity indicates that he is ready to move beyond the single-word response stage. The data for the two-step command activity suggest that this task needs to be modified. Maybe I will try a tactile prompt by placing my hands over his while presenting each command. I will instruct him that he can start responding as soon as I remove my hands from his. For the final consonant task, John needs some kind of cue to improve his performance. What do you think about using a visual prompt that highlights the concept of "final position" like a train that has three parts: an engine, one car, and a caboose? I gave Mom written instructions for homework for the initial and medial /f/ and for prepositions.

CLINICIAN: The articulation work took up a lot of time today, especially the final consonant activity. I need to design the next session so that an equivalent amount of time is spent on the language and articulation activities. I reviewed the audiotape from today's session and I think my feedback to John was immediate and specific to the targets. I think that my ability to accurately judge correct versus incorrect articulation responses is improving. I need to start fading the continuous reinforcement schedule for the tasks on which John is achieving an accuracy rate of 70% or higher.

APPENDIX 1-E

FORM 1–5   DAILY THERAPY PLAN

Client:_____   Clinician: _____

Date: _____   Disorder: _____

Behavioral Objectives	Data/Results

(continues)

OBSERVATION AND COMMENTS

APPENDIX 1-F

FORM 1–6 REPORT OF OBSERVATION HOURS

Name:_____

Semester:_____

KEY:

Age: C = Children,   A = Adults

Category: Select from list below.

Articulation Language Fluency Voice Other
Hearing Evaluation   Selection/Use of Amplification
& Assistive Listening Devices   Aural Rehabilitation

Date	Client's First Name and Initial	Age	Category	Hours		Supervisor Initials
				Diag.	Ther.	
1						
2						
3						
4						
5						
6						
7						
8						
9						
10						
11						
12						
13						
14						
15						
16						
17						
18						
19						
20						
21						
22						
23						
24						
25						

TOTAL OBSERVED HOURS

Number of Speech Hours: _____

Supervisor's Signature: _____

Date: _____

Number of Audiology Hours: _____

Supervisor's Signature: _____

Date:

APPENDIX 1-G

INSTRUCTIONS FOR USING DATA RECORDING FORMS

SESSION DATA LOG: This is an all-purpose data sheet designed to record an individual client's performance within a single session. Determine the type of notational system that will be used to record client responses (e.g., + or −, o or x) and enter this information in the box labeled "Key." Write the name or description of tasks in the left column (up to a maximum of 18). The numbered boxes indicate the number of trials. Record the accuracy of each response in the appropriate box. If the number of trials on a given task exceeds 20, continue to record on the next line of the grid. Calculate the percentage of correct responses and enter this information in the far right column for each task.

SUMMARY DATA LOG: This form is used to summarize information about an individual client's performance across a maximum of 20 sessions. It is designed to display client progress on specific therapy tasks over time. Enter session numbers or session dates in the boxes indicated at the top of the grid. Write the name or description of tasks in the left column (up to a maximum of 17). Retrieve the percentage of correct responses for each task from previous daily sheets (e.g., Session Data Log) and enter this information under each session date or number.

SUMMARY DATA GRAPH: Like the Summary Data Log, this form is used to summarize information about a client's status across a maximum of 20 sessions. The unique aspect of this form is that it allows the clinician to graph a client's progress on one or more objectives. Select a code for each objective that will be used on the graph to plot client performance. The code can consist of lines of different colors or patterns (e.g., solid, dotted, hatched). Enter this information along with a brief description of each task in the Key box. Retrieve performance data for each task from daily data sheets. Enter the session dates on the designated line, beginning with the pretreatment baseline session. Plot percentage of performance on the graph for each date (and for each task), and connect the data points to create a visual display of client progress.

RESPONSE DATA FORM: This is an all-purpose data sheet designed to track an individual client's responses on a single task during one session. It allows the clinician to document the specific stimulus items that are presented to a client during a given activity. Write the behavioral objective, therapy materials, and reinforcement type and schedule on the designated lines. Determine the type of notational system that will be used to record client responses (e.g., + or −, o or x) and enter this information in the Key. Record each stimulus in the left-hand column as it is presented. Note correct versus incorrect responses in column 1. This form can accommodate 20 stimulus items, which can be presented for a maximum of 10 trials each. Count the number of correct and incorrect responses and calculate the percentage of accuracy. Enter this information in the appropriate box at the lower left of the form.

RESPONSE RATING SCALE: This is a general form that can be used to document an individual client's performance within a single session. This form utilizes a scale that allows the clinician to rate the quality of a client's responses along a continuum of accuracy.

(continues)

The continuum is a five-level scale that includes the old error pattern (O), cued responses (C), approximations (A), self-corrections (S), and the new target behavior (T). Enter the task in the left column. The numbered boxes indicate the number of trials. Record the rating for each response (i.e., O, C, A, S, T) in the appropriate box. If the number of trials on a given task exceeds 20, continue to record on the next line of the grid. Calculate the percentage of each response type, and enter this information in the far right columns for each task.

ARTICULATION DATA SHEET: This form is designed to record an individual client's responses during articulation therapy. Determine the type of notational system that will be used to record the client's responses (e.g., + or −, o or x) and enter this information in the box labeled "Key." This form can be used in at least two ways. It can function as a data sheet for a single session, or it can be used to track a client's progress over time. Enter the session date and the therapy activity in the appropriate boxes. All correct and incorrect responses for each activity are recorded in a single box under the appropriate level of difficulty (e.g., Isolation, Syllable, Words). A single box may contain as many as 20 to 30 response notations. The amount of time spent on each activity also can be documented on this form. Count the number of total and correct responses and calculate the percentage of accuracy. Enter this information in the appropriate box.

INDIVIDUAL/GROUP QUICK TALLY SHEET: This form is designed for data collection in individual or group therapy sessions. For individual sessions, enter the client's name in the first box on the left. Assign a code or number (e.g., A or #1) for each activity, and enter this information for the first activity in the same box. As the stimuli are presented, record incorrect responses by making a slash mark through the corresponding number. Correct responses are indicated by the lack of a slash mark. Tally the number of correct responses, and calculate the percentage of accuracy. Enter this information on the appropriate lines. Repeat this tally procedure for each subsequent activity. For group sessions, this form can be used in at least two ways, depending on the size of the group. For groups of three or fewer, enter the name, activity code, and response data for each individual from left to right across the page in the same row. This orientation permits data to be recorded on a maximum of six activities for each group member. For groups with three to six members, enter the data for each client from top to bottom down the page in the same column. This orientation accommodates a maximum of three activities per group member.

GROUP THERAPY DATA SHEET: This form is designed for use in therapy groups that range in size from two to four members. Determine the type of notational system that will be used to record the clients' responses (e.g., + or −, o or x) and enter this information on the line labeled "Response Key." Enter each group member's name on the indicated line. Assign a code or number (e.g., A or #1) for each activity, and enter this information for each group member in the appropriate box. Record the accuracy of each client's responses in the boxes below the numbers. This data form allows for a maximum of 50 trials (per member) to be recorded for each activity. The amount of time each client spends on a given activity also can be documented on this form. Count the number of correct and total responses and calculate the percentage of accuracy for each client. Enter this information in the appropriate boxes.

CLASSROOM DATA FORM: This form is an example of a data sheet used in the classroom to track performance of multiple children on eight curriculum-based language goals. Enter one child's name in each block in the first column. Indicate incorrect responses with slash marks through specific stimulus items. This form can be used to calculate percentage of accuracy for individual children on one or more goals. In addition, performance accuracy of the entire group can be monitored for all eight identified goals.

(continues)

FORM 1–7 SESSION DATA LOG

SESSION DATA LOG

KEY:

Name of Client: _____

Name of Clinician: _____

Date: _____

TRIALS

Task	1	2	3	4	5	6	7	8	9	10	11	12	13	14	15	16	17	18	19	20	% correct

(continues)

Appendix 1-G (Continued)

FORM 1–8 SUMMARY DATA LOG

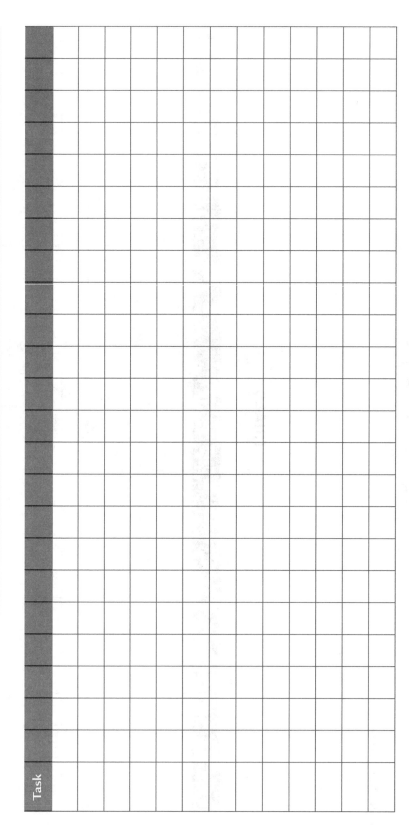

SUMMARY DATA LOG

Name of Client: _____

Name of Clinician: _____

DATE OR SESSION NUMBER

Task

(continues)

FORM 1–9 SUMMARY DATA GRAPH

SUMMARY DATA GRAPH

KEY:

Name of Client: _____

Name of Clinician: _____

Date: _____

PERCENTAGE																					
100																					
90																					
80																					
70																					
60																					
50																					
40																					
30																					
20																					
10																					
0																					
Section # Date	B	1	2	3	4	5	6	7	8	9	10	11	12	13	14	15	16	17	18	19	20

(continues)

FORM 1–10 RESPONSE DATA FORM

RESPONSE DATA FORM

Name of Client: _____   Date: _____

Name of Clinician: _____

Behavioral Objective: _____

Therapy Materials: _____

Reinforcement Type and Schedule: _____

TRIALS

Stimulus Presented	1	2	3	4	5	6	7	8	9	10	Comments
1.											
2.											
3.											
4.											
5.											
6.											
7.											
8.											
9.											
10.											
11.											
12.											
13.											
14.											
15.											
16.											
17.											
18.											
19.											
20.											

Total Number of Responses: _____   KEY:

Total Correct Responses: _____

Total Incorrect Responses: _____

Percent Correct: _____

(continues)

FORM 1–11 RESPONSE RATING SCALE

RESPONSE RATING SCALE

Name of Client: _____

Name of Clinician: _____

Date: _____

KEY:

O = Old behavior   S = Self-correction

C = Cued response   T = Target behavior

A = Approximation

TRIALS

Task	1	2	3	4	5	6	7	8	9	10	11	12	13	14	15	16	19	20	% O	% C	% A	% S	% T

(continues)

FORM 1–12 ARTICULATION DATA SHEET

ARTICULATION DATA SHEET

Name of Client: _____

Name of Clinician: _____

KEY: _____

Date	Activity	Isolated	Syllables	Words	Sentence	Reading	Conversation	Time	Total Resp.	Total Correct	% Correct

(continues)

FORM 1–13 INDIVIDUAL/GROUP QUICK TALLY SHEET

INDIVIDUAL/GROUP QUICK TALLY SHEET

Clinician: ____________ Date: ____________

Name ____________
Activity ____________

1	2	3	4	5
6	7	8	9	10
11	12	13	14	15
16	17	18	19	20
21	22	23	24	25
26	27	28	29	30
31	32	33	34	35
36	37	38	39	40
41	42	43	44	45
46	47	48	49	50

Correct ____________
% Correct ____________

Name ____________
Activity ____________

1	2	3	4	5
6	7	8	9	10
11	12	13	14	15
16	17	18	19	20
21	22	23	24	25
26	27	28	29	30
31	32	33	34	35
36	37	38	39	40
41	42	43	44	45
46	47	48	49	50

Correct ____________
% Correct ____________

Name ____________
Activity ____________

1	2	3	4	5
6	7	8	9	10
11	12	13	14	15
16	17	18	19	20
21	22	23	24	25
26	27	28	29	30
31	32	33	34	35
36	37	38	39	40
41	42	43	44	45
46	47	48	49	50

Correct ____________
% Correct ____________

Name ____________
Activity ____________

1	2	3	4	5
6	7	8	9	10
11	12	13	14	15
16	17	18	19	20
21	22	23	24	25
26	27	28	29	30
31	32	33	34	35
36	37	38	39	40
41	42	43	44	45
46	47	48	49	50

Correct ____________
% Correct ____________

Name ____________
Activity ____________

1	2	3	4	5
6	7	8	9	10
11	12	13	14	15
16	17	18	19	20
21	22	23	24	25
26	27	28	29	30
31	32	33	34	35
36	37	38	39	40
41	42	43	44	45
46	47	48	49	50

Correct ____________
% Correct ____________

Name ____________
Activity ____________

1	2	3	4	5
6	7	8	9	10
11	12	13	14	15
16	17	18	19	20
21	22	23	24	25
26	27	28	29	30
31	32	33	34	35
36	37	38	39	40
41	42	43	44	45
46	47	48	49	50

Correct ____________
% Correct ____________

Name ____________
Activity ____________

1	2	3	4	5
6	7	8	9	10
11	12	13	14	15
16	17	18	19	20
21	22	23	24	25
26	27	28	29	30
31	32	33	34	35
36	37	38	39	40
41	42	43	44	45
46	47	48	49	50

Correct ____________
% Correct ____________

Name ____________
Activity ____________

1	2	3	4	5
6	7	8	9	10
11	12	13	14	15
16	17	18	19	20
21	22	23	24	25
26	27	28	29	30
31	32	33	34	35
36	37	38	39	40
41	42	43	44	45
46	47	48	49	50

Correct ____________
% Correct ____________

Name ____________
Activity ____________

1	2	3	4	5
6	7	8	9	10
11	12	13	14	15
16	17	18	19	20
21	22	23	24	25
26	27	28	29	30
31	32	33	34	35
36	37	38	39	40
41	42	43	44	45
46	47	48	49	50

Correct ____________
% Correct ____________

Name ____________
Activity ____________

1	2	3	4	5
6	7	8	9	10
11	12	13	14	15
16	17	18	19	20
21	22	23	24	25
26	27	28	29	30
31	32	33	34	35
36	37	38	39	40
41	42	43	44	45
46	47	48	49	50

Correct ____________
% Correct ____________

Name ____________
Activity ____________

1	2	3	4	5
6	7	8	9	10
11	12	13	14	15
16	17	18	19	20
21	22	23	24	25
26	27	28	29	30
31	32	33	34	35
36	37	38	39	40
41	42	43	44	45
46	47	48	49	50

Correct ____________
% Correct ____________

Name ____________
Activity ____________

1	2	3	4	5
6	7	8	9	10
11	12	13	14	15
16	17	18	19	20
21	22	23	24	25
26	27	28	29	30
31	32	33	34	35
36	37	38	39	40
41	42	43	44	45
46	47	48	49	50

Correct ____________
% Correct ____________

Name ____________
Activity ____________

1	2	3	4	5
6	7	8	9	10
11	12	13	14	15
16	17	18	19	20
21	22	23	24	25
26	27	28	29	30
31	32	33	34	35
36	37	38	39	40
41	42	43	44	45
46	47	48	49	50

Correct ____________
% Correct ____________

Name ____________
Activity ____________

1	2	3	4	5
6	7	8	9	10
11	12	13	14	15
16	17	18	19	20
21	22	23	24	25
26	27	28	29	30
31	32	33	34	35
36	37	38	39	40
41	42	43	44	45
46	47	48	49	50

Correct ____________
% Correct ____________

Name ____________
Activity ____________

1	2	3	4	5
6	7	8	9	10
11	12	13	14	15
16	17	18	19	20
21	22	23	24	25
26	27	28	29	30
31	32	33	34	35
36	37	38	39	40
41	42	43	44	45
46	47	48	49	50

Correct ____________
% Correct ____________

(continues)

FORM 1–14 GROUP THERAPY DATA SHEET

GROUP THERAPY DATA SHEET

Date: _____

Name: _____

Name of Client: _____

Response Key: _____

Activity						Time						# Correct						Total Responses						% Correct	
1	2	3	4	5	6	7	8	9	10	11	12	13	14	15	16	17	18	19	20	21	22	23	24	25
26	27	28	29	30	31	32	33	34	35	36	37	38	39	40	41	42	43	44	45	46	47	48	49	50

Name: _____

Activity						Time						# Correct						Total Responses						% Correct	
1	2	3	4	5	6	7	8	9	10	11	12	13	14	15	16	17	18	19	20	21	22	23	24	25
26	27	28	29	30	31	32	33	34	35	36	37	38	39	40	41	42	43	44	45	46	47	48	49	50

Name: _____

Activity						Time						# Correct						Total Responses						% Correct	
1	2	3	4	5	6	7	8	9	10	11	12	13	14	15	16	17	18	19	20	21	22	23	24	25
26	27	28	29	30	31	32	33	34	35	36	37	38	39	40	41	42	43	44	45	46	47	48	49	50

(continues)

FORM 1–15 EMERGENT LITERACY DATA FORM

EMERGENT LITERACY DATA FORM

Student's name: _____   Date: _____   Age: _____

Names Letter	Names Sound	Phonological Awareness	Print Knowledge	Reading	Writing Skills
A B C D E F G H I J K L M N O P Q R S T U V W X Y Z	A B C D E F G H I J K L M N O P Q R S T U V W X Y Z	Recognizes rhyme words	Follows left-to-right progression	Sits alone and looks at books	Scribbles
		Says rhyme words	Knows books have a front and back	Pretends to read books	Draws a picture that tells a story
		Identifies first sound in spoken words	Knows how to open/hold books	Recognizes/says familiar words/logos	Prints some letters/numbers
		Knows words can be divided into parts	Moves finger along line of print	Reads a few familiar words by sight	Prints own name
			Points to words in book title		Writes one letter/word for sentence or idea
					Writes strings of random letters
					Uses one to three letters to spell words
Benchmark: _____	Benchmark: _____	Benchmark: _____	Benchmark: _____	Benchmark: _____	Benchmark: _____

APPENDIX 1-H

FORM 1–16 SAMPLE POSITIVE BEHAVIOR SUPPORT PLAN

POSITIVE BEHAVIOR SUPPORT PLAN

Client Name:_____ Date: _____

Clinician Name: _____

Behavior impacting learning is: _____

_____

It impedes learning because: _____

_____

Estimate of current severity of behavior problem: _____

_____

Frequency/intensity/duration of behavior: _____

_____

Current predictors for behavior: _____

_____

What client should do instead of this behavior: _____

_____

_____

What supports the client in using the desired behavior?

Teaching Strategies: _____

_____

_____

Environmental Modifications: _____

_____

_____

(continues)

SAMPLE

SAMPLE POSITIVE BEHAVIOR SUPPORT PLAN

Client Name: Janelle Smith   **Date:** 5/6/15

Clinician Name: Harriet Wilson

Behavior impacting learning is: Janelle exhibits a number of disruptive behaviors including singing, throwing objects, and refusing to participate by pretending to be asleep.

It impedes learning because: (1) It distracts the class's attention from the focus of the teacher's lesson; and (2) thrown objects present a danger to both the teacher and Janelle's classmates.

Estimate of current severity of behavior problem: Moderate

Frequency/intensity/duration of behavior: three to four times per week varying in intensity depending on context with episodes 5 to 10 minutes.

Current predictors for behavior: Janelle is likely to sing, put her head on the desk, or throw books if she does not get enough sleep the previous night, during classes at the end of the day, and most especially during writing tasks (an area of academic weakness for Janelle).

What client should do instead of this behavior: Participate in classroom activities without disrupting others.

What supports the client in using the desired behavior? Consistent verbal reminders from the teacher

Teaching strategies: (1) Implement smaller group instructional format, especially for writing tasks; (2) provide alternative assignments that Janelle can request if the original task is too challenging.

Environmental Modifications: Janelle's mother will notify the school/classroom teacher when Janelle has slept poorly the night before. The teacher can then temporarily reduce expectations for writing assignments on those days.

CHAPTER 2

PHILOSOPHY

The main purpose of clinical reports is to summarize and interpret information regarding a client's performance or status. In this chapter, the term *report* is used to refer to written records that may vary in length from multiple-page documents to brief notations in client charts. (Note: Many facilities are moving to electronic records; thus, the format of reports may be dictated by the electronic platform that is being used.) A well-written document does more than report test scores and performance data. It provides an explanation of each data point and specifies its relation to a client's overall communication profile and needs. Numbers alone do not yield this interpretive information. Inferential statements always must be substantiated by supporting data. Adherence to this philosophy of clinical writing promotes clinician accountability by providing justification for the judgments and decisions that occur throughout the treatment process.

Accountability also requires that reports be written with ethical considerations in mind. Prognosis and recommendation statements, in particular, must be written carefully to ensure that they are not misleading or unrealistic. For example, consider the following prognostic statement for a 60-year-old male with moderate aphasia who suffered a stroke 10 years ago:

> Based on Mr. Hanks's high level of enthusiasm, the prognosis for improvement in therapy is good.

This statement is inappropriate for two important reasons. First, a client's degree of enthusiasm is not a reliable indicator of future success. Moreover, the amount of time that has elapsed since Mr. Hanks's stroke (a more meaningful indicator) may warrant a more guarded statement of prognosis. Ethical considerations also significantly influence the development of treatment recommendations. These statements must be based on client needs and preferences rather than on the type and frequency of service that a particular therapist or facility can provide.

TECHNICAL WRITING STYLE

Clinical reports are formal documents that must be written in an appropriate technical style (Hegde & Davis, 2010). In many cases, written reports may be the first or the only avenue of contact between a speech-language pathologist (SLP) and other professionals. Poorly written reports can severely compromise a clinician's professional credibility. Imagine the reaction of a physician when reading the following section of an SLP's progress report:

> Shirley was initially nervous in the therapy room, particularly when her mother, she thought was going to leave her, she cried. Difficult to illicit spontaneous utterances from her, though she was willing to imitate.

For this reason, the ability to communicate effectively in writing is as important as a clinician's knowledge of communication disorders and their treatment. The following guidelines can assist in the development of professional reports that are clear, concise, and well organized:

- Avoid writing clinical reports in a conversational style (e.g., "He just didn't get the point" versus "He did not appear to understand the task").

- Use correct spelling, grammar, and punctuation, and write in complete sentences.

- Write in the third person (e.g., "The Peabody Picture Vocabulary Test-IV was administered" rather than first person "I administered the Peabody Picture Vocabulary Test-IV").

- Avoid use of contracted verb forms (e.g., isn't, can't, I've).

- Give the full names of tests on first mention, then use acronyms and other abbreviations in the remainder of the report.

- Express information in behavioral terms (e.g., "followed two-step commands" versus "is able to follow two-step commands").

- Present information (particularly case history) in chronological sequence.

- Differentiate clearly between information reported by others and information obtained directly through clinician observation.

- List all data such as test scores, baseline measures, or progress-monitoring measures before providing any interpretative statements. This approach facilitates interpretation of a client's overall profile rather than presenting unrelated descriptions of isolated communication skills.

- Include information about a client's strengths as well as weaknesses in the body of the report.

- In any report, avoid presenting information in the summary section that was not introduced previously in the body of the report.

- Write reports to communicate with colleagues using professional terminology, but include simple explanations and clear examples to make reports meaningful to family members and other nonprofessionals.

- Use language that is specific and unambiguous (e.g., "He demonstrated language skills characteristic of 4-year-old children" rather than "He demonstrated poor language skills").

- Avoid exaggeration and overstatement (e.g., "*completely* uncooperative," "*absolutely* intelligible," "never produces /s/," "*extremely* motivated").

REPORT FORMATS

In the context of intervention, clinical reports serve three main purposes: (1) to outline the intended intervention plan at the beginning of therapy, (2) to document client performance on a session-to-session basis throughout the course of treatment, and (3) to summarize client status periodically and at the end of the treatment program. Report formats for each of these functions can vary greatly among clinicians and service-delivery settings. Regardless of the particular format, however, a basic core of information is important in each of the three types of reports. Following is a framework for each report type.

Initial Therapy Plan

An **initial therapy plan (ITP)** is developed at the beginning of treatment for each client. It specifies long-term goals and short-term objectives based on diagnostic findings and pretreatment baseline results. Following are the basic content and organization of an ITP.

Identifying Information. List identifying information at the top of the report. This section may include a client's name, age, address, type of disorder, date of report, and so on.

Example

Name: José Rodríguez   Date of Birth: July 15, 2007
Parents: Carlos and María Rodríguez   Age: 7 years, 2 months
Address: 1800 Knox Street   Category: Language/Articulation
         College Park, MD 20740   Graduate Clinician: Gary Frost, M.A.
Phone: (301) 555-2379   Clinical Supervisor: Ruth Barr, M.A.,
                                            CCC-SLP

Date of Report: 09/25/14

Background Information/Pertinent History. In paragraph form, state the full name and age of the client, note the location and date of the initial evaluation, and summarize highlights of relevant diagnostic information in a few sentences. If the client was referred from another source, give the date, referral source, and reason for referral. For clients who have received previous therapy, this section should specify the provider, identify the dates of most recent service, and briefly summarize goals and progress.

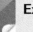

Example

José is a 7-year-old boy who was first seen at the University of Maryland Speech and Hearing Clinic for a diagnostic evaluation in March 2014. At the time of this testing, José demonstrated a number of language and articulation difficulties, including weaknesses in oral expression. José's parents are bilingual, and Spanish is sometimes spoken in the home. However, they identify José's primary language as English. José is currently in the second grade at Maple Elementary School. He is reportedly doing well in school.

Past therapy began on January 15, 2014, in his elementary school, and focused on the production of fricatives (v, z, th), consonant blends, regular plurals, and irregular past tense. These are no longer notable areas of difficulty for José. He did not demonstrate mastery on goals that focused on vowel + /r/ production and irregular plurals.

Goals and Objectives. In outline form, record pertinent speech-language goals and objectives in a hierarchy of complexity ranging from least to most difficult. (Recall that goals are general statements of desired outcomes over the course of the treatment program, whereas objectives specify measurable behaviors that lead to mastery of the long-term goals.) Under each long-term goal, specify relevant test results/baseline data that have been collected and used as the basis for development of the short-term objectives. Baseline data are generally obtained over the initial therapy sessions. Make note of any unusual or clinically significant behavior patterns. Materials and procedures generally are not included as part of this section.

Example

Articulation

Goal I: To improve production of /ɚ/ in spontaneous speech.

Initial Status/Baseline 9/23/14

0% accuracy for spontaneous speech
45% of /ɚ/ productions were at a rating of 2 on a 3-point scale, when produced imitatively in isolation.

Note: Productions were scored on a 3-point scale, where 1 = "uh" and 3 = accurate production.

Objectives

A. Given visual and verbal prompts for correct tongue positioning, José will pronounce /ɚ/ imitatively in isolation at a rating of 3 in 9 out of 10 trials over two consecutive sessions.
B. Given pictures or printed stimuli, José will spontaneously produce /ɚ/ in the initial and final position of words, with a rating of 3 in 9 out of 10 trials over two consecutive sessions.
C. Given pictures or printed stimuli, José will produce /ɚ/ in the initial and final position of words in carrier phrases, with a rating of 3 in 9 out of 10 trials over two consecutive sessions.
D. Given pictures, printed stimuli, or objects, José will produce /ɚ/ in the initial and final position of words in spontaneous sentences during structured activities, with a rating of 3 in 9 out of 10 trials over two consecutive sessions.
E. Given a variety of stimulus prompts (e.g., pictures, objects), José will produce /ɚ/ in the initial and final position of words in structured discourse with a rating of 3 in 9 out of 10 trials over two consecutive sessions.

Language

Goal I: To use irregular plurals in spontaneous speech.

(Target set: *sheep, fish, deer, feet, teeth, children, women, men, geese, mice, knives, loaves, wives, wolves, calves, thieves, halves, shelves, leaves*)

Initial Status/Baseline 9/23/14

15% correct plural form at the single-word level, given picture prompts

Objectives

A. José will provide the correct irregular plural, given a singular word from the target set, with 90% accuracy over two consecutive sessions.
B. José will use irregular plurals in carrier phrases, when given a singular word from the target set, with 90% accuracy over two consecutive sessions.
C. José will use irregular plurals in spontaneous sentences, when given a singular word from the target set, with 90% accuracy over two consecutive sessions.
D. José will use irregular plurals in structured discourse, given a set of singular words from the target set, with 90% accuracy over two consecutive sessions.

Reinforcement. In paragraph form, indicate the type and schedule of reinforcers to be used for shaping target productions and attending behaviors.

Example

A continuous schedule of verbal reinforcement, coupled with token reinforcers, will be used to shape target behaviors. This will be faded to an intermittent schedule as José demonstrates progress. A separate response-cost system will be used to reduce José's tendency to initiate responses prematurely.

Family Engagement. In paragraph form, discuss how family members will be involved in observation of therapy sessions, conferences/counseling, and homework.

Example

Parent(s) will observe José's therapy sessions at least once every two weeks. Brief, informal discussions of José's progress will take place following every session; formal conferences will be held every three months. Periodic training will be provided to help parents participate in homework assignments.

Generalization Plan. In paragraph form, specify strategies for transfer of target objectives to home, school, or work settings.

Example

José will be given weekly homework assignments to facilitate the generalization of target behaviors. Parent will be provided with written instructions for these assignments. The clinician also will contact José's teacher bimonthly to discuss his status and to give suggestions for how therapy objectives can be incorporated into the classroom.

The initial therapy plan can be viewed as the clinician's best prediction of what a client can accomplish in a given amount of time. The client's progress in therapy should be monitored on a periodic basis through the administration of probes to determine whether the plan's original objectives remain appropriate or require modification. (A complete sample ITP is included in Appendix 2-B at the end of this chapter.)

Progress Notes

Once therapy has begun, client performance is documented on an ongoing basis. Progress notes are short and are written during or after each session. They may be filed in a client's medical chart or a client's folder or written on the therapy plan itself. Daily notes serve at least three important functions: (1) they enable the clinician to monitor the treatment program on a continual basis and implement any necessary changes immediately; (2) they provide information on a daily basis to other professionals who also may be working with the client (e.g., occupational therapist, social worker); and (3) they facilitate the continuity of treatment by allowing another clinician to provide services in the event of unexpected clinician absence.

One common format of daily progress notes, particularly in medical settings, is known as SOAP notes. *SOAP* is an acronym that refers to the terms *subjective*, *objective*, *assessment*, and *plan*.

Subjective: Write your opinion regarding relevant client behavior or status in a brief statement.

Objective: Record data collected for each task during the therapy session.

Assessment: Interpret data for current session and compare to client's previous levels of performance.

Plan: Identify proposed therapy targets for the next session.

Example

S: José appeared tired and reluctant to cooperate with the tasks presented.

O: Final /ɚ/ in single words = 85% (17/20); irregular plurals in spontaneous phrases = 50% (20/40).

A: Fading of clinician model to a 5:1 ratio on irregular plural task may have been premature. Today's score of 50% constitutes a decrease in accuracy compared to José's performance of the same task over the two previous sessions (70% and 75%).

P: Continue work on both tasks at the same levels, but increase clinician modeling for the irregular plural task to a 2:1 ratio.

Progress and Final Reports

A report is written for each patient at specific intervals throughout treatment and when intervention services are terminated. These reports also may be referred to as interim summaries, annual reviews, discharge reports, or final summaries, depending on the clinical setting. Progress and final reports document a client's mastery of the goals and objectives outlined in the ITP and implemented over the course of treatment. Following are the basic content and organization of these reports.

Identifying Information. List identifying information at the top of the report. This section may include a client's name, age, address, type of disorder, dates of service, date of report, and so on.

Example

Name:	José Rodríguez	Date of Birth:	July 15, 2007
Parents:	Carlos and María Rodríguez	Age:	8 years, 4 months
Address:	1800 Knox Street College Park, MD 20740	Date of Report:	November 25, 2015
		Disorder:	Articulation and Language
Service Dates:	October 13, 2014 to November 21, 2015	Clinician:	Gary Frost

Background Information/Statement of Problem. In paragraph form, state the full name and age of the client and include the following information: (1) date of first therapy session, (2) client's speech and language status at that time, and (3) session frequency and duration. In some cases, it may be useful to include a brief description of previous therapy goals.

Example

José is an 8-year-old boy, who was first seen at the University of Maryland Hearing and Speech Clinic for a diagnostic evaluation in March 2014. At the time of the initial diagnosis, José demonstrated language and articulation difficulties. He began therapy during the fall semester of 2014 and has continued through the present. He has been seen twice weekly for 50-minute sessions. Past therapy has included the production of fricatives (v, z, th) and consonant blends, regular plurals, and irregular past tense. These are no longer areas of notable difficulty for José. José began therapy for the fall 2014 semester on October 13. Producing vowel + /r/ (e.g., moth*er*) continues to be a target for therapy. Work on irregular plurals was added as a target this semester.

Therapy Objectives and Progress. In outline form, restate all the short-term objectives listed for each goal in the ITP, indicate client's level of mastery for each objective, and cite supporting data for mastery for each objective. Compare the client's current performance levels to the pretreatment baseline data for that target area. Comment on the degree of improvement represented by this comparison (e.g., significant, moderate, minimal). Note any special procedures, strategies, tasks, or cues that facilitated the client's performance.

Example

Articulation

Note: Productions were scored on a 3-point scale, where 1 = "uh" and 3 = accurate production.

Objectives

A. Given visual and verbal prompts for correct tongue positioning, José will pronounce /ɚ/ imitatively in isolation, with a rating of 3 in 9 out of 10 trials over two consecutive sessions (in progress: 89% on 11/18, 86% on 11/20).

B. Given pictures or printed stimuli, José will spontaneously produce /ɚ/ in the initial and final position of words, with a rating of 3 in 9 out of 10 trials over two consecutive sessions. [Not yet addressed]

C. Given pictures or printed stimuli, José will produce /ɚ/ in the initial and final position of words in carrier phrases, with a rating of 3 in 9 out of 10 trials over two consecutive sessions. [Not yet addressed]

D. Given pictures, printed stimuli, or objects, José will produce /ɚ/ in the initial and final position of words in spontaneous sentences during structured activities, with a rating of 3 in 9 out of 10 trials over two consecutive sessions. [Not yet addressed]

E. Given a variety of stimulus prompts (e.g., pictures, objects), José will produce /ɚ/ in the initial and final position of words in structured discourse with a rating of 3 in 9 out of 10 trials over two consecutive sessions. [Not yet addressed]

Comments

José is able to describe where his tongue should be in order to say /ɚ/ correctly. He has made moderate progress in improving his /ɚ/ sounds in isolation, although he continues to need occasional prompting to achieve a rating of 3. On occasion, he can produce the sound accurately at the word level, particularly when /ɚ/ occurs in the final position. José lifts his tongue up at the back of his palate while not holding the sides of his tongue to the hard palate near his teeth. The method José seemed to find most successful in facilitating correct productions was moving from an /i/ sound into an /ɚ/ sound by sliding his tongue back along the palate.

Language

Objectives

A. José will provide the correct irregular plural, given a singular word from the target set, with 90% accuracy over two consecutive sessions (criterion met at 100% accuracy on 10/23 for first half of the set and 11/18 for the second half of the set).

B. José will use irregular plurals in carrier phrases, when given a singular word from the target set, with 90% accuracy over two consecutive sessions (criterion met at 100% accuracy on 10/28 for first half of the set and 11/24 for the second half of the set).

C. José will use irregular plurals in spontaneous sentences, when given a singular word from the target set, with 90% accuracy over two consecutive sessions (criterion met at 100% accuracy on 11/12 for first half of the set and 12/5 for the second half of the set).

D. José will use irregular plurals in structured discourse, given a set of singular words from the target set, with 90% accuracy over two consecutive sessions (criterion met at 100% for all 20 words on 12/7).

Comments

José was familiar with the concept of plurals from previous therapy; however, he was not familiar with plural formation that did not follow the usual rules. Requiring Jose to write down the plural forms of regular plurals and target words from the set helped him differentiate these forms. Once he was familiar with the new words, they were practiced using a variety of game formats. For example, for the carrier-phrase level, José played Go Fish and asked questions such as, "Do you have any *geese*?" When working at the structured-discourse level, José formulated short stories using the target words; this was a particularly functional activity for him because he enjoys telling stories.

Summary and Additional Information. Summarize all the preceding "criterion met" statements. This summary should provide an overall profile of the client's progress over time rather than a simple reiteration of previously stated information. In separate paragraphs, include information about the following:

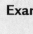 Reinforcement (for both targets and attending behaviors)

 Completion of homework assignments

 Family participation/observation

 Parent/client conferences

 Other pertinent issues such as results of additional testing, significant medical information (e.g., changes in medication), change in educational placement, and so on

---

Example

Overall, José has made moderate progress in improving his pronunciation of /ɚ/ this semester. His knowledge and use of irregular plurals has improved considerably; he learned the set of target words very quickly and was able to generalize to other contexts. From a functional perspective, José's parents report that his general intelligibility seems to have improved based on the increasing number of verbal messages he conveys without adult and peer requests for clarification or repetition.

A continuous verbal reinforcement schedule was used to establish target behaviors. As accuracy improved, an intermittent schedule was introduced. A behavior-management system was implemented, in which José was given 10 tokens at the beginning of each session. He was told that these could be traded in at the end of the session for a small prize. However, one token would be subtracted from his pile for each instance of noncompliant behavior (e.g., off-task talking) during therapy activities.

Homework practice was assigned weekly. Mrs. Rodríguez reported working with José on homework assignments on a daily basis. Mrs. Rodríguez observed a therapy session at least once every two weeks. José's progress was discussed with her informally after each session and formally during parent conferences held every three months.

Recommendations. State whether continued speech-language intervention is warranted. If so, give suggestions for specific goals and objectives. Make any other pertinent recommendations (e.g., psychological testing).

Example

It is recommended that José continue to participate in speech and language therapy primarily to improve his /r/ pronunciation. José learns rules and patterns quickly; therefore, it is felt that specific syntax and word-usage problems that may arise in his spontaneous speech can be addressed successfully in the school setting.

A complete sample progress report is included in Appendix 2-C at the end of this chapter.

TIPS FOR PROOFREADING CLINICAL REPORTS

Students, beginning clinicians, and supervisors can use the following set of proofreading questions to edit and monitor the quality of clinical reports:

- Are spelling, grammar, and punctuation correct?
- Are professional terms used accurately?
- Is there redundancy of word usage or sentence type?
- Are any sentences too lengthy, rambling, or unfocused?
- Is all the important client information included in the report?
- Is information presented only in the germane sections of the report (e.g., no recommendation statements in the background information section)?
- Does the report follow a logical sequence from one section to the next (i.e., from background, to data and interpretation, to summary and recommendations)?
- Are raw data interpreted and not merely reported?
- Are all conclusions and assumptions supported by sufficient data?
- Are speculative statements explicitly identified as such?
- Does the report contain seemingly contradictory statements without adequate explanation?
- Is the wording clear or are some statements vague and ambiguous?
- Is content presented with appropriate emphasis? Has any critical information been overlooked? Has any minor point been overemphasized?
- Is the report written with ethical/legal considerations in mind?

INDIVIDUALIZED EDUCATION PROGRAM

The Education of All Handicapped Children Act (PL 94-142) was passed in 1975 to ensure that all children ages 3 to 21 years with special needs receive a free, appropriate public education (FAPE). Speech-language pathology is a designated special education service under this law. This legislation was most recently reauthorized in 2004 through PL 108-446 and is known as the Individuals with Disabilities Education Improvement Act (IDEA). Final regulations for Part B of this legislation were released in 2006. These regulations pertain to services in school settings.

Each eligible child must have an annual written **Individualized Education Program (IEP)**, which documents the need for the provision of special education services. The purpose of this program is to identify specific areas for remediation. Unlike other clinical reports, the IEP generally does not include a description of the actual intervention procedures that will be used to accomplish the specified annual goals.

The IEP is generated as part of a process that begins with a referral. A comprehensive assessment is then conducted by an appointed team, and the findings are reviewed at a meeting of all involved parties (including therapists, teachers, and parents). The participants develop and approve a written IEP, which is implemented over the subsequent school year and reviewed periodically. When speech-language therapy is the sole or primary special education service to be provided, the SLP may assume principal responsibility for writing the IEP. (For an overview, summary, and questions and answers about IDEA and the IEP process, see the American Speech-Language-Hearing Association's Web site at www.asha.org/Practice-Portal/Professional-Issues/Caseload-and-Workload/IDEA-Influence//H2/IEP Content

To ensure a measure of uniformity and accountability nationwide, federal law requires that all IEPs contain the following basic information:

- *Present levels of academic achievement and functional performance:* This section of the document describes how the disability affects the child's involvement and progress in the general education curriculum. For preschool children, this section describes how the disability affects the child's participation in appropriate activities. For speech-language pathology, test scores and clinical analysis of observed performance are presented.

- *Measurable annual goals:* These goals must be linked to academic and functional performance within the general education curriculum. There is no mandate concerning the number of goals that must be included in an IEP.

- *Progress monitoring:* This section of the IEP describes how the child's progress toward the annual goals will be measured. It also specifies when periodic progress reports will be provided.

- *Special education and related services:* This section identifies the special services needed by the child to achieve the annual goals. Statements about needed supplementary aids, services, and program modifications must be included.

- *Placement recommendation and justification:* This section indicates the specific educational setting into which preschool- or school-aged children will be placed. By law, this setting must be the **least restrictive environment (LRE)** that provides an appropriate education to meet a child's individualized needs. LRE means that, to the maximum extent possible, children with disabilities are educated with children who have no disabilities. Recommendations for placements other than a general education classroom in the child's home school must be accompanied by a written rationale. (Eligibility requirements vary among local educational agencies.) There should be a description of the *extent* to which the child will receive educational services with nondisabled peers. Parents must be participating members of teams that make placement decisions.

- *Individual accommodations:* This section of an IEP describes the accommodations necessary to measure the child's academic achievement and functional performance on state and district-wide assessments. Any recommendation for alternate assessment measures must specify the tools to be used.

- *Initiation and duration of services:* The IEP must state the projected date for the beginning of services/modifications, as well as the anticipated frequency, location, and duration of these services.

These seven categories comprise the basic structure of an IEP. Individual states or local educational agencies may impose additional requirements pertaining to format or content information such as formal or informal plans for transition to postsecondary or employment settings. These plans identify the accommodations/modifications needed by the student to successfully meet expectations within the setting.

Due Process

IDEA (2004) provides legal and procedural safeguards throughout the educational placement process, including timelines for completion of each step, parental notification and consent, and an appeal system to ensure due process for all parties involved. The parent or responsible party must be notified prior to any changes in a child's educational program. The due process system provides a formal mechanism for parents to protest decisions they consider inappropriate or unfair to their child.

INDIVIDUALIZED FAMILY SERVICE PLAN

In 1986, the federal mandate for a free and appropriate education was extended by enactment of PL 99-457 (Part H) to include infants and toddlers with special needs between birth and 3 years of age. Updated in 2011, Part C of this legislation is notable for its emphasis on the importance of early intervention.

This legislation requires the development of an **Individualized Family Service Plan (IFSP)**, which is similar to an IEP. It differs from the IEP in that its main focus is on the family as a unit rather than solely on the child. The written document must include the following components:

- *Statement of child's present level of development:* This section provides information on physical, cognitive, communicative, and social/emotional status.

- *Statement of family resources, priorities, and concerns:* This section includes a statement of the impact that the child's developmental delay has on family functioning. In addition, individual families can specify their desired levels of involvement in the intervention plan.

- *Major outcomes:* This section identifies the goals, criteria, procedures, and timelines anticipated to be achieved for the child and family.

- *Specific early intervention services:* This section provides a statement of the services necessary to meet the child's and family's unique needs. It should include the frequency, intensity, location, and method of service delivery.

- *Natural environment:* This section describes the environments in which services will be provided. The extent to which services will not be provided in authentic settings must be justified.

- *Service coordinator/provider:* The IFSP specifically identifies the individual from the profession most relevant to the needs of the infant and family. This case manager is responsible for the development of the IFSP and for implementation, coordination, and monitoring of all services. The SLP is frequently named as service coordinator for infants and toddlers whose primary developmental delay consists of communication or feeding/oral-motor impairments.

- *Transition plan:* This section outlines the procedures that will be employed to facilitate the transition to services provided under PL 108-446 if the child continues to need special services beyond age 2 years, 11 months.

In addition to the differences just outlined, this legislation extends eligibility to "at-risk" youngsters rather than restricting services to children with recognized disabilities. Moreover, these services can be provided through agencies outside the public school system (e.g., community agencies). PL 108-446 also contains provisions for home-based instruction, as well as family education and counseling. The IFSP is reviewed every six months rather than annually.

504 PLAN

Students who do not meet the eligibility requirements for an IEP often need some assistance to participate fully in school settings. These students may be candidates for a 504 plan authorized through the Americans with Disabilities Act Amendments Act (2008). **504 plans** specify accommodations that allow students to complete the same assignments as their peers without altering the content of tasks or tests. Examples of potential accommodations include the following.

Presentation:	Provide audio recording.
	Provide in large print.
	Reduce number of items per page or line.
	Present instructions orally.
	Provide on-task, focusing prompts.
Response:	Allow for oral responses.
	Allow for answers to be dictated.
	Permit responses to be given via computer.
	Permit answers to be recorded directly into test booklet.
Timing:	Allow frequent breaks.
	Extend allotted time for test taking.
Setting:	Provide preferential seating.
	Provide special lighting or acoustics.
	Provide space with minimal distractions.
	Administer tests in small-group setting or private room.
Test Scheduling:	Administer test over several sessions or days.
	Allow subtests to be taken in different order.

PROFESSIONAL CORRESPONDENCE

In addition to clinical treatment reports, speech-language pathologists often interact with other professionals and agencies through written correspondence. These documents may vary with respect to length, content, and format, but all professional correspondence should be written in a clear, concise manner with correct spelling, grammar, and punctuation. Typically, written correspondence involves authorizing the release of information, making referrals to other professionals, and acknowledging referrals from colleagues.

HEALTH INSURANCE PORTABILITY AND ACCOUNTABILITY ACT

HIPAA is the acronym for the Health Insurance Portability and Accountability Act of 1996. For detailed information on the major components of this legislation, refer to the U.S. Department of Health and Human Services Web site at www.cms.hhs.gov/HIPAAGenInfo/ or www.hhs.gov/ocr/privacy/. The component that addresses standards for privacy of **protected health information (PHI)** is most relevant to discussion in this chapter. PHI is *individually identifiable* health information created, received, transmitted, and/or maintained by health care entities. These standards, which became effective in 2003, are designed to regulate the storage, transmission, and confidentiality of personal patient information, which may include the following:

- Information in a client's file
- Conversations with others about a client's care or treatment
- Information about the client contained in his or her health insurer's data system
- Billing information

Within our profession, HIPAA regulations are applicable to a variety of settings, such as a private practice, school, nursing home, hospital, clinic, and other milieu, including distance services. In general, providers may use PHI for treatment, payment, and health care operations without special permission from clients. Written consent from the client is required for marketing, fundraising, or research activities. If there is a need to share PHI beyond these parameters, the Privacy Rules provide guidelines for how reports should be "de-identified" in order to protect the patient/client. The following list of types of information that should be omitted is adapted from the Department of Health and Human Services Web site at www.hhs.gov/ocr/privacy/hipaa/understanding/coveredentities/ De-identification/guidance.html#rationale. Please refer to this Web site for more detailed discussion and rationales for the de-identification items in the following list.

- Names
- Street address, city, county, precinct, ZIP code, and their equivalent geocodes
- Telephone and fax numbers
- Email addresses and internet protocol (IP) addresses
- Medical record or health plan numbers
- Social Security numbers
- Photographs or other images

Health care providers are required to provide clients with a written description of how confidential information will be handled. This **Notice of Privacy Practices (NPP)** should be reviewed, signed, and dated by the client/legal guardian prior to the initiation of services. Forms 2–1 and 2–2 on the following pages show a sample NPP and acknowledgment statement. Additional information and frequently asked questions (FAQs) on PHI can be found in Appendix 2-A.

The following section contains reproducible release of information authorization forms and sample referral letter and acknowledgment formats.

FORM 2–1 SAMPLE NOTICE OF PRIVACY PRACTICES

NOTICE OF PRIVACY PRACTICES

As Defined by the Privacy Regulations of the

Federal Health Insurance Portability and Accountability Act of 1996 (HIPAA)

PLEASE REVIEW THIS NOTICE CAREFULLY

I. OUR COMMITMENT TO YOUR PRIVACY

The Hearing and Speech clinic at the University of Maryland is dedicated to maintaining the privacy of your protected health information (PHI). PHI is individually identifiable health information about you that relates to your past, present or future physical or mental health or other condition, as well as any related health care services. This Notice of Privacy Practices provides you with the following important information: our obligations concerning your PHI, how we may use and disclose your PHI, and your rights with regard to your PHI.

A. OUR OBLIGATION   The Hearing and Speech Clinic has chosen to abide by federal and state laws requiring that the privacy of your PHI be maintained. By complying with these laws, we are required to provide you with this notice regarding our privacy practices, our legal duties, and your rights concerning your PHI. Except for student records and certain records the University creates or receives in its role as an employer, this Notice of Privacy Practices applies to all records containing your PHI that are created or retained by the Hearing and Speech Clinic. A copy of the Notice of Privacy Practices will be posted in a visible location in the Hearing and Speech Clinic waiting room at all times, and you may request a copy of the Notice at any time.

B. WE MAY USE AND DISCLOSE YOUR PROTECTED HEALTH INFORMATION (PHI) IN THE FOLLOWING WAYS (NOT ALL POSSIBLE SITUATIONS ARE COVERED)

- *For treatment, payment, and healthcare operations, to third-party business associates (e.g., billing services), for health-related services, to individuals involved in your care, under some circumstances for research purposes, when required or allowed by law, with your written authorization*

II. YOUR RIGHTS REGARDING YOUR PHI

You have the following rights regarding your PHI, and you may request any of the following:

- *Confidential communications, restriction of communication to individuals otherwise permitted by law to inspect your PHI, inspection and copies of personal records, amendments to your PHI if you believe the information is incorrect or incomplete, a list of disclosures we have made of your PHI, and a copy of this Notice.*

III. IMPLEMENTATION, COMPLAINTS, AND QUESTIONS

A. IMPLEMENTATION   This Notice provides a general overview of our privacy practices. This Notice and our privacy practices are implemented in accordance with applicable University policies and procedures and the requirements of HIPAA and other federal and Maryland laws, as applicable.

B. COMPLAINTS   If you believe your privacy rights have been violated, you may file a complaint with the Hearing and Speech Clinic. All complaints must be submitted in writing. We will not retaliate against you in any way if you file a complaint with us.

IV. CONTACT INFORMATION

If you have any questions regarding this Notice or our health information privacy practices, please contact:

Director of Hearing and Speech Clinic:_____

Address: _____

E-mail: _____

Phone: _____

FORM 2–2 SAMPLE ACKNOWLEDGMENT OF PRIVACY
PRACTICES NOTICE

ACKNOWLEDGEMENT OF RECEIPT
HEARING AND SPEECH CLINIC NOTICE OF PRIVACY PRACTICES

I acknowledge that I have received a copy of the University of Maryland Hearing and Speech Clinic's Notice of Privacy Practices.

_____   _____   _____

Printed Name   Signature   Date

FOR INTERNAL USE ONLY

Client declined to provide signature for acknowledging receipt of privacy practices

_____

(Clinic staff signature and date)

Client was not able to provide signature for acknowledging receipt of privacy practices

_____

(Clinic staff signature and date)

FORM 2–3 AUTHORIZATION FOR RELEASE OF INFORMATION FROM ANOTHER AGENCY OR PHYSICIAN

The following person has requested the services of our facility: _____.
We understand that this individual has been seen by you. Please forward any hearing, speech, language, medical, psychological, educational, or social records regarding this individual. Below is written authorization for the release of these records. Please send this information to the attention of _____ at the following address:

_____

_____

_____

Thank you for your cooperation.

This will certify that you have my permission to release information concerning

_____
(Client Name)

to the following facility: _____

Signature: _____ Date _____

FORM 2–4 AUTHORIZATION FOR RELEASE OF INFORMATION TO ANOTHER AGENCY OR PHYSICIAN

Name: _____ Date of Birth: _____

I hereby consent to the release of any and all hearing, speech, and language records concerning the above-named individual to:

Name/Agency: _____

Address: _____

_____

_____

_____

Signature: _____ Date: _____

FORM 2–5 REFERRAL LETTER FORMAT

Date: _____

Name of Recipient: _____

Address: _____

Dear _____,

_____ is being referred to you for _____

_____.

He/she was seen at our facility for _____

_____ on/from _____.

His/her communication status is characterized by _____.

I am making this referral because _____

_____. Enclosed please find a copy of _____

_____, along with the client's written authorization for the release of this

information. If you have any questions, please contact me at _____

_____.

Sincerely,

_____
Signature and Title

FORM 2–6 SAMPLE REFERRAL LETTER

April 25, 2015

Timothy Anderson, M.D.

866 Manor Drive

College Park, MD 20742

Dear Dr. Anderson,

Kevin Walters is being referred to you for a laryngoscopic examination. He was seen at our facility for a voice evaluation on April 24, 2015. His communication status is characterized by harsh voice quality, intermittent aphonia, and accompanying throat pain.

I am making this referral to verify Mr. Walter's medical status prior to the initiation of therapy services. Enclosed please find a copy of the diagnostic report, along with the client's written authorization for the release of this information. If you have any questions, please contact me at 301-555-1212.

Sincerely,

Mary Ann Schilling, M.S., CCC-SLP

Speech-Language Pathologist

FORM 2–7 ACKNOWLEDGMENT OF REFERRAL FORMAT

Date: _____

Name of Recipient: _____

Address: _____

Dear _____,

    Thank you for referring _____ to our clinic.

He/she was seen for _____

on/from _____.

    I have enclosed a copy of my full report, including recommendations regarding future services.

If you have any questions, please do not hesitate to contact me at _____

_____.

    We appreciate your referral and look forward to continued collaboration with you.

Sincerely,

_____

Signature and Title

FORM 2–8 SAMPLE REFERRAL ACKNOWLEDGMENT

April 27, 2015

Kitty Davidson, M.D.

31 Rose Lane

Kendall, FL 02113

Dear Dr. Davidson,

Thank you for referring Barbara Hawley to our clinic. She was seen for an initial speech and language evaluation on April 18, 2015.

I have enclosed a copy of my full report, including recommendations regarding future services. If you have any questions, please do not hesitate to contact me at 305-555-1846.

We appreciate your referral and look forward to continued collaboration with you.

Sincerely,

Marian Kirley, M.A., CCC-SLP

Speech-Language Pathologist

ADDITIONAL RESOURCES

Institute of Education Sciences
555 New Jersey Avenue, NW
Washington, DC 20208
(202) 219-1385
Web site: www.ies.ed.gov

Discover IDEA: Supporting Achievement for Children with Disabilities. An IDEA Practices Resource Guide
The package is organized around the key topics in special education in an accurate, easy-to-use format. This resource package brings you immediate access (through the Discover CD) to hundreds of books, handouts, transparencies, and Web links. It provides connections to the centers and programs addressing topical areas in special education, and, in addition, it infuses the IDEA regulations within each area in a strategic and easy-to-follow format.

LinguiSystems
3100 Fourth Avenue
East Moline, IL 61244
Phone: 800-776-4332
Fax: 800-577-4555
Web site: http://www.linguisystems.com/

The SLP's IDEA Companion
A resource for goals and objectives that match the guidelines outlined in the Individuals with Disabilities Education Act (IDEA). Therapy goals link to the classroom curriculum, and appropriate benchmarks for students and levels of performance are determined using the baseline measures provided in the book. Classroom expectations are provided for grades K–12 in the areas of fluency, semantics, syntax, voice, word finding, pragmatics, phonological awareness, oral-motor skills, articulation, and narrative/expository writing.

Pro-Ed
8700 Shoal Creek Boulevard
Austin, TX 78757-6897
Phone: 800-897-3202
Fax: 800-397-7633
Web site: http://www.proedinc.com

Report Writing for Speech-Language Pathologists and Audiologists, Second Edition
This is a resource that describes all the necessary information to be included in reports of various types. There is information about referral acknowledgements, diagnostic evaluation reports, integrated diagnostic reports, treatment plans and reports, IEPs, and progress reports.

Cengage Learning
10650 Toebben Drive
Independence, KY 41051
Phone: 800-354-9706
Fax: 800-487-8488
Web site: http://www.cengage.com

A Coursebook on Scientific and Professional Writing for Speech-Language Pathology, 4th edition
An interactive resource manual designed to help students, clinicians, and instructors master technical writing skills as well as professional writing skills. Includes worksheets of practice exercises for each topic.

Amazon.com, Inc.
Web site: www.amazon.com

What's Best for Matthew?: Version 2.0: Interactive CD-ROM Case Study
Uses a case study of a boy with autism, named Matthew, to help clinicians and teachers develop and write IEPs for students with disabilities. Provides assistance in writing an IEP for Matthew using a step-by-step approach, which can then be used to write IEPs for individual clients. Also includes a special notepad feature that allows the clinician to sort relevant IEP information into categories, such as communication and written language, which can be saved and accessed when needed during the writing process.

APPENDIX 2-A

HEALTH INSURANCE PORTABILITY AND ACCOUNTABILITY ACT (HIPAA)*

FIVE BASIC PRINCIPLES OF THE PRIVACY RULES

1. Consumer Control: Clients have rights to control the release of their medical/clinical information. They should be able to obtain copies of their records and request corrections as needed.

2. Boundaries: A client's information can be used and shared to treat/coordinate care, to pay health care providers, to provide information to family members or others identified by the client, and to protect the public's health and safety. Without the client's authorization, protected health information (PHI) generally cannot be shared with employers or used for marketing, advertising, or research purposes.

3. Security: Health care providers must establish written policies for management of PHI. All clients should be provided with a Notice of Private Practices (NPP) and acknowledge receipt in writing. Reasonable steps should be taken to keep PHI secure (e.g., computer system passwords or locked filing cabinets).

4. Accountability: There are federal penalties for violating HIPAA regulations ranging from monetary fines for accidental disclosures up to prison terms for willful misuse of client records.

5. Public Responsibility: Standards are provided regarding when PHI information should be released to protect public health, investigate fraud abuse, and assist with quality assessment purposes.

WHO MUST FOLLOW HIPAA?

A "covered entity" is anyone who collects, stores, or transmits individually identifiable health information. SLPs and audiologists are generally considered covered entities along with doctors, nurses, hospitals, health insurance companies, and government programs such as Medicare and Medicaid.

MINIMUM NECESSARY RULE

The amount of PHI shared or requested must be limited to only what is needed in a given situation, and employees should have access to PHI on a need-to-know basis.

---

*Some of this information was adapted from the University of Michigan Health System Online HIPAA Training Module (2006) and from P. J. Bonelli at the University of Maryland Department of Hearing and Speech Sciences, http://www.hesp.umd.edu. For additional information on the Privacy Rules, see http://www.hhs.gov/ocr/privacy/hipaa/understanding/summary/privacysummary.pdf.

(continues)

INCIDENTAL DISCLOSURES

PHI may sometimes be disclosed unintentionally to unauthorized individuals. For example, a client's name may be called out or seen on a sign-in sheet in a waiting room. HIPAA regulations refer to this as an "incidental disclosure." Incidental disclosures are allowed if reasonable safeguards are taken to minimize them.

BUSINESS ASSOCIATE AGREEMENTS

Individuals or companies who are not covered entities frequently may be exposed to PHI (e.g., software consultants for a hospital). These vendors should be required to sign a confidentiality agreement to keep PHI secure.

FREQUENTLY ASKED QUESTIONS (FAQS)

Q: Is PHI the same as the medical record?

A: No. HIPAA protects more than the official medical record. A great deal of other information also is considered PHI, such as billing and demographic data. Even the general information that a person is a client is considered PHI.

Q: I work in the hospital and don't need to access PHI for my job, but every now and then a patient's family member asks me about a patient. What should I do?

A: Explain that you do not have access to that information and refer the individual to the patient's health care provider.

Q: What about requests to leave information on voice mail or an answering machine?

A: If you are asked to phone or leave confidential information via voice mail, for example, you should verify with the client or other approved individual that it is okay to leave messages this way. Make sure you confirm the number. Some employers may have more restrictive policies, so check with your supervisor and/or department head. Always leave the minimum possible amount of information.

Q: What if a patient requests that I communicate with him or her via email?

A: Verify the client's identity and have the client fill out a form authorizing email contact. If you receive unexpected requests for PHI via email, contact the client via another method for verification. In general, be careful about sending PHI in response to email requests, due to the difficulty of identifying senders accurately. Disclose the minimum amount of PHI necessary.

Q: What do I do if I receive a request for PHI by fax?

A: If a client, health provider, or payer requests that you fax PHI, confirm that the request is on letterhead, get a specific fax number from the requesting party, and double-check the number before sending. Ask for confirmation that your fax was received. In the event that you find that a fax went to a wrong number, try to contact that party and request that the PHI be destroyed in a secure fashion.

(continues)

Q: What should I do to protect PHI on a laptop, personal digital assistant (PDA), or tablet?

A: Install a hard-to-break password and do not allow others, even family members, to use your equipment. Before selling or otherwise disposing of your electronic device, use a secure erase program to erase PHI.

Q: What's the safest way to dispose of PHI in the office?

A: Paper records containing PHI should be shredded or disposed of in designated confidential recycling receptacles and *not* in the regular trash. In general, follow your employer's secure disposal procedures for using secure disposal bins or shredding documents.

Q: I sometimes run into my client at parties and other social events. Is it okay to talk about therapy with her in these situations?

A: You should not just assume that her participation in therapy is common knowledge, *even if* her communication difficulties are apparent. Keep the conversation social in nature and follow her lead. If she brings up therapy, you can assume that others know, and that she is comfortable discussing it in public. The same goes if you have friends in common. Never discuss your client's therapy, even if mutual friends know that she sees you.

Q: A current client referred her friend to our audiology clinic. When the friend came for his evaluation, he asked how his hearing compares with that of his friend (he was thinking of getting similar hearing aids). Can I tell him?

A: No. While it is possible that your client would not mind sharing that information with her friend, she must explicitly be given the option to consent. Furthermore, this option is typically given when a friend or relative is directly involved in patient care or payment.

Q: I've been in the observation room during a diagnostic test, and we have had to put the speaker on "field" so that all members of the team can hear. Other individuals are typically in the observation room watching therapy sessions. Is this a violation of HIPAA?

A: This would probably be considered "incidental disclosure," which is permissible under HIPAA regulations, provided reasonable safeguards are taken. For example, keep the volume level to a minimum and only use "field" when it is absolutely necessary. During the conference that follows the diagnostic session, it is best to use headphones, because these discussions can be very sensitive.

APPENDIX 2-B

SAMPLE INITIAL THERAPY PLAN

UNIVERSITY OF MARYLAND SPEECH AND HEARING CLINIC

College Park, MD 20742 (301) 405-4218

Initial Therapy Plan

Spring 2014

Name: Andrew Rose

Parents: Jim and Kathy Rose

Address: 2635 Drake Court

       Fairfax, VA 20901

Telephone: (703) 555-9587

Date of Report: February 3, 2014

Date of Birth: February 1, 2006

Age: 8 years

Category: Language, Literacy, and Articulation

Clinician: Ilana Anderson, M.S., CCC-SLP

PERTINENT HISTORY

Andrew is an 8-year-old boy with difficulties in reading/decoding, spelling, word retrieval, and articulation of phonemic /r/, as in "rock" and "rabbit," and vowel plus /r/, as in "early" and "better" (/ɝ/ and /ɚ/, respectively). He began receiving reading and speech therapy at the University of Maryland Speech Clinic on June 11, 2013. Previous therapy goals include production of /r/, /ɝ/ and /ɚ/, segmenting and blending written words, and word retrieval.

Andrew is currently receiving group articulation therapy to improve production of /r/, /ɝ/, and /ɚ/. He also receives individual therapy on a separate day to address reading and word-retrieval difficulties. Each of his two weekly sessions is 50 minutes long. Both sets of goals are included in this report.

SEMESTER GOALS AND OBJECTIVES

ARTICULATION

Goal I: To produce /r/ in the initial positions in spontaneous sentences.

Initial Status/Baseline (as of 01/27/14):

Andrew correctly produces /r/ in the initial position of syllables and words 60% of the time. The remaining 40% of the time Andrew's production of /r/ is slightly distorted, although he does not have a complete /w/ for /r/ substitution pattern. He distorts /r/ by dropping his tongue from the roof of his mouth.

(continues)

OBJECTIVES

A. Andrew will independently produce /r/ in CV syllables (e.g., /ra/ and /ri/) with 90% accuracy over two consecutive sessions.

B. Andrew will produce /r/ in the initial and medial positions at the single-word level with 90% accuracy over two consecutive sessions.

C. Andrew will produce /r/ in the initial and medial positions of words at the phrase level with 90% accuracy over two consecutive sessions.

D. Andrew will produce /r/ in the initial and medial positions of words in spontaneous sentences with 90% accuracy over two consecutive sessions.

Goal II: To produce /ɚ/ in initial and final positions in spontaneous sentences.

Initial Status/Baseline as of 1/27/14:

Andrew correctly produces /ɚ/ in isolation 60% of the time, given visual and tactile cues. Given cues, he produces /ɚ/ in the initial and final position of single words 20% of the time. When he produces /ɝ/ incorrectly, he drops his tongue from the roof of his mouth to produce /ʌ/ (as in up) instead of /ɚ/.

OBJECTIVES

A. Andrew will independently produce /ɚ/ in isolation with 90% accuracy over two consecutive sessions.

B. Given a printed word or picture, Andrew will independently produce /ɚ/ in initial and final positions at the single-word level with 90% accuracy over two consecutive sessions.

C. Given a printed word or picture, Andrew will produce /ɚ/ in initial and final positions of words at the phrase level with 90% accuracy over two consecutive sessions.

D. Given a printed word or picture, Andrew will produce /ɚ/ in initial and final positions of words in spontaneous sentences with 90% accuracy over two consecutive sessions.

LITERACY

Goal I: To segment and blend words of various syllable structures, using knowledge of the alphabetic code.

Initial Status/Baseline as of 1/29/14:

Andrew was asked to segment and blend 16 written real words. He correctly segmented 10 of the 16 words (63% accuracy). Approximately half of his errors consisted of combining consonant clusters (e.g., *fr* in *frog*) as one sound when segmenting. This error type occurred primarily in the initial position, but also in the final position.

(continues)

OBJECTIVES

A. Given no more than two visual and/or verbal cues (e.g., keep the consonants that make one sound together; separate consonants that make two sounds), Andrew will segment and blend written English words and nonsense words of varying syllable structures with 90% accuracy over two consecutive sessions.

B. Given written words, Andrew will independently segment and blend written English words and nonsense words with varying syllable structures with 90% accuracy over two consecutive sessions.

Goal II: To use strategies (e.g., highlighting, previewing questions) effectively to improve reading comprehension skills (e.g., stating the main idea and answering comprehension questions).

Initial Status/Baseline as of 1/20/14:

Andrew silently read two short passages and answered questions about them in an untimed setting. He answered 97% of the questions correctly, but it took him over 20 minutes to answer 18 multiple-choice and short-answer questions. His primary strategy was searching back through the text for answers. He also was hesitant to answer, unless he was absolutely sure his answer was correct.

OBJECTIVES

A. Given direct instruction and verbal prompts/cues, Andrew will use strategies effectively to state the main idea of a paragraph with 90% accuracy over two consecutive sessions.

B. Andrew will independently use strategies effectively to state the main idea of a paragraph with 90% accuracy over two consecutive sessions.

C. Given verbal prompts/cues, Andrew will use strategies to state the main idea of a short story and answer factual questions with 90% accuracy over two consecutive sessions.

SPELLING

Goal I: To spell words of various syllable structures, using knowledge of the alphabetic code.

Initial Status/Baseline as of 1/20/14:

Andrew was asked to spell 14 orally presented English words of varying difficulty, based on the spelling subtest of the *Phonological Awareness Test-2*, which is normed for his age. He spelled 43% of the words correctly. Spelling mistakes were generally on the less common and more difficult items, such as *unicycle*.

(continues)

OBJECTIVES

A. Given oral presentation of the word and verbal cues (e.g., sound-by-sound presentation of the word), Andrew will spell English words and nonsense words correctly with 90% accuracy over two consecutive sessions.

B. Given oral presentation of the word, Andrew will spontaneously spell English words and nonsense words correctly with 90% accuracy over two consecutive sessions.

LANGUAGE

Goal I: To improve word retrieval skills in order to increase verbal fluency.

Initial Status/Baseline as of 1/29/14:

Given 39 target words, Andrew was asked to choose a synonym or antonym for the target word from three choices. He correctly identified 13/19 synonym pairs (68% accuracy) and 15/20 antonym pairs (75% accuracy).

OBJECTIVES

A. Given a set of printed/written target words, Andrew will identify the correct synonym or antonym when presented with a choice of three words with 90% accuracy over two consecutive sessions.

B. When presented with a word(s) in the context of a sentence, Andrew will restate the sentence, replacing the highlighted word(s) with an antonym or synonym with 90% accuracy over two consecutive sessions.

C. Andrew will paraphrase statements, substituting synonyms or descriptions of target words, during spontaneous speech or clinician-directed activities, with 90% accuracy over two consecutive sessions.

REINFORCEMENT

Continuous verbal reinforcement will be used when shaping target behaviors. A token system will be implemented in his group sessions to allow Andrew to earn prizes for good behavior and participation in activities. In addition, activities will be chosen that are intrinsically reinforcing in nature, such as puzzles and games.

PARENTAL ENGAGEMENT AND CARRYOVER

Parent conferences will be held formally during the semester and informally after each therapy session. Andrew will be given homework assignments throughout the semester to facilitate generalization of specific goals. The clinician will review the home program, explain the instructions, and provide demonstrations as needed. Mr. and Mrs. Rose will be encouraged to observe therapy sessions and participate in weekly homework assignments.

APPENDIX 2-C

SAMPLE PROGRESS REPORT

UNIVERSITY OF MARYLAND SPEECH AND HEARING CLINIC

College Park, MD 20742 (301) 405-4218

Semester Progress Report

Spring 2014

Name: Andrew Rose

Parents: Jim and Kathy Rose

Address: 2635 Drake Ct

   Fairfax, VA 20901

Telephone: (703) 555-9587

Number of Sessions: 24 of 27

Date of Report: May 29, 2014

Date of Birth: February 1, 2006

Age: 8 years, 3 months

Category: Language, Literacy, and Articulation

Clinician: Ilana Anderson, M.S., CCC-SLP

PERTINENT HISTORY

Andrew, an 8-year-old boy, began speech and language therapy at the University of Maryland Hearing and Speech Clinic on June 11, 2013. At the beginning of the semester he demonstrated difficulties in reading/decoding, spelling, word retrieval, and articulation of phonemic /r/, as in "rock" and "rabbit," and vowel plus "r," as in "early" and "better" (/ɝ/ and /ɚ/, respectively). He received group therapy to address /r/ and /ɚ/ and individual therapy on a separate day to address reading, spelling, and word-retrieval difficulties. Each of his two weekly sessions was 50 minutes long. Both sets of goals are included in this report.

THERAPY OBJECTIVES AND PROGRESS

ARTICULATION

Goal I: To produce /r/ in the initial and medial positions of words in spontaneous sentences.

A. Andrew will independently produce /r/ in CV syllables (e.g., /ra/ and /ri/) with 90% accuracy over two consecutive sessions. [Criterion met: 90% on 3/15/14]

B. Andrew will produce /r/ in the initial position at the single-word level with 90% accuracy over two consecutive sessions. [In progress: 70% on 4/8/14]

(continues)

C. Andrew will produce /r/ in the initial position of words at the phrase level with 90% accuracy over two consecutive sessions. [Not yet addressed]

D. Andrew will produce /r/ in the initial position of words in spontaneous sentences with 90% accuracy over two consecutive sessions. [Not yet addressed]

COMMENTS

Andrew made fair progress on this goal. Although Andrew demonstrates the ability to accurately produce /r/ in the initial positions of words, his production of /r/ has been inconsistent throughout the semester. For example, on 3/11/14 he correctly produced /r/ in the initial position of words with 85% accuracy. However, on 4/8/14 he produced /r/ correctly in the same set of words with 40% accuracy. When Andrew incorrectly produced /r/, he produced an approximation of /r/, which was slightly distorted but was not a complete /w/ for /r/ substitution pattern. This distortion did not affect Andrew's intelligibility. Andrew benefited from clinician modeling and reminders of correct tongue placement. Although Andrew's production of /r/ was inconsistent, he demonstrated a clear understanding of the mechanics of producing the /r/ sound by his ability to describe and model correct tongue placement.

Goal II: To produce /ɚ/ in initial and final positions of words in spontaneous sentences.

A. Andrew will independently produce /ɚ/ in isolation with 90% accuracy over two consecutive sessions. [In progress: 80% on 3/4/14]

B. Given a printed word or picture, Andrew will independently produce /ɚ/ in initial and final positions at the word level with 90% accuracy over two consecutive sessions. [Not yet addressed]

C. Given a printed word or picture, Andrew will produce /ɚ/ in initial and final positions of words at the phrase level with 90% accuracy over two consecutive sessions. [Not yet addressed]

D. Given a printed word or picture, Andrew will produce /ɚ/ in initial and final positions of words in spontaneous sentences with 90% accuracy over two consecutive sessions. [Not yet addressed]

COMMENTS

Andrew made fair progress this semester. Although he demonstrated the ability to correctly produce /ɚ/ in isolation, he often drops his tongue and produces an approximation of /ɚ/. It should be noted that this approximation is very close to the target sound. A variety of cues and strategies were used throughout the semester to elicit the correct tongue placement for /ɚ/. Tactile cues, such as using a lollipop to stimulate the parts of his tongue and teeth that should touch, were moderately successful. Other successful strategies included maintaining tongue placement on the roof of the mouth and shaping /ɚ/ from both /i/ and /ʌ/. A rating system consisting of thumbs up, sideways, and down was moderately successful in helping Andrew identify

(continues)

his own correct versus incorrect productions of /ɚ/, as well as those made by the clinician and the other clients in the group. Although Andrew did not reach criterion for producing /ɚ/ in isolation, he describes and demonstrates correct tongue placement for /ɚ/.

LITERACY

Goal I: To segment and blend words of various syllable structures, using knowledge of the alphabetic code.

A. Given no more than two visual and/or verbal cues (e.g., keep the consonants that make one sound together; separate consonants that make two sounds), Andrew will segment and blend written English words and nonsense words of varying syllable structures with 90% accuracy over two consecutive sessions. [Criterion met: 100% on 2/19/14 and 2/26/14]

B. Given written words, Andrew will independently segment and blend written English words and nonsense words with varying syllable structures with 90% accuracy over two consecutive sessions. [In progress: 100% on 4/9/14, criterion met 1st time]

COMMENTS

Andrew made significant progress on this goal. He is proficient with sound/symbol (letter) correspondences and became much better at segmenting and blending consonant clusters as two distinct sounds. Andrew was required to segment and blend real words (e.g., *watches* and *fresh*) and nonsense words (e.g., *blemp* and *prishment*). He was presented with the written form and then asked to put a slash between each speech sound and orally blend all the individual sounds together. Written words were presented in a game form, such as tic-tac-toe, and Andrew had to correctly segment and blend the word before earning an X or O. Although Andrew successfully segmented and blended single words, he often guessed instead of segmenting and blending unfamiliar words during reading activities. Therefore, this goal was addressed solely during reading activities as the semester progressed. Andrew was given tokens for words he segmented and blended, but "owed" the clinician a token for words he guessed at or skipped. When Andrew earned a specific number of tokens, he exchanged them for a prize.

Goal II: To use strategies (e.g., highlighting, previewing questions) effectively to improve reading comprehension skills (e.g., stating the main idea and answering comprehension questions).

A. Given direct instruction and verbal prompts/cues, Andrew will use strategies effectively to state the main idea of a paragraph with 90% accuracy over two consecutive sessions. [In progress: 100% on 4/9/14, criterion met 1st time]

B. Andrew will independently use strategies effectively to state the main idea of a paragraph with 90% accuracy over two consecutive sessions. [Not yet addressed]

C. Given verbal prompts/cues, Andrew will use strategies to state the main idea of a short story and answer inferential questions with 90% accuracy over two consecutive sessions. [Not yet addressed]

(continues)

COMMENTS

Andrew made moderate progress on this goal. He learned to use several strategies effectively, including previewing questions, referring back to the text, and highlighting. Previewing questions was most effective when Andrew previewed one question at a time, rather than reading all the questions at once. He would read the first question, then read the text until he came to the answer, answer the question, and then move onto the second question. Toward the end of the semester, Andrew was consistently able to state the main idea of a short story and correctly answer comprehension questions about the story's characters, setting, and plot. He independently used the "referring back to the text" strategy effectively to answer these questions. Age- and grade-appropriate reading passages were used to address this goal; these included short passages on topics that Andrew found interesting, such as sports and sharks. Andrew earned tokens for answering questions correctly, and he exchanged them for a game or prize when he earned a specific number of tokens.

SPELLING

Goal I: To spell words of various syllable structures, using knowledge of the alphabetic code.

A.   Given oral presentation of the word and verbal cues (e.g., sound-by-sound presentation of the word), Andrew will spell English words and nonsense words correctly with 90% accuracy over two consecutive sessions. [In progress: 85% on 4/2/14]

B.   Given oral presentation of the word, Andrew will spontaneously spell English words and nonsense words correctly with 90% accuracy over two consecutive sessions. [Not yet addressed]

COMMENTS

Andrew made some progress on this goal. He was successful with words that are spelled exactly as they sound, but he had difficulty with irregular spellings and was taught appropriate spelling rules for these. For example, the final /k/ sound can be spelled with a "k" or "ck," as in *cake* and *pack*, depending on the vowel sound and neighboring consonants. Written explanations and word lists for each spelling rule taught were given to Andrew in a binder. Activities that elicited word spelling included Jeopardy spelling games and Hangman. Andrew was given tokens for words spelled correctly, and he exchanged them for a game or prize when he earned a specific number of tokens.

LANGUAGE

Goal I: To improve word-retrieval skills in order to increase verbal fluency.

A.   Given a set of target words, Andrew will identify the correct synonym or antonym when presented with a choice of three words with 90% accuracy over two consecutive sessions. [Criterion met: 100% on 2/19/14 and 2/26/14]

(continues)

B. When presented with a word(s) in the context of a sentence, Andrew will restate the sentence, replacing the highlighted word(s) with an antonym or synonym with 90% accuracy over two consecutive sessions. [Criterion met: 100% on 3/5/14 and 3/12/14]

C. Andrew will paraphrase statements, substituting synonyms or descriptions of target words, during spontaneous speech or clinician-directed activities with 90% accuracy over two consecutive sessions. [In progress: 100% on 4/6/14, criterion met 1st time]

COMMENTS

Andrew made excellent progress on this goal. He demonstrated the ability to correctly choose or substitute synonyms and antonyms for target words in a variety of contexts (e.g., multiple-choice questions, written sentences, and in the context of a written story). He was taught the SCUMPS acronym for describing words (S = size, C = color, U = use/used for, M = material/made of, P = parts, S = shape), and effectively used it during therapy activities as a strategy for conveying meaning to the listener when a specific word could not be retrieved. Target words included primarily nouns and verbs. Various games such as charades and Taboo were used to practice the SCUMPS strategies.

SUMMARY AND ADDITIONAL INFORMATION

Andrew made good progress on all of his reading and word-retrieval goals. When prompted, he was able to generalize his segmenting and blending skills to reading and spelling activities. Andrew made fair progress on his articulation goals. A number of strategies proved helpful for eliciting the correct position of /r/ and /ɚ/. He was cooperative during therapy sessions, and a token reinforcement strategy was used to keep Andrew motivated and focused during therapy. Andrew and his "r" group members earned an end-of-semester reward (i.e., going out for ice cream) for good behavior during group therapy. An attempt was made to design therapy activities that were intrinsically motivating, such as games and puzzles. Homework related to Andrew's speech and language goals was assigned and completed weekly starting in February. He was encouraged to do as much as he could independently before asking his parents for help. Often, Andrew reported that he did not need any help with homework assignments, suggesting that skills learned in the therapy room generalized to other environments.

RECOMMENDATIONS

It is recommended that Andrew continue therapy to work on spelling and reading. Therapy goals should include broadening his ability to use strategies to increase his reading comprehension skills, increasing his spelling accuracy, and learning and using strategies to answer inferential questions about a written passage. It is also recommended that Andrew continue speech therapy for production of /r/ and /ɚ/. Specific objectives to be addressed should focus on production of /r/ in the initial position of words, as well as introducing /ɚ/ in the initial and final position of words (e.g., *early* and *father*).

PART TWO

Providing Treatment
for Communication
Disorders

CHAPTER 3

This chapter focuses on the management of articulation and phonological disorders demonstrated by children. An **articulation** model emphasizes the motor component of speech, whereas a **phonologic** orientation stresses the linguistic aspect of speech production. Most articulation approaches focus on the incorrect production of individual phonemes, traditionally classified as substitution, omission, and distortion errors. In contrast, phonological approaches concentrate on rule-based errors that affect multiple speech sounds that follow a predictable pattern. The phonological system governs the ways in which sounds in a language can be combined to form words. Children with phonologically based problems demonstrate difficulty in applying sound-system rules, not necessarily in production of the sounds. These children do not simply possess an incomplete system of speech sounds; rather, their errors have logical and coherent principles underlying their occurrence.

Articulation disorders can be classified as functional or organic in nature. Articulation disorders are considered **functional** when no known pathology is causing the errors. Children with functional articulation disorders demonstrate speech production errors in the absence of any identifiable etiology. These children present with adequate hearing acuity and intellectual abilities and with no signs of significant structural abnormalities or neurological dysfunction. The specific errors displayed vary greatly from one child to the next and are not as readily predictable as those found in organically based disorders. **Organic** disorders result from known physical causes, such as cleft palate, neurological dysfunction, or hearing impairment. Some children may demonstrate both functional and organic deficits.

The information provided in this chapter is based on Standard American English. (See Appendix B at the end of this book for International Phonetic Alphabet symbols.) It is imperative that clinicians take a child's cultural and linguistic background into account in determining whether the production of a given speech sound represents an error or a dialectal difference. (See Chapter 12 for more about multicultural and English language learner treatment.)

TREATMENT APPROACHES

There are a variety of phonetic (i.e., articulation) and phonological (i.e., linguistic rules) approaches to intervention. Williams, McLeod, and McCauley (2010) identified 23 approaches that have been utilized in the treatment of speech sound disorders. Selected examples of classic and more recent remediation approaches are described in the following sections.

Traditional (Van Riper, 1978)

This phonetic approach to intervention is also known as the sensory-perceptual or motor-based approach. It relies on sensory training (i.e., auditory discrimination or "ear-training") either before or concurrently with speech production training to provide the client with an internal standard with which to compare correct versus incorrect productions of sounds. The typical sequence for training in the traditional approach involves: (1) speech sound discrimination training including identification, isolation, and bombardment of specific target sounds; (2) achieving phonetic placement of the articulators for the sound; (3) producing the sound in isolation; (4) producing the sound in nonsense syllables;

(5) producing the sound in the initial, medial, and final positions of words; (6) producing the sound in phrases and sentences; and (7) producing the sound in conversational speech. It incorporates several teaching strategies, such as imitation, multisensory cues for phonetic placement and production, and successive approximation. For more detailed information on this approach, see McDonald (1964) and Rvachew, Nowak, and Cloutier (2004).

Motor-Kinesthetic (Stinchfield-Hawk & Young, 1938)

This phonetic approach emphasizes development of correct movement patterns and requires the clinician to manipulate the articulators to facilitate sound production. This method is based on the assumption that it is possible to establish positive kinesthetic and tactile feedback patterns through direct manipulation of the client's articulators. As a result of the feedback, the client is helped to recognize and then to produce the movements of speech. In this approach, the basic unit of therapy is the isolated sound; only later are words and sentence patterns introduced and established. A more recent iteration of the motor-kinesthetic philosophy concept is PROMPT, which stands for Prompts for Restructuring Oral Muscular Phonetic Targets (Chumpelik, 1984). Originally developed for children with severe speech motor production difficulties, PROMPT is a multidimensional approach that incorporates three main domains: motor-sensory, cognitive-linguistic, and social-emotional. Speech production is facilitated through the use of tactile cues that focus on jaw height, labial/facial positioning, and mylohyoid posture for each sound/word (Grigos, Hayden, & Eigen, 2010; Hayden, Eigen, Walker, & Olsen 2010). The program is highly structured, and therapists must be trained/certified through the PROMPT Institute (www.promptinstitute.com) in order to utilize this therapy approach. In summary, the motor-kinetic method also advocates for the use of tactile, kinesthetic, and proprioceptive cues to facilitate "motor maps" for production of individual speech sounds. For additional information, see Vaughn and Clark (1979) and Dodd and Bradford (2000).

Distinctive Features (McReynolds & Bennett, 1972)

Distinctive feature therapy is a phonological approach based on the theory that speech sounds can be defined in terms of articulatory patterns and acoustic properties. Each phoneme in a language consists of a bundle of binary features, in which the presence or absence of these features is specified (e.g., +voicing/−voicing, +nasal/−nasal, +continuancy/−continuancy; Jakobson, 1968). Some phonemes, such as /t/ and /d/, differ by only one feature contrast, in this case, voicing. Other phonemes, such as /s/ and /g/, differ by many feature contrasts, including voicing, continuancy, placement, and stridency. Table 3–1 presents a complete list of the 11 distinctive features originally identified by Chomsky and Halle (1968). For the purposes of clinical application, however, sounds are usually analyzed according to three basic feature categories: place, manner, and voicing. This breakdown is illustrated in Table 3–2.

The clinician selects a feature for training (e.g., continuancy) and presents syllable or word pairs that contrast presence with absence of the feature (e.g., /fo/ versus /po/). After establishing the feature contrast in auditory discrimination activities, the clinician moves therapy through the traditional speech production hierarchy from isolation/syllables through conversation. For more detailed information, see Blache (1989) and Stevens and Hanson (2013).

TABLE 3–1
Distinctive Feature Analysis Chart

Features	Consonants																								
	k	g	t	d	p	b	f	v	θ	ð	s	z	ʃ	ʒ	tʃ	dʒ	m	n	ŋ	l	r	h	w	j	ʔ
Vocalic	–	–	–	–	–	–	–	–	–	–	–	–	–	–	–	–	–	–	–	+	+	–	–	–	–
Consonantal	+	+	+	+	+	+	+	+	+	+	+	+	+	+	+	+	+	+	+	+	+	–	–	–	–
High	+	+	–	–	–	–	–	–	–	–	–	–	+	+	+	+	–	–	+	–	–	–	+	+	–
Back	+	+	–	–	–	–	–	–	–	–	–	–	–	–	–	–	–	–	+	–	–	–	+	–	–
Low	–	–	–	–	–	–	–	–	–	–	–	–	–	–	–	–	–	–	–	–	–	+	–	–	+
Anterior	–	–	+	+	+	+	+	+	+	+	+	+	–	–	–	–	+	+	–	+	+	–	–	–	–
Coronal	–	–	+	+	–	–	–	–	+	+	+	+	+	+	+	+	–	+	–	+	+	–	–	–	–
Voiced	–	+	–	+	–	+	–	+	–	+	–	+	–	+	–	+	+	+	+	+	+	–	+	+	–
Continuant	–	–	–	–	–	–	+	+	+	+	+	+	+	+	–	–	–	–	–	+	+	+	+	+	–
Nasal	–	–	–	–	–	–	–	–	–	–	–	–	–	–	–	–	+	+	+	–	–	–	–	–	–
Strident	–	–	–	–	–	–	+	+	–	–	+	+	+	+	+	+	–	–	–	–	–	–	–	–	–

– Absence of feature
+ Presence of feature

Vocalic: Oral cavity constriction is less than required for the high vowels /i/ and /u/
Consonantal: Marked constriction in the midline region of the vocal tract
High: Body of the tongue is raised above the neutral or resting position
Back: Body of the tongue is retracted from the neutral or resting position
Low: Body of the tongue is lowered below the neutral or resting position
Anterior: Point of constriction is farther forward than required for /ʃ/
Coronal: Tongue blade is elevated toward alveolar ridge/palate from the neutral position
Voiced: Vocal folds vibrate during sound production
Continuant: Partial constriction of oral cavity; sound can be sustained in a steady state
Nasal: Velum is lowered to allow sound stream to escape through the nose
Strident: Turbulent noise is created by rapid airflow released through a small opening

TABLE 3–2

Place, Manner, and Voicing Chart for English Consonants

Manner	Place	Voiced	Voiceless
Stop	Bilabial	b	p
	Alveolar	d	t
	Velar	g	k
	Glottal	—	ʔ
Fricative	Labiodental	v	f
	Linguadental	ð	θ
	Alveolar	Z	s
	Palatal	ʒ	ʃ
	Glottal	—	h
Affricate	Palatal	dʒ	tʃ
Glide	Bilabial	w	—
	Palatal	j	—
Liquid	Alveolar	l	—
	Palatal	r	—
Nasal	Bilabial	m	—
	Alveolar	n	—
	Velar	ŋ	—

Paired Oppositions—Minimal and Maximal (Weiner, 1981)

These phonologically based approaches target phonemic contrasts (errored versus correct) that signal differences in meaning between two words. No explicit instruction on articulatory placement or sound production is given. Instead, this approach emphasizes the use of the child's communication success or breakdown to teach target sound productions. Minimal opposition pairs differ in only one feature of sound production (e.g., *ban* versus *pan* differ only in voicing) and are generally used with children who demonstrate relatively fewer errors, primarily characterized by sound substitutions. Maximal opposition word pairs differ in several features (e.g., *sad* and *bad* vary in place, manner, and voicing) and are generally used with children who display a larger number of errors that also include omissions and distortions. Four major steps are commonly used with this approach: (1) Client is introduced to pairs through pictures or objects. (2) Client identifies picture/object named by clinician. (3) Roles are reversed and client must request or label picture/object. (4) Client is rewarded by clinician's selection of correct stimulus or is given a chance to repair the communication breakdown caused by inaccurate sound production. Gierut (2001, 2007) has advocated for an intervention strategy to speech production that focuses on across-sound class generalizations to facilitate system-wide phonologic change. In this approach, targets selected for treatment are based on complexity principles would include those that are more complex, later developing, and less stimulable. For more detailed information on oppositions as an approach to treatment, see Barlow and Gierut (2002) and Stoel-Gammon, Stone-Goldman, and Glaspey (2002).

Phonological Processes (Oller, 1975)

This phonological approach to intervention is based on the strategies used by young, typically developing children between 1½ and 4 years of age to simplify the production of an entire class of adult speech sounds (Hodson & Paden, 1981; Khan & Lewis, 2002). For example, young children frequently omit weakly stressed syllables in multisyllabic words (e.g., *ephant/elephant, jamas/pajamas*), reduce consonant clusters (e.g., *bue/blue, dek/desk*), assimilate consonants in words (e.g., *goggie/doggie, chichen/chicken*), and delete final consonants (e.g., *ba/ball, hou/house*). Children who persist in using these processes beyond the age of 4 are frequently referred for speech-language services because their speech is now perceived as difficult to understand. Some children exhibit phonological processes that are not typical of normally developing children. These nondevelopmental processes include (1) backing, the substitution of sounds that are more posterior than the usual place of production (e.g., *koe/toe, mackiz/matches, gipper/zipper*); (2) initial consonant deletion (e.g., *ouse/house, amp/lamp, ellow/yellow*); and (3) glottal replacement, substitution of a glottal stop for a consonant (e.g., *bo?le/bottle, chi?en/chicken, mi?ey/mickey*). Table 3–3 describes the most common phonological processes exhibited by normally developing children.

TABLE 3–3
Selected Developmental Phonological Processes

Process	Definition	Examples
Suppressed by 3 years		
Assimilation (harmony)	A sound becomes similar to or is influenced by another sound in the same word	*guck/duck* *toat/coat* *doddie/doggie*
Final consonant deletion	Omission of the last sound in word	*be/bed* *fi/fish* *so/soap*
Syllable deletion	Omission of weak or unstressed syllable(s)	*nana/banana* *agator/alligator* *zert/dessert*
Suppressed after 3 years		
Cluster reduction	Omission of at least one consonant from a cluster	*top/stop* *mall/small* *net/nest*
Epenthesis	Addition of sounds in a word	*bulack/black* *sthoap/soap* *pulay/play*
Fronting	Substitutions are produced anterior to their usual place of production	*tome/come* *cats/catch* *dum/gum*
Metathesis	The order of sound segments is reversed	*aminal/animal* *flutterby/butterfly* *bakset/basket*

(continues)

TABLE 3–3 *(Continued)*

Process	Definition	Examples
Suppressed after 3 years (Continued)		
Stopping	Fricatives/affricates are replaced by stops	*tun/sun* *dat/that* *dump/jump*
Voicing/devoicing	Voiced consonants replace voiceless sounds in the initial position; in the final position voiced consonants become voiceless	*gup/cup* *doe/toe* *bet/bed*

SOURCES: Based on the work of Bauman-Waengler (2007), Bernthal & Bankson (2009), Hodson (2004), and Shriberg and Kwiatkowski (1980).

Cycles Approach

One of the better-known phonological process intervention programs is the "cycles" approach developed by Hodson and Paden (1983) that is intended for children with highly unintelligible speech. The clinician identifies phonological patterns that are targeted for a designated amount of time (i.e., cycles lasting 5–16 weeks). A typical session sequence includes: (1) auditory bombardment, (2) production training, (3) stimulability probes, and (4) take-home activities for generalization. After approximately 2 to 6 hours of direct intervention, the child is given time to internalize the pattern while the clinician introduces new targets. Thus, the child's progression through the program is not based on achieving a criterion level of mastery. Focus on the original target resumes later in the therapy program. Each cycle is repeated until the target pattern emerges in spontaneous speech. For more detailed information, see Rvachew, Rafaat, and Martin (1999); Stoel-Gammon et al. (2002); Hassink and Wendt (2010); and Hodson (2007).

Core Vocabulary (Dodd, Holm, Crosbie, & McIntosh, 2010)

This approach focuses on functional outcomes in which consistency, as opposed to accuracy, is targeted. The SLP selects 50 to 70 "functionally powerful" words and targets up to 10 at once. Children learn to produce their best pronunciation of the words consistently, both in isolation and connected speech. It targets the ability to generate consistent plans for words; the ability to create a phonological plan is improved by providing detailed, specific feedback about a limited number of words. This approach relies heavily on systematic practice in a drill-like format.

Metaphon

Developed by Howell and Dean (1994), this approach is more accurately labeled a "philosophy" rather than a program; it is designed to provide children with explicit information that will enable them to consciously reflect on the phonemic structure of language. Heavy emphasis is placed on the child's awareness/understanding of the detailed aspects of speech sounds (separately from word meaning) to facilitate accurate sound production. It utilizes a "word-pair" technique to highlight the salient differences between individual sounds in similar words ("deep/keep"). The clinician does not provide specific or corrective feedback regarding the accuracy of the child's tongue placement or manner of sound production. Instead, the environment is deliberately structured to give the child repeated opportunities to distinguish between effective and ineffective communication attempts.

ORAL-MOTOR CONSIDERATIONS

Some children with speech impairments (particularly those with organically based disorders) may exhibit deficits in oral-motor function that affect the neuromuscular control and organization needed for the production of intelligible speech. These deficits may manifest themselves as **hyposensitivity** (reduced reactions to sensation); **hypersensitivity** (overly strong reactions to sensation); and weakness or incoordination of oral structures, including the jaw, tongue, lips, or palate. Please see Appendix D for a schematic of the vocal tract structures discussed in this section. It is important to realize that speech is not an isolated act but the product of a highly complex and synchronized oral-motor system. Further, oral-motor treatment must be conducted with regard for a child's overall neuromuscular profile.

Oral-motor therapy for children with functional articulation disorders generally consists of a variety of tongue, lip, and jaw exercises. Most proponents of this approach subscribe to one or more of the following basic rationales: (1) Speech is founded on earlier-developing nonspeech motor patterns such as sucking and chewing (Marshalla, 1985; Ruark & Moore, 1997). (2) Reduced muscle tone in the oral-facial area results in limited strength of speech articulators (Robin, Somodi, & Luschei, 1991). (3) Normal movement and sensation significantly influence motor learning, a Piagetian construct (Piaget, 1951; Thelen & Smith, 1994). (4) Speech is a highly complex behavior that is more easily learned when broken into smaller components (Magill, 1998). However, controversy exists regarding this approach to intervention. The few controlled studies present correlational rather than causal findings and report no significant connection between nonspeech oral-motor exercises (NSOMEs) and speech sound production (Bunton, 2008; Clark, 2003; Love, 2000; Moore & Ruark, 1996; Nittrouer, 1993). See Forrest (2002); Lass and Pannbacker (2008); and McCauley, Strand, Lof, Schooling, and Frymark (2009) for a comprehensive discussion of the efficacy of oral-motor intervention for functional articulation errors.

Given the scarcity of research-based evidence on this topic, clinicians are encouraged to combine available information with "professional wisdom" (Whitehurst, 2002). Accordingly, the decision to use NSOMEs requires careful consideration and a sound theoretical rationale. We suggest that this rationale serve as the basis for a set of systematic implementation guidelines to be developed by individual practitioners, specific facilities, or regional school districts. These guidelines necessarily include (but are not limited to) the following factors: age, type of disorder, severity of impairment, number and type of speech error, and individual responsiveness to this treatment approach.

The authors of this book do not endorse the use of NSOMEs for any specific clients or groups of clients, especially those with speech sound disorders of nonorganic origin. The remaining coverage of this topic is included for general informational and educational purposes.

Proponents of an oral-motor approach to treatment (Alexander, Boehme, & Cupps, 1993; Mackie, 1996; Morris & Klein, 1987) suggest that children who exhibit the following speech characteristics are potential candidates for such therapy:

- Weak production of bilabials (/p, b, m/) resulting from decreased lip strength and control
- Poor production of sounds requiring tongue elevation (/t, d, n, l/) as a result of decreased tongue strength and coordination
- Poor differential production of midrange vowels (/ɚ, ʌ, ɝ/) as a result of inadequate jaw stabilization
- Weak production of plosives, fricatives, and affricates (/p, b, s, z, ʃ/) in the presence of hypernasality as a result of inadequate velar movement

The basic goals of an oral-motor therapy program for improving speech intelligibility are as follows:

- To heighten conscious awareness of the oral mechanism
- To normalize (increase or decrease) sensitivity to stimulation of the oral area
- To inhibit primitive or abnormal reflex patterns in the oral mechanism, while enhancing normal movement patterns
- To increase differentiation and stabilization of the oral structures
- To refine articulation movements by increasing the strength and range of motion of oral mechanism components

Following is a basic introductory hierarchy of oral-motor treatment steps, along with sample intervention activities.

Hierarchy of Oral-Motor Treatment Steps

1. *Address postural and positioning issues to ensure adequate balance and alignment of the hip, shoulder, neck, and head.*

   Sample activity: Consult with occupational therapist or physical therapist to determine optimal positioning for conducting effective oral-motor therapy.

2. *Normalize oral sensitivity (both hypo- and hypersensitivity).*

   Sample activity: Gradually introduce firm, graded pressure along the child's gums from front to back, using fingertips or a textured implement. If the child reacts negatively, modify the activity by applying the pressure to an area where touch has been tolerated previously.

3. *Increase jaw control to provide a stable base for finely graded movements of the lips and tongue.*

   Sample activity: Place fingers on the child's jaw. Use thumb to quickly pull the jaw down in a firm, gentle manner. Tell the child to try to close his or her mouth while the clinician guides upward movement with his or her index finger.

4. *Strengthen lip movement/increase muscle tone.*

   Sample activity: Use the pads of fingers to stroke diagonally from the child's cheekbones to lips. Tell the child to hold a straw horizontally with lips for at least five seconds. Release and repeat.

5. *Improve tongue control for elevation and lateralization.*

   Sample activity: Place a finger or tongue depressor flat against the child's tongue tip. Instruct the child to try to push his or her tongue tip up against pressure.

Certain general guidelines should be kept in mind when implementing oral-motor therapy:

- Apply stimulation systematically and follow the same sequence of steps each time.
- Begin stimulation with outer body parts and move in toward the midline (e.g., work from the cheeks to the lips to the tongue).
- Use firm, slow touch rather than light, quick strokes.
- Use visual feedback (e.g., mirror) to facilitate the child's ability to categorize new perceptions and improve her or his tolerance of stimulation.
- Explain procedures as each is being implemented (e.g., "Okay, now I'm stroking from your cheek down to your mouth. Good, you let me touch your face.").

TREATMENT EFFICACY AND EVIDENCE-BASED PRACTICE

Gierut (1998) reviewed 64 publications whose subject matter includes intervention effectiveness for functional articulatory/phonological disorders in children. The summary includes mainly small-sample studies that focused on the treatment of consonant sounds. In 2003, Weston and Bain conducted a meta-analysis of 41 peer-reviewed articulation and phonology studies. The studies included descriptive and experimental designs involving children from ages 3 to 8+ years. Similar conclusions were reached in both analyses: (1) Intervention is generally effective in improving correct sound production and increasing speech intelligibility; and (2) No one treatment approach was identified as being more effective than any other. Other factors to consider include the following:

- Minimal pair treatment and cycles approach treatment generally result in phonological gains.

- Computerized instruction is an effective supplement to direct clinical intervention.

- Efficacy data are needed to determine the relative effectiveness of specific treatment procedures as well as their efficiency (i.e., time needed for completion of the therapy programs).

- Clinician and family variables may have an impact on outcomes and should be examined in treatment studies (e.g., level of clinical expertise, parental/family attitudes and motivation).

- Scheduling of treatment (i.e., session frequency and intensity) requires further study as a potential variable in treatment outcomes (Tyler, 2005).

In 2004, Law, Garret, and Nye conducted a meta-analysis of studies focusing on intervention for children with speech-language difficulties. Not surprisingly, the results indicated a significant effect favoring speech interventions compared with no treatment conditions. Courses of therapy lasting less than 8 weeks appeared to be less effective than longer programs. Finally, parent-administered interventions based on receptive auditory techniques (e.g., auditory bombardment) did not significantly affect speech sound production.

An evidence-based practice (EBP) approach to treatment comprises three basic elements: (1) scientific research, (2) clinical expertise, and (3) client/family values. Because the existing literature on treatment efficacy does not clearly identify any gold standard approach to intervention for articulation/phonology deficits, the SLP's clinical judgment becomes the driving force in the EBP process. For this reason, clinicians often adopt a "what works" approach (Stanovich, 2000) to intervention that utilizes the best features of multiple approaches. For more information on SLP's use of evidence-based practices, see Baker and McLeod (2011) and Hoffman, Ireland, Hall-Mills, and Flynn (2013).

TARGET SELECTION FOR INTERVENTION PROGRAMMING

Two primary approaches are used for choosing initial therapy targets for children with articulation/phonological disorders: developmental and nondevelopmental.

Developmental

In this approach, therapy targets are identified based on the order of acquisition in normally developing children. Table 3–4 provides a list of English consonants in the order of their emergence. Table 3–3, earlier in the chapter, outlines the most common phonological processes exhibited by young children.

TABLE 3–4

Age of Acquisition of English Consonants

Consonant	Poole (1934)	Templin (1957)	Prather et al. (1975)	Smit et al. (1990) Females	Males
m	3½	3	2	3	3
n	4½	3	2	3½	3
h	3½	3	2	3	3
p	3½	3	2	3	3
f	5½	3	2–4	3½	3½
w	3½	3	2–8	3	3
b	3½	4	2–8	3	3
h	4½	3	2	7–9	7–9
j	4½	3½	2–4	4	5
k	4½	4	2–4	3½	3½
g	4½	4	2–4	3½	4
l	6½	6	3–4	6	6
d	4½	4	2–4	3	3½
t	4½	6	2–8	4	3½
s	7½	4½	3	7–9	7–9
r	7½	4	3–4	8	8
tʃ	—	4½	3–8	6	7
v	6½	6	4	5½	5½
z	7½	7	4	7–9	7–9
ʒ	6½	7	4	—	—
θ	7½	6	4	6	8
dʒ	—	7	4	6	7
ʃ	6½	4½	3–8	6	7
ð	6½	7	4	4½	7

NOTE: Variability in reported ages of acquisition is partly due to the different criterion levels used across studies to determine mastery of each sound. Poole (1934) = 100%, Templin (1957) = 75%, Prather et al. (1975) = 75%, Smit et al. (1990) = 90%.

Nondevelopmental

In this approach, developmental norms are not used in the selection of target behaviors. Instead, the determining factors fall into two groups. One strategy is client-specific and bases the selection of therapy objectives on several factors:

1. Target(s) that are most relevant to a child or parent (e.g., a sound in the child's name)

2. Target(s) that are most stimulable in a given child's error repertoire regardless of developmental sequence. (It should be noted that several authors take the opposite view and recommend choosing the least stimulable sounds as targets for intervention. They suggest that stimulability is indicative of some degree of phonological knowledge and these sounds may be likely to emerge naturally; in contrast, non-stimulable sounds would benefit most from targeted intervention. For more detailed information, see Baker and McLeod [2011]; Gierut, Elbert, and Dinnsen [1987]; Rvachew [2005]; and Williams [2002].)

3. Target(s) that are most visible when produced (e.g., /θ/ versus /g/)

The second nondevelopmental strategy is based on the degree of perceived deviance associated with a child's errors. This strategy can be applied to both articulation and phonological errors, as follows:

Articulatory

- Omission errors contribute most to unintelligibility, followed by substitutions, and then distortions.

- Errors in the initial position of words contribute most to unintelligibility, followed by medial, and then final.

- Errors that occur on the most frequent sounds in a language contribute significantly to unintelligibility.

Phonological

- Patterns of initial consonant deletion and glottal replacement of medial consonants tend to contribute significantly to listener perception of unintelligibility.

In addition to choosing therapy targets, clinicians must determine the most appropriate "goal-attack strategy" for each client (Fey, 1986). Several strategies can be utilized in the design of a client's therapy program: vertical, horizontal, and cyclical. The basic assumption of **vertical** training is that the best route to target mastery is through intense practice on a limited number of targets. If therapy is being programmed with a focus on motor learning, the clinician is encouraged to design session activities that provide the opportunity for a high rate of responses or **massed practice** (e.g., 150 target productions in 30 minutes). The clinician focuses on one or two targets until the client achieves some predetermined level of mastery, usually at the level of conversation. Therapy then moves on to the next target(s) identified in a hierarchical level of difficulty. This "deep" approach to intervention tends to be most appropriate for clients with relatively few articulatory/phonological errors.

In contrast to training deeply, a **horizontal** strategy attacks goals broadly. It assumes that simultaneous exposure to a wide variety of targets will facilitate a client's ability to produce phonemes or sound patterns. The clinician provides less intense practice on a larger number of targets, even within the same session. This strategy focuses on efficient generalization of target behaviors across the speech sound system and tends to be most appropriate for clients with multiple errors.

Clinicians may choose to combine aspects of the vertical and horizontal strategies into the **cycles** approach. Recall that instead of attacking therapy targets deeply or broadly, this strategy provides a client with practice on a given target for a predetermined amount of time, and then moves on to another target (Hodson & Paden, 1991). This approach gives the client an opportunity to internalize the original sound or pattern while the clinician introduces the new target. Focus on the original target resumes later in the therapy program. This cycle is repeated until the target(s) emerges in spontaneous speech.

EXAMPLE PROFILES FOR FUNCTIONAL ARTICULATION

Disorders

This section presents three commonly seen profiles of childhood articulation problems. These examples have been designed to illustrate the selection of intervention targets as well as specific therapy activities and materials. Most of the chosen activities are easily implemented in either individual or group therapy settings.

For many children, it may be necessary to teach the phonetic placement of target sounds prior to the introduction of actual activities. Appendix 3-A provides specific instructions for establishing the correct placement for consonants that are typically considered difficult to elicit.

The first profile describes a *young child with multiple errors.*

Jill is 3 years old and demonstrates the following articulation errors (error sound/ intended target):

Initial	Medial	Final
d/g	d/g	ʃ/tʃ
j/l	w/r	-/s
b/v	f/θ	-/k
-/s	j/l	-/d
p/f	ʔ/t	s/ʃ
b/m	j/n	-/ŋ
	-/s	

Blends: b/bl, f/fl, w/kl, t/sl, t/skw, fw/kr, b/br, d/dr, w/pr

Selection of therapy targets using a developmental approach. Based on this child's chronological age, the errors to be targeted first are d/g, b/m, p/f, j/n, -/ŋ because these are the earliest emerging sounds, as can be seen in Table 3–4. The second set of target sounds consists of -/k, -/d, and ʔ/t. The remaining errors would not be considered appropriate targets for intervention because they emerge well beyond 3 years of age.

Selection of therapy targets using a nondevelopmental approach. The errors to be targeted are /θ/, /v/, /m/, /f/, /g/, and /s/. The /θ/ and /v/ sounds were chosen despite developmental considerations because Jill was highly stimulable for these sounds in isolation during the diagnostic session. The /m/ and /f/ sounds were selected because they are visible when produced, which facilitates learning of correct articulatory placement. The /f/ and /g/ sounds were included as beginning targets because their status as initial-position errors makes them significant contributors to Jill's overall unintelligibility.

Sample Activities

1. Modify a board game, such as Hasbro® Candy Land™, by requiring a child to produce a target sound in isolation, following the clinician's model, in order to move a game piece. Close approximations, rather than accurate productions, of the target phoneme may be acceptable in the very early stages of therapy. Once the child improves her performance by 30% to 50% over baseline measures, clinician models should be faded. Three consecutive spontaneous productions can then be required for the child to take a turn in the game.

2. Create a game with colored paper fish. Each fish has a picture on it designed to elicit a target sound in the desired position. Attach paper clips to the back of each fish and give the child a "fishing pole" with a magnet on the end of its string. Have the child dangle the magnet over the fish. Instruct the child to respond by producing the stimulus item three times as she lands each fish. The difficulty level of the response can be programmed to vary from single words to lengthy sentences.

3. Assemble twenty-five 4-by-4-inch squares of colored paper with one stimulus picture on each. One of the squares should be marked in a special way (e.g., with a star or a sticker). Cover one wall with the squares so that the stimulus pictures are facing the wall. Tell the child that she is going to pretend to be a detective who has to find the "magic square" in the dark. Hand the child a penlight, turn out the lights, and instruct her to aim the beam at the square that she thinks is the magic one. As each square is lit up, ask the child to produce the target item at the appropriate level of complexity.

4. Assemble the following materials to make two puppets: two glue sticks, two brown paper bags, yarn, two sets of paper cutouts of facial features, and other accessories such as earrings, mustaches, and eyeglasses. Collect 25 pictures containing the targeted therapy sounds and place them in a pile on the table. Explain that the clinician and child will construct puppets using the paper bags and other materials. The clinician selects one picture from the pile, models the correct production of the word, and then glues one feature/accessory to one of the bags. Instruct the child to select the next picture from the pile, produce the word correctly three times, and glue a feature/accessory on the other bag. Alternate turns until both puppets are completed.

The second profile describes a school-age child with *multiple articulation errors.*

Joe is 6 years old and demonstrates the following errors:

Initial	Medial	Final
j/l	j/l	j/l
	s/θ	s/θ
ʃ/tʃ	ʃ/tʃ	ʃ/tʃ
		-/d
ʃ/f	ʃ/f	s/f
b/v	b/v	
w/r	w/r	

Blends: s/sl, b/bl, k/kl, fw/fl, fw/fr, tw/tr, k/skw, fw/kr, t/st

Selection of therapy targets using a developmental approach. Based on this child's chronological age, the errors to be targeted first are -/d, ʃ/f, b/v, and j/l, because these are the earliest emerging sounds as shown in Table 3–4. The second set of targets consists of the remaining sound and blend errors, because all of these are typically acquired by 6 years of age.

Selection of therapy targets using a nondevelopmental approach. The errors to be targeted are /r/, /fr/, /fl/, and /θ/. The /r/ was chosen because it is one of the most frequently occurring sounds in English (see Table 3–5, Frequency of Consonant Occurrence in English). The /fr/ and /fl/ blends were selected because these are the only phonetic contexts in which Joe can correctly produce his otherwise misarticulated /f/ sound. The blends can provide a starting point for facilitating the correct production of /f/ as a singleton. Finally, the /θ/ was chosen because its articulatory placement is highly visible and is therefore relatively easy to approximate.

Sample Activities

1. Draw 10 pictures on a dry-erase board, each containing one instance of a target sound. Give the child a squirt gun and tell him to hit one of the pictures. Instruct the child to produce the stimulus item at the appropriate level of complexity (e.g., single word, carrier phrase, sentence, narrative).

2. For a group activity, gather at least 20 pictures/objects that contain the target sound(s) and place them around the room. Give each child a "suitcase" (box) and tell them that the group is going on a trip. Say, "I'm going to Disney World. I'll take you too if you bring the right things in your suitcase." Have the children take turns retrieving stimulus items from around the room. They may place them in their suitcases upon correct production of the appropriate target sounds.

3. Assemble at least 20 pictures/objects that contain target sound(s) and place them on the table. Introduce a "shopping game" by presenting a carrier phrase such as

"I went to the food store and bought ___ , ___, and ___." Have the child remove the corresponding pictures from the table. Then instruct the child to take a turn at making a shopping list by producing the same carrier phrase with three new food items chosen from the remaining picture stimuli. The type of store named in the carrier phrase can be varied to expose/reinforce the child's ability to organize lexical items into semantic categories (e.g., clothing, toys, pets). Each list can also be written on a dry-erase board or chart paper to emphasize the connection between writing, reading, and speaking. The activity can be easily adapted for small group sessions.

TABLE 3–5
Frequency of Consonant Occurrence in English

Sound	Cumulative Percentage	Percentage of Occurrence
n	12.0	12.0
t	11.9	23.9
s	6.9	30.8
r	6.7	37.5
d	6.4	43.9
m	5.9	49.8
z	5.4	55.2
ð	5.3	60.5
l	5.3	65.8
k	5.1	70.9
w	4.9	75.8
h	4.4	80.2
b	3.3	83.5
p	3.1	86.6
g	3.1	89.7
f	2.1	91.8
h	1.6	93.4
j	1.6	95.0
v	1.5	96.5
ʃ	0.9	97.4
θ	0.9	98.3
dʒ	0.6	98.9
tʃ	0.6	99.5
ʒ	<0.1	99.6

SOURCE: Adapted from "Computer-Assisted Natural Process Analysis (NPA): Recent Issues and Data," by L.D. Shriberg and J. Kwiatkowski, 1983, Seminars in Speech and Language, 4(4), p. 11, www.thieme.com (reprinted with permission)

4. Write each verse of the following song on a sheet of paper. Place clip art or other icons above words containing a targeted sound (e.g., /θ/). Provide a microphone and arrange a spotlight using a flashlight in a darkened room. Explain that in this activity the child will pretend to be on stage. Teach the child to sing the song using any familiar melody.

> I'd rather use a bathtub than a booth
> I'd rather have a toothache than no tooth
> I'd rather have a birthday than a wreath
> I'd rather be an athlete than a thief
>
> *Refrain*
> *Wouldn't you?*
> Yes I would!
> Yes I would!
>
> I'd rather use a thumbtack than a thorn
> I'd rather have a thick one than a thin
> I'd rather have some mouthwash than a bath
> I'd rather be a Matthew than a Keith
>
> *Repeat refrain*

The third profile describes an older school-age child with *persistent /r/ and /s/ substitution errors.*

Sammy is 8 years old and demonstrates the following errors:

Initial	Medial	Final
w/r	w/r	w/r
θ/s	θ/s	θ/s

Blends: Sammy has the same substitution pattern for all /r/ and /s/ blends.

Selection of therapy targets using a developmental approach. A developmental approach for therapy target selection is not relevant in this case. The /r/ and /s/ sounds are typically acquired by 8 years of age, and, therefore, both would be considered appropriate therapy objectives.

Selection of therapy targets using a nondevelopmental approach. The /s/ phoneme is selected as the primary therapy target because Sammy was stimulable for this sound in isolation. It is also considered a particularly relevant objective for Sammy because /s/ is the first sound in his name.

Sample Activities

1. Draw a football field on chart paper with the yard lines (e.g., 10-yard line, 20-yard line, and so on) and end zones clearly delineated. Make a football from colored paper/cardboard and affix masking tape or other adhesive to the back. The therapist and child select team names. The child takes control of the ball at the 50-yard line because he represents the home team. Model stimulus items containing the target sound and instruct the child to repeat the stimulus item five times. He can move the football 5 "yards" toward his end zone for every correct response. If the child produces no correct responses, the clinician gets to move the ball 5 yards toward the other end zone. The difficulty level of this game can be modified in various ways: fading the therapist model, increasing the number of required responses, and increasing the length and complexity of the target response from isolation to complex sentences. This activity also works well in small-group sessions.

2. Design a game sheet with at least six or eight drawings of blank TV/movie screens. Instruct the child to name television shows containing the target sound. A correct production allows the child to draw or write something related to that show on one of the TV sets on the game sheet. For example, for the target sound /r/, the child may name shows such as *Rugrats, Max and Ruby, Ratatouille, Robin Hood,* and *Meet the Robinsons.* Once all the screens are filled in, begin a guessing game in which the child is instructed to describe one of the shows/movies without using the title, and the therapist has to guess its name. All correct spontaneous productions of the target sound during this conversational task should be reinforced. If the child meets a predetermined criterion for accuracy of sound production, a paper "Emmy" can be awarded. Task difficulty can be increased to more complex levels by requiring the child to summarize a show/movie or describe one of its characters in order to fill in a blank screen on the game sheet. This activity is easily adapted for group sessions.

3. On slips of paper, write 25 single words containing the target sound /s/ in initial, final, or medial position. Fold slips of paper and place them in a container or pile them on the table. Affix a Hasbro® NERF™ basketball hoop (or equivalent) to a therapy room wall at least three feet higher than the child's standing height. Explain that this game requires the child to select a slip of paper from the pile and produce a sentence using the word written on the slip. If the target sound is produced correctly, the child is allowed to crumple the paper slip and shoot it at the basketball hoop. If target sound /s/ is incorrectly produced, the slip of paper is returned to the pile or container. The game continues until the pile is depleted and all paper slips have been crumpled and shot.

4. Gather materials to play "detective," including a badge and a small notebook with pencil. Design several simple crime scenarios that contain multiple instances of the target sound. One example of a possible scenario follows:

   > Sue is lying dead on the floor beside a windowsill in a sealed room. Scattered on the floor, there is water and broken glass. Simon is asleep on the sofa across the room. Mr. Soaps, a window washer, spots Sue and calls the police to report his suspicions.

   Tell the child to play a detective and ask questions of the witness, Mr. Soaps (played by the therapist), to solve the crime. The child should be encouraged to ask questions that contain as many instances of the target sound as possible. To facilitate this, all questions could begin with, "Well, Mr. Soaps . . ." Appropriate questions for this scenario include "What sort of clothes was Sue wearing when you saw her?"; "How old is Simon?"; "Where do you suppose the broken glass came from?" (Solution: Sue is a goldfish and Simon is a cat.)

Helpful Hints

1. Do not include more than one error sound in a stimulus word, phrase, or sentence during the initial stages of therapy.

2. Pay attention to the phonetic context of words that contain a child's target sounds. Certain consonant-vowel sequences may facilitate or impede correct production.

3. In some ways, the production of speech sounds is a motor skill like that of playing a piano. Therapy sessions that elicit the greatest number of sound productions will be the most effective in establishing correct production as an automatic behavior.

4. Children with persistent errors that appear to be functional should be evaluated for the presence of oral-motor difficulties.

5. Use books that contain target sounds as immersion activities. The books can be given to parents to use at reading time with their child. For our example child, Sammy, good choices include *Rotten Ralph* by J. Gantos, *Rain Makes Applesauce* by J. Scheer, *Miss Nelson Is Missing* by H. Allard and J. Marshall, and *My Mama Says* by J. Viorst. For further suggestions, see *Books Are for Talking Too!* by J. Gebers (2003).

6. It is important to counsel parents to respond consistently to the content of their child's utterances before pointing out speech errors or modeling correct productions. This is particularly relevant in the early stages of therapy to avoid frustration and other negative feelings.

EXAMPLE PROFILES FOR PHONOLOGICAL DISORDERS

Following are two profiles commonly seen in children with phonological rule problems. The first case depicts a process approach to intervention; the second case illustrates a modified distinctive feature strategy. These examples have been designed to illustrate the selection of intervention targets as well as specific therapy activities and materials. Most of the chosen activities are easily implemented in either individual or group therapy settings.

Gerry is 5 years old and demonstrates the following phonological processes:

1. Final consonant deletion

-/s

-/v

-/p

-/d

-/k

2. Unstressed syllable deletion

   tephone/telephone

   way/away

   tato/potato

   amance/ambulance

3. Cluster reduction

   -t/st

   -m/sm

   p-/pl

   -K/sk

   n-/nd

4. Fronting

   t/k

   d/g

5. Voicing

   b/p

   d/t

   z/s

   v/f

6. Initial consonant deletion

   -/k

   -/l

   -/h

   -/p

   -/t

7. Glottal replacement

   ʔ/t

   ʔ/k

   ʔ/g

Selection of therapy targets. The patterns to be targeted are final consonant deletion, fronting, voicing, and initial consonant deletion. The first five patterns in the preceding list are exhibited by typically developing children and are therefore considered developmental in nature. Final consonant deletion and fronting were targeted because these developmental processes are suppressed from children's speech production repertoires earlier than the other two (by 3 years of age). The last two processes occur much less frequently among typically developing children. Initial consonant deletion was selected as a therapy target because of its severe impact on intelligibility (Khan & Lewis, 2002; Leinonen-Davis, 1988; Yavas & Lamprecht, 1988).

Sample Activities

1. Cut out a large dinosaur (about 3 feet in length) with a very long detachable tail (e.g., Tyrannosaurus rex) from poster board or colored paper and obtain a small paint bottle with a sponge top (bingo marker). Collect a pile of 25 pictures for the child to name. The names should be monosyllabic and contain a variety of singleton final consonants, including examples of his deletion errors as well as any that he might be able to produce spontaneously. Remove the tail from the dinosaur and explain to the child that words have sounds at the ends just like dinosaurs have tails. Instruct the child to select a picture from the pile and name it, making sure to put the ending sound on the word. Following each correct response, illustrate the parallel between the dinosaur's tail and the final sound of the word by allowing the child to reattach the dinosaur's tail and decorate it with one dot of sponge paint. The ultimate goal of this activity is to decorate the dinosaur's tail completely and attach it permanently for the child to take home. This activity can be used effectively up through the level of conversation and narration.

2. Create or collect a deck of picture cards for the game Go Fish, depicting pairs of identical words and minimal contrast words that incorporate the child's fronting errors. Recall that minimal pairs consist of two words that are identical except for a single distinctive feature or phoneme. This approach is designed to emphasize the concept that even small sound contrasts can signal differences in word meanings. Examples include *t*ap and *c*ap, *t*op and *c*op, *d*ate and *g*ate, pi*t* and pi*ck*, be*d* and be*g*. Begin the game by dealing three cards to each player and placing the remainder in a pile in the middle of the table. Explain to the child that the object of the game is to make pairs for all the cards in his hand with *identical* pictures by asking other players, "Do you have any ___?" A correct production allows the child to continue requesting cards. If the child uses a fronting error during a turn at requesting a card, he should be given the picture that corresponds to his actual, not intended, production. For example, if the child says "date" when attempting to match his picture of gate, he will receive the card depicting a date on a calendar and therefore not obtain the match. The clinician should model the intended production for the child to imitate. A correct imitation is rewarded with the desired picture match, but the turn passes to the next player. The player who has the most pairs at the end of the game is the winner.

3. Gather pictures for the parenthesized words in the following sentences and arrange them on a table. Explain that the clinician will say a sentence with a word missing at the end. Instruct the child to finish the sentence by selecting the picture that sounds almost the same as a word in the sentence, except for using "voice on" or "voice off." The clinician reads one sentence at a time with particular emphasis on the italicized word. (Note: The clinician provides the child with a hint that the target word rhymes with one of the words in the sentence.)

The *pig* is ___ (big).

Put the *coat* on the ___ (goat).

The *fan* is in the ___ (van).

I *see* the letter ___ (Z).

Put the *pin* in the ___ (bin).

Don't *tip* over the ___ (dip).

The *girl* has a ___ (curl).

Sue likes the ___ (zoo).

Dan is very ___ (tan).

Go *down* to the ___ (town).

He *came* to play the ___ (game).

Put the *pack* on your ___ (back).

4. Cut out a minimum of 30 colored paper turtles that are approximately 8 inches in length. Two-thirds of the turtles should have their heads protruding out from their shells, whereas the heads of the remaining one-third should not be visible. Place the turtles in an obstacle course–like path around the room so that a child can hop easily from one turtle "stepping-stone" to another. Gather a deck of 20 pictures whose names begin with the child's initial consonant deletion errors. Prepare numerous slips of paper that instruct the child to perform one of the following: (a) hop forward one turtle, (b) hop forward two turtles, (c) hop backward one turtle, or (d) hop backward two turtles. Fold these paper slips and place them in a paper bag. Tell the child that to play the "turtle stepping-stone" game, he has to hop on the turtles and say some words. For each turn, she has to choose a slip of paper from the bag without looking and follow its instruction. As she lands on a turtle, the clinician holds up one card from the picture deck. If the child is on a turtle that has no head, she should name the picture three times without producing its initial consonant sound. If the turtle has a head, the word must be produced five times with its initial consonant sound present. The object of the game is to reach the final turtle on the obstacle course.

Note: It is important to remember that the focus of these activities is on phonological processes rather than the production of particular sounds. For this reason, in the early stages of therapy, the clinician should reinforce any responses that demonstrate a child's use of the targeted phonological process, regardless of the actual phoneme(s) produced. For example, during work on the final consonant deletion process, a child may be reinforced for producing "bat" or "bam" instead of his habitual "ba" when naming a picture of a bag.

Grace is 5 years old and demonstrates the following feature errors:

Manner Errors	Examples
Stops for fricatives:	*zoo* → /doo/, *soap* → /toap/
Fricatives for affricates:	*porch* → /porsh/
Glides for liquids:	*right* → /yight/

Place Errors	
Alveolars for velars:	*tuptake/cupcake, det/get*
Alveolars for palatals:	*sue/shoe, trezure/treasure*

Voicing Errors

Voiced for voiceless:	*gow/cow, doe/toe*
Voiceless for voiced:	*loose/lose, stofe/stove*

For clarity, the examples in the preceding list reflect a single feature contrast between the error sound and the intended target. However, children frequently produce errors that differ from the target by two or more feature contrasts (e.g., *late* → /jet/ differ in both place and manner; *sip* → /gip/ differ in all three features).

Selection of therapy targets.   The first set of therapy targets includes one error contrast from each of the three feature categories. The manner contrast of stop/fricative was selected because fricatives emerge earlier developmentally than the other two sound classes listed under this category (i.e., affricates and liquids). In addition, fricatives have a higher frequency of occurrence in English than affricates. The place contrast of alveolar/velar was chosen because palatals are acquired much later in the developmental sequence than velars. The voiced/voiceless contrast was included because this feature error generally occurs in word-initial position, which contributes heavily to perceived unintelligibility.

Sample Activities

1. Using masking tape, create a hopscotch grid with eight squares on the floor. Draw a long slide on a dry-erase board or piece of paper, and obtain a spinner with numbers. Provide a doll or stuffed animal figure and tell the child that "Harry" uses different types of sounds when playing these two different activities. Demonstrate that Harry produces "short hopping" sounds (stops) such as /b, p, d/ as he jumps on the hopscotch grid. Then demonstrate that Harry produces "long, sliding" sounds (fricatives) such as /s, z, v, f/ as he goes down the slide. Check the child's grasp of the concepts involved by modeling alternating examples of each manner of sound production and asking the child to place Harry on the corresponding activity.

   Start with the hopscotch game and explain that the child will jump from the beginning to the end of the grid while holding Harry. The clinician models examples of stops (such as /t/ or /k/) when the child lands on each square. The child must produce three imitations of the stop before jumping to the next square. After completing the hopscotch grid, move on to the slide activity. Emphasize the feature contrast between stops and fricatives by reminding the child that Harry uses "long, sliding" sounds with this activity. Have the child use the spinner to determine the number of times Harry can go down the slide. The clinician models an example of a fricative sound with exaggerated duration (such as /fffff/ or /sssss/). Tell the child to place Harry at the top of the slide and move him down slowly while imitating the clinician's exaggerated production. Repeat as many times as indicated by the spinner and then have the child spin again for another turn. The clinician should model different fricatives for each turn. Allow the child four more turns with the spinner and then return to the hopscotch game to reinforce the targeted feature contrast.

   Once the child demonstrates mastery at this level, the clinician can introduce more complex stimulus items such as syllables and words.

2. Create a racetrack game board with starting and finishing lines that are connected by 20 squares. Provide a small race car game piece. Make a spinner with numbers, half colored green and half red. Tell the child that the race car moves forward when the spinner indicates a green number and backward with a red number. Explain that whenever the spinner points to a green number, the child will imitate the clinician's model of a "forward" sound (alveolar such as /d/ or /t/), while moving the game piece. If the spinner points to a red number, a contrasting "backward" sound (velar such as /g/ or /k/) will be modeled for imitation. A variety of sounds that highlight the alveolar/velar place contrast should be modeled throughout the game. The object of the game is to cross the finish line.

3. Make a 24-square bingo card (six rows of four squares) and place pictures/stickers of butterflies and bumblebees in alternating columns on the card. Collect a deck of 24 pictures for the child to name. One-third of the names should have voiced consonants in the initial word position (e.g., *boy, girl, duck, zipper, jump*) and the other two-thirds should have voiceless initial consonants (e.g., *soup, table, chair, cat, piano*). Provide 24 game tokens. Explain to the child that bumblebees and butterflies make two different kinds of sounds. The bumblebee uses sounds that buzz, like /zzzzz/, and the butterfly uses sounds that do not buzz, like /sssss/. Then select a picture card from the deck and hold it up. Instruct the child to name the picture and then to categorize the initial phoneme as a bumblebee or butterfly sound. If the child responds correctly to both parts, she is able to place a game token on one of the picture squares that corresponds to the sound category of the target word (i.e., bumblebee versus butterfly). The object of the game is to fill an entire column of squares with tokens.

4. Gather a plastic tablecloth and napkins for a pretend tea party and arrange them on a table in the therapy room. Collect 20 pictures of objects/animals that have easily identifiable front portions and back portions, and cut them in half (e.g., train, horse, car, dog, snake, airplane, pencil, bus, giraffe, fish). Separate the front and back pieces into two piles. Briefly review that certain sounds are made in the front of the mouth (e.g., /p/, /t/) while others are made in the back (e.g., /k/, /g/). Practice a few examples of each with the child.

   Explain that the tablecloth and napkins need to be decorated in a special way for the tea party. Model a front or back sound in a consonant-vowel (CV) syllable and instruct the child to identify it as "front" or "back" and imitate three times. If identification and production responses are correct, the child picks a picture from the appropriate pile and pastes/tapes it to the tablecloth or napkins. Alternate CV models between front and back sounds until all picture pieces have been used as decorations.

Helpful Hints

1. When using a phonological processes approach, it is sometimes useful to teach the underlying concepts in nonspeech activities before moving to speech production tasks.

2. One consideration in the selection of phonological processes for therapy is the relative consistency of their use. Processes that a child demonstrates only occasionally may be more easily modified than those used on a consistent basis.

3. In the initial stages of distinctive feature therapy, selection of target sounds that differ by only a single feature may increase the likelihood of early success.

4. Distinctive feature theory predicts that generalization will most likely occur from trained phonemes to phonemes that share the same feature. Thus, it is important to regularly probe these untrained sounds to determine whether any have been acquired spontaneously and will not require subsequent intervention.

5. Clinicians may need to explain to parents that therapy for phonological disorders focuses on appropriate use of linguistic rules rather than acquisition of correct motor movements. This may eliminate a parent's confusion in the early stages of therapy when the clinician reinforces a seemingly incorrect response (e.g., *toat/boat* when targeting initial consonant deletion) when, in fact, the child is now using the correct rule.

ORGANIC ARTICULATION DISORDERS

Three pathologies associated with severe articulation problems in children are cleft palate, hearing impairment, and childhood apraxia of speech. The selection of initial therapy targets for organic disorders is based on a nondevelopmental approach, because the accompanying speech production deficits are the direct result of structural/neurologic anomalies and are not developmental in nature.

Cleft Palate

This is a congenital malformation of the palate and/or lip that results from the failure of oral structures to fuse at midline during the first trimester of pregnancy (4 to 12 weeks of gestation). A cleft can be unilateral (one-sided) or bilateral. Clefts of the palate have substantially more severe effects on speech intelligibility than do isolated clefts of the lip. Management of children with clefts generally is carried out by an interdisciplinary team that includes a speech-language pathologist. Surgical repair of labial clefts is completed at approximately 3 months of age or earlier; palatal repairs generally occur before the child's second birthday (Kummer, 2008; Peterson-Falzone, Hardin-Jones, & Karnell, 2001; Shprintzen & Bardach, 1995). Pharyngeal flap procedures are considered secondary surgical interventions and involve joining a flap of soft tissue from the posterior pharyngeal wall to the palate, creating a bridge that partially occludes the velopharyngeal space. This procedure is performed primarily for the purpose of facilitating velopharyngeal closure during speech. Speech therapy may begin before surgical repairs are completed but is primarily provided following surgical intervention. Some authors recommend a 3-month postsurgical recovery period before therapy is initiated or resumed.

The most significant speech problem associated with cleft palate is **velopharyngeal incompetence (VPI).** VPI is the inability to close off the oral cavity from the nasal cavity during speech due to inadequate velar movement (Peterson-Falzone, Trost-Cardamone, Karnell, & Hardin-Jones, 2006). This results in audible nasal emission of air, hypernasal resonance, and articulation errors. Audible nasal emission occurs when air flows at an excessive rate through the nasal passages, creating turbulence and generating distracting noise during speech. This leakage of air results in reduced oral breath pressure for the production of pressure consonants (i.e., fricatives, affricates, and plosives). **Hypernasal resonance,** or hypernasality, occurs when the balance between oral and nasal resonance shifts to such a degree that speech is perceived by listeners to be "nasal." This phenomenon is particularly noticeable during the production of vowels, especially when the degree of mouth opening is restricted.

In misarticulations related to VPI, the most frequent errors occur on fricatives, affricates, and plosives. The most common types of errors demonstrated by cleft palate speakers are distortions and omissions, with occasional substitutions in the form of glottal stops and pharyngeal fricatives. In general, the provision of therapy is appropriate only for children who have velopharyngeal (VP) competence or questionable/marginal incompetence, as determined by the cleft palate team (Kuehn & Moller, 2000; Pamplona, Ysunza, & Rami, 2004). Therapy focusing solely on oral direction of the breath stream is not usually recommended for children who demonstrate clear evidence of VPI. It may lead to elevation of the larynx and result in voice disorders.

Following is a profile of the speech sound errors in children with cleft palates:

- The most frequent errors occur on fricatives and affricates, followed by plosives.
- Distortions and omissions are the most common error types, followed by substitutions.
- Singleton fricatives and affricates are most likely to be distorted.
- Consonants in blends are most likely to be omitted.
- Glottal stops tend to be substituted for plosives.
- More misarticulations occur on voiceless consonants than their voiced cognates, especially in young children.
- Most errors occur in the final position, followed by medial and initial positions, respectively.

Example Profile

Following is a typical profile for a child with cleft palate. This example has been designed to illustrate the selection of intervention targets as well as specific therapy activities and materials. The chosen activities are easily implemented in either individual or group therapy settings.

Eddie is 4 years old, has undergone successful palatal repair, and demonstrates adequate VP closure in nonspeech activities. His speech is characterized by audible nasal emission of air, hypernasality, and the following articulation errors:

	Initial	Medial	Final
Distortions	s, z, ʃ	s, z, ʃ	s, z, ʃ
	k, g, p, b	f, θ, k, g	f, θ, k, g
Omissions	-r/pr*	-l/pl*	s-/st*
Substitutions	n/d	ʔ/p, ʔ/b	ʔ/p, ʔ/b
		ʔ/d, ʔ/t	ʔ/d, ʔ/d

*Consonant blends are consistently reduced to singletons in all positions and, therefore, are too numerous to list individually.

Selection of therapy targets. The five main goals of speech therapy with children with cleft palate are (1) correct articulatory placement, (2) achieve light articulatory contacts, (3) attain a greater mouth opening, (4) decrease hypernasal resonance quality, and (5) promote more anterior placement of articulatory production (Golding-Kushner, 2000; Kummer, 2008). Given these goals, the errors to be targeted for intervention are /p/, /b/, /s/, /θ/, /k/, /g/, /t/, /d/, and vowels. The first four sounds were chosen to decrease Eddie's tendency to move frontal articulatory placements to the back of the vocal tract. The /k/, /g/, /t/, and /d/, as well as /p/ and /b/, were selected because pressure consonants are the most effective vehicles for demonstrating light articulatory contact (less forceful movements of oral muscles). Vowels were included because they are the most appropriate targets for encouraging increased or exaggerated mouth opening as a means of improving the balance between oral and nasal resonance.

Sample Activities

Promote anterior placement of speech production

1. Compile a set of 20 pictures that are clear demonstrations of the concept of front versus back (e.g., train, dog, car, house, horse, truck) and cut them in half. (In addition, decorate a blank sheet of paper with 25 drawings or stickers of balloons without strings for later use.) Shuffle the pictures and place them face down on the table. Tell the child that this is a memory game in which he and the clinician will take turns selecting pictures, one at a time, to try to match the pairs that represent the front and back of each object. The child is instructed to identify each picture piece as it is uncovered (e.g., "This is the front of a train"). Each correctly matched pair is given to the player who found both pieces. The player with the most pairs at the end of the game is the winner.

   Once it is established that the child understands "front/back" in relation to everyday objects, explain that this concept also applies to his mouth. Tell him that some sounds are made at the front of the mouth, like /p/ and /t/, and others are made at the back like /k/ and /g/. Sit with the child in front of a mirror and model the anterior placement of simple syllables (i.e., /pa/, /bæ/, /so/, /θi/). Engage the child in a "Simon Says" game in which he has to imitate sounds made by the clinician. For each correct production, the child may draw a string under one balloon on the prepared sheet. The object of the game is to fill the sheet with strings on all of the balloons.

Light articulatory contact

2. Obtain two puppets with easily manipulable mouths. Introduce the puppets to the child. Explain that one uses very hard (forceful) movements of his mouth when he talks, while the other uses gentle (light) movements. The clinician's speech and hand movements should demonstrate forceful versus light contacts as the explanations are given. To ensure the child's understanding of the basic concept, model several exaggerated examples of both articulatory contact types, and have the child point to the puppet that uses that speech pattern. Once the child can reliably discriminate between "hard" and "gentle," hide both puppets in a bag or box, and instruct the child to close his eyes and pull one out and place it on his hand. The clinician provides a model of the type of contact used by the chosen puppet at the

syllable level. Models should focus on pressure consonants in the initial position (e.g., /ka/, /gu/, /ti/, do/, /pa/, and /bæ/). The child is then required to imitate the clinician's stimulus and should be encouraged to use appropriate hand and mouth movements simultaneously. Return the puppet to its hiding place and repeat the activity for 20 or more trials. The level of response complexity can be increased from imitative to spontaneous and also can be programmed to vary from syllables to lengthy sentences.

Increased degree of mouth opening

3. Draw or attach two pictures of frogs to a dry-erase board. One should be depicted as having an exaggerated open-mouth posture, whereas the other frog's mouth is only slightly opened. Instruct the child to throw a beanbag at either of the frogs. The clinician should model a vowel production with the degree of mouth opening that corresponds to the frog that is struck by the beanbag. The child is required to imitate the clinician's model five times for another turn at the game. The vowels /a/, /æ/, /o/, and /e/ are good candidates for the initial phase of training.

Accurate articulatory placement

4. Cut out a 12-inch circle from poster board to use as a "pizza." Use a marker to draw lines dividing the pizza into eight equal slices. Affix three to five small pieces of Velcro to each slice. Gather 24 to 40 small pictures containing targeted therapy sound(s) and attach Velcro strips to each. Explain that the child will decorate the pizza with picture "toppings." Instruct the child to name a picture with emphasis on the target sound. If production is correct, the child can place the topping on the pizza. Repeat this sequence until all toppings have been used.

Helpful Hints

1. Children who show only glottal and pharyngeal place of articulation should have therapy to assess adequacy of fricative and plosive production before any pharyngeal flap surgery is considered.

2. If the child has questionable VPI, delay training of /k/ and /g/ to avoid the tendency to adopt compensatory movements.

3. Children with cleft palates often have persistent dental anomalies that may result in *lateralization* of fricatives and affricates that is not amenable to articulation therapy.

4. In general, speech therapy should be initiated at the earliest possible age to take advantage of sensitive periods in speech development.

5. Self-monitoring skills in children with nasality problems may be strengthened with the use of biofeedback devices such as the Oral & Nasal Listener (SuperDuper, Inc.) and the Nasometer II (KayPentax Corporation). These devices detect nasal emission/resonance and display this information visually or auditorily. The child uses the displayed information to monitor and eventually control velopharyngeal function.

6. The therapeutic process for children with oral-facial anomalies frequently must address the emotional well-being of the child and the family as well as the symptoms of the physical defect.

7. Parents of infants with clefts may require gentle but firm encouragement to engage in natural smiling and vocal interactions with their babies. Parents may need guidance to see beyond the obvious craniofacial defect to bond successfully with their child.

8. Clinicians treating children with cleft palates should be prepared to make referrals to parent support groups or to counseling professionals who have expertise in the area of birth defects.

Hearing Impairment

Hearing impairment refers to a significant loss in auditory acuity. There are two major types of hearing impairments: conductive and sensorineural. A **conductive,** or peripheral, hearing loss refers to a disruption in the mechanical transmission of sounds from the external auditory canal to the *cochlea* or inner ear (Northern & Downs, 2002). Conductive losses do not exceed 60 dB HL (decibel hearing level) and generally are amenable to medical treatment. A common cause of conductive hearing loss in young children is otitis media, an inflammation in the middle ear. A **sensorineural** loss involves a deficit in the neural transmission of sound impulses through the cochlea hair cells or the auditory nerve. Losses of this type usually do not respond to medical treatment and are generally irreversible. A disruption that occurs simultaneously in both pathways is termed a *mixed* hearing loss.

The degree of loss can range in severity from mild to profound. The majority of children with hearing losses are typically labeled hard of hearing (loss of <80 dB HL) and can derive significant benefit from articulation therapy. Children who are profoundly hearing impaired or deaf (loss of >80 dB HL) experience great difficulty acquiring intelligible speech even with intervention. In general, greater degrees of hearing loss result in more severe disruptions of speech development. It is important to note, however, that a loss as mild as 10 to 15 dB HL may be handicapping in the classroom setting with an ambient noise level of 25 to 35 dB. Deficits in speech production may not be marked if the hearing loss is unilateral rather than bilateral. Table 3–6 outlines the effects of different degrees of hearing loss on children's speech production abilities.

TABLE 3–6
Effects of Hearing Loss on Articulation Development

Degree of Loss	Characteristics
Slight (16–25 dB HL)	No noticeable difficulty in relatively quiet listening environments
Mild (26–40 dB HL)	Occasional difficulty with voiceless consonants; vowels and voiced consonants generally intact
Moderate (41–70 dB HL)	Some difficulty with sounds characterized by low intensity, high frequency, or short duration (e.g., final consonant omission, distortion of fricatives and affricates)
Severe (71–90 dB HL)	Significant difficulty in consonant production, with additional confusion of voiced/voiceless consonants and omission of consonants in blends
Profound (91 dB HL)	Global speech production impairment with the addition of neutralization or greater (schwa), substitution, addition, and nasalization of vowels as well as the omission of initial consonants

SOURCE: Adapted from Oller and Kelly (1974). Hudgins and Numbers (1942), Nober (1967), and Clark (1981).

Speech intelligibility is also significantly affected by several other factors, including age of onset, configuration of hearing loss, age of identification, and degree of linguistic complexity (Martin & Clark, 1996; Radziewicz & Antonellis, 2008). With regard to amplification, important factors include the age at which appropriate amplification is fitted, the type and amount of habilitation, and the consistency of device use. Age of onset is a particularly critical factor. Children who are born with or sustain significant hearing losses prior to the critical language learning period (before age 3 years) will have more severe articulation deficits than children whose losses occurred later in life.

Following is a list of the most common types of speech errors exhibited by children with hearing impairment. The first four are characteristic of children whose hearing losses fall in the moderate range. Children who have profound hearing impairment or deafness will likely display all these behaviors.

- Omission of final consonants
- Substitution of voiced consonants for voiceless
- Substitution of stops for nasals, fricatives, and affricates
- Omission of consonants in blends
- Omission of initial consonants
- Substitution of schwa for other vowels (neutralization)
- Insertion of schwa into words or added to the ends of words
- Substitution of vowels for other vowels
- Nasalization of vowels

Educational Approaches. There are three basic approaches to instruction for children with hearing impairment: oral, manual, and total communication. **Oral** programs emphasize spoken language as the primary mode of communication through the use of strategies such as speech reading, amplification, auditory training, and explicit speech-language instruction. A commonly used oral approach is **auditory-verbal therapy.** Auditory-verbal therapy aims to improve the spoken language abilities of a child with hearing impairment to the level of a child with typical hearing by developing his or her listening skills independent of other cues such as speech reading and gestures (Brennan-Jones, White, Rush, & Law, 2014; Jackson & Schatschineider, 2014). **Manual** programs focus on the earliest possible acquisition of a linguistic system, generally via American Sign Language (ASL), finger spelling, and/or manually coded English systems. **Total communication** is a philosophy that encourages any combination of modalities (e.g., speech, writing, signing, gestures, and facial expressions) that is effective in facilitating an individual child's acquisition of language. Recently, a **bilingual/bicultural** model of education has been implemented for children with significant hearing loss. In this approach, children are exposed to ASL as their first language for communication and learn English in the school setting to develop reading and writing skills. Lively debate continues regarding the educational, social, and cultural impact of these different approaches. For comprehensive discussion on this topic, see Lederberg, Schick, and Spencer (2013); and Andrews, Leigh, and Weiner (2004).

The most recent advance in rehabilitation for children with deafness is the use of **cochlear implants (CIs).** The following discussion represents the most current data available at the time of this edition. Because state-of-the-art knowledge in this area is evolving rapidly, clinicians are encouraged to seek out additional, updated information.

Unlike a traditional hearing aid, a CI directly stimulates surviving auditory nerve fibers. One component of the device is a body-worn processor that highlights speech signals and minimizes background noise. These signals are routed first to a receiver implanted in the mastoid bone. Then the signals travel to an array of electrodes implanted in the cochlea, which transfers the sound to the auditory nerve (Niparko, 2009). The CI devices currently approved by the U.S. Food and Drug Administration (FDA) for implantation in children as young as 12 months of age provide multichannel stimulation and continue to evolve technologically. Children implanted at younger ages generally make greater and more rapid strides in vocal development and speech production than those implanted later in life (Ertmer & Goffman, 2011; Ertmer, Young, & Nathani, 2007).

A more recent development is the bilateral implantation of CIs. In a meta-analysis of 16 studies, Schafer, Amlani, Seibold, and Shattuck (2007) examined the relative effectiveness of bilateral and bimodal stimulation (i.e., two cochlear implants versus one cochlear implant and one hearing aid). They found no significant differences in listening performance between bilateral and bimodal stimulation. Based on this information, they recommended bimodal stimulation as the first-order treatment approach for children who can derive benefit from hearing aid use in the nonimplant ear. For additional information on bilateral cochlear implants, see Lammers, van der Heijden, Pourier, and Grolman (2014). Overall, the cochlear implant literature suggests that five important factors are associated with improved speech production skills: age at implantation, years of device use, nonverbal intelligence, oral communication as primary mode after the implant, and number/placement of active electrodes with a wide dynamic range (Chin, Tsai, & Gao, 2003; Geers, 2002; Kirk et al., 2002; Svirsky, Teoh, & Neuburger, 2004; and Tobey et al., 2003).

Example Profile

Following is a typical profile for pediatric hearing loss. This example has been designed to illustrate the selection of therapy targets as well as specific therapy activities and materials. The chosen activities are easily implemented in either individual or group therapy settings.

Sherry is 7 years old, with a congenital moderate-severe bilateral sensorineural hearing loss. She is fitted with binaural hearing aids, and demonstrates the following errors. These errors are illustrative of the misarticulations of children with this degree of hearing impairment.

1. Omission of final consonants

    -/s

    -/z

    -/t

    -/d

    -/k

    -/g

    -/t∫

2. Substitution of voiced for voiceless consonants

v/f

b/p

d/t

g/k

ð/θ

3. Substitutions of stops for nasals, fricatives, and affricates

d/n

g/ŋ

t/s

d/z

d/tʃ

t/ʃ

4. Substitution of schwa for other vowels*

ə/æ (hat)

ə/ɛ (bet)

ə/ʊ (boot)

*Errors of this type may not be found in all children with this degree of hearing loss.

Selection of therapy targets. The errors to be targeted are -/s, -/z, -/t, -/d, ə/æ, ə/ɛ, ə/ʊ, v/f, b/p, and ð/θ. Final consonant omissions and schwa substitutions were identified as priorities because these error types have a significant negative impact on perceived speech intelligibility. The four deletion errors listed (-/s, -/z, -/t, -/d) were chosen because, in the word final position, these sounds also function as plural and tense markers. The æ, ə/ɛ, and ə/ʊ were included because these three substitutions have highly contrastive lip configurations that facilitate differential production. The voiced/voiceless confusion is an appropriate initial target because two of the three critical characteristics of these phonemes (i.e., place and manner) are already present in the child's repertoire, thus increasing the likelihood of early success in therapy. The v/f, b/p, and ð/θ confusions were selected because they are highly visible, which eliminates the need for placement cues and allows training to focus solely on voicing. Production of /ʃ/ also was included as a therapy target because it is the initial sound of Sherry's name. This sound will be programmed at the sentence level, because Sherry demonstrates relatively consistent production at the level of isolated words.

Sample Activities

Final consonant production

1. Draw three "speech flowers" on large pieces of paper, each with a distinct rounded center and 10 petals (similar to daisies). From colored paper, cut 30 loose flower petals that are the same size as the drawn petals and place them in a pile on the table. Write a different consonant-vowel (CV) syllable on every petal and a different final consonant in the three flower centers. The combination of each CV syllable with the final consonant should constitute a real word (e.g., fa + t = *fat*; be + t = *bet*, and so on). Explain to the child that the activity will focus on the production of final sounds

in words. Provide a glue stick or other adhesive. Instruct the child to pick a petal from the pile and fit it in an empty petal on the drawing. The clinician then glides a finger from the top of the petal to the flower center as the child produces the syllable plus final sound and forms a real word. After five correct productions of the target word, the child may glue the petal to the flower. Repeat this sequence until all the CV petals have been attached. The completed flowers can be used for home practice. (This activity can also be used to facilitate language awareness by using rhyming stimuli.)

Contrastive lip configurations for vowel productions

2. Draw three faces on separate pieces of paper or poster board, each depicting distinctly different mouth configurations corresponding to the target vowels. The mouth posture representing /æ/ should be drawn with an exaggerated lowering of the mandible. The /ɛ/ should depict clear lip retraction (similar to a smile), and the /ʊɛ/ drawing should display a pursed, rounded lip position that is slightly opened. For each vowel sound, gather or prepare 10 picture cards representing common monosyllabic words, for a total of 30 cards (e.g., *cat, bag, pen, bed, boot, shoe,* and so on). Draw a gallows on the blackboard in preparation for a Hangman game. Place the three face cue cards on the table and put the shuffled card deck face down in front of the child. Explain the rules of Hangman and emphasize that the game will focus on correct vowel production. Begin the game by having the child turn over the top card of the deck and place it next to the corresponding face cue card. Instruct the child to produce the correct vowel in isolation, making sure to match mouth configuration to the corresponding face, and then name the card five times. Each incorrect production allows the clinician to fill in one part of the hangman drawing. The object of the game is to deplete the picture deck before the hangman is completed.

Voicing contrast

3. With masking tape on the floor, create an outline of a mountain range with at least six peaks. Provide a small toy train or other vehicle and tell the child that the train is going on a long journey up and down the mountain peaks. The clinician introduces a voiced/voiceless cognate pair (e.g., v/f) and instructs the child to produce the voiced sound while moving the train *up* the mountain and to produce the voiceless sound as the train is moved *down* the mountain. Instruct the child to monitor voice onset and offset by placing her free hand on her throat (tactile cue) throughout the journey. Repeat this activity with each target cognate pair.

Production of /ʃ/

4. Engage the child in a hand-clapping or jump-rope activity using the following chant. Explain that the chant emphasizes correct production of the /ʃ/ in lots of different words. Teach one verse at a time to control task difficulty level. Use pictures and/or written words as needed.

   Sheila the fish, fish, fish

   She had one wish, wish, wish

   To have a bowl, bowl, bowl

   Without a hole, hole, hole.

She called up Jo*sh*, Jo*sh*, Jo*sh*

Who said, Oh go*sh*, go*sh*, go*sh*

Do you have a ga*sh*, ga*sh*, ga*sh*

Or a red ra*sh*, ra*sh*, ra*sh*?

She said, Oh *s*ure, *s*ure, *s*ure

Quite an eyesore, sore, sore

My bowl was sma*sh*ed, sma*sh*ed, sma*sh*ed

When the table cra*sh*ed, cra*sh*ed, cra*sh*ed.

Jo*sh* said, Let's ru*sh*, ru*sh*, ru*sh*

Or the water will *gush, gush, gush*

Get the *mesh* net, net, net

So you stay wet, wet, wet.

*Sh*eila the *f*ish, *f*ish, *f*ish

Was plopped in a *dish, dish, dish*

And said, Oh *sheesh, sheesh, sheesh*

I thought I'd be qui*che*, qui*che*, qui*che*.

After a while, while, while

She began to smile, smile, smile

At first slug*gish, ish, ish*

She now goes swi*sh*, swi*sh*, swi*sh*.

Helpful Hints

1. Cued speech can be a helpful tool for teaching place, manner, and voicing in the initial stages of therapy for children with hearing losses greater than 85 dB HL. (For more information and specific techniques, see Cornett [1967] and the National Cued Speech Association Web site [http://www.cuedspeech.org].)

2. Try to incorporate alternative sensory modalities (i.e., visual, tactile, and so on) in the early stages of each therapy task. These cues can be faded out as soon as they are no longer required to elicit a target sound.

3. For school-age children whose hearing losses also result in language impairments, select stimulus words that are related to the classroom curriculum (e.g., spelling words, science vocabulary).

4. Always ensure that the child's amplification system is in working order during therapy sessions to maximize residual hearing capabilities. Good sources for tips regarding troubleshooting hearing aids are Hull (2009) and the Audiology Awareness Campaign Web site (http://www.audiologyawareness.com).

5. Auditory trainers are often used in the classroom environment to facilitate the child's ability to monitor his or her own speech production as well as that of the teacher. Auditory trainers are high-fidelity systems in which the speaker's voice is

fed into a microphone, amplified, and then directed to the child through a receiver. These devices make it possible for the child to receive speech input with minimum background noise (a high signal-to-noise ratio). One widely used system consists of a microphone/transmitter worn by the teacher, which broadcasts directly to an FM receiver worn by the child. Anderson and Goldstein (2004) and Martin (2013) provide an informative discussion regarding the relative benefits of various listening devices.

6. As counselors, clinicians may be asked to provide information regarding a child's academic aptitude and recommendations for appropriate educational placement.

7. Clinicians should anticipate that some children may demonstrate confusion or fear when experiencing sound input for the first time (via devices such as hearing aids and cochlear implants). Comfort with sound stimulation and auditory awareness develops gradually.

8. Given that the number of children with cochlear implants is steadily increasing, SLPs need to develop an ample repertoire of strategies for facilitating auditory perception and speech production skills. Practical clinical ideas can be found in Ertmer (2005).

Childhood Apraxia of Speech

Childhood apraxia of speech (CAS) is a speech-motor planning disorder characterized by a reduced ability to volitionally sequence movements of the articulators for speech in the absence of paralysis, incoordination, or weakness of the oral musculature (dysarthria). (See Appendix 3-B for normative data on diadochokinetic rates for children.) CAS is thought to result from neurologic dysfunction, although currently no definitive evidence of specific brain pathology exists. There is much controversy in the literature as to whether CAS constitutes a discrete clinical entity (e.g., American Speech-Language-Hearing Association, 2007a; Highman, Hennessey, & Leitão 2013; Lewis et al., 2004; McCauley & Strand, 2008; Shriberg, Aram, & Kwiatkowski, 1997a, 1997b, 1997c). Three characteristics have been identified as hallmark indicators of CAS: (1) Vowel errors or distortions may be present, (2) speech production errors are highly inconsistent, and (3) prosodic disturbances are evident, particularly in the appropriate use of stress patterns. This profile of characteristics is generally not observed in children with other articulatory or phonologic disorders.

Following is a list of additional speech production characteristics that have been associated in the literature with CAS:

- Repertoire of phonemes is extremely restricted.
- A reduced ability to imitate sounds modeled by others, especially at the multisyllabic level is present.
- Omission errors predominate; substitution, distortion, addition, prolongation, and metathetic errors (transposition of sounds) also occur.
- A higher percentage of errors in sounds requiring complex oral movements (e.g., fricatives, affricates, consonant clusters) is present.
- Struggling or groping movements of the oral musculature are present.
- The number of errors increases as the length and complexity of utterances increase.

■ The ability to sequence phonemes in words/phrases and diadochokinetic tasks is reduced.

■ More recently, it has been suggested that CAS symptoms include deficits in speech perception and often in literacy-related skills as well.

In general, these children demonstrate receptive language abilities that are significantly superior to their speech production skills and may exhibit an accompanying oral apraxia. Children with CAS can be highly unintelligible; at the most severe levels, these children may be categorized as nonverbal, meaning the near absence of oral expressive output. They frequently demonstrate awareness of and frustration with their reduced ability to communicate.

CAS is noted for its resistance to remediation. That is, CAS does not respond easily to traditional articulation techniques. In fact, there is little scientific support for the effectiveness of therapy approaches for CAS (Morgan & Vogel, 2008; Murray, McCabe, & Ballard, 2012, 2014).

The literature describes several therapy approaches for children who demonstrate CAS. **Integral stimulation** (Milisen, 1954a and b) utilizes a hierarchical cueing procedure that begins with a high level of support characterized by production of slowly spoken simple utterances simultaneously by both client and clinician accompanied by visual and tactile cues. The simultaneous production is gradually faded, and cues are provided until they are no longer needed. The client then produces delayed repetitions of increasingly complex stimulus items. **Dynamic temporal and tactile cueing (DTTC)** is a variation of the integral stimulation approach and is described by Strand, Stoeckel, and Baas (2006) and S. Brienza (personal communication). It retains the same hierarchical structure as just described, but also allows the SLP to use tactile prompts/cues to facilitate correct jaw and lip positions for the initial articulatory configuration. Proprioceptive processing is maximized by having the child maintain the postures for several seconds. Also, DTTC incorporates production of simple consonant-vowel-consonant (CVC) target words, which are slowed down by elongation of the vowel to provide more time to achieve correct phonetic placement. In addition, some approaches target prosodic variables (e.g., loudness, pitch) rather than phoneme production (Ballard, Robin, McCabe, & McDonald, 2010).

Another suggested set of guidelines for implementing therapy for children with CAS was presented by Strode and Chamberlain (2006). Their hierarchy of overlapping steps is based on the principles of motor learning and gradually increases the complexity of the speech task while continuing to utilize repetitive drill and significant cueing:

Level 1: Stabilize existing vowels and consonant sounds

Level 2: Sequence established vowels and consonants in CV and VC syllables

Level 3: Teach new vowel and consonant sounds

Level 4: Produce CVCV and VCVC syllable sequences (emphasis on using established CV and VC syllables from Level 2)

Level 5: Close established CV and VC syllables with an established consonant sound to produce CVC words

Level 6: Produce multisyllabic words from stabilized sounds, syllables, and CVC words

Level 7: Produce consonant clusters and blends in words

Level 8: Produce phrases and sentences (sequencing syllables to form phrases and sentences begins as early as Level 2)

Regardless of the specific approach used, a set of basic factors to be considered in developing treatment programming for this population includes the following:

- Progress in therapy is slow and marked by poor retention and poor generalization of therapy targets across treatment sessions.

- Although repeated practice is an integral component of therapy for all types of articulation disorders, it is important to provide intensive, systematic drill for children with CAS in order for them to master the necessary speech-motor patterns. The random (vs. massed) practice advantage observed in the nonspeech-motor learning literature may not extend to treatment for CAS (Maas & Farinella, 2012).

- Based on the first two factors, sessions that are shorter and more frequent may be helpful in facilitating generalization and avoiding speech-system fatigue (Edeal & Gildersleeve-Neumann, 2011).

- Children with CAS have great difficulty learning articulatory patterns through auditory input alone. For this reason, the use of visual and tactile cues is essential for establishing these sensory-motor patterns.

- Remediation should include an early emphasis on improving children's ability to monitor their own speech production, particularly through tactile and/or kinesthetic modalities (e.g., concentrate on how sounds "feel" and where the tongue is during movement sequences).

- Intervention should incorporate a focus on the melody and rhythm patterns of connected speech.

- For children with extremely unintelligible speech, it may be necessary to use assistive technology (e.g., augmentative/alternative system) to provide the child with a functional means of communication. This option may be temporary in nature or serve as the child's long-term communication mode.

There is relatively little support in the literature for most therapy approaches to CAS. A few meta-analyses/systematic reviews have been conducted and have not reported definitively strong conclusions regarding treatment efficacy for specific approaches in the areas of CAS.

Example Profile

Following is a typical profile of a child with CAS. This example has been designed to illustrate the selection of intervention targets as well as specific therapy activities and materials. The chosen activities are easily implemented in either individual or group therapy settings.

Billy is almost 3 years old and presents with unintelligible speech. His phoneme repertoire is limited to four consonant sounds /b, m, t, d/, which he substitutes for several other sounds. He sometimes produces the same CV syllables for many different words (e.g., /-ba/ for *ball, table, telephone, door,* and *paper*). In addition, Billy demonstrates a significant number of omission errors (sounds and syllables), which occur in all word positions (e.g., /tə/ for *truck*, /ət/ for *dog*, /oh/ for *open*). Billy also demonstrates occasional vowel errors characterized by the substitution of schwa for other vowels, especially diphthongs.

Selection of therapy targets. The primary areas to be targeted are self-monitoring of speech production, restricted phoneme repertoire, and limited speech-sound-sequencing abilities. The self-awareness skills selected for remediation include tongue-tip elevation, tongue lateralization, tongue protrusion/retraction, lip pursing, and lip retraction, because these movements are highly visible. (Children who demonstrate an accompanying oral apraxia may find these tasks very frustrating.) The phonemes /p/ and /f/ were chosen as targets to be added to Billy's consonant repertoire for several reasons. These sounds appear early developmentally, are highly visible, and are sufficiently different from one another to avoid confusion during training. In addition, these consonants are voiceless and therefore require the mastery of one less feature for correct production than do voiced sounds. The complexity level selected for work on sequencing skills was reduplicative CV and VC syllables in which the consonant and vowel remain constant across syllables. The phonemes identified for use in the sequencing tasks were /b, m, t, d/ because these sounds are already present in Billy's consonant repertoire at the single-syllable level.

Sample Activities

Self-monitoring

1. Gather two sets of 5 to 10 items of varying texture, size, shape, and temperature (e.g., ice, tongue depressor, straw, warm liquid, rubber toy). Encourage the child to use each of the objects in a set to engage in oral-exploratory play. Imitate each of the child's play behaviors using the objects in the second set. Establish the child's conscious awareness of oral-motor sensations by commenting on what the child is doing and how it makes the mouth feel. Promote expansion of the number and variety of oral-motor play movements demonstrated by the child. This task is most effective when used as a warm-up activity at the beginning of a therapy session to heighten self-awareness as a building block for monitoring of the child's own speech production.

Visual cueing and massed practice

2. Sit next to the child in front of a large mirror. Tell the child that he is going to play a "clown" game and show him a clown hat and wig made from colored paper and yarn. Instruct the child that this game involves taking turns making funny faces in the mirror. The clinician takes the first turn by putting on the clown hat and modeling a target tongue or lip movement. Have the child imitate the target movement a minimum of five times to earn a chance to be the clown. (In the early stages of therapy, it may be necessary to reinforce any voluntary oral-motor movement that occurs in response to the clinician's stimulus.) Explain that it is now the child's turn to wear the hat and make a funny face for the clinician to imitate. Repeat this sequence with other oral-motor movements that are absent from the child's repertoire. This activity also works well as a warm-up procedure at the beginning of a session (5 to 10 minutes) and may be repeated at intervals throughout the session to reinforce targeted motor patterns. (Refer to the "Oral-Motor Considerations" section at the beginning of this chapter for additional information.)

Intensive short drill

3. Gather four large sacks (pillowcases, trash bags, grocery bags, and so on), fill each one with at least five objects whose names begin with a target sound (avoid blends), and attach the sacks to the wall. For example, objects for the target sound /p/ might include pencil, puzzle, paint, puppet, and pot. Give the child a beanbag and tell him to throw it at one of the sacks. The clinician removes the sack that was hit from the wall and tells the child to close his eyes and pick one object at a time from the sack. The clinician holds the object next to his or her mouth and models the target phoneme in isolation for the child to imitate five successive times. When the sack is empty, take a short break. Then, give the child the beanbag and start the game again.

Intonational contour

4. Cut an egg carton in half lengthwise, turn it upside down, and color or paint each of the six protruding sections a different color. Hide the last three sections from the child's view by covering them with a piece of aluminum foil or other material. Obtain a large plastic dinosaur or other animal with a large mouth opening and collect at least 25 marbles. Explain to the child he is going to play a game in which he has to sing silly sounds in exactly the same way as the clinician to earn a chance to feed marbles to the very hungry dinosaur. The clinician then "sings" a string of three reduplicative CV syllables that are constructed from the identified consonant targets /b, m, t, d/. The clinician produces these strings with a distinctive intonational contour pattern, while simultaneously tapping the egg carton protrusions to pace each CV syllable as it is "sung." Intonational contour patterns might include rising/falling intonation, primary stress on a particular syllable, and increased/decreased loudness on initial/medial/final syllables. Instruct the child to imitate the clinician's syllable sequence using the same intonational pattern and pacing cues as the clinician. Following the successful imitation of at least three different sequences, the child is allowed to feed a marble to the dinosaur. Continue this activity using varied combinations of phonemes and intonation patterns until the dinosaur has eaten all the marbles. The level of difficulty can be modified by increasing the number of syllables in the reduplicative CV/VC strings or by introducing nonreduplicative syllable strings.

Note: This activity represents a simplified adaptation of Melodic Intonation Therapy (Sparks, Helm, & Albert, 1974), in which rhythm and intonation patterns are used to facilitate speech output.

Helpful Hints

1. Oral-motor movements can be used to facilitate articulatory placement for the acquisition of new consonants. For example, after work on tongue-tip elevation, you can add voice to it to produce /l/.

2. Capitalize on an acceptable speech-motor pattern at the moment of its production, when the experience is most recent and vivid in the child's mind. Have the child repeat the utterance immediately for multiple trials to reduce the probability that the articulatory gesture will fade.

3. Early therapy should focus on a child's ability to produce *accurate* responses. As the child improves, the focus can be shifted to *speed* of response by requiring rapid automatic production of the accurate articulatory movements.

4. Rhymes and songs can be used as stimulus materials to facilitate oral-motor sequencing abilities for children who can produce sentence-length utterances.

5. For children at the single-word level, it may be helpful to introduce words that contain reduplicative syllables (e.g., *mama, bye-bye, night-night, dada*). Such utterances highlight the rhythm of speech and can provide a transition to other bisyllabic words (e.g., *cookie, allgone, open*).

6. Given that children with CAS may demonstrate intact language comprehension skills and normal intelligence, there are two commonly occurring counseling issues: (a) the child may be significantly frustrated by the inability to intelligibly convey his or her ideas and thoughts, and (b) parents may inaccurately perceive the inconsistent nature of their child's poor speech production as an indicator of laziness or lack of motivation.

7. Clinicians should make every effort to ensure that therapy remains a positive experience for the child, because intervention with this disorder consists largely of repetitive drill.

8. Incorporating an emphasis on variations in prosody at all stages of therapy can contribute to improved overall intelligibility of speech in children with CAS.

9. Clinicians interested in facilitating parent/family understanding of this disorder are encouraged to consult the series of "Letters to the parent of . . ." by Hall (2000a, 2000b, 2000c, 2000d), which explains the nature, causes, and treatment of CAS in clear, simple language.

CONCLUSION

This chapter has presented basic information, protocols, and procedures for intervention for articulation and phonology at an *introductory* level. This information is intended only as a starting point in the reader's clinical education and training. For in-depth coverage of this area, the following readings are recommended:

Articulation and Phonology

Bernthal, J. E., & Bankson, N. W. (2013). *Articulation and phonological disorders* (7th ed.). Boston, MA: Pearson.

Bleile, K. (2014). *The late eight.* San Diego, CA: Plural Publishing.

Peterson-Falzone, S., Trost-Cardamone, J., Karnell, M., & Hardin-Jones, M. (2006). *The clinician's guide to treating cleft palate speech.* St. Louis, MO: Mosby Elsevier.

Rvachew, S., & Brosseau-Lapre, F. (2012). *Developmental phonological disorders: Foundations of clinical practice.* San Diego, CA: Plural Publishing.

Secord, W. (2006). *Eliciting sounds: Techniques and strategies for clinicians.* Independence, KY: Cengage Learning.

Strode, R., & Chamberlain, C. (2006). *The source for childhood apraxia of speech.* East Moline, IL: LinguiSystems.

Oral-Motor Dysfunction

Alexander, R., Boehme, R., & Cupps, B. (1998). *Normal development of functional motor skills: The first year of life.* Tucson, AZ: Therapy Skill Builders.

Bahr, D. C. (2001). *Oral motor assessment and treatment: Ages and stages.* Boston, MA: Allyn & Bacon.

Marshalla, P. (2004). *Oral motor techniques in articulation and phonological therapy.* Everett, WA: Marshalla Speech and Language, Inc.

Morris, S. E., & Klein, M. D. (2000). *Pre-feeding skills: A comprehensive resource for feeding development.* Tucson, AZ: San Antonio, TX: Psychological Corp.

ADDITIONAL RESOURCES

Articulation

Super Duper Publications
P.O. Box 24997
Greenville, SC 29616
Phone: 800-277-8737
Fax: 800-978-7379
Web site: http://www.superduperinc.com

Webber Articulation Cards (Sets I, II, and III)
Decks of cards with colored pictures designed to elicit 15 target phonemes in all word positions; duplicate cards are included to make the decks suitable for many children's card games.

Artic Pix CD-ROM and Resource Guide
This guide allows you to create board games and flash cards for 18 different sounds. Also includes instructions for 50 additional easy-to-make games using the Artic Pix CD-ROM.

Funny Flips: /ch, k, l, r, s, sh, g/
The books contain over 46,000 sentence combinations in the initial, medial, and final positions, plus blends. Color-coded tabs make it easy to practice just one sound position, or the whole book can be used to practice sounds in any position.

Month-by-Month Artic Carry-Over Fun
Open-ended pages that can be customized for any sound. Each month contains two types of activity pages: four-part pages with separate topics that can be completed in different ways and full-page sheets with word scenes, fill-in blanks, etc. Parent letter included.

Artic Chipper Chat
Sixty different game boards, each filled with sound-loaded pictures. Students pick a question card and search their boards for the correct picture answer. As they answer questions, they fill up their boards with magnetic chips. The game focuses on 12 different sounds, targeting the initial, medial, and final position and/or combinations.

Pro-Ed
8700 Shoal Creek Boulevard
Austin, TX 78757-6897
Phone: 800-897-3202
Fax: 800-397-7633
Web site: http://www.proedinc.com

The Big Book of Sounds, Fifth Edition
A 246-page book of drill-based activities with sections for initial, medial, and final position. Includes syllable drills, syllable rhymes, word lists, word rhymes, short sentences, and word list enhancements for each sound.

The Speech Bin
P.O. Box 922668
Norcross, GA 30010-2668
Phone: 800-850-8602
Fax: 800-845-1535
Web site: http://www.speechbin.com

Photo Articulation Library
1,085 real-life photos arranged by sounds and word positions, 350 cards in each set, suitable for all ages. Twenty-seven categories include events, communication, actions, games and toys, occupations, transportation, and more, organized by consonants, vowels, and word position.

Apraxia Uncovered Book
The *Apraxia Uncovered Book* shows how to develop consonants and vowels by facilitating 39 specific respiratory, articulation, phonology, and oral-motor methodologies. It presents a systematic plan of phoneme development for children who have apraxia and other severe expressive speech disorders.

LinguiSystems
3100 Fourth Avenue
East Moline, IL 61244
Phone: 800-776-4332
Fax: 800-577-4555
Web site: http://www.linguisystems.com

Click and Create Articulation Board Games Software
Create customized articulation therapy materials with this tool. This easy-to-use program contains thousands of words and pictures that represent all articulation sounds.

HELP for Articulation
This resource gives you a variety of target sounds and activities that use the HELP format to improve articulation skills. It includes Individualized Education Plan (IEP) goals for each lesson and offers suggestions for the use of stimulus materials at each level.

No-Glamour Articulation Cards

This picture card set provides 400 pictures for articulation practice. They can be used for flash-card drills or to expand language and transition articulation skills to conversation with the question directions printed on the back of each card.

Sally's Circus: An Articulation Game

For ages 4–9. The stimulus items provide articulation practice in a variety of speaking contexts. Students practice using their target sounds in three levels of production: short phrases, sentence completion tasks, and silly rhymes or tongue twisters. Contains 300 game cards to target these sounds in all positions: *k, g, l, s, z, r, ch, sh, j,* and voiced and voiceless *th.*

50 Quick-Play Articulation Games

More than 50 creative, fun, interactive games on reproducible sheets for ages 5–10. Games target these sounds in all positions: *p, b, m, k, g, t, d, f, v, sh, ch, j, s, z, r, l, l* blends, *r* blends, *s* blends, and voiced and voiceless *th.* There are 50 path games, 15 card games, 11 noncompetitive games, plus a *Make Your Own Game* path and a *Target the Stars* motivational sheet.

Artic Shuffle

Fifty-two different pictures per deck to give students tons of articulation practice by playing Go Fish, Crazy Eights, or a memory-type board game. Students match suits, numbers, and face cards so there is no need for picture pairs. Ten card decks cover 12 sounds plus sounds in blends.

Just for Kids: Apraxia

This systematic approach uses the alphabet as the basis for organizing apraxia therapy sessions and goes through five phases to help children develop intelligible speech.

The Source for Childhood Apraxia of Speech

This resource provides tips for clients who are resistive to therapy, have developmental delays or autism, or are very young. It contains comprehensive information on the neurologically based disorder, as well as goals and techniques to facilitate both speech and language skills simultaneously.

Easy Does It for Apraxia and Motor Planning

This program includes techniques from traditional articulation therapy and phonology therapy and emphasizes developing sound sequencing skills and closed syllables in tasks of increasing complexity.

Phonology

Pro-Ed
8700 Shoal Creek Boulevard
Austin, TX 78757-6897
Phone: 800-897-3202
Fax: 800-397-7633
Web site: http://www.proedinc.com

Minimal Pair Cards

Four decks of illustrated 3-by-5-inch cards remediate five common phonological processes—stopping, fronting, gliding, cluster reduction, and final consonant deletion—and develop vocabulary, language, and game-playing skills in children grades K–3. There is the option to purchase the whole set or individual decks.

LinguiSystems
3100 Fourth Avenue
East Moline, IL 61244
Phone: 800-776-4332
Fax: 800-577-4555
Web site: http://www.linguisystems.com

Just for Kids: Phonological Processing

A set of 22 lessons that target six phonological processes: velar fronting, final consonant deletion, syllable reduction, cluster reduction, liquid gliding, and stridency deletion. Each lesson includes reproducible materials, such as target word lists and picture cards.

Cengage Learning
5 Maxwell Drive
Clifton Park, NY 12065
Phone: 800-998-7498
Fax: 800-487-8488
Web site: http://www.cengage.com

Sourcebook of Phonological Awareness Activities

This book includes training materials to be used in conjunction with popular books such as *The Hungry Caterpillar*. It also introduces the concept of phonological awareness and its relationship to reading skills.

Super Duper Publications
P.O. Box 24997
Greenville, SC 29616
Phone: 800-277-8737
Fax: 800-978-7379
Web site: http://www.superduperinc.com

Giant Book of Phonology

This book contains reproducible pictures to practice phonological processes with target words, phrases, and sentences.

Have You Ever . . . ?

A collection of interactive books that allow clients to place the pictures onto the pages as they practice reducing the occurrence of phonological processes at the word, phrase, sentence, and conversational levels.

Oral-Motor Dysfunction

LinguiSystems
3100 Fourth Avenue
East Moline, IL 61244
Phone: 800-776-4332
Fax: 800-577-4555
Web site: http://www.linguisystems.com

Oral-Motor Activities for Young Children

Uses simple snack foods to achieve oral-motor function and stimulate accurate speech production.

Easy Does It for Articulation

Includes specific techniques to develop better oral-motor control, precision, strength, and coordination for accurate speech sound placement.

The Speech Bin
P.O. Box 922668
Norcross, GA 30010-2668
Phone: 800-850-8602
Fax: 800-845-1535
Web site: http://www.speechbin.com

Whistle Kit & Blow Toy Kit

The Whistle Kit is a nine-piece collection of motivating whistles featuring moving parts. The Blow Toy Kit gives you colorful toys to encourage prolonged blowing without sound with ocular tracking.

Miscellaneous

Smit, A. B. (2004). *Articulation and phonology resource guide for school-age children and adults.* Clifton Park, NY: Cengage Learning.

APPENDIX 3-A

PHONETIC PLACEMENT INSTRUCTIONS
FOR DIFFICULT-TO-TEACH SOUNDS

/ ɚ /

1. Open your mouth and put your tongue up like this (model tongue tip in center of mouth almost touching hard palate, using mirror). Close your mouth until teeth are almost clenched and say /ɚ/.

2. Open your mouth and get ready to say /k/ (or /g/). Put your tongue tip up and say /ɚ/.

3. Say /θ/ while raising your tongue tip to produce /ɚ/.

4. Raise the tip of your tongue toward the roof of your mouth just as you do for /l/. While making the /l/ sound, curl your tongue tip back toward your throat to make the /ɚ/ sound.

5. Stick out your tongue. Touch edges of client's tongue with tongue depressor to show him where the tongue should be touching the teeth. Bring your tongue back into your mouth, touching its edges to the teeth. Raise the tongue tip slightly and say /ɚ/.

6. Pretend you are a puppet. I am going to pull an imaginary string attached to the back of your head. You should raise the back of your tongue slightly and say /ɚ/ as I pull the string.

7. Spread the sides of the child's mouth with your fingers. Make a really long /n/ sound, while curling the tip of your tongue toward your throat to produce /ɚ/.

8. Make a long /i/ sound with your lips really tight, like a big smile. While continuing to make the sound, relax your lips and move your tongue back gradually to produce /ɚ/.

/ s, z /

1. Make a long /ð/ sound and slowly draw the tip of your tongue back behind your teeth to produce /s/.

2. Position your tongue for the /t/ sound. Hold the /t/ sound and drop your tongue tip slightly to produce /s/.

3. Move a tongue depressor or straw down the midline of the child's tongue to indicate the appropriate pathway of the airflow. Hold the sides of your tongue against the edges of your upper side teeth. Point your tongue tip toward the exact center of your upper front teeth and blow the airstream straight out the middle of your tongue to make the /s/.

(continues)

4. Draw a picture of the two upper and two lower central incisors in contact with one another. Make a circle on the picture to show the small center opening where the four teeth meet to indicate the correct direction of the airstream. Make your top and bottom teeth touch the same way as in the picture. Use your tongue to seal off all the way around your mouth except the very small center opening between your middle front teeth, like the circle in the picture. Let the /s/ sound come out only from that small opening in a very fine stream, just as if you poked a tiny little hole in a water hose.

5. Make a little smile with your teeth nearly closed. Hide your tongue behind your teeth. You can keep the tip of your tongue up or down. Rest the sides of your tongue against the inside of your top teeth. Let the airstream come out the front to make the /s/ sound.

/θ, ð/

1. Put your tongue between your top and bottom teeth so that it peeks out a little bit. Rest the sides of your tongue against the sides of your top teeth. Blow air out the front of your mouth to make the /θ, ð / sound.

2. Make a long /s/ sound and slowly stick out your tongue tip slightly to make the /θ, ð / sound.

3. Use a mirror to contrast the articulatory placements for /θ, ð/ with the child's sound substitution. For example, show the child that the /θ, ð / are made with the tongue placed slightly between the front teeth, while /f/ requires the upper teeth to touch the lower lip.

/ʃ, ʒ/

1. Hold your index finger straight up and touch it to your lips as if to make a hushing sound and say /ʃ, ʒ/.

2. Make a long /s/ sound and gradually round your lips, letting a little extra air rush out the front of your mouth.

3. Elevate tongue tip toward hard palate and allow the lateral edge of the tongue to touch the side teeth and blow air out centrally.

/tʃ, dʒ/

1. Produce /t/ and then /ʃ/. Repeat these two sounds more and more rapidly until they blend into one /tʃ/ sound.

2. Make the sound of a train coming down the tracks by saying "choo-choo." This takes advantage of children's tendency to produce nonspeech sounds without the errors evidenced in their real word productions.

3. Make a long /n/ sound and add /sh/. Repeat this combination stronger, louder, and faster until it blends into /tʃ/.

(continues)

/l/

1. Put the tip of your tongue on the bumpy part behind your upper front teeth and drop it while saying /a/.

2. For w/l substitutions, contrasting the lip postures using a mirror is particularly helpful. For /w/, explain and show the child that the lips are visibly rounded and protruded, whereas /l/ is made with the lips separated at the corners and somewhat lax.

3. Close your mouth, put your tongue behind your top teeth, and open your mouth while keeping your tongue up. Now let your tongue down as you say /la/.

/k, g/

1. Put the back of your tongue up against the roof of your mouth and hold your breath for a second. Drop your tongue quickly and release your breath with a coughing sound to produce /k/.

2. Pretend you are a puppet with an imaginary string attached to the back of your head. As I pull the string, raise the back of your tongue against the roof of your mouth. Drop your tongue quickly to allow a sudden escape of air to say /k/ as I let go of the string.

3. Use a tongue depressor to hold down the tongue tip while at the same time pushing the tongue backward and upward until it comes into contact with the soft palate. When I remove the tongue depressor, quickly lower the back of your tongue to say /k/.

Note: All of these instructions can be adapted for the voiced cognates by directing the child to "turn your voice on" or "make your throat buzz." In addition, a mirror can be used to highlight sounds whose articulatory placements are visible (e.g., /θ/, /p/, /l/).

APPENDIX 3-B

DIADOCHOKINETIC RATES FOR CHILDREN

Age/Years	pʌ*	tʌ	kʌ	pʌtəkə**
6	4.0–5.6	3.9–5.9	4.6–6.4	7.2–13.4
7	3.8–5.8	4.0–5.8	4.3–6.3	7.4–12.6
8	3.5–4.9	3.7–5.1	4.1–5.5	6.2–10.4
9	3.4–4.6	3.5–4.7	3.9–5.3	5.8–9.6
10	3.3–4.1	3.4–4.2	3.8–4.8	5.6–8.6
11	3.0–4.2	2.9–4.3	3.4–4.6	5.1–7.9
12	3.0–3.8	3.0–4.0	3.3–4.5	4.8–8.0
13	2.7–3.9	2.8–3.8	3.1–4.3	4.3–7.1

*Scores represent time range (in seconds) required for 20 repetitions of single syllables (i.e., pʌ, tʌ, kʌ).
**Scores represent time range (in seconds) required for 10 repetitions of trisyllables (i.e., pʌtəkə).

SOURCE: Adapted from Fletcher (1972); Kent, Kent & Rosenbek (1987).

INTRODUCTION TO CHAPTERS 4 AND 5

Chapters 4 and 5 focus on the treatment of childhood language disorders. Childhood language disorders affect a diverse group of children who present with differing profiles of language impairment. Intervention with this population is the subject of an enormous amount of literature that covers the age span from infancy through adolescence. To organize this body of information in a manner that is clinically useful for the reader, this section of the book begins with overview material that is germane to the entire range of child language disorders. Chapter 4 then presents specific intervention information for children from birth through the preschool years. Intervention information for school-age children and adolescents is the subject of Chapter 5.

The information in these chapters is provided as general guidelines regarding language acquisition and treatment. The relative applicability of this material will depend on a host of factors, including the sociocultural background of any particular client and family.

A **language disorder** can be defined as the abnormal acquisition, comprehension, or use of spoken or written language. This includes all receptive and expressive language skills. The disorder may involve any aspect of the form, content, or use components of the linguistic system. Children with language disorders are a heterogeneous population in several respects, including the following:

- *Primary versus secondary disorder:* For some children, the reduced ability to acquire language is their primary deficit in the relative absence of impairment in other developmental areas. For other children, the language deficit occurs in association with other impairments (e.g., intellectual disabilities).

- *Developmental versus acquired:* Developmental language disorders are present from birth or occur prior to the onset of typical language acquisition. Acquired disorders involve the loss or interruption of language function due to illness or trauma.

- *Delayed versus aberrant/unusual acquisition:* Children with delayed language proceed through the same sequence of acquisition as typically developing children but at a substantially slower rate. In contrast, children with aberrant language development demonstrate acquisition patterns that are deviant and differ significantly from the normal developmental sequence.

- *Range of severity:* The severity of language deficits can range along a continuum of mild to profound impairment.

CLASSIFICATION OF LANGUAGE DISORDERS

A disorder can involve both the comprehension and production of language. Language **comprehension** (receptive language) refers to the ability to derive meaning from incoming auditory or visual messages. Language **production** (expressive language) involves the combination of linguistic symbols to form meaningful messages. Language disorders are generally classified according to the major components of the linguistic system: semantics, morphology, syntax, pragmatics, and phonology.

Semantics involves the meaning of individual words and the rules that govern the combinations of word meanings to form meaningful phrases and sentences. Impairments in this subsystem can take the form of reduced vocabulary and depth of word knowledge, restricted semantic categories, word-retrieval deficits, poor word-association skills, limited word-definition skills, and difficulty with figurative (nonliteral) language forms such as idioms, metaphors, and humor.

Morphology involves the structure of words and the construction of individual word forms from the basic elements of meaning (i.e., morphemes). Deficits in this component are manifested as difficulties with inflectional markers such as plurals, past tense, auxiliary verbs, possessives, and so on.

Syntax involves the rules governing the order and combination of words in the construction of well-formed sentences. Syntactic deficits are characterized by problems with simple and complex sentence types such as negatives, interrogatives, passives, and relative clauses, as well as occasional word-order difficulties.

Pragmatics involves the rules governing the use of language in a social context. Pragmatic impairments can include a reduced repertoire of communicative intentions, poor shared/joint attention, reciprocal turn-taking difficulties in conversation, an inability to repair messages that are not understood by the listener, and difficulty with narrative discourse such as storytelling and personal narratives.

Phonology involves the particular sounds (i.e., phonemes) that make up the sound system of a language and the rules that govern permissible sound combinations. (For a discussion of phonological impairments, see Chapter 3.)

Language disorders can affect the development of basic language skills and/or higher-order *meta*linguistic knowledge in any of the previously mentioned components. In addition to language deficits, children may demonstrate certain associated behavioral characteristics, the most common of which are defined in Table 1.

TABLE 1
Behavioral Characteristics Associated with Language Disorders

Behavior	Definition
Inattention	Impairment of concentration characterized by difficulty with completing tasks, attending to details, following through on instructions, and tuning out distracting stimuli
Impulsivity	The abrupt performance of actions without sufficient deliberation or consideration of the consequences
Hyperactivity	An excessively high level of activity accompanied by a reduced ability to inhibit the activity volitionally
Attention deficit disorder (ADD)	Disorder characterized by one or more of the above features: inattention, impulsivity, or hyperactivity
Perseveration	Inappropriate and often involuntary continuation of a motor or verbal response when it is no longer relevant
Echolalia	Excessive and developmentally inappropriate repetition of the speech of others, generally with the same intonation; may be immediate or delayed; may be communicative or noncommunicative

RELATIONSHIP BETWEEN ORAL LANGUAGE AND LITERACY

It is now recognized that speech-language pathologists (SLPs) play a significant role in the acquisition of literacy. Literacy involves the development of reading and writing skills. From a basic perspective, reading consists of two component processes: word recognition and comprehension. Word recognition includes decoding and reading fluency. Decoding is the ability to assign sound–letter correspondences to printed symbols (the alphabetic principle), whereas reading fluency refers to the speed, accuracy, and automaticity of reading words and connected text. Comprehension involves the ability to derive meaning from printed text at the word, phrase, sentence, or text level. Writing involves the acquisition of spelling and the ability to compose text at the sentence level and beyond. Spelling is the ability to construct words using the conventional orthography (i.e., written symbols) of a given language, and composition is the formulation of coherent units of connected language, including narrative and expository texts.

Oral language serves as the basis for the development of reading and writing skills, beginning with the period known as *emergent literacy*, which extends from birth through the preschool years. **Emergent literacy** is a child's increasing awareness of the world of print and an understanding of the functions of literacy. During the preschool period, children develop foundational knowledge about print through everyday, naturally occurring experiences in their home and preschool/daycare environments. These experiences prepare them for the formal literacy instruction (learning to read and write) that begins in the early elementary school grades. For this reason, emergent literacy skills are considered the developmental precursors to children's achievement of skilled reading and writing.

Of the oral language skills studied thus far, metalinguistic awareness is the area that has been most closely linked to literacy acquisition. **Metalinguistic awareness** is the explicit knowledge of and ability to manipulate aspects of the linguistic system independently of the meaning conveyed by the message. Phonological awareness is a metalinguistic skill that involves manipulation of the sound structure of language through tasks such as rhyming, blending, and segmenting of words, syllables, or phonemes. In particular, a child's control of sounds at the phoneme level (*phonemic awareness*) is highly predictive of decoding and spelling skills. A common example of a phonemic awareness task is asking a child to say a word such as *fat* and then to say it again without the /f/. In turn, acquisition of decoding skill leads to subsequent improvement of phonemic awareness ability. (Note: *Phonics* is the written language counterpart to this ability and focuses on sound–letter correspondences.)

Children and adolescents with language and learning impairments demonstrate considerable difficulty with phonemic awareness tasks. There is evidence that these children can benefit from direct phonological awareness instruction (Malani, Barina, Kludjian, & Perkowski, 2011; Torgesen, Wagner, & Rashotte, 1994).

Intervention in this skill area is most effective when delivered in conjunction with training on the alphabetic principle and results in measurable gains in reading and spelling (Torgesen & Davis, 1996). See Table 2 for scope and sequence information on phonological awareness instruction, organized in a progression from least to most difficult.

Other aspects of oral language that are associated with literacy development are vocabulary knowledge, word retrieval, and morphological awareness. Vocabulary size during the toddler years appears to be related to a child's ability to accurately decode single words in the first and second grades (Scarborough, 1998; Scarborough & Dobrich, 1990).

TABLE 2
Scope and Sequence for Phonological Awareness Intervention

Phonological awareness skills

1. Rhyming/alliteration

2. Blending

3. Segmenting

    a. Categorization (e.g., Which one begins with a different sound: *feet, five, soup, fat?*)

    b. Deletion (e.g., Say *trip* without the /t/.)

    c. Substitution (e.g., Replace the /m/ in *man* with /f/.)

    d. Manipulation (e.g., Say the word *stop*. Now move the /s/ to the end of the word and say it again.)

Task mode

1. Matching (e.g., Show me the one that rhymes with *hat*.)

2. Elimination (e.g., Show me the one that doesn't rhyme with the other two words.)

3. Judgment (e.g., Do *hat* and *bat* rhyme?)

4. Production (e.g., Tell me a word that rhymes with *hat*.)

Stimuli level for segmenting/blending

1. Sentences into words

2. Words into syllables (Compound words such as *blackboard* are easier than noncompound words such as *finger*, because each syllable is a common word.)

3. Syllables into phonemes such as "c-a-t" (Polysyllabic words and/or consonant clusters increase task difficulty.)

Phoneme class for segmenting/blending

Continuant sounds such as fricatives and nasals are easier than noncontinuant sounds such as stops. (Continuants are longer in duration and acoustically more discrete; they can be produced in isolation and emphasized by overarticulation.)

SOURCE: Adams, Foorman, Lundberg, and Beeler (1998); Blachman, Ball, Black, and Tangel (2000); Roth, Troia, Worthington, and Dow (2002); Roth, Troia, Worthington, and Handy (2006); Swank and Catts (1994); Troia, Roth, and Graham (1998); van Kleeck and Schuele (1987).

Once a child reaches the middle elementary school years, the focus of reading shifts away from decoding or word recognition, and vocabulary size becomes predictive of reading comprehension skill (Stanovich, 1986; Baker, Simmons, & Kameenui, 1998). With regard to word retrieval, naming accuracy is predictive of current and future decoding skill, whereas naming speed has been found to be strongly related to reading comprehension (Scarborough, 1998; Wolf, 1984, 1991). Morphological awareness is linked to both word reading and reading comprehension, as it reflects a child's familiarity with the meanings of words and their parts (e.g., prefixes, suffixes) as well as the ability to apply this knowledge to decipher the meaning of written words and text (Carlisle & Goodwin, 2014). Importantly, deficits in vocabulary and word retrieval are among the most common characteristics of language impairment throughout childhood and adolescence.

Role of the Speech-Language Pathologist in Literacy

The traditional scope of practice for SLPs has evolved over the past several years to incorporate more emphasis on literacy-related issues. Accordingly, in 2000, the American Speech-Language-Hearing Association (ASHA) developed a position statement, guidelines, and several other documents to address the roles and responsibilities of SLPs in serving children and adolescents with reading and writing difficulties. These documents clearly indicate that "SLPs play a critical and direct role in the development of literacy for children and adolescents with communication disorders . . . " (p. 1) and are based on the following premises:

- Oral language is the basis for the acquisition of reading and writing.
- There is a reciprocal relationship between oral and written language in that each builds on the other.
- Children and adolescents with oral language deficits often have difficulty acquiring the ability to read and write (and vice versa).
- Reading and writing deficits can involve any of the subsystems of language: phonology, morpho-syntax, semantics, and pragmatics.
- SLPs have knowledge of typical and atypical patterns of language development, as well as experience in assessment and intervention for children and adolescents.
- Literacy development requires an interdisciplinary approach in which SLPs participate collaboratively with other professionals, families, and students.

The ASHA guidelines also identify the various roles and responsibilities that SLPs may undertake to foster literacy development. These include, but are not limited to:

- *Prevention:* Promote opportunities to participate in oral and written language experiences that facilitate literacy (e.g., shared book reading, alphabet/letter exposure, adult modeling of reading and writing).
- *Identification:* Provide screening/early detection of children with or at risk for reading and writing problems as a result of oral language difficulties.
- *Assessment:* Evaluate reading and writing abilities in relation to oral language skills, using a comprehensive battery of norm-referenced and descriptive measures.
- *Intervention:* Implement evidence-based instruction for reading and writing problems, which emphasizes the reciprocal relationships between oral language and literacy and utilizes curricular subject matter.
- *Other roles:* Collaborate/advocate for effective language-based literacy practices in general and special education settings, promote family involvement in literacy activities, and advance the knowledge base regarding the relationship between oral language and literacy through clinical research and continuing education.

THEORETICAL MODELS OF INTERVENTION

There are different theoretical orientations to language intervention. These arise, in part, from different philosophies about the nature of normal language acquisition and differing viewpoints regarding the application of normal language acquisition to children with language disorders. Theoretical models differentially stress the primacy of cognitive, linguistic, or behavioral variables (e.g., Chomsky, 1965; Piaget, 1954; Pinker, 1989, 1996; Skinner, 1957; Vygotsky, 1962). Other models propose an integrative/connectionist approach and incorporate elements of several philosophies (Bates & MacWhinney, 1987; Bruner, 1974; MacWhinney, 2001, 2002). Still others use computational analyses (statistical probabilities) to make predictions that quantify the ease of acquisition of linguistic constructions (Hsu, Chater, & Vitanyi, 2011). Regardless of theoretical perspective, intervention practices should be informed by evidence. Clinicians implement effective strategies and procedures in conjunction with their own judgment and knowledge acquired through professional experience.

These models lead to different strategies of language intervention. In general, a behavioral orientation results in a nondevelopmental approach to therapy. Language targets may be selected without consideration of prerequisite skills, and behaviors are taught solely through the use of stimulus-response-consequence procedures. In contrast, other models are associated with developmental strategies in which target selection is determined by known sequences of acquisition, whether cognitively, linguistically, or pragmatically based. (See Appendix 4-A for major developmental language milestones.) For most children who present with a profile of delayed language, a developmental treatment strategy is generally utilized. A nondevelopmental approach may be adopted for atypical patterns of language acquisition (e.g., children with severe-profound intellectual impairment).

TREATMENT EFFICACY/EVIDENCE-BASED PRACTICE

Two comprehensive reviews have examined peer-reviewed studies on evidence-based practice (EBP) in the area of child language. Law, Garrett, and Nye (2004) conducted a meta-analysis of 13 studies, and Cirrin and Gillam (2008) systematically reviewed 21 articles. All studies selected met criteria for reliable and valid experimental design (see Table 1-3 in Chapter 1 for an evidence rating hierarchy). The overall findings indicate that language intervention is effective for preschool, kindergarten, and first-grade children, especially in the areas of phonology, expressive vocabulary, simple syntax/morphology, and phonological awareness. Neither of these reviews located high-quality studies of language intervention for older children and adolescents.

Significant gaps in the professional literature were identified by both investigations; the gaps include the following:

- studies on receptive language
- experimentally controlled studies
- studies of relative effectiveness of different treatment approaches for the same therapeutic targets
- studies on higher-order language skills (e.g., figurative language, narrative discourse)
- studies on pragmatic language skills
- studies examining intervention characteristics (e.g., duration, dosage, delivery model)
- investigations of the effects of language intervention with general/special education curriculum
- studies of maintenance of treatment effects

Cirrin et al.'s (2010) work focused on the effect of different service-delivery models (e.g., pullout, classroom-based, indirect consultation) on speech-language intervention outcomes for students of elementary school age. These authors conducted a systematic review of evidence-based studies published during the past 30 years and found that only five studies met the review criteria and addressed the effectiveness of service-delivery models. Even within this small sample, results were mixed, revealing large gaps in our knowledge of the relative effectiveness of different service-delivery models.

Kamhi (2014) argues there often is a disconnect between the findings of efficacy research and clinical practice implementation. Two examples are *treatment intensity* and *distributed practice*. Most efficacy studies suggest that that a higher dose of instruction (e.g., four 50-minute sessions/week) will result in better learning outcomes than a lower dose (e.g., two 30-minute sessions/week; Bellon-Harn, 2012). Yet, evidence shows that "more is not always better." Studies suggest that many children show learning plateaus and threshold effects for early reading intervention (e.g., Denton et al., 2011), expression of communicative intentions (Fey, Yoder, Warren, & Bredin-Oja, 2013), and print referencing instruction (McGinty, Breit-Smith, Fan, Justice, & Kaderavek, 2011). Beyond a point, the quantity or quality of the intervention has little effect on language and literacy outcomes. Another example involves *massed practice* versus *distributed practice*. Research findings on *spacing effects* (long intervals between learning episodes) show that distributed learning resulted not only in in short-term gains but also in better retention of newly learned behaviors. In fact, Yoder, Fey, and Warren (2012) suggested that the spacing and distribution of teaching episodes may have a greater influence on learning outcomes than treatment intensity. Taken together, these findings demonstrate the need for further study of the instructional elements that impact language learning and development.

There also are a number of smaller studies that examine the value and benefits of specific treatment protocols. For example, a growing body of emergent literacy literature indicates that read-alouds, shared/interactive book reading, and print referring are efficacious approaches for at-risk preschool children with and without language impairments and can be used successfully in home-based programs (e.g., Justice, McGinty, Piasta, Kaderavek, & Fan, 2010; Justice, Skibbe, McGinty, Piasta, & Petrill, 2011; Pelatti, Justice, Pentimonti, & Schmitt, 2013).

Finally, the efficacy of the term "auditory processing disorder/central auditory processing disorder" (APD/CAPD) has been questioned with respect to whether APD/CAPD can be differentiated from (specific) language impairment. From a clinical perspective, the term *APD* frequently is used indiscriminately by professionals in different contexts to mean different things. The label APD has been applied (often incorrectly) to a wide variety of difficulties and disorders. As a result, there are some who question the existence of APD as a distinct diagnostic entity and others who assume that the term *APD* is applicable to any child or adult who has difficulty listening to or understanding spoken language (see, e.g., www.asha.org/public/hearing/Understanding-Auditory-Processing-Disorders-in-Children/). ASHA convened an ad hoc committee to examine this controversial issue (Richards, 2011). The results provided inconclusive support for APD. Based on these findings, Fey et al. (2011) concluded that current research does not provide the SLP with adequate guidance for treating children diagnosed with APD.

CHAPTER 4

INTERVENTION WITH INFANTS (BIRTH TO 3 YEARS)

During this early developmental period, the infant masters the cognitive, social, motor, and communicative behaviors that underlie the acquisition of the linguistic system. (See Appendix 4-A for major developmental language milestones, Appendix 4-B for gross and fine motor skills milestones, and Appendix 4-C for stages of cognitive development.) In this view, language is one aspect of the baby's developing system and requires the clinician to look across developmental systems when planning and implementing language interventions. This perspective also promotes a team-based, coordinated approach rather than a series of fractured interventions by the speech-language pathologist (SLP), occupational therapist (OT), physical therapist (PT), and other professionals.

It is generally agreed that early intervention is crucial for infants who do not demonstrate these prerequisite skills within the typically expected time frame. Early intervention also is critical for children who are considered at risk for developing language difficulties due to factors such as prematurity, low birth weight, family history, medical complications, and so on (e.g., Dawson & Bernier, 2013; Diamond, Justice, Siegler, & Snyder, 2013; Guralnick, 1997, 2011, 2012, 2013; Paul & Roth, 2011). For at-risk children, intervention can be provided indirectly through monitoring of developmental progress or directly through infant stimulation and family enrichment programs. Some programs extend this focus to the concept of prevention, in which attempts are made to reduce or eliminate the risks and conditions that ultimately may result in communication disorders. Intervention provided during the first 2 years of life is thought to be extremely productive because it capitalizes on the rapid neural growth and learning potential of the young brain.

ASHA Early Intervention Guidelines

According to the American Speech-Language-Hearing Association (ASHA, 2008), **early intervention (EI)** refers to a broad range of services, including the following:

- Prevention
- Screening
- Evaluation and assessment
- Planning, implementing, and monitoring intervention
- Consultation with and education for team members, including families and other professionals
- Service coordination
- Transition planning
- Advocacy

EI is characterized by a primary emphasis on family involvement and education Ingber & Dromi, 2010; Wilcox & Woods, 2011). A family-centered approach addresses the child's needs within the sole relevant context for the child—the family unit. This model acknowledges the cultural, social, economic, and values or belief factors that may affect family dynamics. EI services promote children's participation in their natural environments, which can include home- or center-based settings (Caesar, 2013; Banerjee & Luckner, 2014). Although the term *natural environment* has often been assumed to refer to a child's home, it actually encompasses all settings and individuals with whom the child has regular contact. With infants and toddlers, more than with any other single age group, the clinician will likely work in an interdisciplinary or transdisciplinary model of service delivery. In an interdisciplinary model, each team member functions within his or her specific discipline and shares information with other team members through established channels such as team meetings. In contrast, members of a transdisciplinary team cross traditional professional boundaries. They receive training in other disciplines and interchangeably provide services as needed by the child and family. These collaborative approaches to intervention are highlighted in Part C of the Individuals with Disabilities Education Act (IDEA, 2011, idea.ed.gov) and emphasize the need for a team of professionals to be involved in the Individualized Family Service Plan (IFSP) process (Paul & Roth, 2011).

The goal of EI is the development of basic skills thought to be critical to successful speech, language, and communication learning. Repeated, interactive exposure to **authentic learning experiences in natural environments** and **modeling/stimulation** are the primary therapy strategies for infants. (Additional strategies relevant to this population are presented later in this chapter.) The main therapy targets for infant intervention programs comprise the following prelinguistic and early language skills.

Localization. Infants demonstrate awareness of sounds in their environment by turning toward and visually searching for the source of a sound. This auditory–visual association marks the beginning of an infant's conceptual grasp of cause–effect relations.

A clinician can enhance the localization behaviors of an infant by presenting a sound stimulus (e.g., rattle or other noisy object) outside the baby's visual field. This will require an observable head turn for the baby to locate the sound source. If this response is not observed, the clinician can gently turn the infant's head toward the sound to reinforce the auditory–visual association. The following developmental sequence can be used as a guideline for the appropriate response level for a given infant.

3 to 4 months:	Primitive attempt to turn head
4 to 7 months:	Localization to side only
7 to 13 months:	Localization to side or below
13 to 21 months:	Localization to side, below, or above
21 to 24 months:	Direct localization to any angle

Joint/Shared Attention. A shared focus underlies successful communication. Joint attention between an adult and infant highlights the relationship between the adult's utterances and the objects, actions, or concepts they represent. In this context, the adult and infant are focused on the same referent in the environment (e.g., a rattle). According to Bruner (1977), joint visual attention is the prerequisite for all subsequent communication. One effective method for facilitating joint attention or shared reference is to place an attractive or noisy object in front of the infant, look at it, and comment on it. The adult may point to the object, shake it, or gently turn the infant's head to encourage eye contact with the object. Sometimes, it may be necessary to follow the infant's gaze to a particular object and then point to and label it to promote joint visual regard.

Mutual Gaze. This eye gaze pattern is a characteristic of early communicative development in which the infant and caregiver look at each other during social interactions. It is thought to form the basis for attachment/bonding between infant and caregiver

(Lloyd, & Masur, 2014; Rossetti, 2001) and serves as a basic building block for later development of the important skill of turn-taking in conversation (Owens, 2013). Immediate parental response to the infant's initiation of eye contact increases the baby's motivation to communicate and ultimately results in more frequent and varied interactions (Zero to Three, 2012). Establishment and maintenance of mutual gaze with infants can be enhanced when adult eye contact is accompanied by smiling and other facial expressions, touching, and novel or entertaining vocalizations.

Joint Action and Routines. Joint action between an adult and infant occurs in play sequences known as sound–gesture games or routines such as peekaboo, patty-cake, or "I'm gonna get you." A **routine** is a prepackaged or ritualized exchange between an adult and infant. It has a definite structure with a clearly marked beginning, middle, and end, with clearly specified positions for appropriate vocalization or verbalization. This structure allows for the anticipation of events and increases the potential for successful adult–child interaction. It ensures that each partner knows what to expect from the other, thus making the order of events highly predictable. Ratner and Bruner (1978) point out that the semantic content of the mutual play is highly restricted and within the conceptual repertoire of the child. It is generally believed that the regularity and invariance of these routines allow the infant to make his or her first attempts at "cracking the linguistic code" and acquiring the first words (Ferrier, 1978; Newson, 1979). Many investigators also believe that these routines facilitate turn-taking behavior and role shifting in dialogue, both important building blocks of conversational exchanges.

Clinicians can initiate these playful routines in therapy and select the target response for an infant based on the following typical acquisition sequence for young children:

- At approximately 6 months, infants show enjoyment and pleasure (i.e., change in facial expression or body posture) when a parent initiates a sound–gesture routine.
- By 7 months, the infant anticipates the game when the adult produces the verbal component alone (independent of any gesture).
- The 8- to 9-month-old baby initiates as well as participates in the game (e.g., crawls behind the door and peeks his head out while smiling).

For slightly older babies, the clinician can utilize the "Picture-Book-Reading Routine" (Ninio & Bruner, 1978) with the baby seated next to or on the adult's lap. Select an enjoyable picture book and follow this sequence:

Adult: Say "Look" (attentional vocative) and point to picture

Child: Touches or looks at the picture (response)

A: Say "What are these?" (query)

C: Vocalizes, smiles, or names the picture (response)

A: Say "Yes, that is a ___" or "No, that's not a ___, it's a ___" (feedback)

Vocalizations. The first year of life is characterized, in part, by rapid physical growth and neuromuscular maturation. As a result, the infant gains increasing control over the speech mechanism and exhibits significant expansion in the quality and variety of vocalizations. Infant vocalizations proceed through a series of predictable developmental stages, as outlined in Table 4-1.

TABLE 4–1
Stages of Vocal Development in Infancy

Age	Behavior	Description
0–2 months	Reflexive	Undifferentiated crying and vegetative sounds (e.g., coughing, burping, sighing)
2–4 months	Cooing	Vocal signs of pleasure, primarily vowel and vowel-like sounds
4–6 months	Laughter	Sustained combination of cooing and crying features to produce audible "ha ha ha"
	Vocal play	Exploration of mouth with tongue, producing sounds such as squeals, growls, lip smacking, raspberries, and clicks
	Early babbling	Self-initiated sound play; combines stop consonants with vowels to produce isolated CV or VC syllables (e.g., /bo/ or /ok/)
6–8 months	Reduplicative babbling	Series of CV or VC syllables each identical to the other and frequently initiated with a /ə/ (e.g., /ədadada/)
8–10 months	Nonreduplicative babbling	Consonants and vowels may differ from one syllable to the next within a single string (e.g., /bawada/)
10–12 months	Jargon	Conversational intonation contours are imposed on longer strings of sound combinations; real words may be interspersed
	Protowords	Invented sound sequences that are used consistently to refer to a specific item or event (e.g., /na/ used to mean "Give [object] to me")

SOURCE: Adapted from Oller, D. (1980). The emergence of the sounds of speech in infancy. In G. Yeni-Komshian, J. Cavanaugh, & C. Ferguson (Eds.), Child Phonology: Vol. 1. Production (pp. 93–112). New York, NY: Academic Press. Stark, R. (1980). Stages of speech development in the first year of life. In G. Yeni-Komshian, J. Cavanaugh, & C. Ferguson (Eds.), Child Phonology: Vol. 1. Production (pp. 73–92). New York, NY: Academic Press.

Expansion of an infant's vocal repertoire can be promoted by increasing the frequency, variety, or quality of the vocalizations produced by the infant. The clinician can stimulate vocalization by talking to the infant, singing, humming, cuddling, tickling, or playing sound–gesture games such as peekaboo. Clinicians may also imitate the infant's vocalization in a playful manner to initiate a repetitive imitative exchange. Action-identification tags are playful sounds that infants enjoy listening to and may attempt to reproduce, such as the motor sound ("vroom"), cow sound ("moo"), telephone ("dingaling"), dog barking ("ruff ruff"), or car horn ("beep beep").

Communicative Intentions. The meaning that a speaker wishes a message to convey is known as a **communicative intention.** At about 9 months of age, infants discover intentional communication and begin to express their communicative intentions through gesture and vocalization (see Table 4-2). Requests and statements are among the earliest communicative intentions to emerge. Requests represent the infant's intentional use of a listener as an agent or tool in achieving some end (e.g., a desired object). Statements are the infant's attempts to direct an adult's attention to some event or object in the environment. As children begin to acquire an initial vocabulary, they express communicative intentions

TABLE 4–2

Preverbal Communicative Intentions

Intention	Descriptive Example
1. Attention-seeking	
a. To self	Child tugs on adult's jeans to secure attention.
b. To events, objects, or other people	Child points to airplane to draw adult's attention to it.
2. Requesting	
a. Objects	Child points to toy animal that he wants.
b. Action	Child hands book to adult to have story read.
c. Information	Child points to usual location of cookie jar (which is not there) and simultaneously secures eye contact with mother to determine its whereabouts.
3. Greetings	Child waves "hi" or "bye."
4. Transferring	Child gives mother the toy that he was playing with.
5. Protesting/ rejecting	Child cries when mother takes away toy. Child pushes away a dish of oatmeal.
6. Responding/ acknowledging	Child responds appropriately to simple directions. Child smiles when parent initiates a favorite game.
7. Informing	Child points to wheel on his toy truck to show mother that it is broken.

SOURCE: Categories are derived, in part, from: Bates, E., Camaioni, L., & Volterra, V. (1975). The acquisition of performatives prior to speech. Merrill-Palmer Quarterly, 21, 205–224. Escalona, S. (1973). Basic modes of social interaction: Their emergence and patterning during the first two years of life. Merrill-Palmer Quarterly, 19, 205–232. Halliday, M. A. K. (1975). Learning how to mean: Explorations in the development of language. London: Edward Arnold. Wetherby, A., Cain, D., Yonclas, D., & Walker, V. (1988). Analysis of intentional communication of normal children from the prelinguistic to the multi-word stage. Journal of Speech and Hearing Research, 31, 240–252.

through single-word utterances (see Table 4-3). Evidence suggests that the *rate* of preverbal communication in young children with developmental delays is a strong predictor of later vocabulary usage (Brady, Marquis, Fleming, & McLean, 2004; Calandrella & Wilcox, 2000; McCathren, Yoder, & Warren, 1999). The *frequency* of intentional communication is also predictive: Higher rates of nonverbal intentional communication during the preverbal stage are associated with better language outcomes 1 to 2 years later (Paul & Roth, 2011; Watt, Wetherby, & Shumway, 2006; Woynaroski, Yoder, Fey, & Warren, 2012).

Intervention in the area of communicative intentions may be aimed at (1) increasing the number of different types of intentions a child can understand or express and/or (2) increasing the variety of forms (e.g., vocalization, gesture, word) understood or used to express a given intention. To elicit specific communicative intentions, the clinician should provide facilitating environments in which the intentions are obligatory or at least highly likely to occur (Paul, 2007; Roth, 1999; Spekman & Roth, 1984). Following are examples of facilitating environments for selected intentions:

Requests for action:	Introduce toys that cannot be operated without assistance from the clinician, such as a windup toy.
	Place highly desirable toys where child cannot gain access to them without assistance from the clinician.
	Present incomplete or broken materials such as puzzles with missing pieces or paints without brushes.

TABLE 4–3
Communicative Intentions Expressed at the Single-Word Level

Intention	Definition
1. Naming	Common and proper nouns that label people, objects, events, and locations.
2. Commenting	Words that describe physical attributes of objects, events, and people, including size, shape, and location; observable movements and actions of objects and people; and words that refer to attributes that are not immediately observable such as possession and usual location. These words are not contingent on prior utterances.

3. Requesting object
  a. Present
  b. Absent
	
	Words that solicit an object that is present in the environment.
	Words that solicit an absent object.

4. Requesting action	Words that solicit that an action to be initiated or continued.
5. Requesting information	Words that solicit information about an object, action, person, or location. Rising intonation is also included.
6. Responding	Words that directly complement preceding utterances.
7. Protesting/rejecting	Words that express objection to ongoing or impending action/event.
8. Attention-seeking	Words that solicit attention to the child or to aspects of the environment.
9. Greetings	Words that express salutations and other conventionalized rituals.

SOURCE: Adapted from Dale, P. S. (1980). Is early pragmatic development measurable? Journal of Child Language, 8, 1–12. Dore, J. (1974). A pragmatic description of early language development. Journal of Psycholinguistic Research, 3, 343–350. Halliday, M. A. K. (1975). Learning how to mean: Explorations in the development of language. London: Edward Arnold.

Requests for information:	Introduce novel or enticing toys for which the child is likely to request a label or information regarding its function, operation, or construction, such as a transformer, spinning top, or a talking book.
Attention-seeking:	Pretend not to hear the child so that he or she must use the clinician's name, raise vocal pitch or intensity, or move closer to the clinician.

Nonsymbolic Play and Symbolic Play. Children learn through play and often practice their new acquisitions in play. Infants gain experience in how both receptive and expressive language function by participating in play sequences. In addition, play is the most important context for the development of social communication skills and the natural context for early language learning (Johnson, Christie, & Yawkey, 1987; Katz, 2001; Norris & Hoffman, 1990; Rivkin, 1986; Rogers & Sawyers, 1988). In early types of play, children use objects for their intended purposes (functional play) or engage in exploratory play such as dropping, mouthing, or transferring objects) and do not require the use of symbolic agents. Additional examples of functional play include activities such as running, filling and emptying receptacles, driving toy cars, and water play. Later, symbolic forms of play emerge, where, the child substitutes objects or events for other objects/events. Examples include pretending to talk on the telephone or using a stick as a sword. (See Appendix 4-D for stages of play development.)

Following are some suggested themes and activities for facilitating play, arranged developmentally:

- Exploring common objects such as blocks, rattles, spoons, pots, and pans, through banging, mouthing, manipulating, and visual inspection

- Using toys appropriately, such as a busy box or Fisher-Price See 'n Say®

- Pretending to act out familiar single actions such as eating, sleeping, and drinking

- Manipulating a doll to perform familiar activities such as kissing, dancing, and waving bye-bye

- Pretending to act out sequences of familiar actions such as pouring liquid into a cup, taking a sip, and then spilling the liquid onto the floor

- Using dough or clay to create "pretend" food such as hot dogs or pancakes

- Using miniature people, cars, or dishes to act out daily routines such as taking a bath, going to the store, or having a birthday party

Initial Vocabulary/First Lexicon. Infants begin to understand a few familiar words between 6 and 8 months of age. Production of first true words occurs around the first birthday. Early vocabulary development can be stimulated at the receptive and/or expressive level (Beck, McKeown, & Kucan, 2013; Bloom, 2000; Tomasello, 2003; Whitehurst et al., 1991). Intervention aimed at the facilitation of a child's *receptive* vocabulary generally consists of repeated presentation of a target word as well as the use of gestures and exaggerated/varied vocal intonation patterns to highlight salient aspects of an object or event. Following are two sample activities that can be used to stimulate comprehension of early vocabulary for a 12- to 24-month-old child with a language impairment:

- Engage the child in play with a large, lightweight ball. Demonstrate and say the following to the child:

  "Can you *throw* the ball to me? Put two hands over your head and throw it to me. That's right, let go and *throw* it over here. Great, you did it."

  "Now can you *drop* the ball? I'll drop it first and then you drop it again. Let me see you *drop* the ball. Good job."

  "Let me see you *kick* the ball. *Kick* the ball with your foot. *Kick* the ball as hard as you can. Good for you, you kicked the ball."

- Engage the child in play using a surprise box such as Playskool's Busy Poppin' Pals. Say to the child:

  "Can you find Monkey's *banana*? Guess what? I see a *banana* right here. Do you see Monkey's *banana*? That's not Monkey, that's Panda. Point to Monkey's *banana*."

The early *expressive* vocabularies of young children are not arbitrary. Initial lexicons are highly selective because children communicate about the social and physical events that are within their conceptual grasp and immediate environment. A grammatical classification of a typical initial lexicon is presented in Table 4-4. Expressive vocabulary growth is charted in Table 4-5.

Researchers also agree that children's early vocabularies express a basic set of semantic functions or intentions (Bloom, 1973; Brown, 1968; Nelson, 1973). Strategies for facilitating the acquisition of early lexical items are frequently based on semantic function rather than grammatical classification. Three main considerations in the selection of

TABLE 4–4

Grammatical Classification of the First 50 Words Produced

Grammatical Function	Percentage of Vocabulary	Examples
Nominals	50	*milk, dog, car*
Action words	11–14	*give, do, up, bye-bye*
Modifiers	14–19	*mine, no dirty*
Personal/social	10	*no, please*
Functional	4	*this, for*

Source: Based on Benedict, H. (1979). Early lexical development: Comprehen-sion and production. Journal of Child Language, 6, 183–200. Nelson, K. (1973). Structure and strategy in learning to talk. Society for Research in Child Development Monographs, 38, (1–2 Serial No. 149). (Reprinted in part in Mussen, Conger, & Kagan, Readings in child development and personality, (3rd. ed.). Harper & Row, 1975.)

TABLE 4–5

Expressive Vocabulary Growth

Age	Number of Words
15 months	4–6
18 months	20–50
24 months	200–300
3 years	900–1,000
4 years	1,500–1,600
5 years	2,100–2,200

Source: Adapted from Bates, E., Marchman, V., Thal, D., Fenson, L., Dale, P., (1994). Developmental and stylistic variation in the composition of early vo-cabulary. Journal of Child Language, 21, 85–123.

target vocabulary are: (1) words that can be used in many different contexts during the child's daily activities; (2) words that are important to the child, such as names of significant others or types of favorite foods or toys; and (3) words that represent dynamic rather than static states, especially referents that can be acted on or manipulated directly by the child such as a ball or a spoon, rather than a tree or a wall. Following are suggested contexts/activities that can be used to stimulate different types of semantic intentions at the single-word level.

Existence/naming:	Introduce a container filled with interesting objects and reveal them to the child one at a time.
Nonexistence:	Expose an attractive object to the child and then hide it from view.
Recurrence:	Initiate a desirable activity and then stop.
Action:	Engage the child in an activity such as making pudding that will elicit a number of different actions (e.g., open, pour, stir, mix).
Possession:	Place a combination of the child's and clinician's belongings in a box, pull them out one at a time, and sort into separate piles.
Locative:	Engage the child in play with trucks or cars using props such as a Fisher-Price Garage or Little Peoples Wheelies Race Track that encourage changes in location.
Rejection:	Offer objects or activities that are known to be unappealing to the child.
Denial:	In a playful manner, intentionally misname objects or body parts that the child already knows.

One evidence-based strategy to promote simultaneous development of receptive and expressive vocabulary is reading books together. Clinicians should regularly engage in shared book reading with their young clients and encourage parents to read books to their children. (See the section on emergent literacy later in this chapter for more information.) Ideal books for infants include things to touch, language that repeats over and over again, and colorful pictures of objects and words to match.

The following case example illustrates several of the main principles of EI for infants and toddlers.

Mina is an 18-month-old girl from a bilingual family (Spanish is her first language [L1]). Mina has a complex medical history of prematurity and seizures, and is at significant risk for delayed language. In addition to SLP services, Mina is receiving PT, OT, and physician care through the county health department. The parents have a relatively good grasp of English, their second language (L2), but a language barrier remains. For example, they have difficulty understanding the specific nature of her language delay and the likelihood that Mina will continue to have language-learning problems. Their English language comprehension also interferes with their ability to understand the SLP's initial suggestions for stimulating language and communication at home and in daily activities. Both parents work outside the home and Mina is cared for by her grandmother (who only speaks L1) during the day. The family wants to know how to interact more effectively with their daughter in everyday situations and provide Mina with opportunities to interact more frequently with other children. They are also interested in learning more about the development of language/communication and reasonable expectations for their daughter at different stages of development.

Clinical strategy. As part of the EI team, the SLP initiated a family-centered approach that includes several areas of focus:

- The clinician refers Mina to an infant–toddler social interaction group at the county health department that is staffed by members of the EI team.

- The clinician also makes biweekly home visits with Mina's family to demonstrate behaviors for encouraging adult–child interactions (e.g., modeling, expansions) and directly engages Mina's family in the planning and implementation of these activities. The clinician consults with the family to select recommended developmentally supportive play activities and routines, toys, and books that Mina would likely enjoy that are consistent with the family's culture and interests to increase family–child engagement and build Mina's communication skills.

- The clinician recommends that the family participate in an ongoing support group for families of children with significant handicaps, which are coordinated by EI professionals at the county health center. These sessions provide information on early development, stress the importance of adult–child interactions in facilitating language learning, and offer ways to increase positive and relaxed adult–child engagement, because several of the family members expressed difficulties relating to their children with delays.

To ensure coordination of services across disciplines, the EI team meets regularly with one another and with the family. The SLP's main role is to provide information about language intervention targets, with expressive vocabulary being a primary focus. She also describes the cues/prompts/strategies that were most and least successful in stimulating Mina's vocabulary. The team discusses how the target vocabulary and strategies will be incorporated by the teacher of the interaction group, in OT and PT sessions, and at home. The SLP emails a weekly updated log of goals, strategies, and Mina's progress to the team, and updates the hard-copy binder that she maintains for the family and the teacher. At the end of each week, the EI team logs on to the Web-based forum or chat site at a designated time to share updates, concerns, and next steps. (Mina's family requested that the SLP attend these weekly meetings on their behalf because of their work schedules.)

As children approach the third birthday, a **transition plan** is developed for those youngsters who are going on to other services. The transition plan is typically prepared at the last IFSP meeting before the transition occurs. It includes the steps needed to prepare the child and family for the new setting. It also outlines the steps for preparing the professionals who will be providing the special education services at the new setting.

Helpful Hints

1. Clinicians may want to incorporate some of the main characteristics of *motherese*, or child-directed speech, in their speech to young children. These include exaggerated intonation, short utterance length, simple vocabulary and syntactic structures, frequent repetition of utterances, and talking about topics in the "here and now."

2. Clinician (CL) responses to child (CH) utterances should be framed in a way that encourages the exchange to continue and keeps the child in the interaction (sometimes referred to as **turnabouts**). For example:

   CH: dat?

   CL: Kitty cat. What does it say?

   vs.

   CH: dat?

   CL: It's a kitty.

3. Clinicians can maximize the effectiveness of intervention activities by selecting toys and materials that are developmentally supportive for a particular child. (See Appendix 4-E for a developmental toy list.)

4. Clinicians need to be aware that many infants with communication impairments may exhibit concomitant impairments in other areas. Intervention programs must accommodate the infant's overall developmental profile. For example, tactile stimulation often elicits abnormal primitive reflexes in children with cerebral palsy and can significantly interfere with therapeutic programming.

5. Clinicians should be prepared to address skepticism of other professionals and families/caregivers regarding the merits of language intervention with infants and very young children.

6. The clinician can provide families with the treatment steps that are followed, and address their concerns and questions.

INTERVENTION WITH CHILDREN (3 TO 5 YEARS)

During this developmental period, children acquire the major portion of the linguistic system. This period is characterized by rapid growth in vocabulary. After the age of 18 months, children add approximately 9 to 10 new words to their lexicons each day, or 3,000 words per year (Graves, 1986). Average utterance length continues to increase, and the acquisition of syntax has its onset as children begin to impose word order on their two-word combinations. Morphological forms emerge and become solidified, although complete mastery is not attained until the early elementary school years. This developmental period also is marked by children's ability to understand and produce a variety of simple and complex sentence forms. In addition, children in this age range demonstrate substantial development in the area of emergent literacy through exposure and interaction with print. See Tables 4-6 through 4-14 for a review of mean length of utterance (MLU) stages, two-word semantic intentions, acquisition of grammatical morphemes, auxiliary verb development, negation development, question development, sentence-type comprehension progression, hallmarks of literacy development, and the developmental stages of early writing.

TABLE 4–6
Stages of Mean Length of Utterance Development

Stage	MLU (morphemes)	Approximate Age
I	1.0–2.0	18–24 months
II	2.0–2.5	2–2½ years
III	2.5–3.0	2½–3 years
IV	3.0–3.5	3–3½ years
V	3.5–4.0	3½–4 years

SOURCE: Adapted from Brown, R. (1973). A first language. Cambridge, MA: Harvard University Press.

TABLE 4–7
Two-Word Semantic Relations

Relation	Examples
Agent + action	Daddy eat, mommy drive
Action + object	Eat cookie, throw ball
Agent + object	Daddy shoe, grandma hat
Attribute + entity	Big doggie, pretty lady
Possessor + possession	Daddy car, baby bottle
Recurrence	More juice, more cookie
Nonexistence	No bed, allgone milk
Demonstrative + entity	This cup, that doggie
Entity + location	Daddy chair, toy floor
Action + location	Go home, sit horsie

SOURCE: Adapted from Bloom, L. (1973). One word at a time: The use of single-word utterances before syntax. New York, NY: The Hague Mouton. Brown, R. (1973). A first language. Cambridge, MA: Harvard University Press. Schlesinger, I. (1971). Production of utterances and language acquisition. In D. Slobin (Ed.), The ontogenesis of grammar (pp. 63–101). New York, NY: Academic Press.

TABLE 4–8
Brown's 14 Grammatical Morphemes: Order of Acquisition

Morpheme	Example	Stage
Present progressive -ing (no auxiliary verb)	Daddy sleeping	I–II
In/on	Doggie on table	II
Regular plural −s	Me have two shoes	I–III
Irregular past	Drank, came, fell, broke, ate	I–IV
Possessive 's	Daddy's chair	I–IV
Uncontractible copula (used as main verb)	This is hot.	II–IV
Articles (a/the)	Open the door.	II–V
Regular past -ed	Mommy walked the dog.	I–Post V
Regular third person -s	Mommy works.	I–V
Irregular third person	Does, has	II–Post V
Uncontractible auxiliary	The doggie was running.	II–Post V
Contractible copula	He is tall.	II–Post V
Contractible auxiliary	Daddy is coming home.	II–Post V

SOURCE: Adapted from Brown, R. (1973). A first language. Cambridge, MA: Harvard University Press.

TABLE 4–9
Auxilitary Verb Development

Category	Form/Examples	Stage
Contracted form of is	's	Early II
Forms of to be	is, am, are, was	Late II
Early infinitives (catenatives)	hafta, gonna, wanna	Late II
Early modals	can, do, may, will	Stage III on
Subjunctive modals	could, would, should, might	Stage III on
Mood of obligation modals	should, must, have to	Stage IV on
Perfective	have . . . -en	Stage V or later
Double expansion of auxiliary	has been, might have	Stage V or later

TABLE 4–10
Development of Negation

MLU Stage	Form	Example
I	Negative + utterance Utterance + negative	No drink; not hungry Mommy no; doggie not
II–III	Subject + negative + main verb Unanalyzed don't/can't (not true auxiliary forms)	Me no drink; he not sit Don't hit; You can't go
III–IV	Subject + auxiliary + negative + main verb	He is not running; Mommy cannot go

SOURCES: Adapted from Bellugi, U. (1967). The acquisition of negation (Unpublished doctoral dissertation). Harvard University, Cambridge, MA. DeVilliers, P. A., & DeVilliers, J. G. (1979). Early language (The developing child). Cambridge, MA: Harvard University Press.

TABLE 4–11
Development of Question Forms*

MLU Stage	Form	Example
I		
Yes/no	Rising intonation	Me go? See hole?
Wh-	What NP doing?	What daddy doing?
	Where NP going?	Where mommy going?
	Wh-word + NP	What that?
II–III		
Yes/no	Rising intonation in longer utterances	You see red ball?
	Wh-word + sentence	Who you draw in book?
III–IV		
Yes/no	NP and auxiliary verb	Can I go? Do you see me?
	Inversion of subject	
Wh-	Wh-word + subject NP + auxiliary + main verb	Why he can ride?
IV–V		
Yes/no	Remains the same in longer utterances	Should I throw it over there?
Wh-	Wh-word + auxiliary verb + subject NP + main verb	Why can he ride?

Source: Adapted from Klima, E., & Bellugi, U. (1966). Syntactic regularities in the speech of children. In J. Lyons & R. J. Wales (Eds.), Psycholinguistics papers. Edinburgh, UK: Edinburgh University Press. Valian, V. (1992). Categories of first syntax: be, be+ing, and nothingness. In J. M. Meisel (Ed.), The acquisition of verb placement: Functional categories and V2 phenomena in language development. Dordrecht, Netherlands: Kluwer.
*Note: Wh-words emerge in the following sequence: (a) what, where; (b) who; (c) when, how, and why, in variable order. NP = Noun phrase.

TABLE 4–12
Developmental Sequence of Sentence Comprehension

Syntactic Structure	Example	Age of Comprehension between 75% and 90%
Simple imperative	Stop!	4–6 to 6–0
Negative imperative	Don't touch the stove!	5–6 to 7–0
Active declarative		
Regular noun and present progressive	The girl is walking.	3–0
Irregular noun and present progressive	The deer are running.	6–6 to 7–0
Past tense	The dog chased the cat.	5–6 to 7–0+
Past participle	The lady has spoken.	6–0 to 7–0+
Future tense	She will play the piano.	7–0 to 7–0+
Reversible	The man kisses the lady.	6–6 to 7–0+
Perfective	Daddy has been working.	7–0+

(continues)

TABLE 4–12 *(Continued)*

Syntactic Structure	Example	Age of Comprehension between 75% and 90%
Interrogative		
Who	Who is on the bed?	3–0
What	What do we wear?	3–6 to 5–0
When	When do you sleep?	3–6 to 5–6
Negation	The man isn't swimming.	5–6 to 7–0+
Reversible passive	The dog is chased by the cat.	5–6 to 6–0
Conjunction		
If	If you're a teacher, point to the dog.	7–0+
Then	Look at the third animal, then point to the dog.	7–0+
Neither/nor	Show me the one that is neither the ball nor the dog.	7–0+

Source: Adapted from Scarborough, H. (1989). Index of productive syntax. Applied Psycholinguistics, 11, 1–22.

TABLE 4–13
Hallmarks of Literacy Development

Stage	Description
Early Emergent	Awareness of some print conventions (e.g., front versus back of books; left-right directionality of writing; words versus pictures) Shows sustained interest during book reading Recognizes familiar environmental print (e.g., logo for fast food restaurant) Engages in random drawing and scribbling
Later Emergent	Pretends to read and write Demonstrates a sense of "story" (i.e., beginning/middle/ending) Recognizes and produces predictable language patterns of familiar stories Attempts to write letters using scribbles and wavy lines

(continues)

TABLE 4–13 *(Continued)*

Stage	Description
Early Beginning Reader	Attempts to read words by matching each letter to its corresponding sound (early decoding)
	Begins to develop a sight-word vocabulary which consists of highly familiar words
	Attempts to write words using primarily beginning and ending letters
Later Beginning Reader	Decodes familiar print easily; may struggle with new material
	Demonstrates large sight-word vocabulary
	Engages in self-correction during reading and writing
	Spells most familiar words accurately
	Shows awareness of writing conventions such as punctuation
Independent Reader	Reads fluently and focuses on understanding the meaning of text
	Uses text-based strategies such as predicting, summarizing, re-reading, and paraphrasing
	Demonstrates consistent use of spelling rules and writing conventions such as punctuation, paragraphing, and topic versus supporting sentences

SOURCE: Adapted from Salinger, T. (2001). Assessing the literacy of young children: The case for multiple forms of evidence. In S. B. Neuman & D. K. Dickinson (Eds.), Handbook of early literacy research (pp. 390–418). New York, NY: Guilford Press.

TABLE 4–14

Developmental Stages of Early Spelling

Stage	Description/Example
Drawing	Child scribbles using wavy and circular lines
Pre-phonemic	Random combination of pictures, squiggles, letters, and numbers with no connection between letters and sounds (e.g., Az4Esu7)
Semi-phonemic	Writes 1–3 letters to stand for a word (e.g., P = piano, PTE = pretty)
Phonetic/letter name	Spells words the way they sound (e.g., LETL = little, EGL = eagle)
Transitional	Within-word patterns include vowels in each syllable (e.g., EGUL = eagle)
Conventional	Basic rules of spelling are mastered (e.g., EAGLE = eagle)

SOURCES: Adapted from Bear, D., & Templeton, S. (1998). Explorations in spelling: Foundations for learning and teaching phonics, spelling, and vocabulary. The Reading Teacher, 52, 222–242. Gentry, J. R. (2000). A retrospective on invented spelling and a look forward. The Reading Teacher, 54, 318–332.

TREATMENT APPROACHES FOR INFANTS, TODDLERS, AND PRESCHOOLERS

There are a variety of approaches to language intervention, most of which can be implemented with children across a wide range of ages and stages of development. These approaches emphasize the provision of intervention in naturalistic contexts. This means that children/students are engaged in authentic, meaningful activities that are functionally linked to their daily activities. Several basic remediation approaches are described in the following sections. They can be used in combination and are appropriate for a variety of service models, including Response to Intervention (RTI), other collaborative approaches, and small-group/individual therapy.

Focused Stimulation (Fey, 1986). In this approach, the clinician provides concentrated exposure to a target form in a variety of contexts (e.g., individual words, embedded in sentences or short stories). The clinician preselects a linguistic target and produces it in high concentration throughout natural and meaningful adult–child interactions. Because the focus is on comprehension, the child is not required to produce the linguistic form. This approach can encompass a wide variety of targets, including vocabulary, grammatical morphemes, and syntax.

Incidental Teaching (Hart & Risley, 1974; Hart & Rogers-Warren, 1978). This is a naturalistic approach that encourages a child to initiate communication by arranging the environment to increase the likelihood that the child will produce a verbal or nonverbal intervention target. The child's successful communicative attempts are rewarded through natural consequences such as a requested object or event. The clinician also responds to the child's communicative attempts with requests for expansion or elaboration. Variations of incidental teaching include milieu (Kaiser & Warren, 1986) and time-delay approaches (Halle, Marshall, & Spradlin, 1979).

Floortime/Developmental, Individual Difference, Relationship-Based (DIR; Greenspan, 1998). This approach to intervention focuses on building the foundations of social, emotional, and intellectual capacities in young children rather than targeting isolated behaviors or skills. It encourages socially appropriate child-initiated interactions with emphasis on developmental milestones, individual differences, and the relationship between the child and others in the environment. A critical component of this model is family engagement.

Family-Centered (Manolson, 1985; Schopler & Reichler, 1971). This approach trains parents and other caregivers to foster the development of language and communication in naturalistic contexts such as the home setting. The SLP functions in an indirect or educational capacity with family members, helping them become the "change agents" for their child. These programs may focus on improving the child's communication skills and/or improving the adult family members' ability to engage in mutually reinforcing communicative interactions with their child.

EMERGENT LITERACY INTERVENTION (BIRTH THROUGH PRESCHOOL YEARS)

The overall goal of emergent literacy intervention is to promote oral and print-knowledge skills that are associated with the ability to successfully learn reading and writing skills. This goal addresses the significant reciprocal relationship between early intervention and academic achievement. SLPs may play a variety of direct and indirect roles in this area of intervention. Clinicians can work directly on providing emergent literacy intervention to children with identified communication disorders. Indirect roles encompass collaborative consultation with others, professional staff development, parent/community education, and curricular policy recommendations regarding the critical nature of emergent literacy skill acquisition for all children. From an RTI/multi-tiered perspective, all areas of emergent literacy skill can be integrated into Tiers 1, 2, or 3.

There are several other components of emergent literacy, each of which can be used as an avenue to increase a child's print knowledge. Following are five main areas, accompanied by instructional guidelines (Roth & Baden, 2001).

Shared Book-Reading and Sense of Story

- Engage in dialogic reading. It's important to ask questions throughout the reading activity about what has been read and what might happen next. See Whitehurst, Arnold, Epstein, and Angell (1994) and Whitehurst and Lonigan (1998) for helpful guidance on the use of this technique.

- Expose the child to quality literature that is developmentally supportive with respect to complexity and content. A variety of text genres should be incorporated into intervention, including fiction, informational formats, poetry, and others.

- Select predictably patterned stories with repetitive themes and well-developed plot structure.

- Direct the child's attention to the printed words rather than focusing solely on the pictures. Engage in *print referencing*, an interactive reading style in which adults highlight specific aspects of print in storybooks and other genres (e.g., alphabet or informational books) verbally with comments and questions and nonverbally through gestures and tracking print while reading.

- Encourage the child to recount familiar experiences that occur in routinely in daily life (e.g., scripts), such as grocery shopping or getting dressed.

- Encourage the child to recount personal event narratives, which are event sequences experienced by someone else (e.g., Daddy cooking dinner).

Phonological Awareness

- Recite fingerplays (e.g., "Itsy-Bitsy Spider" and "I'm a Little Teapot").

- Sing songs and chants (e.g., "This Old Man" and "Teddy Bear, Teddy Bear").

- Engage in alliteration and rhyming (e.g., "dad, dad, stick, stad").

- Point out words that begin with the same sound.

- Say simple words such as "cat"; have the child think of one or two words that start with the same initial sound.

Application of phonological awareness instruction is clearly demonstrated in a program such as **Promoting Awareness of Speech Sounds (PASS**; Roth, Worthington, & Troia, 2012). PASS is a comprehensive and explicit phonological awareness curriculum that was originally designed for preschool children who may be at risk for literacy problems, including children with speech and language impairments or other learning disabilities. PASS also can be used with typically developing preschoolers and early elementary-aged children with and without disabilities. PASS consists of three instructional units—Rhyming, Blending, and Segmentation—that can be used together or in isolation, depending on a child's current phonological performance profile.

In each unit, there are a series of highly structured lessons based on a developmental sequence of learning objectives: each lesson follows an identical format of opening activity, guided instruction, and closing activity. Each lesson can be taught in approximately a half hour, and the program is designed so that two to three lessons per week will permit a youngster to complete all three units in approximately 6 months. Evidence-based practices are embedded in the scripted lessons, and the program provides assessment/progress-monitoring procedures and forms. All lesson stimuli and materials are included, as are nine children's books such as *Mouse Mess* (Riley); *Polar, Bear, Polar, What Do You Hear?* (Alhern); and *Dogs Don't Wear Sneakers* (Numeroff). PASS is intended to be used in conjunction with letter–sound correspondence training because phonemic awareness instruction has most impact on early reading when accompanied by alphabetic principle training.

PASS has demonstrated efficacy and effectiveness with several child populations, including preschool children with and without speech and language disabilities, preschool children at risk for literacy difficulties, and children who are English language learners (ELLs). Further, research findings show that this instructional program is effective when implemented in several different contexts: as a whole-class activity, in small-group instruction, in one-on-one instruction, and in tier-based models of instruction such as RTI (e.g., Roth, Troia, Worthington, & Dow, 2002; Roth, Troia, Worthington, & Handy, 2006; Roth, Worthington, & Troia, 2009).

Three lessons are presented in Appendix 4-F that represent different levels of task difficulty:

- The Rhyming lesson demonstrates a receptive task at the level of Matching and Recognition: Choosing two pictures that rhyme from a set of three.

- The Blending lesson utilizes a yes/no judgment task in which a child is given a word phoneme by phoneme (e.g., b-a-t) and then a whole word. The child is required to indicate whether the whole-word version is the same as or different from the unblended version.

- The Segmentation lesson requires a child to produce a word using its individual sounds (e.g., when given the word "bat," the correct response is "b-a-t").

Alphabetic Letter Name and Sound Knowledge

- Program instruction hierarchically in the following order: letters in which the sound represents the beginning of the letter name (e.g., b, p); letters in which the sound represents the end of the letter name (e.g., f, l); and, finally, letters in which the sound is not related to the letter name (e.g., w, y). (*Note:* The order in which alphabetic letters are introduced varies across curricula. The order presented here is one example.)

- Call attention to the way letters are formed by the mouth (e.g., lip rounding for /w/ or tongue tip elevation for /t/).

- Call attention to the sounds that each letter makes (e.g., "em" is the letter's name, whereas /mmmm/ is the sound it makes).

Adult Modeling of Literacy Activities

- Provide frequent opportunities for the child to observe adults engaged in reading and writing in natural contexts (e.g., preparing a grocery list, following written instructions to assemble a toy).

- Engage the child as a "helper" in everyday activities (e.g., hunting for items in a catalog or following a simple recipe to prepare a favorite food).

- Engage the child in interaction with various kinds of written materials (e.g., menus, shopping lists, recipes, books)

Experience with Writing Materials

- Provide materials that permit children to write by themselves (e.g., pens, pencils, markers, crayons, rudimentary keyboarding).

- Facilitate all forms of writing (e.g., drawing, scribbling, basic letter formation). (See Table 4-13 for stages of writing development.)

- Encourage child to dictate a "story" given visual stimuli (e.g., wordless picture books, cartoon frames).

Example Profiles

Following are two typical profiles of preschool children with language disorders. These examples have been designed to illustrate the selection of intervention targets, as well as a variety of service models, specific therapy approaches, activities, and materials. Most are easily implemented in either individual, small group, or classroom settings.

Austin is a 3-year, 1-month-old male child who presents with moderate delays in receptive and expressive language skills. Birth and developmental history are unremarkable, and hearing acuity is within normal limits. The results of a recent speech-language evaluation indicate that Austin's language comprehension abilities approximate the 24-month level, whereas expressive language skills fall at the 18- to 20-month level. Numerous articulation errors also were noted. Family members and the preschool teacher report that Austin is a socially interactive child who understands simple directions and communicates mainly through single words and occasional gestures.

Selection of therapy targets. The areas to be targeted are the comprehension of two-step commands, production of action + object utterances, and comprehension of early developing wh- questions. These targets were selected for two primary reasons: (1) These behaviors represent the next logical steps in the normal developmental sequence and (2) they are highly relevant to the majority of Austin's daily activities. In addition, shared book reading was selected as an instructional focus to enhance the development of emergent literacy.

Sample Activities

Following Directions

1. Gather 20 common objects with which the child is familiar. Develop a list of 10 two-step commands, each containing four linguistic elements in verb + object (V + O) constructions (e.g., "*Give me the car and push the spoon*"). Place three objects at a time on the table in front of the child. Verbally present the corresponding two-step command and encourage the child to perform each part as it is spoken. If the child is successful, repeat the same stimulus but instruct the child to refrain from responding until the entire two-stage command has been presented. Following are sample commands:

   Pick up the cup and give me the shoe.

   Throw the spoon and wave bye-bye to the doggie.

   Give me the cup and push the car.

   Drop the spoon and point to the ball.

   Give me the brush and pick up the shoe.

   Push the doggie and throw the ball.

   Open the book and drop the cup.

   Close the box and give me the car.

   Hug the doggie and bang the spoon.

   Pick up the block and close the book.

Two-Word Utterances

2. Develop a list of 20 two-word action + object utterances containing vocabulary words that are already part of the child's spontaneous expressive repertoire. Try to develop sets of two or three utterances that are topically related to one another, to provide a meaningful context. Examples include the following:

open juice	throw ball
pour juice	kick ball
drink juice	roll ball
open book	wash baby
read book	brush hair
close book	kiss baby

   Gather toy replicas of each of the objects and any other toy props that may be required to perform the action sequences (e.g., for the utterance, "pour juice," a juice container and a cup will be needed). Place the objects in a large bag or pillowcase. Shake the bag to solicit the child's attention. Instruct the child to close or cover his eyes and to pull one of the objects from the bag. Depending on the child's abilities, either label the object or ask the child to name it. Then ask the child to perform one of the actions on the object (e.g., "Open the juice") and say, "What are you doing?" or "What's happening?" Following the child's correct production of the target utterance "open juice," reinforce the response with a comment such as "I like the way you opened the juice so carefully" or an expansion such as "You opened the juice." Then ask the child to perform another action with the same object (e.g., "Pour the juice"). Repeat the same training sequence with the other action + object combinations. If the child does not produce a verbal response or responds with a single-word utterance (e.g., "open"), model the target two-word utterance and repeat the item. After two unsuccessful attempts with a given utterance, model the target response and proceed to the next item.

Understanding wh- Questions

3. Obtain a theme toy such as a farm, house, car wash, airport, or hospital and four toy people that can serve as a "mommy," "daddy," "sister/brother," or "baby," based on the composition of the child's family. Place the theme toy (e.g., house) on the floor in front of the child and put the "family" in front of the house. To ensure understanding of the lexical items, ask the child to point to each of the locations in and around the house and the family members when named. Examples of locations include the following:

kitchen	patio
bedroom	stairs
bathroom	laundry room
den/family room	backyard
basement	dining room

Instruct the child to place one of the people in a location about the house (e.g., "Put mommy in the living room") and say, "Who is in the living room?" Following the child's correct response, query the child: "Where is mommy?" Reinforce a correct response with a comment, expansion, or other scaffolding utterance. If the child responds incorrectly to either or both of the wh- questions, provide a prompt such as "Who? Mommy. That's who is in the living room. Mommy." Then ask: "Who is in the living room?"

Shared Book-Reading

4. Select a simple story from children's literature (e.g., "The Three Bears") to read to the child. Throughout the reading of the book, engage the child in the PEER picture-book-reading routine (Burns, Griffin, & Snow, 1999):

P = *Parent*/adult initiates exchange about the book (e.g., "What are the three bears doing?")

E = Parent/adult *evaluates* child's response (e.g., "Yes, Papa Bear is tasting the porridge.")

E = Parent/adult *expands* child's response (e.g., "And what is Momma Bear doing?")

R = Parent/adult *repeats* initial question to check child's comprehension (e.g., "What are the three bears doing? Do you remember?")

Keisha is a 5-year, 7-month-old female child who demonstrates a mild receptive language delay and a moderate expressive impairment. Birth and medical history are unremarkable except for chronic middle ear infections during the first 2 years of life. At present, Keisha exhibits normal hearing acuity bilaterally. Her current communicative status is characterized by a 6- to 9-month delay in most areas of language comprehension. Her language production abilities are more impaired, approximating the 3- to 3½-year level and consisting primarily of three-word utterances that tend to be telegraphic in nature (e.g., "It my book"; "Daddy sleeping bed"). Keisha's pragmatic use of language is essentially age appropriate and her speech intelligibility is judged to be good.

According to her kindergarten teacher, Keisha seems to understand most classroom activities but experiences a great deal of difficulty with emergent literacy skills such as sound-letter correspondence.

Selection of therapy targets. The areas to be targeted are the auxiliary verb *is*, regular plural *-s*, and rhyme recognition. This auxiliary form was chosen for two reasons: (1) the progressive *-ing* form is already occasionally observed in Keisha's spontaneous speech and (2) the productive use of this auxiliary form would significantly decrease the telegraphic quality of her utterances. The plural marker *-s* was selected because Keisha grasps the concept of plurality but lacks the means for coding this information linguistically. Finally, rhyme recognition was targeted because it is a basic phonological awareness skill that contributes to early reading success. The SLP and the classroom teacher will work together to reinforce these learning objectives in the classroom setting.

Sample Activities

Present-Progressive-Tense Marker

1. Collect 20 pictures or drawings of single agents performing various actions and attach each picture to an index card or other durable surface. Appropriate actions may include the following:

eating	kissing
drinking	reading
sleeping	hugging
laughing	painting
crying	washing
kicking	driving
throwing	swimming

   Cut basic shapes of laundry items (e.g., shirts, pants, socks) out of colored paper and mark an X on several of them. Loosely attach one picture card to the back of each laundry item cutout. String a clothesline between two chairs and hang the cutouts on the line with clothespins. Explain that the laundry items will be removed from the line one at a time. As the child removes an item from the line, the clinician models an appropriate sentence incorporating the *is ___ ing* construction (e.g., "The boy is swimming"; "He is sleeping") and instructs the child to imitate it. Following a correct response, the child can remove the picture card from the cutout to look for an X on the back of the laundry item. If an X is found, the child receives a sticker or other reinforcer. Repeat this sequence for all 20 action pictures.

Plurals

2. Gather materials including paper, marker, small paint bottle with sponge top (i.e., bingo marker), pictures or drawings of 10 single and 10 multiple objects, index cards, and a Colorforms kit. Using the marker, make a 20-square bingo board template (four rows of five squares each) on a large piece of paper. Laminate the pictures to the index cards and stack them randomly in a deck. Instruct the child to select the top card from the deck and name it three times. Remind the child that plural *s* must be added to the end of a word whenever more than one object is pictured (e.g., shoes). If all three productions are correct, the child uses the bingo marker to place a dot in one of the squares on the bingo board. Each time a row of five dots is completed, the child is given a Colorform® piece. After the final row is completed, the child is allowed to create a picture using all of the accumulated Colorform pieces.

Rhyme Recognition

3. Write the numbers 1 to 10 on 3-by-5-inch index cards. Construct a list of 20 word-rhyme pairs, two of which rhyme with each number (adapted from B. Baden, personal communication, March 1994). Examples of rhyme pair stimuli are as follows:

1 = sun done	6 = kicks-fix
ton-won	mix-sticks
2 = clue-blue	7 = heaven-leaven
shoe-moo	Evan-Kevin
3 = see-knee	8 = date-gate
tree-free	wait-mate
4 = store-pour	9 = dine-line
sore-wore	fine-mine
5 = dive-hive	10 = men-pen
chive-drive	then-den

Review the concept of rhyming with the child by explaining that rhymes are words that end in the same way. Give some examples of words that do and do not rhyme (e.g., hat-bat, shoe-blue, map-cap, cat-cow, top-tall), explaining why each does or does not rhyme. Place the number cards in a row on the table or floor in front of the child. Ask the child to name each of the numbers aloud. Explain that the clinician will say words that rhyme with or sound like the numbers on the cards. Instruct the child to listen carefully as the clinician says each rhyme pair and to hold up or point to the corresponding rhyming number. For example, the clinician says "store-pour" and the child holds up the number 4. Following a correct response, say, "That's right, store-pour-four all rhyme with each other." Instruct the child to repeat the verbal sequence.

Note: A variation of this activity is to substitute color words for number words with children who have reliable color word vocabularies.

Helpful Hints

1. It may be useful to teach the agent + action and action + object semantic relations sequentially because it generally provides an easy transition into three-word utterances (i.e., agent-action-object constructions).

2. Clinicians can encourage families to engage children in activities to promote emergent literacy. These may include the following:

   - Reading aloud to a child who is in a comfortable position. Ideal books for children at this age range include objects to identify, language that repeats and has rhymes, and activities that are highly familiar to the child.

   - An adult reads a story and has the child draw a picture to go with it.

   - Have the child plan a party for four to six people. Look in the food section of the newspaper for ideas of what to serve.

   - Adult and child look through newspapers and clip out articles about events in different parts of the world and attach each article to its location on a map or globe.

   - Create a "sound-activity" calendar to promote phonological awareness skills. Each day on the calendar identifies a short, fun activity that families can easily incorporate into daily activities (e.g., On Monday, "Tell me three words that start with the sound /b/"; on Tuesday, "Do *bat* and *cat* rhyme?"; on Wednesday, "What would the word *cupcake* sound like if we didn't say the *cup* part?"; on Thursday, "Guess the word I'm trying to say *ba...na...na*"; on Friday, "Which word doesn't belong: *make, take, boot?*"). These can be repeated several times throughout the day in a wide variety of contexts (e.g., bath time, grocery store, car trip).

3. It may be more effective to repeat or expand a child's utterance than to directly correct the child's form.

4. Encourage parents to use daily activities (e.g., putting away toys; put clothes in hamper) to practice one- and two-step instructions. Model activity as needed and provide praise for a job well done.

5. Many of the language and communication activities in *RTI in Action: Oral Language Activities for K–2 Classrooms* (Roth, Doughtery, Paul, & Adamczyk, 2010) are appropriate for preschool children.

6. Parents of children with severe language impairments often overestimate their child's level of ability, particularly in the area of language comprehension. Effective counseling may require that the clinician carefully guide parents to a more realistic perception of their child's true language skills.

CONCLUSION

This chapter has presented basic information, protocols, and procedures for intervention for early childhood language disorders at an *introductory* level. This information is intended only as a starting point in the reader's clinical education and training. For more in-depth coverage of this area, the following readings are recommended:

Nelson, N. W. (2010). *Language and literacy disorders: Infancy through adolescence.* Boston, MA: Allyn & Bacon.

Owens, R. E. (2013). *Language disorders: A functional approach to assessment and intervention* (6th ed.). Needham Heights, MA: Allyn & Bacon.

Paul, R., & Norbury, C. (2012). *Language disorders from infancy to adolescence: Assessment and intervention* (4th ed.). Boston, MA: Mosby.

Schwartz, R. (Ed.). (2012). *The handbook of child language disorders.* New York, NY: Taylor and Francis.

ADDITIONAL RESOURCES

Pro-Ed
8700 Shoal Creek Boulevard
Austin, TX 78758-9965
Phone: 800-897-3202
Fax: 800-397-7633
Web site: http://www.proedinc.com

Early Communication Games
These games encourage infants from birth to 24 months to develop beginning communication skills. They also include reproducible handouts and a set of goals for the child's development, making it an ideal resource for bridging the gap between assessment and development of functional goals on the IFSP. Separate lists of skills are provided for children functioning at a developmental level of 0–12 months and for those functioning at 12–24 months.

Books Are for Talking Too!, **3rd Edition**
A compendium of suggested books for preschool through 12th grade. For each book, the following information is provided: (1) synopsis of the book, (2) the target area for therapy, (3) suggested strategies for teaching targets, and (4) suggested grades and interest level.

LinguiSystems
3100 Fourth Avenue
P.O. Box 747
East Moline, IL 61244
Phone: 800-776-4332
Fax: 800-577-4555
Web site: http://www.linguisystems.com

Maxwell's Manor: A Social Language Game

This game teaches students the social skills needed to get along with others, be more accepted by their peers, and be successful in the classroom. A dog named Maxwell leads the way as students practice positive social language skills. Six card decks offer practice in nonverbal communication, conversational skills, being a friend, practicing self-control, being polite, and following the rules.

Take Home: Preschool Language Development

This illustrated resource augments therapy objectives through interaction techniques and fun activities that enhance speech and language development at home. The take-home language development activities are easily modified to meet individual needs.

Preschool Vocabulary Cards: Actions, Concepts

These age-appropriate cards can be used to expand younger clients' receptive and expressive vocabularies as well as help them make requests and construct sentences. The full-color illustrations reflect the vocabulary and experiences that preschoolers are exposed to every day.

Speech and Language Activities for Young Learners

This literacy-based intervention program uses multisensory information to help develop articulation and phonology skills. Each chapter is based on a well-known children's book and the activities relate to the story and reinforce story concepts. The articulation, phonological awareness, and phonological pattern activities focus on critical skills needed to become a successful speaker and reader.

Just for Me! Series: Concepts

Teaches basic concepts in four areas: spatial, attributes, quantity, and temporal. The activities include coloring, cutting, and creating an example of each concept.

The Speech Bin
P.O. Box 922668
Norcross, GA 30010-2668
Phone: 800-850-8602
Fax: 800-845-1535
Web site: http://www.speechbin.com

Practicing Individual Concepts of Language (PICL)

Board game that reinforces skills in language content and use. Two to six players learn target structures in 30 categories, including vocabulary, qualitative concepts, pronouns, plurals, and verb tenses.

Silly Sentences

Card games to learn: subject + verb agreement, subject + verb + object (S + V + O) sentences, humor and absurdities, speech sound articulation, questioning and answering, and present progressive verbs. Includes three color-coded decks of 40 cards each.

Creatures and Critters: Barrier Games for Referential Communication

These language barrier games use dinosaurs and other "critters" to teach children how to take turns, listen for details, follow and give directions, and understand listeners' needs. Five decks of full-color cards, a manual, and data sheets are included.

Speech and Language Handouts

These are two-sided fact sheets to answer parents' questions about speech/language development at specific ages and regarding topics along several speech/language parameters, such as developing pragmatic skills, fostering listening skills, increasing vocabulary, keeping a healthy voice, reading to your child, and so forth.

Super Duper Publications
P.O. Box 24997
Greenville, SC 29616
Phone: 800-277-8737
Fax: 800-978-7379
Web site: http://www.superduperinc.com

Webber® Photo Cards: Everyday Go-Togethers

This deck has card pairs that are ideal for memory-based, matching, and Go Fish games. All cards are 3 by 4 inches, and the deck has content/game idea cards in six languages: English, Spanish, Japanese, Chinese, French, and German.

Webber Classifying Cards

This large, colorful card pack comes in carrying tote with seven decks, including animals, food, around the home, occupations, clothing, transportation, colors, shapes, and numbers.

Look Who's Listening

For ages 3 and up, this includes 10 auditory games in one. Included are auditory skill card decks to target auditory discrimination, auditory memory, and auditory integration. Students take turns listening carefully, following card directions, rolling the die, and placing tokens on the game board.

Interactive Sing-Along Big Books

These books teach early reading skills through music. All books come preassembled and include a music CD with two recordings of all songs. One track uses a slower pace to help children learn the song. The second track has a more natural pace for children after they have learned the song.

Brookes Publishing
P.O. Box 10624
Baltimore, MD 21285-0624
Phone: 800-638-3775
Fax: 410-337-8539
Web site: http://www.brookespublishing.com

Road to the Code

This developmentally sequenced 11-week program is designed to give kindergarten and first-grade students repeated opportunities to practice and enhance beginning reading and spelling abilities. Contains 44 lessons, each featuring three activities.

Miscellaneous

Burns, M. S., Griffin, P., & Snow, C. E. (1999). *Starting out right: A guide to promoting children's reading success.* Washington, DC: National Academy Press.

> Clinician- and parent-friendly guide to the development of reading and spelling skills in young children. Includes specific activities to promote emergent and early literacy from infancy through mid-elementary school.

Griffith, L., & Olsen, M. A. (1992). Phonemic awareness helps beginning readers break the code. *The Reading Teacher, 45,* 516–523.

> This article contains a list of books that involve sound play for young children.

Torgesen, J. K., & Bryant, B. R. (1994). *Phonological awareness training for reading.* Austin, TX: Pro-Ed.

> Focuses on training in four areas: sound blending, sound segmenting, reading, and spelling. Skills are taught in a sequential manner through a variety of games.
> It includes a detailed description (script) for each activity as well as precise instructions for implementation.

Yopp, H. K. (1992). Developing phonemic awareness in young children. *The Reading Teacher, 45,* 696–703.

> This article focuses on the use of songs and melodies for training phonological awareness and provides specific suggestions.

Yopp, H. K., & Yopp, R. H. (2000). Supporting phonemic awareness in the classroom. *The Reading Teacher, 54,* 130–143.

> This article provides sample phonological awareness activities appropriate for preschool, kindergarten, and first-grade classrooms within a developmental hierarchy of difficulty.

APPENDIX 4-A

DEVELOPMENTAL LANGUAGE MILESTONES: BIRTH TO 5 YEARS

Age	Milestones
Receptive	
1 month	Startle response to loud or sudden sound
	Sound arrests activity; human voice usually has quieting effect
	Generally looks at speaker
2 months	Alert to surroundings
	Direct regard of speaker's face
	Visually and auditorily recognizes mother
	Beginning response to human voice
	Anticipates bottle
3 months	Localization: turns head when hears a voice; may not be in direction of sound
	Frightened by angry voices
	Excited when favorite toy is presented (increased kicking, arm waving)
	Resists adult who playfully tries to remove toy from grasp
	Aware of strange people and situations
4 months	Cessation of crying upon hearing human voice
	Reciprocal gaze (4–8 months)
	Responds to name by turning head (4–6 months)
5 months	Localization: horizontal plane to right or left depending on sound source
	Responds to "no" when said with inflection
	Distinguishes meaning of warning, anger, and/or friendly voices (changes in facial expression and/or body gestures)
	Responds to gesture stimulus with a gesture response (e.g., come up)
	Recognizes familiar environmental sounds (e.g., doorbell, running bath water)
	Reciprocal gaze (4–8 months)
	Responds to name by turning head (4–6 months)

(continues)

Age	Milestones
6 months	Localization: two-step behavior, horizontal scan then vertical scan (6+ months)
	Begins to understand a few familiar words such as *mommy, daddy, bye-bye*, and phrases such as "Daddy's coming," "Do you want the bottle?" (change in behavior)
	Responds to name by turning head (4–6 months)
	Reciprocal gaze (4–8 months)
8 months	Responds to "no" said without inflection
	Ceases activity when name is called
	Recognizes names of a few common objects
	Responds to scary faces; "stranger anxiety"
	Pats image in mirror
	Reciprocal gaze (4–8 months)
9 months	Gives toy in hand on request
	Follows simple verbal directions when accompanied by a gesture (e.g., "Get ball," "Open door")
	Uses gesture in response to a verbal *bye-bye* stimulus
11 months	Responds to music with body movements
	Says "bye-bye" on request
12 months	Responds to simple commands without an accompanying gesture (e.g., "Get ball," "Come here")
	Identifies one body part
	Selects object in a two-way object discrimination task
	Understands up to 10 words
14 months	Responds to verbal direction "Give me + object" without an accompanying gesture cue
15 months	Pats pictures in a book
	Points to common objects when named
16 months	Identifies object in a four-way object discrimination task
18 months	Completes one-stage commands containing two linguistic elements in a four-way object discrimination task (e.g., "Throw the car")
	Responds to some question forms: What-doing? Where-object? (18–24 months)
	Points to three body parts
	Attends to pictures and identifies one or more
	Understands up to 50 words
21–22 months	Understands some personal pronouns

(continues)

Age	Milestones
24 months	Follows one-stage commands containing three linguistic elements in four-way object discrimination task ("Give me the car and the spoon") Responds to some question forms: What-doing? Where-object? (18–24 months) Points to at least four body parts Points to five or more pictures Understands prepositions *in* and *on*
3 years	Follows two-stage commands containing four linguistic elements in a four- to five-way object discrimination task (e.g., "Give me the spoon and push the car") Understands some simple wh- questions Recognizes basic colors Understands concepts of same and different Categorizes items into basic groups (e.g., toys)
4 years	Understands 5,600 words Responds correctly to most questions about daily activities Uses word-order strategy to understand message Understands most wh- questions Understands concept of rhyming and alliteration
5 years	Understands 9,600 words Understands temporal concepts (e.g., before/after; yesterday/tomorrow) Follows three-stage commands with six linguistic elements in a four- to five-way object discrimination task (e.g., "Throw the shoe, give me the baby, and kiss the cup") (4–5 years) Recognizes some alphabet letters Understands short paragraph-length material
5½ years	Understands 13,500 words Understands subordinating conjunctions *if, because, when,* in most contexts Understands most simple and some complex sentence constructions; understands reversible passive sentences (e.g., "The dog is chased by the cat").
Expressive	
1 month	Produces undifferentiated crying and vegetative sounds (e.g., cough, sneeze, burp) (0–1½ months) Produces differentiated cry (e.g., pain, anger, hunger) (1½–2 months) Cries if adult removes pacifier

(continues)

Age	Milestones
2 months	Gurgles and coos when played with
	Produces two or more syllables
	Produces vowels with consonant-like sounds (*gu, nu*) that are one second in duration
	Cries if adult removes toy
	Does not cry if adult removes pacifier
	Social smile (2–4 months)
3 months	Vocalizes in response to speech
	Produces pleasure sound (e.g., nasal "mmm")
	Coos without external stimulus
	Social smile (2–4 months)
4–5 months	Produces early babbling sounds; frequently heard consonants: p, b, d, h, w
	Produces some intonation during sound making
	Produces vocal play when playing with toys (e.g., squeals, growls, raspberries, trills: sounds produced in front of mouth)
	Produces approximately four different sounds
	Produces a displeasure sound
	Social smile (2–4 months)
	Takes turns with sounds
6 months	Produces reduplicative babbling
	Responds to name 50% of the time by vocalizing
7 months	Vocalizes upon seeing bottle
	Produces more consonant sounds such as t, n, d
8 months	Vocalizes to threaten, persuade
	Produces five or more consonants
	Shakes head for "no"
9 months	Produces "uh oh" exclamation
10 months	Produces nonreduplicative babbling
	Tries to imitate sounds
11 months	Produces three or more words or protowords
	Produces and imitates sounds and correct number of syllables

(continues)

Age	Milestones
12 months	Produces five or more words (12–14 months) Produces true words during sound play Uses voice and gesture to get objects (12–14 months) Uses jargon; mixes words with jargon Most words are one and two syllables (12–18 months) Speech is 25% intelligible to the unfamiliar listener (12–18 months) Imitates animal noises (12–15 months)
14–16 months	Produces four to seven words Communicates using gesture + words/vocalizations Uses jargon and words in conversation Most words are one and two syllables (12–18 months) Speech is 25% intelligible to the unfamiliar listener (12–18 months)
16–18 months	Produces 6 to 12 words Uses words to express wants and to communicate Imitates most words Uses jargon Most words are one and two syllables (12–18 months) Speech is 25% intelligible to the unfamiliar listener (12–18 months)
18–24 months	Produces 10 to 20 words Begins to combine words into two-word utterances Uses jargon Names one picture in a book Imitates two- and three-word sentences Names some body parts Enjoys humming and singing
20–22 months	Produces 20 to 30 words Uses question intonation (e.g., "Me go?")
22–24 months	Produces most vowels and the consonants: m, b, p, k, g, w, h, n, t, d Uses 50 to 200 words by 24 months 65% of speech is intelligible Uses two- and three-word combinations to express a variety of semantic relationships Names at least three of these objects: car, chair, box, key, fork Says "no" Uses some pronouns but not necessarily correctly

(continues)

Age	Milestones
3 years	Produces 900 to 1,200 words Produces multiword utterances Routinely uses subject-verb-object forms Asks what, where, and who questions Overregularizes past tense (e.g., "goed") Begins to use complex sentences
4 years	Produces 1,500 to 1,600 words Names primary colors; counts to five Uses complex sentence constructions more frequently Uses personal pronouns more accurately Uses negative and question forms correctly Uses conjunctions (e.g., *and, but*) correctly Uses relative pronouns (e.g., *who*)
5 years	Produces 2,100 to 2,200 words Has mastery of most syntactic rules and can converse easily Formulates short, well-structured stories Uses past and future verb tenses correctly
5½ years	Produces 2,300 words Continues to master irregular morphological and syntactic forms

APPENDIX 4-B

GROSS AND FINE MOTOR DEVELOPMENTAL MILESTONES

Age Range	Description and Examples
Gross Motor	
Birth	Newborn is flexed or semi-flexed at rest in all positions; poor head control General inability to move against gravity
1 month`	Lifts head in prone (stomach); turns side to side with bobbing motion
2 months	Holds head up briefly in prone, but bobs
3 months	Attains good head control when picked up; turns heads freely to look around Turns from side to back (supine) Props in prone on forearms and raises head
4–6 months	Sits with support for short periods when put in sitting position Sits without support momentarily by leaning forward Turns head in all positions hands Assumes "swimming" position (supports weight on stomach and wiggles arms and legs off surface [e.g., floor, mattress]) Rolls from prone to supine Props in prone on elbows and reaches with arm Plays with feet; brings feet to mouth
6–8 months	Attains independent sitting without support when placed in sitting position May try to creep/crawl; sometimes backwards Engages in segmental rolling (effortless rotation of the trunk and body, with weight shifting, and coordinated movements of the head, neck, and upper body) Assumes "plantigrade" position (pushes up on hands and feet and rocks back and forth in a continuous motion) May exhibit "belly crawling"
8–9 months	Pulls to stand on furniture
9–11 months	"Comes to sit" (gets in and out of sitting from any position) Stands alone briefly Crawls easily Sits from a standing position Shifts weights from one foot to the other while standing Cruises sideways along furniture, shifting weight laterally End of period: stands alone, but collapses when balance is threatened

(continues)

Age Range	Description and Examples
12–15 months	Stands alone Walks alone with hands in "high guard" (hands raised above shoulders)
15–18 months	Walks with rapid gait Throws ball over and under hand
18–20 months	Motorically very active Walks smoothly Walks *up* stairs with assistance, 1 foot at a time Runs stiffly Throws and catches ball Jumps with 2 feet without falling
21–23 months	Walks up *and* down stairs with support Jumps, runs, and climbs Kicks large ball
2 years	Runs smoothly Walks up and down stairs without alternating feet
3 years	Walks up and down stairs without assistance Walks backward Stands alone on 1 foot—balancing momentarily Rides tricycle/scooter Catches smaller ball and throws it
4 years	Jumps over objects Hops on 1 foot
5 years	Shows good gross motor control and body awareness
Fine Motor	
Birth–4 weeks	Reflexive finger closure (around rattle, ring, or pacifier)
2 months	Opens and closes hand
3 months	Reaches and grasps Swipes at objects
4 months	Begins thumb opposition Manipulates and lifts objects Puts objects in mouth
5–6 months	Begins evolution of ulnar grasp (uses of 4th and 5th digits to grasp cube) Cube grasp progresses from the ulnar grasp → palmar grasp (mid fingers; 7–8 months) → radial grasp (use of thumb and forefinger; 9–10 months)

(continues)

Age Range	Description and Examples
7 months	Transfers object from hand to hand
	Begins evolution of the "pellet grasp"; picks up pellet (small round object) with thumb and forefingers opposed without using thumb)
	Thumb is used as a stabilizer and child secures objects by flexing fingers toward the palm; called a primitive raking grasp
8–9 months	Manipulates objects to explore
	Drops and throws objects
	Puts objects in containers
	Holds bottle
10 months	Holds cup for drinking
11 months	Begins to feed self with spoon
12 months	Points with index finger
	Demonstrates mature thumb opposition ("superior pincer grasp"); enables thumb to move to tip of index finger. This grasp develops in 3 stages:
	(1) raking (8 months) → (2) scissors (aka inferior pincer grasp) (object is held between thumb and forefinger) → (3) superior pincer (12 months)
	Uses spoon, cup
	Holds crayon, marker
	Removes socks
	Imitates adult's use of objects
12–18 months	Uses fork or spoon when eating, inefficiently
	Turns 2—3 pages at a time
	Scribbles lines (15 months)
	Drinks unassisted (18 months)
	Scribbles in circles (18 months)
21 months	Unzips
	Fits puzzle pieces (easy ones)
2–3 years	Turns pages one by one
	Opens door and turns on faucet
	Folds paper in half
	Effectively eats with utensil
3–4 years	Unbuttons, but has difficulty buttoning
	Cuts with scissors
	Takes apart objects
	Copies block letters

(continues)

Age Range	Description and Examples
5 years	Cuts food with knife
	Colors well within lines
	Prints simple words
	Dresses without assistance
	Has established hand preference

SOURCES: Adapted from Gallahue, D. L. (1994). Motor development. In J. Winnick (Ed.). Adapted physical development and sports. Champaign, IL: Human Kinetics. Piper, M. C., & Darrah, J. (1994). Motor assessment of the developing infant. Philadelphia, PA: Saunders. Robertson, M. A., & Halverson, L. E. (1984). Developing children—Their changing movement. Philadelphia, PA: Lea & Febiger.

APPENDIX 4-C

STAGES OF COGNITIVE DEVELOPMENT

Stage	Age	Name and Description
Sensorimotor	Birth–2 years	
Stage 1	birth–1 month	*Random and Reflex Actions*: Hunger cry and reflexive sucking
Stage 2	1–4 months	*Primary Circular Reactions*: A patterned action that produces feedback which then re-elicits the same action. These are natural cycles of repetition (i.e., circular). At first, these actions occur by chance and lead to an interesting result (e.g., brings thumb to mouth). The infant immediately tries to reinstate/rediscover the behavior. After a process of trial and error, the infant succeeds. The behavior is usually part of the infant's existing repertoire (e.g., sucking, grasping). This is the first time the infant shows *voluntary* action, and the action is centered around the baby's own body.
Stage 3	4–10 months	*Secondary Circular Reactions*: Called secondary because these reactions involve events/objects in the external environment.
		Infant's horizon has expanded since crawling and manipulating objects. For example, infant accidentally kicks hanging mobile; then reinstates the event to watch it move. *Imitation* emerges at this stage; infant can only imitate actions that he or she can see and already can perform (e.g., clenched and unclenched fist).
Stage 4	10–12 months	*Coordination of Secondary Schemes*: Represents an advance in *intentionality:* has goal in mind from outset and directs his or her behavior toward a desired outcome (e.g., pushes away truck to get ball); attains *object permanence* (at 12 months): concept that an object no longer ceases to exist when it disappears from baby's visual field. Imitation advances; baby imitates actions he or she cannot observe, and can imitate new models that are not too different from own (e.g., facial expressions).

(continues)

Stage	Age	Name and Description
Stage 5	12–18 months	*Tertiary Circular Reactions*: Now walking, child searches for novelty and has "curiosity about the world for novelty's sake"; he or she explores objects and what can be done with them. Child uses *new means to an end* (e.g., if pushing an object fails, child tries pulling object instead). What is distinct about this stage is that child varies his or her actions, trying new actions rather than repeating actions already known. Final stage of imitation: Imitation becomes more systematic and adept; child can now modify his or her actions to make them exactly like the model.
Stage 6	18–24 months	*Inventions of New Means Through Mental Combinations*: Onset of symbolic/representational behavior; by symbolic behavior frees child from immediate present and child can re-present reality, which is demonstrated in several areas: deferred/delayed imitation, mental imagery (e.g., drawing), pretend play, and combinatorial language (i.e., syntax).
Pre-Operational	2–7 years	Child demonstrates perceptual thought; child's thinking is influenced by attributes of objects (i.e., irreversibility)
Concrete Operational	7–11 years	Child demonstrates symbolic (logical) thinking; thinking no longer influenced by attributes of objects because child can now think conceptually.
Formal Operations	11–adult	True abstract thinking emerges; child solves complex verbal problems and hypothetical thought (e.g., develop and test hypotheses).

Sources: Paget, J. (1962). The language and thought of the child. London: Routledge & Kegan Paul. Piaget, J. (1928). The child's conception of the world. London: Routledge & Kegan Paul. (London: Kegan Paul. Piaget, J. (1952). The origins of intelligence in children. New York: International University Press. Piaget, J. (1962). Play, dreams and imitation in childhood. New York: Norton, 1962.

(continues)

APPENDIX 4-D

STAGES OF PLAY DEVELOPMENT

Age Range	Description and Examples
6–8 months	Exploratory play: nonmeaningful manipulation of objects (e.g., mouthing, banging, dropping).
9–12 months	Functional play: purposeful exploration of objects. Child shows knowledge of the appropriate use of objects (e.g., bangs toy drum; winds up jack-in-the-box).
12–18 months	Self-related symbolic play. Play behavior mimics daily activities involving only the child and uses only real objects (e.g., child picks up an empty cup and pretends to drink).
18–24 months	Other-related play. Child's symbolic play behaviors begin to involve other recipients of actions, but still uses only real objects (e.g., child uses his spoon to feed a doll). At the end of this period, the child begins to combine action sequences by (1) performing a single action on a variety of different recipients (e.g., feeding a doll, then feeding mommy, and finally feeding self) and (2) performing a series of actions on a single recipient (e.g., feeding a doll, putting it to bed, and kissing the doll good night).
24–30 months	Planned symbolic play. Play behaviors are characterized by (1) child using one object to represent another (e.g., a stick for a spoon); (2) evidence of planning prior to engaging in the play sequence (e.g., child verbalizes or searches for props before initiating play schema); and (3) use of a doll or other object as the agent of the play action (e.g., the doll feeds the baby).
3–5 years	Sociodramatic play. Pretend play sequences involve at least two or more children who (1) select a theme (e.g., going to the doctor); (2) assign roles (e.g., nurse, patient, doctor); and (3) use language appropriate to the different roles. (At this point, language begins to become an integral part of symbolic play.)

SOURCES: Adapted from Nicholich, L. (1977). Beyond sensorimotor intelligence: Assessment of symbolic play through analysis of pretend play. Merrill-Palmer Quarterly, 23, 89–101. Katz, J. R. (2001). Playing at home: The talk of pretend play. In D. K. Dickinson & P. O. Tabors (Eds.), Beginning literacy with language (pp. 53–73). Baltimore, MD: Brookes.

APPENDIX 4-E

DEVELOPMENTAL TOY LIST

Birth to 3 Months
rattles
stuffed animals
textured materials (i.e., smooth, scratchy, fuzzy, and
    soft objects) for rubbing on hands, arms, or feet
mobiles
plate designs (pictures or drawings on paper plates)

3 to 6 Months
rattles
stuffed animals
textured objects that the baby can hold on to
mobiles
mirrors
play gym
dolls
book of faces

6 to 9 Months
blocks
rings on a cone
stacking cubes
vinyl books

9 to 12 Months
ball
containers (to put objects in and take out)
small switches, dials, and slides
busy box
bath toys

12 to 15 Months
pull and push toys
ball
book
floating water toy
playdough
large boxes

15 to 18 Months
toy garage set
zoo set
telephone
bubbles
tape recorder and tapes
toy boats

18 to 24 Months
books
containers that open and close
puzzles
indoor slides
farm set
mini sandbox
pretend painter's set
push and pull toys
water toys

24 to 36 Months
tricycle/Big Wheels
interlocking block systems
puzzles
Lego bricks
toy house
tea set
kitchen set
cars, trucks, road signs
windup plane

36 to 48 Months
tricycle
wagon
board games (Candy Land, Hi-Ho
    Cherry-O)
shape sorter
wooden beads for stringing
medical kit
swings, slides
sandbox
concentration picture matching game

48 to 60 Months
ball
magnetic letters
dominoes
alphabet game
musical instruments (drum, tambourine,
    castanets, bells)
playing cards
art materials

SOURCE: Adapted from Schwartz, S., & Miller, J. E. (2004) (3rd ed.). *The new language of toys: Teaching communication skills to special-needs children.* Bethesda, MD: Woodbine House.

APPENDIX 4-F

EXAMPLES OF LESSONS FROM "PROMOTING AWARENESS OF SPEECH SOUNDS" (PASS)

This appendix contains sample lessons from each of PASS's three instructional units:

Rhyming
Segmentation
Blending

The corresponding progress-monitoring (data-collection) forms also are included.

(continues)

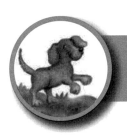

Lesson 5: Instructional

Goal

To develop rhyming skills

Objective

Choose two pictures that rhyme

Task

Recognition

Tips

Use exaggerated volume and articulation for rhyming words throughout the lesson.

Steps

Opening Activity: Gross Motor Song

1. Using Goldie, say, *We are going to sing a song called "Pat-a-Cake." We will move our bodies while we sing it. In the song there are lots of rhyming words. Rhyming words are words that sound the same at the end. Watch me and Goldie.*

2. Model the song once using exaggerated volume, articulation, and movements for rhyming words: man, can, G, me.

> Pat-a-cake, pat-a-cake, baker's **man,**
> Bake me a cake as fast as you **can,**
> Roll it, pat it, and mark it with a **G,**
> And put it in the oven for Goldie and **me.**

Say, *Now, let's do it together!* Then sing the song with movements.

Materials

- Goldie, the dog puppet

- **Student Flip Book**

- **Progress Monitoring Form**

(continues)

3. Say, *Let's sing it again together.* Then, sing it once for each child, substituting his or her name and initial for the yellow highlighted information.

Guided Instruction

4. Say, *It's really important now that you turn on your ears and try very hard to hear the rhymes.*

5. Open the **Student Flip Book** to page 23. Ask the children to name each picture on the page. (Remember to tell children the name of the picture if needed.)

6. Say, *Remember, rhyming words are words that sound the same at the end. Look at the* chair (point to the chair). *Now I want you to look at these two pictures* (point to and name bear *and* brush) *and point to the one that rhymes with* chair.

 If correct, say, **Good,** bear **and** chair **rhyme because they end with** air.

 If incorrect, say, **Brush and** chair **don't rhyme because they don't sound the same at the end. Now let's try** bear**. Oh yes,** bear **and** chair **rhyme because they both end with** air.

For both correct and incorrect responses, say, *Let me tell you what else rhymes with* chair *and* bear. Provide three or four examples of rhyming words without pausing between each word (e.g., care, dare, snare).

7. Follow this procedure, substituting items 2–20 for the yellow highlighted information. Have the children take turns responding and note their responses on the **Progress Monitoring Form.**

Sample	Picture 1	Picture 2
1. chair	bear	brush
2. hat	milk	bat
3. pail	nail	egg
4. carrot	parrot	hammer
5. cake	horse	snake
6. feet	rug	meat
7. phone	mouse	bone
8. duck	truck	wheel
9. mitten	kitten	flower
10. swing	ball	king

(continues)

Sample	Picture 1	Picture 2
11. car	star	spoon
12. rain	bus	plane
13. slipper	zipper	button
14. hole	sun	bowl
15. can	man	corn
16. glue	zoo	cage
17. toe	ice	snow
18. brick	hill	stick
19. fish	fork	dish
20. goat	coat	train

Closing Activity: Gross Motor Song and Fingerplay

8. Say, *Now let's sing "Pat-a-Cake" with Goldie like we did before. Remember, "Pat-a-Cake" has lots of rhyming words. We just learned about rhyming words. Rhyming words sound the same at the end. So listen carefully for the rhyming words. Now let's sing it together!*

   Sing the song with movements and use exaggerated volume, articulation, and movements for rhyming words: man, can.

9. Say, *Let's sing it again together.* Sing it once for each child.

(continues)

Rhyming Progress Monitoring Form

☐ **Lesson 3**   ☐ **Lesson 4**   ☐ **Lesson 5**   ☐ **Lesson 6**

Date: _____

Students: _____   _____

_____   _____

Directions: Indicate correct responses with a plus (+) and incorrect responses with a (–).
Total responses and calculate a percentage correct.

	Example	**Picture 1**	**Picture 2**	**Child 1** Name	**Child 2** Name	**Child 3** Name	**Child 4** Name
1	chair	bear	brush				
2	hat	milk	bat				
3	pail	nail	egg				
4	carrot	parrot	hammer				
5	cake	horse	snake				
6	feet	rug	meat				
7	phone	mouse	bone				
8	duck	truck	wheel				
9	mitten	kitten	flower				
10	swing	ball	king				
11	car	star	spoon				
12	rain	bus	plane				
13	slipper	zipper	button				
14	hole	sun	bowl				
15	can	man	corn				
16	glue	zoo	cage				
17	toe	ice	snow				
18	brick	hill	stick				
19	fish	fork	dish				
20	goat	coat	train				
			Total	/	/	/	/
			Percentage				

Plan of Instruction:

(continues)

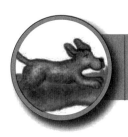

Lesson 25: Instructional

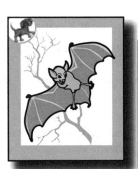

Goal

Develop segmenting skills

Objective

Segment a word into sounds (phonemes)

Task

Production

Tips

Use exaggerated volume and articulation for segmented words throughout the lesson.

If at any time during this lesson a child appears to be unfamiliar with a pictured item, make every effort to ensure that the child learns the vocabulary item before proceeding with the task.

When a letter appears within the slashes (e.g., /m/), **say the sound the letter makes.** Be careful to not add a vowel sound to the letters when you pronounce them (e.g., say /b/ rather than /bu/). Note that the long o, as in row, is represented as /o/.

Steps

Opening Activity: Baby Puppy Game

1. Put the following picture cards face down on the table: soup, bell, cup, ball, man, shark, coat. Have the doggie biscuits and Goldie's dish on the table as well.

2. Say, *Remember, when Goldie was little, she talked like a baby puppy. She was funny because she left the first sound off of her words. When she wanted to play with her ball, she would say all instead of ball. Let's have fun with*

Materials

- Goldie, the dog puppet

- 14 picture cards: soup, bell, cup, ball, man, shark, coat, beach, boot, jeep, mop, ice, bat, duck

- Goldie's dog dish

- 7 doggie biscuits

- **Student Flip Book** (pages 227–248)

- 3 animal game pawns

- **Progress Monitoring Form** (Appendix E)

(continues)

Goldie. Here are some picture cards. You pick a card. Then pretend to be Goldie as a baby puppy and leave the first sound off the word. Let's see if Goldie can figure out what you are saying. If Goldie figures it out, let's give her a doggie biscuit.

3. Be certain the children know the names of the pictures. Have them take turns picking a picture, and then saying the word without the **first** sound while Goldie listens. Have Goldie say the whole word. Let the children judge if Goldie was correct and then give Goldie a doggie biscuit for good listening. If a child has difficulty deleting the initial sound, say the whole word, then say it again without the first sound. Have the child imitate you.

   soup   **b**ell   **c**up   **b**all   **m**an   **sh**ark   **c**oat

Guided Instruction

4. Say, *It's really important now that you turn on your ears and listen well.*

5. Open the **Student Flip Book** to page 227. Place the three animals game pawns in front of the children.

6. Say, *I'm going to show you pictures in this book. The pictures have squares below them. We will be putting one of these animals on each square as we say each sound in the word. Let's try one together for practice.*

7. Point to the demo item in the Student Flip Book. Say, *This is a picture of row. I'll put one dog on the first square and then I'll say the first sound /r/. Now you put an animal in the last square and say the last sound in the word row. That's right, the last sound is /o/.*

8. Point to each animal and say each sound in row, /r/, /o/. Have the children imitate you. Then ask the children what sound each animal stands for when you point to it. Praise the children for correct responses. If the responses given are incorrect, have the children imitate you saying each sound and pointing to the corresponding animal.

9. Repeat this procedure with item 1 in the Student Flip Book. Say, *Look at this picture* (point to the picture of saw) *and the squares below it. This is a picture of saw Put an animal in the first square as you tell me the first sound in the word. Now put an animal in the next square and tell me the next sound.*

 If the child responds by correctly segmenting the sounds in the word, say, ***Good, /s/ is the first sound in saw and /aw/ is the second sound.***

 If the child responds by incorrectly segmenting the sounds in the word, say, ***Oops, /s/ is the first sound in saw and /aw/ is the second sound.***

(continues)

10. Follow this procedure substituting items 2–4 for the text highlighted in yellow. Have the children take turns responding and note their responses on the **Progress Monitoring Form.**

> 1. saw
> 2. knee
> 3. two
> 4. sew

11. Refer to the next demo item in the Student Flip Book. Say, *Now let's try another one. This is a picture of* rope. *I'll put an animal on the first square and say the first sound,* /r/. *Now I'll put an animal on the next square and say the next sound,* /o/. *Now you put the animal on the last square and say the last sound in the word* rope. *That's right, the last sound is* /p/.

12. Point to each animal as you say each sound in rope, /r/, /o/, /p/. Have the children imitate you. Then ask the children what sound each animal stands for when you point to it. Praise the children for correct responses. If the responses given are incorrect, have the children imitate you, saying each sound and pointing to the corresponding animal.

13. Repeat this procedure with item 5 in the Student Flip Book. Say, *Look at this picture* (point to the picture of news) *and the squares below it. This is a picture of* news. *Put an animal in the first square as you tell me the first sound in the word. Now put a dog in the next square and tell me the next sound. Now put an animal in the last square and tell me the last sound.*

 If the child responds by correctly segmenting the sounds in the word, say, ***Good,*** /n/ ***is the first sound in*** news, /oo/ ***is the second sound, and*** /z/ ***in the last sound.***

 If the child responds by incorrectly segmenting the sounds in the word, say, ***Oops,*** /n/ ***is the first sound in*** news, /oo/ ***is the second sound, and*** /z/ ***in the last sound.***

14. Follow this procedure, substituting items 6–20 for the text highlighted in yellow. Have the children take turns responding and note their responses on the **Progress Monitoring Form.**

(continues)

5. news	13. fish
6. comb	14. log
7. five	15. rake
8. sit	16. tub
9. knot	17. witch
10. shave	18. mail
11. dime	19. ham
12. web	20. sun

Closing Activity: Baby Puppy Game

15. Put the following picture cards face down on the table: beach, boot, jeep, mop, ice, bat, duck. Have the doggie biscuits on the table as well.

16. Say, *Remember, Goldie talked like a baby puppy. She was funny because she left the last sound off of her words. Let's have fun with Goldie again. Here are more picture cards. You pick a card. Then pretend to be Goldie as a baby puppy and leave the last sound off the word. Let's see if Goldie can figure out what you are saying. If Goldie figures it out, let's give her a doggie biscuit.*

17. Be certain the children know the names of the pictures. Have them take turns picking a picture, and then saying the word, without the **last** sound, while Goldie listens. Have Goldie say the whole word. Let the children judge if Goldie was correct and then give Goldie a doggie biscuit for good listening. If a child has difficulty deleting the final sound, say the whole word and then say it again without the last sound. Have the child imitate you.

1. bea**ch**
2. boo**t**
3. jee**p**
4. mo**p**
5. i**ce**
6. ba**t**
7. du**ck**

(continues)

Blending Progress Monitoring Form

☐ **Lesson 11**   ☐ **Lesson 12**   ☐ **Lesson 13**   ☐ **Lesson 14**

Date: _____

Students: _____   _____

_____   _____

Directions: Indicate correct responses with a plus (+) and incorrect responses with a (–).
Total responses and calculate a percentage correct.

	Segmented Word	Target Word/Foil	Correct Answer	Child 1 Name	Child 2 Name	Child 3 Name	Child 4 Name
			CV-C (Final)				
1	bea-ch	beach	Y				
2	ma-d	mad	Y				
3	fo-g	fog	Y				
4	di-me	leash	N				
5	key-s	run	N				
6	kno-t	knot	Y				
7	co-mb	yell	N				
8	che-ck	check	Y				
9	wa-sh	nip	N				
10	t-ap	lick	N				
			C-VC (Initial)				
11	v-ote	vote	Y				
12	s-ign	beg	N				
13	sh-ave	shave	Y				
14	p-aint	wood	N				
15	t-ub	tub	Y				
16	g-ame	game	Y				
17	l-ump	chin	N				
18	f-old	name	N				
19	p-ost	post	Y				
20	b-ay	fool	N				
			Total	/	/	/	/
			Percentage				
Plan of Instruction:							

(continues)

Segmentation Progress Monitoring Form

☐ **Lesson 25**   ☐ **Lesson 26**   ☐ **Lesson 27**   ☐ **Lesson 28**

Date: _____

Students: _____   _____

_____   _____

Directions: Indicate correct responses with a plus (+) and incorrect responses with a (–).
Total responses and calculate a percentage correct.

	Word	Child 1 Name	Child 2 Name	Child 3 Name	Child 4 Name
1	saw				
2	knee				
3	two				
4	sew				
5	news				
6	comb				
7	five				
8	sit				
9	knot				
10	shave				
11	dime				
12	web				
13	fish				
14	log				
15	rake				
16	tub				
17	witch				
18	mail				
19	ham				
20	sun				
Total		/	/	/	/
Percentage					

Plan of Instruction:

(continues)

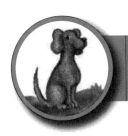

Lesson 12: Instructional

Goal

To develop blending skills

Objective

Judge blending

Task

Judgment without Pictures-Recognition

Tips

Use exaggerated volume and articulation for segmented words throughout the lesson.

When presenting items, be sure to say each segment at one-second intervals.

If at any time during this lesson a child appears to be unfamiliar with a pictured item, make every effort to ensure that the child learns the vocabulary item before proceeding with the task.

Steps

Opening Activity: Dinner with Goldie

1. Place these picture cards face up on the table: fish, ham, rice, meat, corn, soup, and cheese. Set Goldie's dog dish on the table too.

2. Say, *Today we are going to make dinner for Goldie. Everyone gets to be the chef and make different meals for her. We have all this food on the table. I'll say the name of a food for dinner in small parts. Blend the parts in your head and find the matching picture. If you're right, you get to feed Goldie. You can put her food in her dog dish.*

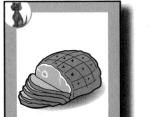

Materials

- Goldie, the dog puppet

- Goldie's dog dish

- 14 picture cards: fish, ham, rice, meat, corn, soup, cheese, cake, chip, juice, peach, shake, nut, gum

- **Progress Monitoring Form** (Appendix D)

(continues)

3. Segment the following words as indicated. Have the children take turns blending the words and feeding Goldie.

> fi-sh (fish)
> ha-m (ham)
> ri-ce (rice)
> mea-t (meat)
> cor-n (corn)
> sou-p (soup)
> chee-se (cheese)

Provide appropriate feedback, say, *You're all doing so well blending word parts!*

Guided Instruction

4. Say, *It's really important now that you turn on your ears and listen well.*

5. Say, *We are going to play a yes/no game. Goldie will tell you a word in small parts and then I will say a word. I want you to tell me if our words match. You say, "Yes" if Goldie's word matches my word, and "No" if they don't match. She'll say the word in small parts, in puppy code, so you will have to listen carefully.*

6. Have Goldie present the segmented word bea-ch. Then, ask, *Did Goldie say beach?*

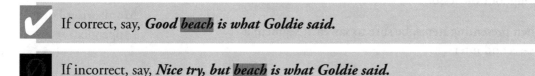

✔ If correct, say, **Good beach is what Goldie said.**

⊘ If incorrect, say, **Nice try, but beach is what Goldie said.**

7. Follow this procedure, substituting items 2–20 for the yellow highlighted information. The first 10 items are segmented as consonant vowel-consonant (CV-C); the last 10 items are segmented as C-VC. Have the children take turns responding and note their responses on the **Progress Monitoring Form.**

	Segmented Word	Target Word/Foil
CV-C	bea-ch	beach
	ma-d	mad
	fo-g	fog
	di-me	leash
	key-s	run

(continues)

	Segmented Word	Target Word/Foil
CV-C	kno-t	knot
	co-mb	yell
	che-ck	check
	wa-sh	nip
	t-ap	lick
C-VC	v-ote	vote
	s-ign	beg
	sh-ave	shave
	p-aint	wood
	t-ub	tub
	g-ame	game
	l-ump	chin
	f-old	name
	p-ost	post
	b-ay	fool

Closing Activity: Dinner with Goldie

8. Place these picture cards face up on the table: cake, chip, juice, peach, shake, nut, and gum.
    Set Goldie's dog dish on the table too.

9. Say, *Now Goldie wants dessert. Everyone gets to be the chef again. We have all these desserts on the table. I'll say the name of a dessert in small parts. Blend the parts in your head and find the matching picture. If you're right, you get to feed Goldie. You can put her dessert in her dog dish.*

10. Segment the following words as indicated. Have the children take turns blending the words and feeding Goldie.

    c-ake (cake)
    ch-ip (chip)
    j-uice (juice)
    p-each (peach)
    sh-ake (shake)
    n-ut (nut)
    g-um (gum)

CHAPTER 5

The initial portion of this chapter provides a description of the developmental language characteristics of two major age groups: 5- to 10-year-olds and 10- to 18-year-olds. These sections are followed by a discussion of several treatment approaches that can be appropriately used across both age ranges. Example profiles and sample activities are then presented for each age group. *The reader is encouraged to review the joint introduction to Chapters 4 and 5 for important information on the following:*

- *Definition of a language disorder*
- *Classification of language disorders*
- *Behavioral characteristics associated with language disorders*
- *Relationship between oral language and literacy*
- *Role of a speech-language pathologist (SLP) in literacy*
- *Theoretical models of intervention*
- *Treatment efficacy/evidence-based practice*

CHARACTERISTICS OF STUDENTS AGES 5–10 YEARS

Several advancements in oral language occur during this period. Children's vocabularies increase in size and in depth of word knowledge (e.g., shades of meaning: *red* versus *crimson*; *run* versus *sprint*). Utterance length increases by an average of one word per year until about 9 years of age, when the length of oral language utterances begins to taper off. Syntactic growth is marked by the increased use of low-frequency structures (e.g., passive sentences) and an increased use of complex sentences (e.g., relative clause constructions).

Another important advance in oral language development during this period occurs in the area of *metalinguistic awareness*. Metalinguistic awareness involves explicit knowledge and the ability to manipulate the structural aspects of language independently from the meaning conveyed by the message. Many language activities require this ability to focus on language as an entity unto itself, including the phonological awareness tasks of segmenting and blending speech sounds or syllables (metaphonology); provision of formal definitions; appreciation of humor, metaphors, idioms, and other figurative language forms (metasemantics); and the ability to make grammatical judgments (metasyntax).

Of particular significance is the refinement of children's phonological awareness knowledge to the level of phonemic awareness (i.e., the ability to segment and blend *individual* speech sounds in words). It has been determined that phonemic awareness, and specifically the ability to segment words into phonemes, is the strongest predictor of early reading and writing skills (Torgesen, Wagner, & Rashotte, 1994; Wagner & Torgesen, 1987; Wagner, Torgesen, & Rashotte, 1994). Thus, there is a developmental relationship between oral language skills and literacy, and further, this relationship is reciprocal. That is, phonemic awareness skills promote early reading ability, and early reading skill furthers the development of phonemic awareness (see Chapter 4 for additional information regarding phonological awareness and its development).

In addition to progress in oral language, children acquire basic literacy skills during the elementary school years as they begin to receive formal instruction in reading and writing. In reading, they first learn to *decode* printed words (and nonwords) by making sound–letter correspondences (i.e., use the alphabetic principle). As children gain word-recognition accuracy, their reading *fluency* improves and they begin to read connected text with greater ease and automaticity. By middle elementary school, the focus of reading and reading instruction shifts to *reading comprehension*, or reading for meaning. Thus, third to fourth grade represents a critical transition because "learning to read" becomes "reading to learn." See Table 5-1 for definitions and stages of reading development.

Third to fourth grade is also the point at which children's writing development progresses in both *spelling* and written *composition* (writing at the text level). By mid to late elementary school, children reach the stage of conventional spelling and can correctly spell a large number of words automatically (see Chapter 4 for the developmental stages of spelling) and can spell with enough fluency to compose sentence-length text. Thus, they display advances in both the processes and products of writing. According to Hayes and Flower (1987), *writing processes* include:

- Planning (prewriting)—generating and organizing ideas about the topic, taking into account both the goal and target audience
- Drafting/composing—putting ideas into words and text
- Revising—reviewing and evaluating content to reorganize, consolidate, and develop new ideas
- Editing written text—polishing the flow and format of the composition

For skilled writers, these process are overlapping and continuous until the final composition is generated. The following *writing products*, the output of writing processes, occur at the word, sentence, and text levels (Dockrell, 2014; Nelson, 2014):

- Word selection and spelling (word level)
- Grammatical complexity and morphological forms (sentence level)
- Cohesion devices that link sentences together (text level)
- Discourse type such as persuasive essay vs. compare-and-contrast composition (text level)
- Capitalization and punctuation (across all levels)

The development of written text structures proceeds from the narrative form to various types of expository writing. Narrative discourse involves story or story-like forms in which the events occur in a chronological order. Expository texts present nonchronologically sequenced events and generally convey information that is novel to the reader. Examples of different types of expository text structures are description, comparison/contrast, and persuasion/argumentation. See Table 5-2 for the differences between narrative and expository texts and see Table 5-3 for different types of text structures and their characteristics. In addition to narrative and expository texts, there are persuasive essays. The main difference between them is that an expository essay explains and provides clarifying information, while persuasive pieces argue for a particular point of view on a debatable topic.

TABLE 5–1

Definitions of Reading Processes and Stages of Reading Development

Terms	Definition/Description
Decoding	Knowledge of letter–sound correspondences (alphabetic principle) to convert print into words
Word recognition and fluency	Rapid and automatic identification of written words
Comprehension	Processes by which printed language is understood and interpreted
Stages of Development	
Word-Level Reading	
Logographic/ Pre-alphabetic	Association of spoken words with environmental print without knowledge of letter–sound correspondences (alphabetic principle); for example, logos, brand names, street signs
Transitional	Partial knowledge of sound–letter correspondences; for example, use of initial or final letter to guess the word; sight-word vocabulary for highly familiar words
Alphabetic	Full knowledge of alphabetic principle; that is, ability to decode both familiar and unfamiliar words
Orthographic	Use of spelling patterns to recognize and pronounce commonly recurring letter patterns as units (e.g., root words, prefixes, suffixes, syllables); builds large reading vocabulary
Automatic word recognition	Proficient and fluent reading of most words by sight
Text-Level Reading	
Phase 1, 4th–6th grade	Can read familiar content (i.e., narratives); consolidates reading fluency and speed; not reading to gain new information so can concentrate on the print
Phase 2, 7th–8th grade	Reads text to learn new information (reading becomes a source of ideas); reads materials that contain one point of view to obtain facts, concepts, how to do things, rather than for nuance; begins to bring prior knowledge and experience to written text; growing importance of vocabulary/word meanings
Phase 3, 9th–12th grade	Can read multiple points of view, can read more than one set of facts, and can acquire new concepts and viewpoints from text (textbooks, reference works, mature fiction, newspapers, magazines)
Phase 4, 12th+ grade	Mature reading stage; reads for greater detail and completeness; reading becomes more qualitative, as reader constructs own knowledge using analysis, synthesis, and evaluation of information from different sources; reads at different levels to obtain desired level of detail, such as skimming versus studying text

TABLE 5–2
Narrative and Expository Text Difference

Narrative	Expository
Purpose to entertain	Purpose to inform
Familiar schema content	Unfamiliar schema content
Consistent text structure	Variable text structures
Focus on character motivations, intentions, goals	Focus on factual information and abstract ideas
Often requires taking multiple perspectives, understanding the points of view of different characters	Expected to take the perspective of the writer of the text
Can use pragmatic inferences, that is, inference from similar experiences	Must use logical-deductive inferences
Connective words not critical—primarily *and, then, so*	Connective words critical—wide variety of connectives, for example, *because, before, after, if-then, therefore*
Each text can stand alone	Expected to integrate information across texts
Can use top-down processing	Relies on bottom-up processing

SOURCE: Adapted from Westby, C. E. (2012). Assessing and remediating text comprehension problems. In A. G. Kamhi & H. W. Catts (Eds.) &, Language and reading disabilities (3rd Ed) (pp. 154–223). Boston, MA: Pearson.

TABLE 5–3
Expository Text Types and Characteristics

Text Type	Function	Key Words
Descriptive	Does the text tell me what something is?	none
Sequence/procedural	Does the text tell me how to do or make something?	*first . . . next . . . then; second . . . third . . .; following this step; finally*
Cause/effect	Does the text give reasons for why something is or happens?	*because, since, then, therefore, for this reason, results, effects, consequently, so, in order, thus, then*
Problem/solution	Does the text state a problem and offer solutions to the problem?	*one problem is; a solution is*
Comparison/contrast	Does the text show how two things are the same or different?	*different, same, alike, similar, although, however, on the other hand, but, yet, still, rather than*

SOURCE: Adapted from Westby, C. E. (2012). Assessing and remediating text comprehension problems. In A. G. Kamhi & H. W. Catts (Eds.) &, Language and reading disabilities (3rd Ed) (pp. 154–223). Boston, MA: Pearson.

CHARACTERISTICS OF ADOLESCENTS 10–18 YEARS

Adolescence is the developmental period during which youngsters (1) develop a stable identity, (2) acquire independence from family, (3) develop career plans, and (4) develop moral and ethical values consistent with those of society (Erikson, 1968). There are three main stages of adolescence, and the intervention goals for each stage differ slightly. In early adolescence (10 to 14), the primary focus is on developing communication skills for academic and personal-social purposes. The goals for mid-adolescence (14 to 16) involve facilitation of communication skills for academic, personal-social, and vocational aims. By late adolescence (16 to 20), language intervention is concentrated on developing communication skills for personal-social and career purposes.

In the adolescent period, communication skills are refined and higher-order language abilities undergo significant development as the child's linguistic system reaches the adult form. Significant growth occurs in the metalinguistic area of nonliteral or figurative uses of language, including idioms, metaphors, proverbs, and humor. These are considered higher-order language forms because they require the ability to go beyond the conventional meaning of language for correct interpretation or use. Figurative language forms increasingly appear in both oral and written language materials beginning in middle and upper elementary school years. In fact, by eighth grade at least 20% of teacher talk and written text consist of nonliteral uses of language (Nippold, 1998; Nippold, Hesketh, Duthie, & Mansfield, 2005).

During adolescence, continued development also occurs in conversational maturity, utterance length, the comprehension/production of complex sentences and linguistic cohesion devices (see Appendix 5-A for types), and low-frequency syntactic structures (language forms that occur in literate texts, spoken and written, with greater frequency than in oral conversational speech, such as expanded noun phrases and expanded verb phrases). Semantic knowledge also undergoes further growth with respect to both vocabulary size and depth of word knowledge. Word knowledge reflects an increased understanding of multiple meaning words (e.g., block, cold) and the literate lexicon (words that commonly occur in scholarly contexts such as textbooks, lectures, and seminars).

In addition to oral language, students demonstrate advances in the written language domain as they become mature readers and skilled writers by the end of this developmental period. Students are reading longer and more complicated texts (see Table 5-1 for stages of reading development) and can increasingly concentrate on obtaining and synthesizing new information from a variety of print materials (i.e., textbooks, essays, poems, reference sources). In both reading and writing, there is a shift in focus from content facts (simple propositions conveyed by a text, such as information about a character in a story or facts about mammals) to content schema (macrostructures that represent the organization of a text structure, such as a story or a compare/contrast essay). Schema knowledge provides structure that allows the reader to do the following:

- Organize sets of facts (content knowledge)
- Assimilate new text information (e.g., new facts)
- Make inferences necessary for accurate and full comprehension (e.g., predict what's coming next; understand what is not explicitly stated)
- Search for information from memory in an orderly fashion
- Improve in the reconstruction and summarization of text

Adolescents' written expression shows steady gains in the use of planning and organizational strategies; the ability to reflect on and revise/edit initial drafts for grammar, punctuation, and word choice; and the ability to meet the organizational and structural demands of different discourse genres. See Table 5-3 for different types of text structure and their characteristics.

Older students with **language learning disabilities (LLD)** frequently demonstrate significant difficulties with both the processes and products of writing. The primary process characteristics of students with LLD are as follows:

- Lack of planning

- Reduced use of background knowledge

- Lack of revision and editing

- Composition does not align with genre

- Reduced sense of audience (understanding audience perception)

Primary characteristics of the writing products of students with LLD are the following:

- Shorter texts

- Reduced sentence complexity (both semantic and syntactic)

- Fewer cohesive ties and less accurate use of cohesion

- Higher proportion of grammatical errors

- Higher proportion of punctuation errors

A final area of importance during this developmental period is **metacognitive/ executive functioning**. Metacognitive abilities involve an awareness of one's own problem-solving abilities and include self-regulation behaviors that are used to guide, monitor, and evaluate the success of one's performance (Baddeley, 2007; Barkley, 1996, 1997). They include planning, attending selectively to certain aspects of a situation, shifting attention as necessary, inhibition of behavioral impulses, setting goals, and organizing/modifying one's behavior and work. Metacognition/executive functioning has been aptly described as "the brain's air traffic control system" (see, e.g., www.developingchild.harvard.edu). Students show marked advances in metacognitive functioning beginning at about fourth grade, and as a result, they gradually become more strategic learners. Metacognition is considered a higher-order ability area because these "meta" strategies must be invoked from the outset of a task and require task analysis and a great deal of planning. Metacognition also requires "mindfulness": skills that allow for intentional, adaptive, and flexible learning. Students with these higher-order difficulties often have difficulty with overall organization, in setting and attaining goals, planning according to the task demands, identifying errors in their own work, and initiating alternative approaches to a task (making behavioral adjustments). Knowledge of metacognitive development and deficits is necessary for SLPs because these skills and strategies are largely mediated through language, and they are not generally taught explicitly in the classroom. In traditional educational settings, students implicitly are encouraged/expected to engage in "self-talk" throughout the school day about the nature of a task/assignment, how and why they are doing it, the effectiveness of their strategies, and ways to change their behaviors and strategies.

Students with language and learning disabilities often seek postsecondary education, employment or career opportunities. Many of these individuals continue to need accommodations to function effectively in these advanced settings (Association on Higher Education and Disability [AHEAD], 2008). Qualifying for these supports requires transition documentation of a disability. Unfortunately, there is no uniformity across settings as to the type or rigor of documentation needed. For example, in some environments, the emphasis is on the "history" of disability and its functional limitations rather than a current diagnosis of the disability. In other cases, such as most 2- and 4-year academic institutions, a "recent" diagnosis is required, where "recent" is defined as not longer than the prior 3 years. SLPs, other professionals, and families need to be aware that documentation is required, that it can be burdensome, and that it takes planning and preparation. For example, if an institution, training program, or job site requires recent documentation of a diagnosis, then the SLP can plan to complete an exit evaluation accordingly.

INTERVENTION CONSIDERATIONS FOR SCHOOL-AGE CHILDREN AND ADOLESCENTS

Intervention for school-age students revolves, in large part, around the relationship between oral language and literacy. Language therapy goals are programmed to address the demands and expectations of the educational curriculum. Therefore, service delivery is often accomplished through a variety of models, including classroom consultation and collaboration in addition to more traditional individual therapy sessions. Cirrin et al. (2010) focused on the effect of different service-delivery models (e.g., pullout, classroom-based, indirect consultation) on speech-language intervention outcomes for elementary-school-age students. These authors conducted a systematic review of evidence-based studies published during the past 30 years and found that only five studies met the review criteria and addressed the effectiveness of service-delivery models. Even within this small sample, results were mixed, revealing large gaps in our knowledge of the relative effectiveness of difference service delivery models.

Approaches to goal selection still may include a developmental focus, especially for younger school-age children. However, strategies designed to facilitate *functional* performance are used increasingly with preteens and adolescents. Many approaches to language therapy have been designed for the wide variety of communication deficits exhibited by this population. Regardless of theoretical orientation, all intervention goals should be guided by well-designed studies that demonstrate their instructional effectiveness. See Stone, Silliman, Ehren, and Wallach (2014) for a compendium of research-based practices in language instruction/intervention. Clinicians should remain sensitive to the cultural and linguistic background of each student throughout all stages of the intervention process.

For intervention to be successful with the adolescent, the teen has to be a fully cooperative partner in the therapy program. The teen should be consulted regarding the selection of specific therapy objectives, and the clinician must clearly explain the rationale for each target behavior. This allows the student to take ownership of the problem, take primary responsibility for achieving the goals, and recognize that he or she is the one who will lose out if follow-through does not occur. At least two potential problems may be encountered when working with adolescents: (1) resistance to dependent relationships with adults because they are striving to achieve and demonstrate their own independence and (2) rejection of the idea of being flawed or different in any way from their peer group.

The Common Core State Standards

The Common Core State Standards (CCSS) were developed in 2010 to improve the college and career readiness of high school graduates. These national standards outline/map the hierarchy of knowledge and skills in English language arts and mathematics that students should develop within grades K–12 to be competitive in a global workforce/society. Led by state education organizations, the goals of the standards are to improve U.S. educational outcomes and provide equivalent educational opportunities for all students. They are a defined set of increasingly complex standards that are internationally benchmarked (see Table 5-4 for an example of the K–12 "staircase" of complexity for the Reading—Literature standard). The CCSS clearly require that the standards be taught using high-quality, research-based instruction that reflects best practices (www.corestandards .org/). Most states have adopted the CCSS and are in various stages of implementation in K–12 classrooms.

Table 5–4

Example of Increased Complexity of CCSS Across Grade Levels for the Domain of Reading—Literature

Grade Level	Reading for Key Ideas and Details
K	With prompting and support, ask and answer questions about key details in a text.
1	Ask and answer questions about key details in a text.
2	Ask and answer such questions as *who, what, where, when, why*, and *how* to demonstrate understanding of details in a text.
3	Ask and answer questions to demonstrate understanding of a text, referring explicitly to the text as the basis for the answers.
4	Refer to details and examples in a text when explaining what the text says explicitly and when drawing inferences from the text.
5	Quote accurately from a text when explaining what the text says explicitly and when drawing inferences from the text.
6	Cite textual evidence to support analysis of what the text says explicitly as well as inferences drawn from the text.
7	Cite several pieces of textual evidence to support analysis of what the text says explicitly as well as inferences drawn from the text.
8	Cite the textual evidence that most strongly supports an analysis of what the text says explicitly as well as inferences drawn from the text.
9–10	Cite strong and thorough textual evidence to support analysis of what the text says explicitly as well as inferences drawn from the text.
11–12	Cite strong and thorough textual evidence to support analysis of what the text says explicitly as well as inferences drawn from the text, including determining where the text leaves matters uncertain.

SLPs have significant roles in helping students meet CCSS expectations, particularly in the English language arts (ELA) domain. The ELA standards are comprised of four areas: Reading, Writing, Speaking, and Listening and Language, all of which are central to the roles and responsibilities of SLPs professionals for several reasons:

1. Language and communication underlie all of the ELA standards.

2. Language competencies are essential to successful academic, social, and career/ employment outcomes.

3. All students need communication skills to participate meaningfully in the classroom, to learn to read and write, and interact with peers and adults.

4. Developing subject-area knowledge (i.e., disciplinary literacy) depends on the integrity of language skills (the ability to comprehend, generate, and respond to material presented by teachers or contained in texts).

5. At-risk students and students with disabilities generally do not have the requisite language and communication skills to be successful in classroom environments.

Following are examples of specific ELA standards that require language and communication skills and knowledge:

- Ask and answer questions about **unknown words** in a text.

- Describe **characters in a story** (e.g., their traits, motivations, or feelings) and explain how their actions contribute to the sequence of events.

- Determine the **meaning of words and phrases** in a text relevant to grade-level topic or subject area.

- Speak in **complete sentences** when appropriate to task and situation in order to provide requested detail or clarification.

- Follow **agreed-upon rules for discussions** and carry out assigned roles.

- Write **narratives** that recount two or more appropriately sequenced events, include some details regarding what happened, use of **temporal words to signal event order**, and provide some sense of closure.

- **Ask and answer questions** about information from a speaker, offering appropriate elaboration and detail.

- Write opinion pieces on topics or texts . . . and **use linking/transition words and phrases** (e.g., *because, therefore, since, for example*) to connect opinion and reasons.

- Write narratives about experiences or events **using temporal words and phrases to signal event order**.

- Demonstrate understanding of **figurative language, word relationships, and nuances in word meanings**.

- **Adapt speech to a variety of contexts and tasks**, demonstrating command of formal English when indicated or appropriate.

- Determine or clarify the meaning of **unknown and multiple-meaning words and phrases** based on grade-level reading and content, choosing flexibly from a range of strategies.

- **Use common, grade-appropriate Greek or Latin affixes and roots** as clues to the meaning of a word (e.g., audience, auditory, audible).

Many school districts are implementing CCSS within a Response to Intervention (RTI) framework, using multi-tiered instruction to improve student performance in the general education setting. (See Chapter 1 for a description of RTI.) Linking the CCSS with a multi-tiered system facilitates ongoing monitoring of student progress and prevents/reduces learning and behavior problems. It also provides a means to identify students who may be eligible for special education services.

Implementing the CCSS in an RTI framework requires "shared responsibility" among educators. SLPs, general education teachers, special education teachers, other professionals, and students must *collaborate* to develop and implement instructional/intervention approaches that are coordinated, strategic, and deliberate if students in all classrooms are to achieve academic goals. Teachers and SLPs bring distinct but complementary skills sets. Working together, SLPs and teachers can give students support needed to develop and strengthen oral language and literacy skills. For example, SLPs can communicate information about areas of language to teachers (e.g., figurative language; multiple-meaning words, linguistic cohesion; complex syntax), whereas teachers know effective methods for teaching these linguistic areas to students using classroom-wide instructional activities. Following are examples of collaboration opportunities for clinicians:

- Identify initial status and progress-monitoring data to identify at-risk students.
- Develop techniques for classroom-wide implementation of standards.
- Implement team-teaching or demonstration lessons in general or special education classrooms.
- Share responsibility for providing differentiated or increasingly intense instruction for smaller groups or individual students who require additional support.

Although intended for *all* students, the CCSS do not address the needs of students with learning difficulties, including those with identified language-learning disabilities or English language learners. SLPs and teachers have to translate/adapt the standards-based curriculum to specific goals and objectives for Individualized Education Programs (IEPs). This includes identification and implementation of instructional strategies and scaffolds (accommodations and supports) to maximize the learning of each student. Moreover, SLPs and other educators must recognize that implementation of the CCSS does not preclude the need to teach functional skills to students with language-learning and communication difficulties.

TREATMENT APPROACHES FOR SCHOOL-AGE CHILDREN AND ADOLESCENTS

There are a variety of approaches to language intervention, most of which can be implemented with students across a wide range of ages and stages of development. These approaches emphasize the provision of intervention in naturalistic contexts. This means that children/students are engaged in authentic, meaningful activities that are functionally linked to their daily or classroom activities. The basic remediation approaches described here are often used in combination and align with the expectations of the CCSS. The approaches also are appropriate for a variety of service models, including RTI (or other multi-tiered support systems [MTSSs]), other collaborative curriculum-based approaches, as well as small-group/individual therapy.

Previewing. This is a planning strategy that is used to prepare students for upcoming lessons. For oral material, it may involve topic identification, pertinent vocabulary review, and a brief synopsis of information to be presented. In addition to these components, previews of written material may involve identification of section headings and photo captions to provide a "big picture" of the structure/content of a reading selection. The final step in previewing generally involves pausing at the end of a section to check comprehension by restating the information and ideas in the oral/written material.

Predicting. In this approach, knowledge of the subject matter is used to make predictions about content and vocabulary and to check comprehension. Different kinds of knowledge can be the focus of a prediction strategy. For example, information about the genre allows predictions about discourse structure. Information about the *author* can be used to make predictions about writing style, vocabulary, and content.

Think-Aloud. This is a strategy for improving comprehension and monitoring of oral and written material. It focuses on both literal and inferential comprehension. Students are encouraged to engage in self-talk throughout a learning task. Clinicians orally describe their own thought processes while engaged in a difficult comprehension or problem-solving task, in order to model the target behavior. For example, "I am very frustrated because I cannot understand the directions given by the teacher for my homework assignment. What can I do to help me understand it? I will use the strategy: 'Ask again and take notes.'"

K-W-L Procedure. (Ogle, 1986). This approach focuses on improving comprehension of oral or written language, using a three-column chart: K = What we KNOW; W = What we WANT to know; L = What we have LEARNED. The first two columns give clinicians information about students' present knowledge and what needs to be explicitly taught and emphasized. As a new topic/concept is introduced and previewed, students brainstorm everything they know about the topic (prior knowledge) and the clinician records this information in the K column. Then the students generate ideas about what they want to know at the completion of the lesson (W column). Following the lesson, the L column is completed as students identify what they have learned and compare this knowledge to the first two columns.

Metacognitive Stems. This strategy provides students with a structure to improve their organization skills and completion of an assignment. Clinicians teach the steps necessary to complete a task in the correct chronological sequence. As students progress through the steps, they are asked to complete phrases such as: *I'm thinking, I'm picturing, I'm noticing, I'm wondering,* and *I'm feeling,* A visual aid (e.g., poster with written thinking stems) often is provided as a reminder.

Discussion-Oriented Approach. (Ebbers & Denton, 2008). This strategy offers a forum (in classroom or smaller groups) where word meanings are talked about and explained in a conversational context. Students are provided with opportunities to share their background knowledge, ask questions, make predictions about word meanings and correct contexts for use, and validate/modify their predictions.

Social Stories. (Gray, 1995). The main focus of this approach is to improve pragmatic language skills. The clinician develops written scripts that provide explanations of appropriate communicative interaction behaviors in given social situations. These "stories" typically contain both descriptive and directive statements. Descriptive statements provide the specific words, phrases, and sentences that are appropriate in that context, whereas directive statements identify more socially appropriate alternatives to the child's current behavior. For children who cannot read, pictures and other visual supports can be used.

Computer-Driven Therapy. These approaches to language and literacy intervention utilize personal computers to present therapeutic stimuli and feedback. They are generally student-paced and move sequentially through a predetermined hierarchy of difficulty levels. The clinician's primary role is to monitor and facilitate the student's learning progress rather than providing direct teaching. Two examples of computer-driven programs are FastForward (www.scilearn.com) and Earobics (www.earobics.com).

Instructional Strategies for Writing

In 2007, a meta-analysis of different approaches to writing instruction identified the most effective strategies (Graham & Perin, 2007). The report's general findings are summarized as follows:

1. Provide exemplary models that are explicitly contrasted with weak examples.
2. Use strategy-based approaches that are aimed at increasing the quantity and quality of students' background knowledge, knowledge of characteristics of good writing, and knowledge of different text structures.
3. Use repeated revision (e.g., "I will revise my composition three times").
4. Use the spelling editing strategy: Have students read their essays backward, because they are less likely to "fill in the gaps" and more likely to focus on the actual words.
5. Use flash drafting: Have students draft a small portion of text and revise, and then draft the next section followed by revision (this approximates the writing process of skilled writers).
6. Use graphic organizers to highlight the different elements of expository text (see Table 5-3 for details).
7. Provide extended time periods (minimum of 30 minutes) for student writing, with encouraging, constructive feedback provided throughout the writing activity.
8. Combine reading and writing instruction that simultaneously focuses on text comprehension of text and expressing the knowledge in written form.

There are a wide variety of strategy-based approaches to writing instruction. Selected examples of effective strategies are described next.

Self-Regulated Strategy Development (SRSD; Graham & Harris, 1989; Graham, Olinghouse, & Harris, 2009). This approach is used for teaching both narrative and expository texts. It focuses on both processes and products of writing and employs peer-mediated teaching as an instructional technique. It consists of six steps:

1. Develop background knowledge (brainstorm).
2. Discuss/explain the steps.
3. Model the steps (think-alouds).
4. Memorize and rehearse (through self-talk and self-evaluation to facilitate self-monitoring of own progress).

5. Support it (graduated scaffolding: students and instructor collaborate and students write with assistance).

6. Perform independently (scaffolds are faded).

SRSD employs a Think (who will read this?), Plan (what to say), and Write (and say more) strategy to help students plan and generate a sufficient amount of text in their essays.

Genre-Specific (Wong, 2000). This five-step program focuses on teaching specific genres of expository writing such as compare/contrast, cause/effect, and opinion essays. The program provides a rubric for each genre that includes anchors such as clarity, organization, and relevance of information. Prompt cards are used for different essay types and include introductory phrases (e.g., "This paper explains . . ."; "The cause of . . ."), explanatory phrases (e.g., "The reasons for . . ."; "As a result of . . ."), and concluding remarks (e.g., "To sum up the reasons for . . .").

Compensatory Strategies (MacArthur, 2000, 2009). This category of approaches generally involves some form of assistive technology (AT) for struggling writers to supplement, but not replace, explicit instruction. In addition to word processing, examples of AT include: voice-to-text speech-recognition software, word-prediction software, hypermedia (multimedia presentations of materials), and electronic concept map software.

Example Profiles

Following are four typical profiles of children and adolescents with language disorders. These examples have been designed to illustrate the selection of intervention targets, as well as a variety of service models, therapy approaches, activities, and materials. Most are easily implemented in either individual, small-group, or classroom settings.

Willy is an 8-year, 3-month-old male student with normal nonverbal intelligence who demonstrates a moderate broad-based language impairment. His receptive language is notable for a reduced vocabulary, difficulty understanding complex sentence constructions, and difficulty monitoring the adequacy of a speaker's message. Willy's expressive output is characterized by use of simple sentences; omission of grammatical markers; overuse of nonspecific referents; and difficulty relating information in a logical, sequential order. Willy's teacher reports that he continues to experience significant problems with basic grade-level reading materials and word problems used in mathematical instruction (i.e., addition and subtraction).

Selection of therapy targets. Due to the broad-based nature of Willy's language impairment, multiple components of the linguistic system will be targeted for treatment:

- In the area of semantics, categorization skills will be taught to strengthen Willy's vocabulary and concept knowledge.

- Coordinating conjunctions will be targeted to facilitate his use of syntactically more complex utterances.

- Present, past, and future verb-tense markers will be included in the therapy program because Willy consistently omits these morphological forms in his spontaneous speech (although he evidences understanding of the time concepts).

- In the area of pragmatics, therapy will focus on increasing Willy's ability to recognize inadequate messages from other speakers and implement appropriate repair strategies.

- Instruction also will be provided in the metalinguistic area of phonemic awareness (i.e., sound blending) to facilitate the acquisition of early reading skills (i.e., decoding).

- Finally, specific vocabulary will be taught to address Willy's curriculum goals in mathematics.

Sample Activities

Semantic Categorization

1. Collect 15 picture cards depicting items in each of two semantic categories (e.g., clothes and birds) and 10 unrelated picture cards to serve as foils (e.g., book, car, horse). Provide the student with a simple definition of both target concepts. For example: A bird is an animal that has feathers, two legs, and two wings; clothes are things that you wear to cover your body, arms, and legs. Shuffle the cards and place them in a deck on the table. Instruct the student to sort the cards into two piles according to category (e.g., "Find all the birds"). As each card is sorted by the student, the clinician explains why the card belongs in either the birds or clothes category (e.g., "It's a bird because it has wings"). For unrelated foils, the clinician explains why the item should be excluded from the two primary categories (e.g., "It doesn't have feathers, and you can't wear it.").

Note: The categorization activity can be made conceptually more sophisticated by modifying the task according to the following progression:

   a. Sort objects by function (e.g., things we eat, things we use as furniture, things we play with, things we use in a hospital).

   b. Sort objects according to semantic relationships (e.g., "What goes together?"— bat and ball, milk and cookies, hammer and nail).

   c. Sort objects by dimensions or attributes such as size, shape, color, or texture (e.g., big versus little, round versus square).

   d. Sort objects within a single category according to whether they are central or peripheral instances of the concept (e.g., robin versus emu, shirt versus scarf).

Coordinating Conjunctions

2. Develop a list of 20 sentences, each of which contains the coordinating conjunction *and*, *or*, or *but*. Print each sentence on a long strip of paper (approximately 2 inches by 11 inches) with the conjunction word represented by a blank line. Write each of the three conjunction words on small triangular pieces of paper. Following are example sentences:

   The waitress said, "You can order salad, rice, ___ a potato with your meal."

   Ed likes basketball, ___ he likes baseball more.

Which one do you want: soda, hot chocolate, ___ lemonade?

For breakfast, you can have an omelette ___ scrambled eggs.

John ___ Billy went to the movies together.

For lunch, Dion had a hamburger ___ french fries.

Mary had to decide whether to go to New York by train ___ plane.

The dentist drills ___ fills cavities in teeth.

Rita wants to go to the movies ___ she has no money.

Bill wants to be a lifeguard ___ he cannot swim that well.

We ate all the donuts ___ one.

Place sentence strips face-down in a pile in the center of the table. Position the conjunction triangles in a row in front of the student. Define the conjunctions by explaining when each is used:

And is used to connect things together.

Or is used to indicate a choice of one thing over others.

But is used to mean "except," "with the exception of," or "on the other hand."

Instruct the student to turn over one sentence strip. The clinician reads the sentence aloud and instructs the student to choose the triangle that best finishes the sentence and place it on the blank line. The clinician then reads the completed sentence aloud and instructs the student to imitate the model.

Task difficulty can be increased by eliminating the conjunction triangles, thereby changing the multiple-choice format to a spontaneous generation task.

Verb-Tense Markers

3. Print 25 third-person singular active sentences on separate index cards. Develop three cue cards for present progressive, past, and future verb tenses in the following manner:

Yesterday	*Right Now*	*Tomorrow*
-ed	is ___ ing	will

Place the cue cards in a row on the table approximately 3 inches apart in the order illustrated. Place the deck of sentence cards on the table. Instruct the student to read each of the cue words aloud or to repeat each word following the clinician's model. Review the three verb tense forms with the student. Explain as follows:

a. When something has already occurred and is no longer happening, we attach -*ed* to the end of the action word. For example, you would say "Yesterday, the boy order*ed* the pizza."

b. When something is happening right now, we say "is" before the action word and attach -*ing* to the end of the action word. For example, you would say "The boy *is* order*ing* the pizza."

c. When something has not yet happened but will happen in the future, we say the word "will" before the action word. For example, you would say "Tomorrow, the boy *will* order the pizza."

Instruct the student to select the top card from the sentence deck and to inflect the sentence correctly as the clinician points to each of the cue cards. Example sentences include the following:

The girl talks on the phone.

Jose plays his guitar.

Sam walks to school.

The dog chases the cat.

Daddy paints the house.

The teacher points to the world map.

Jamie washes her hair.

Maria wishes for a puppy.

Joey kicks the football.

Mom picks apples from the trees.

Lee cheers for his team.

Monique laughs at the funny clown.

Tim practices his spelling words.

Grandma cooks dinner for the family.

The dog barks at the mailman.

As the student begins to master the past and future tense markers, the cue cards can be modified to include other lexical items that denote these concepts (e.g., *last week, when I grow up, next summer, 2 days ago*).

Recognition of Inadequate Messages

4. Prepare a list of 20 directions for completing a variety of simple tasks and gather the necessary props. Some directions should contain ambiguous, incomplete, unintelligible, or absurd information, whereas others are clearly worded. Examples may include the following:

Direction	*Context*
Give me the red block.	There are no red blocks on the table.
Give me the pencil with the eraser.	All three pencils on the table have erasers.
Give me the #$%$#% (unintelligible).	There are three different objects on the table.
Place the pencil next to the book.	There are a book and a pencil on the table.
Put the money in the brown wallet.	There are three wallets on the table, none of which are brown.
Give me the ingredients for making pizza: dough, sauce, cheese, picture frame.	All these objects are on the table.
Cut a big hole in the white piece of paper.	There are red and white pieces of paper on the table, along with scissors and tape.
Give me three (*mumble rest of message*).	There are three paper clips, six pencils, and five pennies on the table.

Explain that the student will be asked to carry out directions using props and that some of the messages will be inadequate and require more information. This activity focuses on two strategies for obtaining this additional information: (a) asking for repetition of the direction (e.g., "Huh?" or "What did you say?") and (b) requesting clarification of the message (e.g., "Which book?" or "What color?"). Instruct the student to listen to the clinician's messages and think carefully about what is being said. After each direction is presented, instruct the student to identify whether the message was "OK" or inadequate. If the direction is identified as unclear, instruct the student to request a repair using one of the two target strategies. The clinician then revises the original message according to the type of repair requested and the student performs the task. If the student does not recognize the need for repair, prompt with one or more of the following: "Is that clear?", "Did I say that right?", or "Do you get it?"

Phonemic Awareness

5. Print a list of 25 monosyllabic words with initial continuant sounds on index cards and segment each word into phonemes (see following examples). Draw a game board of a bridge that consists of 20 blank spaces and draw a pot of gold at the end of the bridge. Place a small, wrapped "prize" on the pot of gold. Shuffle the cards and place them face-down in a pile in the center of the board. Obtain a game piece that can be moved from space to space on the board and place it at the footpath to the bridge. Explain to the student that, in this game, there is a troll who lives under the bridge and who talks in a very funny way; he says all his words one sound at a time (Lundberg, Olofsson, & Wall, 1980). Tell the student that he has to figure out the words and say them to move his game piece to the end of the bridge and find the hidden prize. Instruct the student to pick up the top card and give it to the clinician. The clinician plays the role of the troll and produces the segmented word, phoneme by phoneme. (Always produce the actual sound rather than the alphabet letter name.) The student blends the sounds together and "guesses" the troll's message. Following a correct guess, the clinician repeats both the segmented word and the whole word. The student is then permitted to move the game piece one space on the board. Following are some sample words:

f—or—k

s—u—n

z—oo—m

v—o—te

m—a—p

s—ou—p

v—e—s—t

n—o—se

f—u—ll

m—a—tch

Curriculum-Content Vocabulary: Math

6. Make two lists of the following words/phrases on separate poster boards and attach to the wall.

Addition Words	*Subtraction Words*
in all	how many more
more	how many are left
altogether	difference
sum	less
total	fewer

Write 10 to 20 simple word problems, half of which require addition and half subtraction, on 3-by-5-inch index cards. (Examples of these follow these instructions.) Obtain two containers into which the cards can be sorted. Label one container with a large plus (+) sign; label the other container with a large minus (−) sign. Provide a highlighter and game board. Explain to the student that the words on the two wall charts are clues for solving math word problems. Review each clue word on the addition chart and remind the student that these are "adding" words; then review each clue word on the subtraction chart and remind the student that these are "take away" words. Shuffle the index cards and place them face-down in a pile on the table. Explain that the top card should be turned over and read aloud. Instruct the student to highlight any clue words that are recognized from the wall charts and state whether the problem requires addition or subtraction. Then have the student place the index card in the correct container. Repeat this procedure for all cards in the deck.

Example Addition Problems

a. Juan has 3 jelly beans and Eddie gives him 3 more. How many does Juan have altogether?

b. Ilana has 5 pencils on the desk and Eli put 4 more on the desk. What's the total number of pencils on the desk?

c. There were 7 birds sitting on a fence. Five more birds joined them. How many birds are there in all?

d. Mary put 6 blue beads on a string. Kayla put 5 red beads on the string. What is the total number of beads on the string?

e. Ali drove 8 blocks to Steve's house and then both boys drove 9 blocks to the store. Find the sum of the blocks they drove.

Example Subtraction Problems

a. Kate has 10 stickers and Shawna takes 4. How many are left?

b. John has 5 green crayons and Daron has 9 yellow crayons. How many more yellow crayons are there?

c. Marsha put 12 cards in a pile and Kim put 7 in another pile. What's the difference between the two piles?

d. Kathy has 9 books and Stacy has 6 fewer books. How many books does Stacy have?

e. Jean drank 14 cups of water. Nan drank 8 cups of water. How much less water did Nan drink?

Note: This activity can be repeated using a game board with spaces color coded for plus and minus. The student rolls the dice and moves a game piece the appropriate number of spaces. If the piece lands on an "addition" space, instruct the student to remove a card from the (+) container and solve the problem. Follow the same procedure for subtraction.

Vivian is a 9-year, 1-month-old female student with normal nonverbal intelligence who has been diagnosed with a learning disability. She demonstrates a significant reading deficit characterized by the inability to decode written words. Weaknesses in the area of receptive language include comprehension of connected oral text, such as stories. Expressively, Vivian experiences notable difficulty with assignments that require formulating definitions for vocabulary known to be within her receptive repertoire. According to the classroom teacher, these difficulties are exacerbated by Vivian's inability to sustain focused attention. As a consequence, her academic performance across the entire fourth-grade curriculum is adversely affected.

Selection of therapy targets. Vivian's profile of oral language and literacy deficits warrants intervention in a variety of areas necessary to effectively learn from teacher discourse and textbook information:

- In the area of semantics, the structure and elements of formal definitions will be targeted to strengthen Vivian's network of higher-order semantic knowledge.

- The framework of narrative structure will be taught to promote recall, comprehension, and production of oral and written text-level material often incorporated into fourth-grade curricula.

- Finally, intervention will target the phonemic awareness skill of sound segmentation in conjunction with letter-sound correspondence training (alphabetic principle) to improve Vivian's reading decoding ability.

Sample Activities

Definitions

1. Create a Jeopardy! game, including stimulus cards, a buzzer, and play money. Use curriculum materials (e.g., textbooks, homework assignments, educational software) to develop a list of 10 to 15 familiar vocabulary words in three or four different semantic categories (see the following sample list with definitions).

Science

a. microscope: A *microscope* is an *instrument* that makes *small objects look bigger.*

b. solar system: A *solar system* is a *group of planets* that *revolve around a sun.*

c. volcano: A *volcano* is a *mountain* that *explodes with lava and ash.*

Math

a. number: A *number* is a *symbol* that *shows how many.*

b. fraction: A *fraction* is a *number* that *compares small pieces or parts to the whole.*

c. calculator: A *calculator* is a *machine* that *does arithmetic.*

English/Language Arts

a. paragraph: A *paragraph* is *two or more sentences* about *a single idea.*

b. topic sentence: A *topic sentence* is a *statement* that *gives the main idea of a paragraph.*

c. comma: A *comma* is a *mark* that *shows a small break between parts of a sentence.*

Miscellaneous

a. bicycle: A *bicycle* is a *vehicle* that has *two wheels.*

b. dog: A *dog* is an *animal* that *barks.*

c. house: A *house* is a *building* that *people live in.*

For each category, print the words on the face of index cards and write increasing dollar values on the back (e.g., $100, $200, $300). Attach the cards to a wall in category columns with the dollar amounts facing out. Construct a wall chart that shows the three key elements of a formal definition, which are the word, the superordinate category name, and a relevant function/attribute of the referent, in a style that the student can understand.

Explain to the student that this activity is a Jeopardy game, in which the student will select a category and dollar level. The clinician will read the vocabulary item and the student must sound the buzzer and respond using the formal definition structure. Correct responses receive play money in the amount listed on the back of the card; incorrect responses result in the subtraction of specified dollar amounts from the total.

Teach the student that a definition explains the meaning of a word by (a) stating the word, (b) identifying the larger category it belongs to, and (c) describing how it looks or what it does. Encourage the student to use the wall chart as a visual cue to remember all three components. For example:

Student: I'll take "living things" for $200, please.

Clinician: Spider.

Student: A *spider* is a *bug* that has *eight legs.*

Clinician: Great definition. You win $200. What category do you want next?

Note: The activity works particularly well in a small group setting.

Narrative Discourse (Oral and Written)

2. Write or identify a short story that contains at least one episode. The story should clearly illustrate the following components:

Setting: Information regarding characters and physical, social, and/or temporal environment

Problem: Occurrence that influences the character(s) to act; precipitating event

Actions: The character's overt attempt to solve the problem

Resolution: The character's success or failure in solving the problem and resultant thoughts or feelings

See the following sample story:

The Cookie Jar Incident

Once there was a stubborn young lady named Leigh-Anne who lived in New York City. Late one afternoon, she was really hungry and wanted a chocolate chip cookie. She knew that she wasn't allowed to eat sweets before dinner, but that didn't stop Leigh-Anne. She sneaked into the kitchen, stood on her tiptoes, and reached for the cookie jar. As she grabbed it, the jar fell on the floor and broke into a thousand pieces. As she heard her mother's footsteps, Leigh-Anne felt guilty about doing something she wasn't supposed to do.

Setting

Character: Leigh-Anne

Environment: New York City

late afternoon

Problem

hungry

no cookies before dinner

Actions

sneaked

stood

reached

grabbed

Resolution

jar broke

felt guilty

Obtain a large poster board and small self-stick notes. Draw a story map like the one in Figure 5-1. Explain that this map will help the student identify the main parts of a story. Using the definitions provided previously, teach the student each of the four story parts and where they belong on the map. Instruct the student to listen as the clinician reads the story

FIGURE 5–1
Story Map

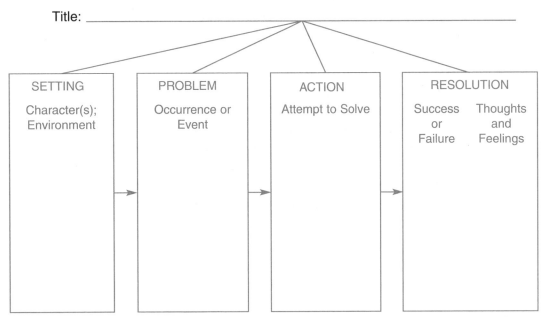

Title: _____

SETTING	PROBLEM	ACTION	RESOLUTION
Character(s); Environment	Occurrence or Event	Attempt to Solve	Success or Failure — Thoughts and Feelings

SOURCE: Adapted from Thomas, P. (1971). "Stand back, said the elephant. I'm going to sneeze." New York, NY: Lothrop, Lee and Shepard.

aloud. Upon completion, ask the student to identify the components of each story part on the map, beginning with the setting and ending with the resolution. The clinician writes each of the student's responses on a self-stick note and has the student place it on the map in the correct box. Then jointly retell the story using the map as a visual guide. Finally, have the student write the story in his or her own words using the story map components in a "beginning-middle-end" format.

Note: The difficulty level of this activity can be adjusted in a variety of ways. To branch down to an easier level, the response mode can be a multiple-choice format, in which the student's task is to select the appropriate piece of story information from an array of completed self-stick notes. To branch upward, the clinician can increase the number of episodes in a given story.

Phonemic Awareness and Alphabetic Principle

3. Make a list of 30 two- and three-phoneme words that are picturable and within the student's expressive vocabulary repertoire. To incorporate exposure to the alphabetic principle, choose words with consonant-vowel (CV), VC, or CVC patterns. Avoid words that involve digraphs (e.g., h*ea*t; *s*o*ap; th*ief*) and silent vowels (e.g., gat*e*; bon*e*; sam*e*). Following is an illustrative word list:

top	cab	up	van	mop	no
cup	bus	in	fog	nut	ma
sad	sit	hi	Dad	nap	me
mat	tag	go	dot	pot	us
jam	red	on	bag	pig	he

Attach the picture for each word to a "playing card." Gather six small blocks and individual alphabet letters (can be written, plastic, or cut from foam).

Tell the student that this game involves breaking words down into smaller parts. Explain that the point of the game is to figure out which words have more sounds. The cards are dealt into two equal decks. The clinician and student simultaneously turn over the top card from each deck (clinician = Deck 1; student = Deck 2). The clinician verbally segments the word from Deck 1 and lines up one block for each sound. Instruct the student to do the same for the card from Deck 2. Tell the student to identify which of the two words has more sounds. The clinician then adds the appropriate alphabet letters on top of the blocks and sounds out that word again. If the student correctly chose the word with the most sounds, the student wins both cards and sets them aside. If the choice was incorrect, the clinician wins both cards. Repeat this sequence until all cards from both decks have been played. (If the two words have the same number of sounds, each player wins one card.) The player with the most cards at the end of the game is the winner.

Note: The difficulty level of the activity can be increased or decreased according to the hierarchy in Table 2, Scope and Sequence for Phonological Awareness Intervention, in the introduction to Chapters 4 and 5.

Pedro is a 12-year, 6-month-old male who presents with a moderate language-learning disability. He demonstrates particular difficulty with higher-order language skills. Specifically, Pedro performs poorly on confrontational naming tasks and tasks that require the comprehension of figurative language forms. His oral and written narratives and expository essays omit essential information and lack a logical sequence. According to direct observation and teacher report, Pedro exhibits difficulty initiating and maintaining conversational exchanges, as evidenced by his tendency to talk about inappropriate topics and interrupt ongoing conversations. Although some minor grammatical errors were observed during timed tasks, comprehension and production of syntax and morphology were noted to be relative strengths.

Selection of therapy targets. Based on Pedro's overall profile, the areas to be targeted involve semantics, narrative discourse, expository writing, and conversational discourse.

- With respect to semantics, idioms were selected because they are among the earliest developing forms of figurative language.

- In addition, word finding was chosen to accommodate the increasing demand at the middle school level for accurate retrieval of specific vocabulary words in different academic subject areas.

- Narrative discourse was targeted to improve Pedro's knowledge of the organization of extended text, because text is the primary vehicle for transmitting academic knowledge.

- Expository writing instruction will focus on the processes of planning and composing for "compare-and-contrast" essays.

- The area of conversational initiation was selected to address the negative effects/perceptions that Pedro's verbal interaction style has on peers and adults in his environment.

Sample Activities

Figurative Language: Idioms

1. Select five idioms and write three different short story contexts for each. For each story, include three written alternative response choices (see following examples). Duplicate these materials for the student. Define an idiom for the student by explaining that idioms are expressions in which a new meaning is given to a group of words that already has a meaning. For example, the expression "over the hill" can be interpreted literally *or* as an idiom meaning that someone is old. Explain that the clinician will be reading stories containing idioms and that the student will be asked to select the most appropriate meaning from three choices. Recite the first short story aloud as the student reads along silently. Depending on the student's skill level, instruct him or her to listen to or read the choices and select the response that best fits the context of the story. After the three stories for a particular idiom have been successfully completed, ask the student to brainstorm at least one personal experience to which the specific idiom could have been applied. Examples include the following:

Kick up our heels:

1. John made the football team. He was so happy and excited. He wanted to kick up his heels.

   Does this mean? He wanted to celebrate.

   　　　　　　　He kicked his feet in the air.

   　　　　　　　He was upset.

2. Hannah sat in her classroom and waited for the announcement. The principal finally came on the public-address system and said: "Students, the winner of the school spelling contest is Hannah Smith. Congratulations!" Hannah felt like kicking up her heels.

   Does this mean? She took off her shoe.

   　　　　　　　She was thrilled.

   　　　　　　　She was very disappointed.

3. Larry wanted to get an A in math. He was a good math student but always got Bs. The final exam was last week and he studied harder than ever. When the mail came, Larry ran to see his report card. He opened it up, saw an A next to math, and felt like kicking up his heels.

   Does this mean? He did not do well in math.

   　　　　　　　He lifted his legs in the air.

   　　　　　　　He wanted to cheer.

Shake a leg:

1. Sue forgot to set her alarm for the swim meet. Her mom woke her up and said, "We have only 10 minutes to get to the pool, so shake a leg."

   Does this mean? Sue has to hurry.

   Sue's leg is hurting.

   Sue's mom shook her leg.

2. Bobby wanted to win the bicycle race. He had trained hard for it all summer. But now he was in fourth place with just 1 mile to go. He told himself that he'd better shake a leg if he wanted to win.

   Does this mean? Bobby has to slow down.

   Bobby has to ride faster.

   Bobby does not want to win.

3. Mom and Dad are going out to dinner for their anniversary. It's time to go, but Dad is still shaving. Mom says, "Honey, shake a leg; our reservation is in 20 minutes."

   Does this mean? They will probably be early.

   Dad should move his leg while shaving.

   Dad should hurry up.

A fish out of water:

1. Mariah was very excited about the school dance. She wanted to look really cool. She decided to wear her new faded blue jeans and her favorite flannel shirt. When she walked into the gym, all of the girls were wearing party dresses. Mariah felt like a fish out of water.

   Does this mean? Mariah doesn't like to swim.

   Mariah was not wet.

   Mariah felt different from everyone else.

2. Joan was going to sleep-away camp for the first time. She kissed her parents good-bye after checking in. When she walked into her cabin, all the other girls seemed to know each other. They laughed and talked like old friends. Joan felt like a fish out of water.

   Does this mean? Joan felt like she didn't fit in the group.

   Joan wanted to go swimming.

   Joan likes to go fishing at the lake.

3. Jason just moved to the city and was starting his senior year in high school. Jason rode his bike on the first day of school. As he entered the parking lot, he noticed that all the seniors were driving cars. Jason felt like a fish out of water.

   Does this mean? He felt like he couldn't breathe.

   He felt like he didn't belong.

   He felt very happy.

All thumbs:

1. Jack was helping his dad build a birdhouse in the maple tree. Jack hammered the nail into the wood but kept missing it. His dad said, "Son, you're all thumbs today."

   Does this mean? Jack was clumsy.

           All of Jack's fingers look like thumbs.

           Jack put his thumb on the nail.

2. Kate and Nika decided to bake some chocolate chip cookies. Nika took the eggs out of the refrigerator and dropped one on the floor. Then she spilled the flour all over the table and knocked over the milk. She said to Kate, "I guess I'm all thumbs."

   Does this mean? Nika was finished with the cookies.

           Nika was klutzy.

           Nika's thumbs were all sticky.

3. The period bell rang and David raced to his locker to get his English book before the next class. He held his books in one hand and turned the combination, but the lock wouldn't open. He tried again and dropped all his books onto the floor. He said to himself, "I'm all thumbs."

   Does this mean? David wished that all his fingers were thumbs.

           David's locker opened easily.

           David was clumsy.

Word Retrieval

2. Develop a list of 20 names of objects or people. Write a synonym, category name, or other semantic cue for each word on an index card. In addition, write the initial sound (not letter) of each word on another set of index cards. Examples include the following:

Word	Semantic Cue	Phonological Cue
cook	chef	/k/
gloves	mittens	/g/
jacket	coat	/dʒ/
comb	brush	/k/
tissues	Kleenex	/t/
van	vehicle	/v/
pencil	writing utensil	/p/
shoe	sneakers	/ʃ/
lamp	light	/l/
soda	Coke	/s/
hat	cap	/h/
purse	handbag	/p/
painting	picture	/p/
carpet	rug	/k/

car	automobile	/k/
notebook	binder	/n/
jeans	clothing	/dʒ/
backpack	knapsack	/b/
sailboat	kind of boat	/s/
dollar	money	/d/

Explain that the student will be asked to guess a specific word based on two clues provided by the clinician. Further explain that the two clues represent different strategies that the student can use when trying to retrieve specific vocabulary words. Instruct the student to use the first clue to create a visual image of the object and the second clue to identify what the mystery word sounds like. For example, the clinician says, "I'm thinking of a word. It's like a 'chef' and starts with /k/." Encourage the student to refrain from responding quickly, but rather, to pause reflectively and think about the cues. After each item, instruct the student to produce the target word in a sentence that describes its function.

Narrative Discourse

3. Write the *main elements of a story* on separate index cards along with short definitions of each part (Stein & Glenn, 1979). For example:

Setting: The main characters in the story (who the story is about) and where the story takes place

Problem: The main event or problem that the main character faces

Response: The way that the main character feels about the problem

Attempt: What the main character actually does to try to solve the problem or achieve the goal

Outcome: What happens at the end of the story; whether or not the character achieves the goal

Reaction: How the main character feels about the outcome (success or failure at attaining the goal)

In addition, write one or more *question* cues for each of the main story parts on separate index cards. For example:

Setting: Who is the story about?

              Where does the story take place?

Problem: What happened to the main character?

              What caused the main character to act?

Response: How does the main character feel about the problem?

Attempt: What does the main character do to solve the problem?

Outcome: What happens at the end of the story?

              Does the main character achieve the goal?

Reaction: How does the main character feel at the end of the story?

First, review the story element definition cards with the student. Then explain that the clinician will tell a short story aloud as the student follows the written text.

Example Story

Once upon a time, there was a 12-year-old boy named Jacob who lived in a town called Wallston. He lived about one mile from school and rode his bike there every day. Last week for his birthday, his parents gave him a new bike, the one he'd been asking for since June. On Wednesday morning, Jacob grabbed his backpack and headed for school. As he approached the front gate, he immediately noticed that his new bike was gone. Jacob thought to himself, "Oh no! I forgot to chain the bike last night. Somebody probably stole it. Mom will ground me for a month. I promised to take care of it." Jacob thought all day about what to do. After school, he went to the police station and spoke to one of the officers. The police officer suggested that Jacob put up signs in lots of places such as the police station, the post office, and in store windows. The signs should include Jacob's name, telephone number, and a description of the bike. So Jacob made the signs, put them up all over town, and walked home to wait by the telephone. At about 5:30 P.M., it rang and Jacob jumped up to answer it.

A woman named Mrs. Ramirez said, "I just saw a bike at the grocery story that matches the description on the signs." Jacob thanked the lady and ran to the market as fast as he could. Sure enough, it was his bike. His initials were on the bottom of the seat just as he had scratched them on. Jacob was so happy and relieved. As he rode home, he promised himself that he would never leave his bike unlocked again.

After the story is completed, instruct the student to answer the cue card questions either verbally or in writing. Review and discuss each answer with the student to ensure a correct response.

Then instruct the student to use the cuing questions to construct a story of his or her own. During the initial stages of therapy, the clinician may want to provide the student with a set of choices for each part of the story to facilitate story construction. For example, the clinician might say: "Your story needs a setting. Do you want it to be about a boy named Joe or a teacher named Mr. Petry?"

Task difficulty can be increased by requiring the student to generate a spontaneous story and use the question cues as a self-monitoring strategy to check the quality of the finished product. The task also can be made more sophisticated by decreasing the number and specificity of question cues. A final set of questions might include the following:

a. Are all of the story parts included?

b. Does my story have a beginning, middle, and end?

c. Are the story parts in the correct order?

Note: This activity can be adapted to facilitate the student's production of written narratives. Mnemonic devices are effective tools for helping clients remember and sequence ideas in a logical manner (e.g., SPACE: *S*etting, *P*roblem, *A*ction, *C*onsequent *E*vent; Harris & Graham, 1996). Other acronyms can be used to revise and/or proofread written text (e.g., COPS: *C*apitalization, *O*verall appearance, *P*unctuation, *S*pelling; Schumaker et al., 1982).

Expository Writing: Descriptive Essay

4. With eyes closed, the student should brainstorm descriptive details about a favorite place. Encourage the student to identify what the place looks like and how it sounds, smells, and feels. Create a written list of the comments the student produces. Introduce the parts of a descriptive essay and explain each:

Topic/thesis statement: What the essay is about and why this topic was chosen.

Content paragraphs: The particular qualities/characteristics that the student wants to focus on

Transitions: Words and phrases that provide logical connections between ideas

Conclusion: Brief summary of essay content

Conversational Initiation

5. Tell the student that today's session will focus on how to start a conversation. Explain that there are four sequential steps in initiating a conversation: (a) choosing the setting, (b) selecting the topic, (c) getting the listener's attention, and (d) introducing the topic. Design at least six scenarios, most of which are conversationally inappropriate, for each of the four steps. Explain that the clinician will read the scenarios for each step aloud. Instruct the student to show a thumbs-up or thumbs-down gesture to identify the appropriateness of each event. Example scenarios include the following:

Choosing the Setting

Your friend is on a cell phone. (thumbs down)

Your friend is sitting next to you on the bus. (thumbs up)

Two classmates are sitting in the corner and whispering to each other. (thumbs down)

You are watching a movie in a theater. (thumbs down)

A new classmate is sitting by himself in the cafeteria. (thumbs up)

You are in science class during a lecture. (thumbs down)

Selecting the Topic

Do you have any brothers or sisters? (thumbs up)

Why is your hair so short? (thumbs down)

What kind of music do you like? (thumbs up)

I heard that your parents are getting a divorce. (thumbs down)

Does your father make lots of money? (thumbs down)

You're not invited to my graduation party. (thumbs down)

Getting the Listener's Attention

Saying: "Hey, how's it going?" to the church pastor. (thumbs down)

Saying: "Good morning, Mr. Web" to the school principal. (thumbs up)

Saying: "Know what?" to a group of teachers in the hallway. (thumbs down)

Saying: "Get over here" to an upperclassman. (thumbs down)

Saying: "Excuse me" to an adult who is reading a book. (thumbs up)

Saying: "Here I am" to a group of classmates talking in the cafeteria. (thumbs down)

Introducing the Topic

Starting a conversation with: "Did you see where he went?" (thumbs down)

Starting a conversation with: "I wanted to talk to you about, you know, the assignment we . . . Remember what Ms. Jones said yesterday . . . You know what I'm talking about?" (thumbs down)

Starting a conversation with: "Everyone says that you didn't make the school play." (thumbs down)

Starting a conversation with: "I lost my doohickey, the thing I need to do the math homework problems." (thumbs down)

Starting a conversation with: "Can I talk to you about the party on Saturday night?" (thumbs up)

Starting a conversation with: "Wanna shoot hoops after school with me?" (thumbs up)

Paul is a 17-year-old high school junior with a long-standing history of language deficits and persistent academic difficulties in the absence of overall intellectual impairment. He presents as an outgoing and friendly individual who demonstrates basic conversational competence in the areas of semantics, syntax, and morphology. Significant deficits are noted in his knowledge of higher-level abstract language forms, especially multiple-meaning words, metaphoric uses of language, and inferential comprehension. Recent test results indicate that Paul is reading and writing at approximately the eighth-grade level. According to classroom observation and teacher report, Paul is "disorganized" and demonstrates ineffective study habits and test-taking strategies, poor time management, and poor follow-through on class assignments. These traits are indicative of limited metacognitive functioning (i.e., the awareness of one's own problem-solving strengths and weaknesses, how to apply them, and when to use them effectively). Recently, Paul met with his guidance counselor to discuss his academic status and explore his options following graduation. He expressed a clear preference for career training over college education.

Selection of therapy targets. The areas to be targeted are metalinguistics, metacognition, social communication skills, inferencing, writing processes and products, and language-mediated study skills.

- In the area of metalinguistics, metaphors were selected because this figurative language form occurs frequently in the academic environment.

- Metacognitive training will focus on goal setting, self-monitoring, self-evaluation, goal outcomes, and reflection.

- Both Paul's age and current academic status indicate that he would benefit from therapy activities that focus on social-communication skills in a vocational setting.

- Inferencing was chosen as a means of improving Paul's ability to derive intended meaning from oral and written material.

- Finally, the intervention program will target language-mediated study skills to provide Paul with the requisite tools for improving his academic performance.

Sample Activities

Figurative Language: Metaphors

1. A metaphor is a nonliteral use of language in which one element (**topic**) is compared to another element (**vehicle**) on the basis of one or more common features (**ground**). Develop a list of metaphors and write each on an index card. Each should contain an explicitly stated topic, vehicle, and ground. Each card also should contain two alternative meanings for each metaphor. Following are examples, with the incorrect choice indicated by an asterisk (Nippold, Leonard, & Kail, 1984).

   The sun was a basketball sitting in the sky.

   This means that the sun:

   a. was orange and round.

   b. was very hot.*

   The giraffe was a flagpole living at the zoo.

   This means the giraffe:

   a. was tall.

   b. was on top of the flagpole.*

   The skater was a top spinning on the ice.

   This means the skater:

   a. was twirling very fast.

   b. had a top next to her on the ice.*

   David's nose was a grapefruit sitting on his face.

   This means that David's nose:

   a. was big.

   b. was bleeding.*

   The girl's smile was a ray of sunshine on a cloudy day.

   This means that the girl's smile:

   a. was bright.

   b. was big.*

The man was a pumpkin walking down the street.

This means that the man:

    a. was fat.

    b. was orange.*

Matt's arms were broom handles hanging at his sides.

This means that Matt's arms:

    a. were long and skinny.

    b. were hairy.*

John's teeth were kernels of corn growing in his mouth.

This means that John's teeth:

    a. were yellow.

    b. were chipped.*

The soldiers were cornrows going down the road.

This means that the soldiers:

    a. were in straight lines.

    b. were tall.*

The runner was a jet plane flying in the sky.

This means that the runner:

    a. was fast.

    b. was getting on an airplane.*

Explain that a metaphor is a comparison between two things that are alike in some way. For example, in "The girl's hair is spaghetti," the two things that are being compared are "hair" and "spaghetti." Both are thin and long. So this metaphor means that the girl's hair is thin and long. Explain that the student will read each metaphor aloud and, along with the clinician, identify the two things that are being compared. The student will then be presented with two choices and asked to pick the "best" meaning.

Note: Similes are easier to understand than metaphors because they have the syntactic markers *like* or *as* to signal the comparison. These markers can be used as a transition to metaphors (e.g., "The sun was [like] a basketball sitting in the sky").

Metacognition: Executive Functioning

2. Explain that this activity is designed to help the student approach problems or tasks in a systematic, organized manner. Jointly review the student's current course requirements and select a relevant assignment. For example, a civics class assignment might be a group project to develop a campaign to change some aspect of school board policy or local government ordinance. This student's group chose to petition the county council to install a stop sign at a busy intersection. As a group member, the student's responsibility is to write a persuasive letter to the appropriate government officials.

Goals and Target Behaviors	Self-Questions
a. Goal-Setting/Planning Think before acting/speaking/writing.	What do you want to do? What message do you want to send? How do you want this to come out?
b. Self-Monitoring Think about how the task is coming along. Are you devoting enough time/effort/attention?	How does your work look? Are there any problems? Do you need new or different strategies? How is your progress?
c. Self-Evaluation Rate the overall quality of the finished product and effectiveness of your performance.	Did you solve the problem(s)? Were the strategies useful? Was your work correct? Was it efficient?
d. Goal Outcome Evaluate the result of your work.	Did you achieve the goal? Was the goal realistic? Should it have been modified in some way?
e. Reflection Think about what the experience taught you.	Would you do things differently next time? What did you learn about your ability to solve problems?

Gather two 5-by-7-inch index cards in each of five colors for a total of 10 cards. Write goals and target behaviors from the list on one card of each color. Follow color coding and write corresponding self-questions on the remaining cards.

Introduce and discuss each of the goals and target behaviors in the order in which they were listed. Provide several examples for each component. Then have the student generate additional examples. Once the student demonstrates reliable recall of the five goals and target behaviors, begin the task by implementing the first goal (planning). Introduce the self-questions as instructional cues to facilitate achievement of the target behavior. When goal-setting is finalized, proceed to each subsequent component in the hierarchy using the self-questions to support the student's performance at each phase.

Note: The ultimate aim of this metacognitive training procedure is for the student to internalize the self-questions and use them as strategies for problem-solving across tasks.

Social Communication

3. Teach social communication skills in the context of vocational settings by using the training sequence of explanation, demonstration, and role-playing. As each activity is mastered in the therapy session, the clinician can ask school personnel to participate in simulated work environments to provide the student with practice and promote generalization of the newly learned skills. For example, the school media specialist, principal, or cafeteria staff could play the role of "employers" or "potential employers" to provide the student with opportunities to practice the skill in quasi-work environments (i.e., library, office, restaurant).

Debriefing sessions can be held on a regular basis to review performance and improve the student's self-monitoring skills. Following are suggested tasks/contexts:

Telephoning to request a job interview

Undergoing a job interview

Accepting a suggestion from an employer

Accepting criticism from an employer

Providing constructive criticism to a coworker

Explaining a problem to a supervisor

Complimenting a coworker

Accepting a compliment from a coworker

Inferencing

4. Develop 20 situations that have clear logical inferences and write each on the top portion of an index card. Explain that an inference is a conclusion reached by using information that you know to be true to make a "good guess" about what is also likely to be true. For example, Mr. Jones made several jokes in class today, so I *inferred* that he was in a good mood. Instruct the student to read each situation and write one logical inference. After each response, discuss with the student the reason that it was a correct/incorrect inference. Examples include the following:

The principal usually makes the announcements, but today the vice principal gave them.

Tyler blushed when he saw Emily.

Tony picked up his baseball bat and walked out to the plate.

Joe hammered the nail and yelled "Ouch!"

Ken walked into his apartment and his laptop and iPod were gone.

Chad walked by his best friend Steve without saying "Hello."

Hank rented a tuxedo for Saturday night.

Ashley is making a salad for dinner. Her eyes are stinging and tears are rolling down her cheeks.

Noah made sure to put on gloves and a hat.

Wanda put the book down after reading only half of it.

The boss walks by and gives you a pat on the back.

Alex looked at the clock and ran out of the room.

The sand burned Madison's feet.

Danny took one bite of the apple and threw it away.

Mrs. Jensen frowned as she handed Tim his math exam.

Jack smiled as he left his basketball game.

Allison took the cookies out of the oven and threw them in the trash.

Sam walked into the backyard to get some tomatoes and peas.

Mia could hear the waves from her bedroom window.

Fred searched for some change and called a tow truck driver.

Compare/Contrast Essay Structure

5. Brainstorm writing topics of great interest to the student. (The clinician can provide some examples, such as baseball and football, or different types of transportation, such as a skateboard and roller blades.)

   ■ Explain to the student that the compare-contrast essay identifies how things are alike and different. Briefly define each term (i.e., *comparison* refers to how two things are alike, whereas *contrast* refers to how they are different).

   ■ Review/teach examples of vocabulary that signal the compare-contrast structures. Base selection of words on curricula content materials and content area learning objectives.

   Vocabulary for comparing: *similar, like, still, likewise, in the same ways, in comparison, at the same time, in the same manner.*

   Vocabulary for contrasting: *however, on the other hand, but, yet, nevertheless, conversely, rather, on the contrary, nonetheless, in contrast.*

   ■ Make a list of salient characteristics for each of the subjects (e.g., football and baseball). Use a highlighter to indicate characteristics that are found under each subject header.

   ■ Use the list as an aid to compose a compare-and-contrast essay in the following suggested format:

   Paragraph 1: Introduction: Begin with a sentence that will catch the reader's interest. This might be a question, or a reason people find the topic interesting/important. Then, name the two subjects and say they are very similar, very different, or have many important (or interesting) similarities and differences.

   Paragraph 2: The next paragraph(s) describe features of the *first* subject. Do not mention the second subject.

   Paragraph 3: Begin this section with a transition word showing you are comparing the second subject to the first. For each comparison, use a cue word such as *like, similar to, also, unlike, on the other hand.* Be sure to include examples that clearly demonstrate that the similarities and/or differences exist. (Note: Some students may benefit from writing a paragraph about the characteristics of the second subject prior to this paragraph.)

   Final paragraph: Write a conclusion by giving a brief, general summary of the most important similarities and differences. End with a personal statement, a prediction, or another snappy clincher.

Study Skills

6. The development of language-mediated study skills is particularly critical for successful academic performance at the middle and high school levels. A compendium of important skill areas is included in Table 5-5. Training can be accomplished most effectively by using the students' actual curricular materials (e.g., lecture notes, textbook readings, homework assignments, and term projects). One effective school-based service delivery model for study skill training is the provision of a course that meets regularly and is taken for academic credit.

TABLE 5–5

Language-Mediated Study Skills for Older Students and Adolescents

STUDY SKILLS

1. *Time Organization*
   Budgeting time for completion
   Establishing daily homework and study schedules
   Breaking assignments into smaller units
   Planning for deadlines
   Organizing notebook/planner

2. *Text Analysis*
   Table of contents
   Glossary
   Legends, maps, diagrams, tables

3. *Note-Taking*
   Importance of taking notes
   Different methods: mapping, outlining, abbreviating, summarizing, webbing

4. *Study Strategies*
   Active thinking method
   Scanning versus skimming versus reading
   Memory strategies: mnemonic devices, chunking, acronyms, brainstorming, visualizing

5. *Test-Taking Strategies*
   Preparation: establishing study schedule; inquiring as to type of questions that
      will be on test
   Review terms often used on tests: for example, prove, review, summarize, compare,
      contrast, criticize
   Strategies for different types of tests: fill-ins, multiple choice, matching, true/false, essay

6. *Reference Skills*
   Library and media center skills: alphabetical order, online catalogue skills,
      cross-referencing
   Review different types of reference sources: Internet searches, dictionary, atlas,
      thesaurus

CRITICAL THINKING

1. *General Thinking Behaviors*
   Observing and describing
   Developing concepts
   Hypothesizing
   Generalizing
   Predicting outcomes
   Explaining an event
   Offering alternatives
   Inferencing

(continues)

TABLE 5–5 *(Continued)*

2. *Problem-Solving*
   Teach steps in decision making: define problem, break into small parts, develop options, choose option, predict outcome, critique decision made

3. *Higher Thinking Skills*
   Inductive and deductive reasoning
   Solving analogies

LISTENING/READING

1. *Prelistening/Previewing*
   Strategies for "getting ready" to listen/read, for example, reviewing material beforehand

2. *Listening/Reading*
   Teach recognition of organizational cues and phrases, for example, *in the beginning, the first point, the key point, three main areas are, in summary*
   Reading: teach identification of topic sentence, supporting sentences, details

3. *Evaluative Listening*
   Teach distinction between fact and opinion in various materials: propaganda, commercials, prejudices, absurdities

ORAL AND WRITTEN EXPRESSION

1. *Organization*
   Ways in which to ask questions
   Strategies for organizing paragraphs
   Teach forms of expository writing: description, explanation, compare/contrast

2. *Craftsmanship*
   Sentence and paragraph construction: S-V agreement, tense agreement, topic versus supporting sentences, coherence
   Editing
   Proofreading: spelling, peer proofing

SOURCE: F. Roth and E. Fye, personal communication, July 1991.

Helpful Hints

1. Whenever possible, conduct phonological awareness activities in a group setting to encourage interaction and avoid a sense of drill/rote memorization. In addition, a group setting is beneficial because it encourages interaction and participation.

2. Whenever appropriate, supplement an activity with the provision of written word or sound cues as an indirect means of facilitating word-recognition skills in students who are beginning readers.

3. Visualization is an effective strategy for some students to enhance semantic categories. For example, a student might be instructed as follows: "Close your eyes and imagine that you are in (*a particular location*; e.g., classroom, supermarket). Look all around and tell me all the things you see."

4. A referential communication task is a good instructional mechanism for facilitating the development of a variety of pragmatic skills. It involves a speaker who is responsible for describing something (e.g., objects, shapes) so that a listener can identify the correct object or replicate the pattern. This task can be manipulated in numerous ways to focus on communicative intentions, perspective taking, and conversational discourse abilities. (See Spekman & Roth, 1984, for specific intervention suggestions.)

5. Another aspect of metalinguistic skills that can be trained is humor. One common type of humor is riddles. The appreciation of riddles require the ability to detect ambiguity. There is a developmental progression that the clinician can keep in mind when programming targets in this area:

   Phonological (6 to 9 years): A sound sequence can be interpreted in more than one way

   Example: Why was the doctor upset? He was out of patience (patients).

   Lexical (9 to 12 years): A word has more than one meaning

   Example: Why didn't the skeleton cross the road? It didn't have the guts.

   Syntactic (13+ years): Words in a sentence can be grouped differently

   Example: What is the difference between a running dog and a running man? The man wears trousers and the dog pants.

6. The information-giving aspect of counseling may involve educating families about the purpose and procedures of the IEP process so that they can effectively participate in decision making for appropriate educational placements and services.

7. An important aspect of counseling with this age group often is apprising the family of the potential impact of oral language disorders on the acquisition of early reading and writing skills.

8. Story frames can facilitate a student's generation of a well-formed story. See the following examples:

   Once upon a time ___

   Suddenly ___

   Luckily ___

   In the end ___

9. With adolescents, it is important to use written materials that are relevant and age appropriate (e.g., blogs, magazines, emails, or Web sites on topics of interest, advertisements, bus/metro routes and schedules). Also, engage the student in relevant writing tasks such as making shopping lists, copying recipes, writing letters of inquiry jobs, preparing résumés, practicing interviewing skills.

10. When using role-playing as a technique for fostering the development of social skills, it may be useful to portray examples of both appropriate and inappropriate behaviors to highlight the differences between more and less socially acceptable behavior.

11. To facilitate peer relationships through small-group settings, it may be helpful to include a normally achieving peer who can model appropriate skills. This strategy

may also buffer the effects of low acceptance and rejection that may occur in larger peer groups.

12. Inferencing can be trained in the context of paragraph-length material using a multiple-choice response format. For example:

> Hal was watching a movie on TV. It was about a man who was crossing a desert. Hal could almost feel the hot sun. Soon, Hal ran to get something he wanted very much. What do you think it was?

> a. Something to ride on

> b. Something to drink

> c. Something to play with

13. To reinforce meaning and foster generalization over time, it is preferable to use several different contexts for the same figurative language form rather than introducing several different expressions.

14. Introduce new figurative language forms in matching and multiple choice tasks because they are easier than explanation tasks.

15. Certain types of idioms, metaphors, and so on are easier to understand than others because their meaning is more transparent or closer to the literal meaning. For example, the idiom "keep a straight face" is more explicit than "come apart at the seams." The following examples are from Schweigert (1986, pp. 33–45):

Examples of Transparent Idioms	*Examples of Opaque Idioms*
hit the road	asleep at the switch
pain in the neck	has a green thumb
burned out	big frog in a small pond
coast is clear	piece of cake
over his head	shout from the housetops
hit the sack	build a fire under
have a ball	paddle his own canoe
on the tip of his tongue	clip his wings
up the creek without a paddle	know which side his bread is buttered on

16. Begin with predictive metaphors because they are easier to understand than proportional metaphors. **Predictive metaphors** are based on similarity and contain only one topic and vehicle. **Proportional metaphors** contain two topics and two vehicles and express an analogical relationship, usually with one topic left unstated (e.g., The bird's nest was a piggy bank that had no coins). The analogy is: *nest* is to *piggy bank* as *eggs* are to *coins* (leaving the topic of eggs to be inferred).

17. Dictionaries of English figurative language forms are commercially available. Two examples are the *Dictionary of American Slang and Colloquial Expressions* (2005; New York: McGraw-Hill) and the *Cambridge Dictionary of American Idioms* (2003; New York: Cambridge University Press).

18. Adolescents may demonstrate significant behavioral problems that are, in fact, related to their language impairment. Clinicians may need to provide counseling to help students function more effectively in classroom as well as clinical settings. Clinicians also may recommend that families seek services from specialized counseling professionals.

19. Instruction that addresses linguistic cohesion devices can significantly improve a student's comprehension and production of oral and written text. See Appendix 5-A for examples of the most common types of cohesion.

CONCLUSION

This chapter has presented basic information, protocols, and procedures for intervention for childhood language disorders at an *introductory* level. This information is intended only as a starting point in the reader's clinical education and training. For more in-depth coverage of this area, the following readings are recommended:

Nelson, N. W. (2010). *Language and literacy disorders: Infancy through adolescence.* Boston, MA: Allyn & Bacon.

Owens, R. E. (2013). *Language disorders: A functional approach to assessment and intervention.* Needham Heights, MA: Allyn & Bacon.

Paul, R., & Norbury, C. (2012). *Language disorders from infancy to adolescence: Assessment and interventions.* St. Louis, MO: Elsevier.

ADDITIONAL RESOURCES

Super Duper Publications
P.O. Box 24997
Greenville, SC 29616
Phone: 800-277-8737
Fax: 800-978-7379
Web site: www.superduperinc.com

Granny's Candies
This board game expands vocabulary skills with question cards from one of eight semantic areas, such as "What belongs in this group?" and "How are they alike?"

Core Curriculum Vocabulary Cards
These 200 color-coded and research-based cards will help your students learn tier-two, high-frequency vocabulary words by matching a word to its definition. It targets words students need to know for success in the early grades in the areas of language arts, science, social studies, and math.

Language Strategies: For Little Ones (grades K–1), for Children (grades 2–5), and for Older Students (grades 5–8)
These resources contain a series of curriculum-based lessons that focus on language comprehension, oral expression, and story grammar knowledge. The reproducible lessons

reinforce listening, questioning, categorizing, sequencing, reasoning, and vocabulary skills. Each unit integrates whole-language philosophy, classroom curriculum concepts, literature-based intervention techniques, and strategies for self-prompting.

500 Prefixes, Suffixes, and Stems Super Fun Deck

This deck presents 500 illustrated prefixes, suffixes, and stems. One side of each card presents a word part and its meaning, along with two words (using the word part) and their definitions. Knowing the meaning of various word parts can greatly expand vocabulary and help to figure out the meaning of words that have never been seen or heard before. The other side is a flash card to test knowledge of the word's meaning.

Ten Steps to Writing Better Essays

This standards-based guide provides lessons for older students who have difficulty organizing their thoughts and materials before writing expository essays.

LinguiSystems

3100 Fourth Avenue
East Moline, IL 61244
Phone: 800-776-4332
Fax: 800-577-4555
Web site: www.linguisystems.com

No Glamour Grammar

Each skill is broken down into small increments of learning. The pages have few visual distractions and a consistent format so students know what to expect. Units progress in difficulty with the mastery of each grammar skill. Includes pretests and posttests for each unit to chart progress.

HELP for Auditory Processing

This workbook is designed to foster the skills necessary to receive, interpret, and internalize language. The hierarchy of activities is broken down into smaller tasks so you can see where processing breakdowns occur. Exercises for processing information in word classes, following directions, picking out important details, using information to make inferences, answering and asking questions, sequencing information by features, processing details from stories, and listening for sounds in words.

101 Language Activities

These varied language activities promote the skills necessary to communicate effectively in the classroom. They provide motivational language and reasoning tasks using curricular topics and vocabulary.

Blooming Speech and Language Activities

This resource contains interactive lessons that elicit speech and language targets naturally. Play, craft, and food activities are used to teach vocabulary, concepts, language, phonological awareness, and thinking skills.

Tasks of Problem Solving: Elementary

These activities are designed for students with impairments in language and problem-solving skills. The tasks incorporate test-taking strategies, comprehension activities, and classroom decision-making skills. They also improve metacognitive skills by teaching students the vocabulary and language to describe how they are thinking.

Sounds Abound Series

This series includes several resources, such as Bingo and Storybook Activities, that aim to enhance phonological awareness. Each resource also helps to develop pre-reading skills by teaching students the sounds of their language and the letters that represent them.

Amazon
Web site: www.amazon.com

100% Writing

Shows students how to organize random thoughts into cohesive, interesting writings. The step-by-step procedures and complete lessons eliminate guesswork, as each skill builds upon the previous skill. The writing topics and practice pages provide scenarios for students to write about. There are separate editions for persuasion, exposition, narration, and compare and contrast.

Multiple Meanings for the Young Adult

This resource has a set of exercises that help older students build a meaningful vocabulary. It focuses on common words that have many different meanings and is designed for older, mature students who are reading at approximately a second- or third-grade level.

Language Development, Differences, and Disorders

This text provides a unique collaborative approach between general and special educators and a speech-language pathologist. It approaches teaching children with language differences and disorders by focusing on their access to the general education curriculum. It is divided into four sections, including one on strategies for classroom-based assessments and interventions for students with language problems.

PATHS: Phonological Awareness Training and Help for Students

A reproducible resource that helps older students understand sound systems and functions. It targets academic skills such as phonological awareness, phonemic processing, phonemic relationships, listening, and memory. It also teaches the linguistic rules needed by students who have experienced difficulty in reading, writing, and spelling.

Pro-Ed
8700 Shoal Creek Boulevard
Austin, TX 78758-9965
Phone: 800-897-3202
Fax: 800-397-7633
Web site: www.proedinc.com

Books Are for Talking Too!, **3rd ed.**
A compendium of suggested books for preschool through 12th grade. For each book, the following information is provided: (1) synopsis of the book, (2) the target area for therapy, (3) suggested strategies for teaching targets, and (4) suggested grades and interest level.

Workbook for Synonyms, Homonyms, and Antonyms
This workbook has reproducible activity pages as well as specific suggestions for supplemental teaching activities appropriate for use with individual students, small groups, or an entire class. Activities are presented in order of increasing difficulty, with easy-to-follow instructions, including choosing word pairs, completing sentences, matching words to definitions, unscrambling words, rhyming riddles, and solving crossword puzzles.

Dormac Inc.
P.O. Box 1699
Beaverton, OR 97075-1699
Web site: https://openlibrary.org/publishers/Dormac,_Inc
For school-age children and adolescents, this series of workbooks facilitates the comprehension and use of idioms, including:

Raining Cats and Dogs
Monkey Business
Sticky Fingers
In the Dog House

Academic Communication Associates
Publication Center, Department IN-20
P.O. Box 4279
Oceanside, CA 92052-4279
Phone: 888-758-9558
Fax: 760-722-9593
Email: acom@acadcom.com
Web site: www.acadcom.com

Developing Language for Literacy
This resource targets strategies for using linguistic knowledge to learn basic reading skills for children ages 5 through 10. It includes a discussion of the interrelationship between language learning and the acquisition of reading skills. Topics range from the importance of prediction strategies to facilitating development of phonological awareness. It also emphasizes pragmatic activities and strategies for working with bilingual/multicultural populations.

Exercises for Descriptive Language Skills
For ages 4 to 10 years, this collection of activities targets skills such as sequencing story pictures and retelling stories, describing details using precise vocabulary, describing similarities and differences, creating stories and finishing incomplete stories, and giving explanations. It also includes reproducible pictures and worksheets.

Laureate Software
110 East Spring Street
Winooski, VT 05404
Phone: 800-562-6801
Fax: 802-655-4757
Email: laureate@laureatelearning.com
Web site: www.laureatelearning.com

The Language Activities of Daily Living Series: My School

This talking instructional computer software program was designed to help clients understand and express the language they encounter during daily routines. Each program has four different activities designed to increase understanding of object names and their functions or descriptions: discover names, identify names, discover functions, and identify functions. In this program, a classroom, playground, library, cafeteria, art/music room, and school hallway are included. There are also programs for activities of daily living pertaining to an individual's house and to his or her town.

Mobile Education Store
Web site: http://mobile-educationstore.com/

Cracking the Books Interactive Science Books

This series of digital books is designed for use with upper-elementary-school-aged children. Lessons are written to align with core curriculum standards and universal design parameters. The lessons can be adjusted to meet the needs of students on varying reading levels (covering first- through eighth-grade reading levels) without altering the content for these students. Book topics include geography, anatomy, U.S. history, and weather. The books have interactive features such as imbedded videos, pop-up definitions, voice-over options, and quizzes/tests.

Paul H. Brookes Publishing Company
P.O. Box 10624
Baltimore, MD 21285-0624
Phone: 800-638-3775
Fax: 410-337-8539
Web site: www.brookespublishing.com

Road to the Code

This developmentally sequenced 11-week program is designed to give kindergarten and first-grade students repeated opportunities to practice and enhance beginning reading and spelling abilities. Contains 44 lessons, each featuring three activities.

Miscellaneous

Bear, D.R., Invernizzi, M., Templeton, S, & Johnston, F. (2011). *Words their way: Word study for phonics, vocabulary, and spelling instruction* (5th ed.). Boston, MA: Allyn & Bacon.

> This clinician and teacher guide provides evidence-based activities for teaching phonological awareness, vocabulary, spelling, alphabetic principle, and reading decoding skills.

Beck, I. L., McKeown, M. G., & Kuckan, L. (2013). *Bringing words to life: Robust vocabulary instruction* (2nd ed.). New York: Guilford.

This book provides practical vocabulary instruction strategies for early, intermediate, and later grades. It also identifies specific children's books with corresponding target vocabulary words.

Burns, M. S., Griffin, P., & Snow, C. E. (1999). *Starting out right: A guide to promoting children's reading success.* Washington, DC: National Academy Press.

This is a clinician- and parent-friendly guide to the development of reading and spelling skills in young children. Includes specific activities to promote emergent and early literacy from infancy through mid-elementary school.

Glazer, S. (1990). *Creating readers and writers.* Newark, DE: International Reading Association.

This book contains a section that describes the types of books that are appropriate for children in four different age ranges between infancy and 12 years of age.

Marzano, R. J. (2004). *Building background knowledge for academic achievement.* Alexandria, VA: Association for Supervision and Curriculum Development.

This book provides specific steps for building students' general and subject-specific background knowledge. It contains helpful vocabulary lists organized by 11 subject areas (e.g., math, science, social studies, etc.) and grade levels from kindergarten through 12th grade.

Rooney, K. J. (2010). *Strategies for learning: Empowering students for success. Grades 9–12.* Thousand Oaks, CA: Corwin.

This text presents practical strategies to help adolescent learners access curricula content across subject areas and meet the performance demands of secondary educational settings.

Roth, F. P., Worthington, C. K., & Troia, G. A. (2012). *Promoting Awareness of Speech Sounds (PASS): A phonological awareness intervention program.* Verona, WI: Attainment, Inc.

This book focuses on training in three areas: rhyming, sound blending, and sound segmenting. Skills are taught in a sequential manner through a variety of games. It includes a detailed description (script) for each activity as well as precise instructions for implementation.

Scott, C. (2012). Learning to write. In A. Kamhi & H. Catts (Eds.), *Language and reading disabilities* (3rd ed., pp. 244–268). Boston, MA: Pearson.

This text focuses on the differences between spoken and written language disabilities. This chapter covers writing skills and provides information on writing texts for specific genres.

Torgesen, J. K., & Bryant, B. R. (2013). *Phonological awareness training for reading* (2nd ed.). Austin, TX: Pro-Ed.

This book focuses on training in four areas: sound blending, sound segmenting, reading, and spelling. Skills are taught in a sequential manner through a variety of games. It includes a detailed description (script) for each activity as well as precise instructions for implementation.

Yopp, H. K., & Yopp, R. H. (2000). Supporting phonemic awareness in the classroom. *The Reading Teacher, 54,* 130–143.

This article provides sample phonological awareness activities appropriate for preschool, kindergarten, and first-grade classrooms within a developmental hierarchy of difficulty.

APPENDIX 5-A

TYPES OF COHESION

Cohesion: Linguistic devices for connecting sentences to one another so that text is coherent and "hangs together" (Halliday & Hasan, 1975).

ELLIPSIS: Redundant words are eliminated from the utterance.

Examples: The *roses* were red. There were twelve.

Have you been swimming? Yes.

CONJUNCTION: Connective words link two independent clauses.

Examples: She was never happy here. *So* she's leaving.

Harry left *because* the party was over.

Sally ran downstairs, *but* she missed the bus.

LEXICAL: General nouns or repetitions link two sentences.

Examples: Joe stayed awake three nights in a row. The *man* is crazy.

There was a caterpillar in the forest. The *caterpillar* was green.

REFERENCE: Pronouns, demonstratives, the definite article, and comparative terms are used to refer back to a referent.

Examples: John went to the store. *He* bought a sweater.

I went to New York City. Guess what I did *there*?

My grandfather had a clock. *The* clock had chimes.

Two birds sat in a tree. *Another* came along.

CHAPTER 6

OVERVIEW OF AUTISM SPECTRUM DISORDER

Autism spectrum disorder (ASD) is a complex disorder, and its study is rapidly evolving. The original term "early infantile autism" was used by Kanner (1943) to describe children who showed extreme self-isolation, lack of social interaction, impaired language, and "insistence on the preservation of sameness." Asperger (1944) published an account of children with impaired communication and interaction skills whose language and intelligence were in the average to above-average range. The name for the disorder described by these researchers and others changed to "autism" during the 1970s–1980s. And in the 1990s, the "spectrum" terminology was added to capture the range and severity of impairment along a continuum from mild to profound. In this chapter, the authors have made a decision to include material that is widely known in the field and do not specifically endorse particular treatment strategies.

The fifth edition of the *Diagnostic and Statistical Manual of Mental Disorders* (DSM-5; American Psychiatric Association [APA], 2013) was released in May 2013, and it contains several *significant changes* to the definition and criteria for diagnosis of autism. First, the overall category name, "pervasive developmental disorder" has been replaced with "autism spectrum disorder," and all of the subcategories (e.g., "Asperger's PDD-NOS") are no longer used. According to the DSM-5, this change was due primarily to the lack of evidence for discrete categories. Second, the criterion related specifically to oral language development has been removed. Now the diagnosis of ASD as a neurodevelopmental disorder is based on the demonstration of two basic symptoms prior to the age of 3 years: (1) *persistent deficits in social communication and social interaction* and (2) *restricted or repetitive patterns of behavior, interests, or activities that cause significant impairments in daily functioning*. Children who meet these criteria will be given a diagnosis of ASD with varying levels of severity: mild, moderate, or severe (see Table 6-1). These children also can receive an accompanying diagnosis of language and/or intellectual impairment. About 50% of children with ASD have below-average intelligence (Centers for Disease Control and Prevention [CDC], 2014). This represents a significant shift from 10 years ago, when only one-third of children with ASD scored above the IQ cut-off for intellectual disability/impairment (Dykens & Lense, 2011). Thus, children diagnosed with moderate to severe ASD are likely to exhibit significant intellectual deficits. Guidelines from the American Speech-Language-Hearing Association (ASHA) state that speech-language pathologists (SLPs) play a critical role in the diagnosis of ASD, typically as part of an interdisciplinary/collaborative team (see the ASHA position statement at www.asha.org/policy/PS2006-00105/). In addition, the DSM-5 states that diagnoses are most valid and reliable when based on multiple sources of information, including clinician observations, caregiver history, and, when possible, self-report (APA, 2013, p. 53).

The authors of this text do not agree with the omission of language as one of the defining characteristics of ASD. Disorders of language are a hallmark of ASD and include deficits in the comprehension and expression of phonology, morphology, semantics, syntax, and use, at both the verbal and nonverbal levels. There are 40 years of research literature demonstrating the centrality of language to a diagnosis of ASD. Moreover, language development is often an early indicator of ASD. Many children with ASD are nonverbal, but even those who are verbal often have not internalized the rules for generating and understanding novel utterances. The verbal repertoires of other individuals with ASD may

TABLE 6–1
Levels of Severity for Autism Spectrum Disorder

Severity Level	Social Communication	Restricted, Repetitive Behaviors
Level 3 "Requiring very substantial support"	Severe deficits in verbal and nonverbal social communication skills cause severe impairments in functioning, very limited initiation of social interactions, and minimal response to social overtures from others. For example, a person with few words of intelligible speech who rarely initiates interaction and, when he or she does, makes unusual approaches to meet needs only and responds to only very direct social approaches.	Inflexibility of behavior, extreme difficulty coping with change, or other restricted/repetitive behaviors markedly interfere with functioning in all spheres. Great distress/difficulty in changing focus or action.
Level 2 "Requiring substantial support"	Marked deficits in verbal and nonverbal social communication skills; social impairments apparent even with supports in place; limited initiation of social interactions; and reduced or abnormal responses to social overtures from others. For example, a person who speaks simple sentences, whose interaction is limited to narrow special interests, and who has markedly odd nonverbal communication.	Inflexibility of behavior, difficulty coping with change, or other restricted/repetitive behaviors appear frequently enough to be obvious to the casual observer and interfere with functioning in a variety of contexts. Distress and/or difficulty in changing focus or action.
Level 1 "Requiring support"	Without supports in place, deficits in social communication cause noticeable impairments. Difficulty initiating social interactions, and clear examples of atypical or unsuccessful responses to the social overtures of others. May appear to have decreased interest in social interactions. For example, a person who is able to speak in full sentences and engages in communication but whose to-and-fro conversation with others fails, and whose attempts to make friends are odd and typically unsuccessful.	Inflexibility of behavior causes significant interference with functioning in one or more contexts. Difficulty switching between activities. Problems of organization and planning hamper independence.

consist mainly of echoed speech, stilted speech, or strictly literal language. Thus, omitting language in the definition of ASD renders a fundamental mischaracterization of this disorder. Because of this omission, SLPs will need to advocate for inclusion of language in the Individualized Education Plans (IEPs) and intervention plans for children and adolescents with ASD.

Incidence

ASD is one of the most common developmental disabilities in the United States, and is marked by gender differences, with males representing a significant majority of children diagnosed with the disorder. Over recent decades, there has been a steep increase in estimated incidence figures:

> 1 of every 125 children in 2004
>
> 1 of every 110 children in 2006
>
> 1 of every 88 in children in 2011/12
>
> 1 of every 68 children in 2014 (CDC, 2013, 2014)

Several reasons for this increased incidence have been proposed, including:

1. More children may have ASD (i.e., the true frequency of autism has increased).
2. There is increased awareness of the condition by health care and educational professionals as well as the general public.
3. The diagnosis may be applied more broadly than before the concept of "spectrum" was added to the definition.
4. Diagnosis is being made at increasingly early ages.
5. Better diagnostic tools are increasingly available.

Jick and Kaye (2012) examined data from three countries to clarify the reasons for the sharp increase in the diagnosis of autism in the 1990s. They compared 250 case pairs of boys with and without a diagnosis of autism in the 1980s and 1990s. Those in the nonautistic group had diagnoses of developmental delays. Several factors were compared across the two populations, including exposure to drugs, maternal rubella, pre-existing medical illness of children or their mothers, vaccinations, and pregnancy history. No material differences were found, causing the authors to conclude that (1) a major cause of the steep increase in the number of boys diagnosed with autism in the 1990s is probably due to changing diagnostic practices; and (b) in the 1980s, these same children would have been diagnosed with developmental disabilities rather than autism. In summary, the factors driving the dramatic increase in incidence of diagnosis as well as the shift in the intellectual profile of children with ASD continue to be debated in this rapidly evolving communication disorder.

Etiology

The cause of autism is unknown and somewhat controversial. Most researchers agree that there is not a single etiology, and multiple clinical phenotypes exist. Overall, many researchers and clinicians believe that genetic vulnerabilities/predispositions interact with environmental risk and resilience (protective) factors to alter the development of brain structure and function, thus compromising the child's ability to learn. In addition to genetic influence, other commonly proposed contributing factors include infectious agents (e.g., maternal rubella), brain structure abnormalities (hemisphere asymmetries), physiologic brain abnormalities (e.g., deficits in coordination among neural areas), and metabolic diseases (e.g., phenylketonuria). Several well-done studies (e.g., Plotkin, Gerber, & Offit, 2009) have ruled out vaccinations (e.g., DPT, MMR) as causative factors.

In an effort to increase our understanding of the developmental mechanisms underlying the disorder, Jones, Gilga, Bedford, Charman, and Johnson (2013) published an article that focused on mapping how ASD evolves from birth. Using a novel methodology, they reviewed numerous prospective studies of infants with familial history of ASD. These "high-risk" infant siblings were followed until 2 to 3 years of age, when diagnosis of ASD is usually made. A low-risk control group composed of children who have a **typically developing (TD)** older sibling and no family history of ASD was similarly followed. According to the authors, this methodology may help to identify **early markers** of ASD and facilitate prediction of clinical outcome. The studies reviewed involved several different methodologies: observation in more than one context, standardized tools, eye-tracking tasks, and neuroimaging. This design also allowed for the identification of a **broader ASD phenotype (BAP),** which consists of a collection of subclinical traits/characteristics that are present at an elevated rate in individuals with ASD. Importantly, Jones et al. (2013) found that most of the preverbal impairments emerge during the second year of life (e.g., lower number and variety of communicative gestures, combine eye gaze with gesture to communicate). Also, social communication deficits are not always the earliest symptoms of ASD and frequently do not precede impairments in other areas (e.g., sensory, ritualistic behaviors; Elsabbagh & Johnson, 2010; Rogers, 2009; Yirmiya & Charman, 2010).

CHARACTERISTICS OF CHILDREN WITH ASD

The myriad characteristics of autism spectrum disorder can be divided into three major groups of "core" deficits: (1) persistent failure to develop effective social communication; (2) language impairments; and (3) restricted/repetitive patterns of attention, interest, and behaviors (including fine and gross motor movement). It is important to realize that not all children with ASD will demonstrate every characteristic and not to the same degree. Behavior may vary on a daily basis.

Social Communication

Children with ASD fail to establish reciprocal social interactions with others in their environment. Rather, they tend to remain self-isolated and detached. This lack of awareness/disinterest is evidenced in their failure to anticipate arrival of parents or recognize their voices, failure to develop natural kiss and cuddle routines, and lack of social imitation (e.g., waving bye-bye). Significantly, these children do not develop joint attention, which is the ability to focus/share eye gaze with another person on the same object (Bruner, 1983). Each individual must understand that the other individual is looking at the same object and realize that there is an element of shared attention. This ability to engage in the "same line of regard" is the prerequisite for the development of referencing (e.g., pointing and other gestures). Further, children with ASD demonstrate significant difficulty with simple and more abstract forms of play. For example, when given a toy car, the child is likely to spin the wheels rather than rolling the toy along the floor. In addition, pretend/symbolic play is frequently absent from the child's repertoire. Play that appears symbolic may actually be overlearned or rote behavior. These children show a lack of curiosity about the world, which is manifested, in part, as a resistance to learning new things.

Finally, emotional development is severely compromised. Children with ASD have difficulty understanding and expressing feelings, and lack empathy. In 1985, Baron-Cohen, Leslie, and Frith introduced the concept of "**Theory of Mind (ToM)**" or "mindblindness," which they defined as the ability to take the perspective of others, especially when that perspective is different from one's own. This includes the ability to understand that others have feelings and emotions of their own. It also includes the ability to differentiate between different emotions, and label and recognize one's own emotional states. ToM is mediated by language; it begins to develop during in early childhood, at about 2 to 3 years of age. This "other awareness" is thought to affect social, emotional, communication, and language development. For example, a child might laugh when his classmate falls down at recess and scrapes his knee. The same child may not be able to select "happy" when shown pictures of "happy" and "sad" faces. Joint attention is a prerequisite skill for developing ToM; so, before any ToM strategies (e.g., perspective taking) can be meaningfully expected/introduced, a child must have first developed joint attention (Baron-Cohen et al., 1985).

Language

Although oral language development is no longer a DSM criterion for the diagnosis of ASD, it is important to understand that children with ASD exhibit significant quantitative and qualitative language impairments. The pattern of development and language use described in ASD is often strikingly different from TD children and children with other developmental disabilities. Sometimes, their language development is characterized as aberrant rather than "delayed." That is, their language development does not follow a typical developmental pattern and does not represent any stage of typical language development. Most often, these children demonstrate a failure to acquire spoken language, demonstrating significant language comprehension and production problems. For children with ASD who are verbal, their use of language is often inappropriate and out of context (e.g., failure to stay on topic during a conversation, irrelevant responses to requests/questions) and conveys a significantly lower proportion of communicative intentions than the language of nonimpaired peers and peer with other kinds of disabilities (Shumway & Wetherby, 2009). They also have difficulty understanding the nonverbal communication of others (e.g., gestures, facial expressions) and do not use meaningful gestures to communicate. A notable feature characteristic of these children's expressive language is pronoun reversal. For example, a child who is asking for juice will likely say: "You want juice" rather than the conventional "I want juice," or "He eat cookie" in response to the question: "What are you eating?" In addition, proper nouns are commonly used to refer to oneself, as in "John wants juice" rather than "I/me want juice." These individuals often recite long passages of verbal material (entire poems, weather reports, news articles) without comprehension; this is because they have excellent "recording memory," but cannot chunk linguistic information into meaningful units.

One of the hallmark characteristics of ASD is the use of echolalia, which is the partial or full repetition of the speech of others (Prizant & Duchan, 1981). This linguistic behavior can be described according to when it occurs (i.e., immediate vs. delayed) or according to the function it is intended to serve (i.e., communicative vs. noncommunicative). In general, delayed echolalia is often viewed as a self-stimulatory behavior, whereas immediate echoes tend to be used when the child does not know what is expected in terms of verbalization (e.g., turn-taking filler or searching for the correct response). Although the traditional view of echolalia characterized it as an aberrant behavior that should be eliminated, Prizant (1983) found that the echoes can serve a variety of different communicative functions, such as requesting, protesting, or commenting. Some children with ASD demonstrate use of both communicative and noncommunicative echolalia. This verbal behavior is not unique to autism; children with other disabilities such as intellectual impairment, fragile X syndrome, and childhood schizophrenia may exhibit echolalia (Tager-Flusberg, Paul, & Lord, 2005). However, compared to these other populations, a much larger proportion of children with ASD (approximately 85% of verbal communicators) produce echolalic utterances, the length of their echoed utterances are longer, and their echoes include more precise replication of the original utterance with regard to factors such as intonation, coughs, and accents (Rydell & Prizant, 1995). Table 6-2 summarizes the different aspects of echolalia.

Elimination/extinction of echolalia should not be considered an initial, appropriate, or even necessary intervention goal. Many children with ASD use echoes communicatively to request, comment, or respond to others. Echolalia may be a significant portion of the child's communicative repertoire. In some cases, it may be the primary or sole means of communication and will continue throughout the life span, particularly in stressful situations. In other cases, echolalia can be a transitional step/phase prior to or during therapy to facilitate development of spontaneous spoken language. In general, echolalia decreases significantly as the child acquires greater receptive and expressive language skills.

Emergent Literacy and Literacy

In both emergent literacy and literacy, children with ASD show strengths in form and weakness in meaning. Some children demonstrate *hyperlexia*: an advanced ability to recognize the written word in the presence of delayed or deviant language development (Mehegan & Dreifuss, 1972; Silberberg & Silberberg, 1967). Hyperlexia also has been characterized as a compulsive preoccupation with the written word.

At the emergent literacy stage, children can name letters, but not understand what people read and write (Lanter, Watson, Erickson, & Freeman, 2012; Lindgren, Folstein, Tomblin, & Tager-Flusberg, 2009). At the literacy stage, the same pattern is seen. Decoding and spelling are strengths for children with ASD, whereas reading comprehension is quite challenging. Specifically, children with high-functioning ASD perform as well as or even better than typically developing peers (matched for age and IQ) on word-reading and spelling tasks, whereas their reading comprehension is very poor. Moreover, children who demonstrate accurate reading comprehension at the word level often experience severe difficulties at the passage level for both reading accuracy and comprehension (Arciuli, Stevens, Trembath, & Simpson, 2013).

In addition to communication and language deficits, children with ASD demonstrate speech impairment in the presence of good speech articulation skills. The main speech impairment occurs in speech prosody (melody or rhythm of speech), and this characteristic is observed even in adolescents with no discernible language impairment (Grossman, Bemis, Skwerer, & Tager-Flusberg, 2013; Rapin & Dunn, 1997).

TABLE 6–2
Examples of Different Types of Echolalia*

Type	Example and Context/Intent
Immediate/ Noncommunicative	Adult: Where did you go yesterday? Child: Where did you go yesterday? Adult: Wash your hands. Child: Wash your hands.
Delayed/ Noncommunicative	Child: Don't throw the doll off the balcony. (Child is repeating an utterance heard 2 years previously for no apparent reason.) Child: Give this to John. Give this to John. Give this to John. Give this to John. (No referent in sight. Said intoning a melody.)
Mitigated	Adult: Why are you crying? Child: Why are you screaming? Adult: Do you want to watch *Snow White*? Child: You want to watch *Snow White*. (Meaning, "Yes, I do.")
Immediate/ Communicative	Adult: Do you want a sandwich? Child: Do you want a sandwich? Yes. (Meaning that the child wants a sandwich.) Adult: Soup's on. Child: Soup's on. (Meaning that the child wants a bowl of soup.)
Delayed Communicative	Child (When child is tired): It's been a long day kids, but you've done a great job. (Child is repeating a line from a Tonka Truck computer game.) Child (When child is asked to do a difficult task): And in other news. . . . Child (Whenever child breaks something): Can we fix it? Yes, we can! (Child is repeating a line from *Bob the Builder*.)
Immediate/Mitigated	Adult (Pointing to a gingerbread house that was hit by a peer): It's smooshed into pieces. Child: It broke into pieces.
Delayed Mitigated	Child (Whenever sees classmate crying): It's not easy being green. (Child is repeating a line from the Muppets characters.)

Source: Portions are adapted from I. Betz and E. Brady (personal communication, 2014).

Grossman et al., (2013) showed that high-functioning adolescents with autism performed as well as typically developing peers on receptive tasks that required them to perceptually differentiate stress patterns in speech (e.g., HOTdog versus hotDOG) as well as affective prosody (happy, sad, neutral), but demonstrated significant differences in the production of prosody. Specifically, their production of two-syllable words was atypical, with noted exaggerated pauses between syllables, especially for second-syllable-stress items. This labored and slow enunciation pattern was in stark contrast to the briefer, more fluid productions of their typically developing peers. These abnormal prosody production patterns also have been noted by Paul, Augustyn, Klin, and Vollkmar (2005).

Other characteristics often observed in the speech of children with ASD include:

- Monotone inflection at the utterance level
- Instances of singing interspersed into the child's production of connected speech
- Repetition and perseveration on individual sounds as well as some sound sequences

Repetitive/Restricted Behaviors, Interests, and Activities

In addition to social and language impairments, children with ASD also exhibit other significant deficits. Again, the reader is reminded that every child with ASD does not exhibit all of these characteristics and not to the same degree.

- Non-goal-directed behaviors (i.e., self-stimulatory behaviors such as rocking back and forth, pacing, hand waving)
- Self-injurious and aggressive behaviors (e.g., head banging, biting)
- Obsessive behaviors: Remaining fixated on a particular stimulus (e.g., learning how a vacuum cleaner works) and ignoring other stimuli (aka over-selected attention)
- Difficulty developing/following important routines (e.g., feeding/sleeping), probably as a result of inability to cope with even the smallest changes in the environment
- Hypo-/hypersensitivity to stimuli (e.g., high tolerance for pain, extreme reactions to everyday sounds, aversion to certain food or fabric textures)
- Extreme food selectivity (aka "food fetishes"): Child restricts his or her intake to one or two very specific foods (e.g., Dannon strawberry yogurt; strawberry Twizzlers) and rejects all others. This can result in significant developmental and health consequences. Another eating problem is pica, ingesting or chewing on nonedible substances such as dirt, paper, wood, or plastic.
- Stimulus oveselectivity: Focus on isolated aspects of objects or people (e.g., fascination with sensory experiences such as lights or visual patterns)
- Difficulty integrating auditory and visual information simultaneously (e.g., hold hands over ears to reduce confusion between the senses)
- Attentional difficulties: Orienting, sustaining, and shifting attention, especially when a rapid shift of attention is required (transitions)
- Situational-specific learning (aka "local learning"): Learning a skill in one context but not recognizing the skill in another context

Medications

About 70% of children with autism are prescribed psychoactive medications to ameliorate disruptive behaviors, which range from impulsivity to self-injury to overt aggression to mood disorders. SLPs need to understand the potential side effects of medication and be able to differentiate these effects from the actual symptoms of ASD. Side effects are not well understood. Efficacy data for most classes of drugs are increasing, but they are still somewhat limited. Classes of drugs that are commonly used in the ASD population include:

- *Antipsychotics:* Risperdal, Haldol
- *Stimulants:* Ritalin, Cylert
- *Nonstimulants:* Stratera
- *Secretin and serotonin re-uptake inhibitors (SSRIs):* Prozac, Paxil
- *Anti-seizure medication:* Ativan, Keppra
- *Complementary and alternative medicine (CAM) interventions:* insufficient evidence about effectiveness or adverse effects

Outcomes

Language skills and IQ are the strongest predictors of a child's outcome (Gotham, Pickles, & Lord, 2012; Pellicano, 2013; Witwer & Lecavalier, 2008). Specifically, a good outcome is best predicted by attainment of meaningful communication and demonstration of normal nonverbal IQ by 5 years of age.

In addition to overall prognosis and outcome, researchers have traced the development of specific skill areas in small samples of individuals with ASD over time and examined how change in one area affects another. One area of focus is metacognition/executive functioning with children/adolescents in the average or high-functioning range of intelligence between 4 and 19 years old (Bennett et al., 2013; Pellicano, 2012). Metacognitive/executive functioning abilities involve an awareness of one's own problem-solving abilities and include self-regulation behaviors that are used to guide, monitor, and evaluate the success of one's performance (Baddeley, 2007; Barkley, 1996, 1997). Findings suggest a positive link between executive functioning, ToM development, and language development. Overall, children/adolescents with the strongest executive functioning skills (planning, carrying out complex tasks) demonstrated the strongest ToM (taking the perspective of another). These findings suggest that intervention focused on executive functioning and ToM may yield overall developmental benefits, including advances in language and communication. Because these studies involved small sample sizes, the results must be viewed as promising, but preliminary.

Autism is a lifelong developmental disorder, but most of the research studies are cross-sectional (e.g., Kalk, Law, Landa, & Law, 2010). A few longitudinal studies followed large samples of children with ASD over two decades and provide insight into the trajectories for ASD from early identification through adolescence and into adulthood. The findings of Lord and her colleagues (2012) are representative. These authors followed 300 children from age 2 to 21 years and found three distinct subgroups:

- About 10% of children showed dramatic improvement by middle adolescence (i.e., live independently, self-supporting, professional careers, marry).
- Another 10% worsened over time.
- Eighty percent continue to demonstrate significant deficits over time with regard to core symptoms/severity.

These subgroups remained surprisingly stable over time, with little variability within or across the groups.

In summary, most children with ASD continue to demonstrate significant deficits throughout life and may not be able to live independently. But even those with the mildest symptoms have residual deficits in the social domain (viewed as "eccentric"), exhibiting highly stereotypic interactions (e.g., scripts), difficulty in turn-taking and reciprocal conversations, poor coordination of eye contact and speech, and unusual speech patterns. These limitations may affect their ability to adjust to new social demands in academic, vocational, and community settings. When working with adolescents, SLPs may need to include transitional objectives and functional outcomes to prepare these individuals for employment in highly structured jobs such as computer programming, sorting/assembling materials, or stocking shelves.

TREATMENT EFFICACY/ EVIDENCE-BASED PRACTICE

The unprecedented increase in the prevalence of ASD in the U.S. population has fueled a strong demand for information on evidence-based practices with this group of individuals. Given the wide range of intervention approaches that have been developed over the past 60 years (e.g., behavioral, dietary, educational, etc.), combing through the existing ASD treatment literature can be daunting for the practicing clinician. Fortunately, there have been several systematic reviews of intervention practices published within the past decade.

The National Standards Project conducted a comprehensive review of intervention studies completed by 2007 for children and adolescents with ASD (National Autism Center, 2009b). The National Standards Project found 5 practices for which researchers demonstrated no effects, 22 practices that were characterized as "emerging," and 11 practices that were identified as evidence-based.

The National Professional Development Center on ASD (NPDC) also performed a systematic review of intervention articles published between 1997 and 2007 (Odom, Collet-Klingenberg, Rogers, & Hatton, 2010). This group found that 24 focused intervention practices met criteria for being identified as "evidence-based." In an attempt to directly translate this scientific information into practice, the NPDC investigators/staff developed online training modules for clinicians, which can be accessed via the NPDC website (autismpdc .fgp.unc.edu/content/autsim-internet-modules-aim).

The NPDC recently updated its comprehensive review of the ASD intervention literature to include articles from 1990 through 2011 (Wong et al., 2013). This review identified 27 focused intervention practices as meeting criteria for being judged as "evidence-based." These practices were characterized as achieving a range of 3 to 11 outcomes in a set of 12 identified areas, such as social, communicative, cognitive, behavioral, and others. They found that some practices (e.g., antecedent-based intervention, prompting, video modeling) could be characterized as having strong support based on the number of studies in the literature, especially if single-subject designs are considered. Other practices (e.g., social narratives, technology-aided instruction, and visual supports) were supported by a combination of single-subject and group-design studies. Still, other practices (e.g., auditory integration training, music therapy, reciprocal imitation training) were judged to have some support in the literature, but not a sufficient amount to earn the designation of "evidence-based."

Given the complex and sometimes controversial nature of intervention in ASD, clinicians are strongly encouraged to become acquainted with the breadth of practices available and the extent to which they are supported in the current literature. When combined with the SLP's clinical judgment and the needs/values of the child/family with ASD, this will ensure that intervention is individualized for each client and programmed and implemented in the most efficacious manner possible.

TREATMENT FOR AUTISM

Theoretical Models

Two primary theoretical orientations underlie the treatment of autism: developmental and functional/behavioral:

- *Functional/behavioral (Lovaas, Koegel, Simmons, & Long 1973):* This framework places primary emphasis on improving a child's effectiveness as a communicator. Intervention does not follow any developmental sequence and is not limited to verbal speech. Target behaviors are selected based on individual need/skill as well as instructional/ family priorities.

- *Developmental (Tager-Flusberg et al., 2009):* This framework focuses on spoken language skills and moves away from terminology related to "functional speech and language." It uses benchmark criteria based on typical language development as a rubric for language intervention programming. The hierarchy progresses from meaningful gestures/vocalizations, to single words, to phrases/sentences, and culminates with complex language forms.

These two philosophical orientations are not mutually exclusive and are frequently combined to varying degrees (i.e., hybrid). In general, selection of a model is heavily influenced by the client's cognitive profile. Developmental approaches are usually appropriate for children with mild or no cognitive impairment, whereas functional approaches are appropriate for children whose cognitive abilities are severely compromised. These theoretical models can be implemented in different settings or contexts (e.g., location, communicative partner, activity). The degree to which programming is child-directed or clinician-directed may vary across settings or over time. Before specific treatment approaches are presented, the particular pattern of language, communication, and social development demonstrated by these children necessitates discussion of important programming considerations:

- *Universal design principles for learning (UDL):* All instruction and intervention should align with UDL, in terms of providing the child/adolescent with multiple means of access to the curriculum, multiple means of expressing knowledge, and multiple opportunities for meaningful practice of the newly learned skills to sustain motivation for learning.

- *Early intervention (EI):* The environment has greatest influence on brain structure and function during the first few years of life. Thus, maturation coupled with early, appropriate stimulation capitalizes on neural plasticity. Another benefit of early intervention often is minimization of the emergence of the maladaptive behaviors and behavioral difficulties that are frequently part of the developmental course of ASD (Boyd, Odom, Humphreys, & Sam, 2010; Paul, 2008).

- *Comprehensive and intensive intervention:* Because of the pervasiveness of ASD, it is recommended that intervention programming address multiple areas of deficits, across all of a child's daily settings and activities, with an intensity of 25 to 40 hours/week (National Autism Project, National Autism Center, 2009). This comprehensive approach should be implemented over extended periods of time because ASD is a life-span disorder (Boyd et al., 2010).

- *Structure versus flexibility:* Children with ASD function best in environments that are predicable—where rules and expectations are clear and consistent. However, excessive reliance on structure has the potential to become a hindrance and even an obstacle to learning new skills and adapting to changes in daily routines. These children need some degree of flexibility to learn new skills. SLPs are encouraged to use small, incremental changes/transitions (e.g., new materials; new location in room; order of activities), and to let students know of these changes in advance.

- *Generalization:* Children with ASD learn in situation-specific ways, and thus do not generalize spontaneously to other contexts. Target behaviors need to be explicitly taught across all daily environments and activities, including home, school, daycare, and community settings. A pull-out model may create an artificial context that does not provide the child with consistent connections to real-life contexts (e.g., Wetherby & Prizant, 2000).

- *Behavior and emotions:* Individuals with ASD often emulate the emotion of their communication partner. If a question, direction, or request is given in a directive, strident, or loud manner, distress is a likely result, and this negativity can escalate rapidly. Clinicians are encouraged to use a positive, soft, and even tone when interacting with their clients, even when the intended message is disapproving.

- *Visual supports:* Many individuals with autism spontaneously convert spoken/verbal messages into sequences of visual images; that is, they are visual thinkers (Grandin, 2010). These children benefit from strategies that utilize their strength in visual processing, such as picture schedules, behavior graphing, and so on. Visual supports also help children transition from one activity/context to another.

- *Interdisciplinary/collaborative team:* The nature of ASD necessitates an integrated approach to intervention in which there is coordinated and cooperative involvement of the SLP, classroom teacher, parents/families, and other professionals. The team also may include:

  - Occupational therapist for teaching fine motor and self-care skills, and sensory integration (e.g., food texture sensitivities).

  - Social worker to help families access to available resources, self-help, and support groups. Moreover, a family-based strategy recognizes the impact that this impairment has on the entire family dynamic. It also emphasizes that "improvements" must be measured in terms of family adjustment as well as child progress (Woods & Brown, 2011).

  - Physician for managing seizures and psychiatric co-morbidities—most common are anxiety disorders and depression.

- Psychologist/psychiatrist for addressing management of behaviors such as self-injury and severe tantrums.

- Psycho-pharmacologist to prescribe medications, especially if problematic behaviors are severe, chronic, and unresponsive to behavioral interventions (Self, Hale, & Crumrine, 2010).

Treatment Approaches

This section presents information on a variety of intervention models and techniques for ASD. The approaches selected for discussion are based on a combination of factors, including orientations that have a primary focus on communication, those that have evidence supporting their efficacy and effectiveness, and those that are commonly used by SLPs in clinical and instructional settings. The authors do not endorse any particular orientation, and have ourselves utilized a variety of different approaches and combinations of approaches according to the needs of individual children and their families. The reader is encouraged to develop a large repertoire of treatment strategies to maximize the effectiveness of treatment programming for each child. This chapter does not discuss comprehensive treatment models that address the broad range of deficit areas exhibited by children with ASD, such as Learning Experiences and Alternate Programs for Preschoolers and Their Parents (LEAP; Strain & Hoyson, 2000), More Than Words (Carter, et al., 2011), Preschool Autism Communication Trial (PACT; Green et al., 2010), and the Early Start Denver Model (Dawson et al., 2010; Rogers, Hall, Osaki, Reaven, & Herbison, 2000). For additional information on these and other comprehensive models, refer to Odom, Boyd, Hall, and Hume (2010).

For children with autism who are nonverbal, an alternative or augmentative system of communication (AAC) is frequently adopted. It may be used as a step toward useful speech or it may serve as a child's main form of communication. AAC is used to supplement, enhance, or replace spoken language. It has many forms, including no-tech (e.g., signs, gestures), low-tech (e.g., pictures, photographs), and hi-tech (electronic devices, computerized speech).

Some of the approaches discussed in the next section clearly align with a particular theoretical model, whereas others cross philosophical or conceptual categories, and can be adapted for use within more than one theoretical orientation. It is important to remember that age of onset of treatment and treatment intensity are more important than use of a specific treatment program or model (Warren et al., 2011).

The approaches are presented in alphabetical order rather than any potential author preference. This strategy was adopted to ensure objectivity of the discussion.

Treatment & Education of Autistic and Related Communication-Handicapped Children (TEACCH; Mesibov & Shea, 2010; Schopler & Reichler, 1971). The **TEACCH** approach was originally developed in 1971 as a home-based approach. It has evolved to include a classroom-based focus, and the current version is described here. TEACCH can be used with children at a wide range of ages and can incorporate **assistive technology (AT) or AAC** for children who are nonverbal. The structured classroom-based approach to teaching is based on the premise that children with autism are predominantly visual learners. Structured teaching involves four components:

1. Organize the physical environment to maximize learning and to minimize distractions.

2. Use visual teaching to capitalize on the child's relative strength in visual/spatial information processing (e.g., photographs, schedule boards, written words).

3. Individualize goals and activities to engage the child's attention (e.g., use stimuli related to the child's favorite superhero when teaching turn-taking).

4. Facilitate meaningful child-initiated communication (e.g., provide opportunities for the child to make choices versus prompted responses).

Applied Behavioral Analysis (ABA). **Applied behavior analysis** (ABA) represents a class of interventions that apply behavioral science principles to address behavior problems and learning in children with autism and other developmental disorders. All ABA approaches are based on Skinner's (1957) behavioral principles of operant conditioning: a stimulus, or antecedent event, is presented to elicit a target response, which is immediately followed by a consequent event (reward or punishment) to increase desired behaviors or decrease unwanted behaviors. The proper implementation of ABA requires objective observation and analysis of behavior. ABA has several forms, some of which focus on the reduction of disruptive behaviors (e.g., self-injury, aggression, repetitive, ritualistic mannerisms), whereas others are aimed at increasing adaptive behaviors, communication, and spoken language. All ABA approaches break complex tasks, actions, and behaviors into smaller sequential parts for easier access by the child. Most ABA approaches are intensive, consisting of 30 to 40 hours of one-to-one therapy per week. Emphasis also is placed on the role of parents as primary intervention agents.

Discrete Trial Training (DTT), a form of ABA therapy developed by Lovaas et al., (1973), is based on the learning principle that if a behavior is rewarded, it is more likely to be repeated. Although ABA is sometimes referred to as the "Lovaas method," this version, DTT, is one specific type of ABA. The clinician presents a stimulus (e.g., question or request to stand up), along with the correct response. Following each correct response, the child is rewarded with consequent events such as praise, food, or other incentives. Incorrect responses are ignored. This immediate schedule of reinforcement for correct behaviors is used to clearly establish the expected behavior and provide immediate feedback to the child about the accuracy of his or her response.

Pivotal Response Teaching (PRT) is an ABA approach developed in the 1970s by Koegel and Koegel that uses naturalistic procedures that focus primarily on two "pivotal" areas: motivation to learn and initiation of activities. As such, PRT is specifically designed to increase a child's motivation to participate in learning new skills. Target behaviors are selected based on each child's developmental level and may include social skills (e.g., turn-taking), adaptive behaviors (dressing, feeding), and language-learning skills. The intent of PRT is to increase and generalize skills in language, play, and social interaction in a child-directed format.

Reciprocal Imitation Therapy (RIT) is a variation of PRT developed by Ingersoll and Lalonde (2010) for teaching play skills. Within the context of a play environment, it is specifically aimed at teaching spontaneous, reciprocal imitation skills to young children with autism. The clinician imitates actions and/or vocalizations of the child in an obvious manner and then the child is rewarded for any subsequent attempted imitative behavior. Assistance is provided through prompting, modeling, and physical guidance.

Social Stories. (Gray, 1994, 1998; Gray & Garand, 1993). The **social stories** approach is designed for higher-functioning children and adolescents with autism (i.e., children whose cognitive status ranges from mild intellectual disabilities to above-average intellectual function). "Scripts/stories" are written for each child that provide explanations of appropriate behaviors in social situations with which the individual is having difficulty. The scripts are tailored to the client's level of language comprehension.

Most stories contain three sequential statements: descriptive statements, perspective statements, and directive statements. Descriptive statements are intended to help a child understand a particular situation and provide words, phrases, or sentences for a situation that child cannot generate on his or her own. Perspective statements facilitate the child's ability to verbally identify the feelings, wants, and motivations of other people. Directive statements provide specific social cues that tell the children what they could do in a situation that would be more socially appropriate than their current responses. For children who cannot read, visual scripts and visual modeling serve as the social stories. Social stories also foster executive functioning skills, particularly in the areas of planning and self-monitoring. Role-playing and repeated reading are common strategies used to teach social stories, along with traditional techniques of prompting, modeling, imitating, and other types of cues. Typical examples of social story topics include joining a game, praising others for accomplishments, waiting your turn in an activity, raising your hand in class, or monitoring one's own production of inappropriate/disruptive vocalizations.

Social-Communication, Emotional Regulation, and Transactional Support (SCERTS). The **SCERTS** program (Wetherby & Prizant, 2000) focuses on the core deficits of children with ASD and emphasizes communication, social relatedness, and sensory domains using a family-centered model (Prizant, Wetherby, Rubin, & Laurent, 2003). Intervention occurs in an integrated manner because, according to the authors, the difficulties presented by children with ASD do not occur in isolation, and therefore must be treated as a whole. For example, mealtime is a daily activity that involves skills from each of these areas. Intervention planning is individualized according to the strengths, natural motivations, and needs of each child and the priorities of the family. Family involvement, support, and education are deemed essential to enhance a child's development and progress.

The main elements of the SCERTS model are:

- *Communication and language:* A social-pragmatic approach to language therapy is used that focuses on the functional use of preverbal and verbal communication skills in natural and semi-structured interactions. Nonspeech communication systems such as the Picture Exchange Communication System (PECS) and picture symbols often are incorporated to facilitate communication initiation and responsiveness. Both ABA and developmentally based strategies are used.

- *Social relatedness and social-emotional reciprocity:* Greenspan's DIR/Floor Time® approach is the approach of choice to treat deficits in these areas because of its emphasis on developmental progressions in naturalistic contexts. (See later section on DIR for further information.)

- *Sensory processing:* Sensory integration therapy and environmental modifications, adaptations, and supports are integral parts of SCERTS because many children with autism have motor planning problems and difficulties with daily living skills (e.g., feeding, dressing).

Picture Exchange Communication System®. The **Picture Exchange Communication System** (PECS), developed by Bondy and Frost (1994), is a structured AAC system that promotes symbolic communication in nonverbal children with autism (or children with limited speech), encouraging spontaneous initiations. Its overall goal is to help children begin to discover/understand the power of communication. It uses a combination of incidental teaching and behavioral methods to foster meaningful communication interactions. It starts with a basic goal: to develop the concept of how to use a picture/object (symbol) to obtain a desired item or action. It progresses through six phases, beginning with simple requests and moving to single words, phrases, comments, and answering questions. At all steps of the program, children make choices/decisions that allow them to have more control over their world through the use of communication. In a typical early session, the clinician places an item (object or picture) on the table for which the child has previously shown desire. When the child reaches (makes a physical request) for the item, the SLP places it in the child's hand and helps the child to "exchange" the item (symbol) for the desired object. The immediacy of the exchange demonstrates the social interactive nature of communication in a highly concrete and functional way. This is important because children with autism often are not reinforced by typical social rewards associated with the act of communication, such as eye contact, a smile, or praise. Some children using PECS later develop speech, others may move to a more sophisticated AAC system, and still others continue to use PECS as their major form of communication both at home and at school.

Video Modeling (Charlop & Milstein, 1989). This is an instructional technique that uses a video format to teach a variety of social and communication behaviors to children with autism (Bellini & Akullian, 2007). Target behaviors are scripted and videotaped by the clinician (referred to as an *other-as-model method*). The child watches repeated videotaped presentations of adults or peers engaging in exchanges using appropriate communicative behaviors. **Video modeling** can be used to teach basic communication skills (e.g., establishing joint attention during play) and more complex communication behaviors (e.g., increasing utterance length during conversational exchanges). It also can be effective for improving a variety of emotional, behavioral, and daily living skills in children with ASD. For older and more advanced children, a "self-as-model" procedure can be used where the client acts as his or her own model. The clinician then edits the video so that only desired behaviors are shown.

Relationship Development Intervention (RDI) (Gutstein & Sheely, 2002). This approach is a home-centered treatment program for young children with ASD and is a parent-implemented method. Developed by Gutstein in the 1990s, it is based on his theoretical construct of "dynamic intelligence," which Gutstein defines as the ability to think flexibly. Flexible thinking includes the ability to take the perspective of others, adapt to changes in the environment, and integrate information from a variety of sources (e.g., auditory, visual, tactile). The main premise is that individuals with autism can participate in authentic social and emotional relationships if they are exposed to them in a gradual, systematic way. The goal of **RDI** intervention is the gradual development of a child's reciprocal social communication that underlies the ability to form emotional bonds and interpersonal connections/relationships. Parents receive formal training in behavioral methods to slowly and systematically change/shape the interaction patterns between themselves and their children in everyday activities and settings. RDI has several core objectives to foster flexible thinking, such as emotional referencing (the ability to learn from the emotional and subjective experiences of others), social coordination (the ability to control one's behavior to successfully participate in social relationships), declarative language (the ability to use verbal and nonverbal communication to express curiosity, invite interactions, share perceptions and feelings, and coordinate with others), and relational information processing (the ability to solve problems that lack clear-cut solutions).

In a typical session, parents or other caregivers use an ordered set of developmentally sensitive objectives based on routine daily activities. For example, in the early stages of training, spoken language may be limited to encourage eye contact, joint attention, and other forms of nonverbal communication. The objectives gradually expand as the child's abilities increase.

Functional Communication Training (FCT) (Durand, 1990; Franzone, 2009).

FCT is aimed at replacing a child's disruptive behaviors with more appropriate and effective communication behaviors or skills. FCT is a highly systematic and structured program that utilizes the basic principles of operant conditioning (antecedent event-response-consequent event). The clinician first identifies the function of the interfering behavior (e.g., biting classmates to get a wanted toy) and then teaches a more conventional replacement behavior (e.g., pointing) that serves the same communicative purpose as the interfering behavior. The replacement behavior should allow the child to obtain his or her goal just as easily or more easily than the disruptive behavior. The replacement behavior can be nonverbal (e.g., pointing, sign, informal gestures) or verbal (e.g., "Please"; "I want the truck"; "Want"). The clinician structures each session to elicit several instances of the interfering behavior to provide the child with numerous opportunities to practice using the replacement behavior.

DIR/Floortime® (Developmental, Individual Difference, Relationship-Based) (Greenspan, 1990).

DIR is a framework developed by Greenspan (1990) that identifies six developmental milestones for healthy emotional and intellectual growth: (1) attending, (2) relating, (3) purposeful communication, (4) problem-solving interactions, (5) using ideas creatively, and (6) using ideas logically. This model emphasizes identification of each child's individual differences in the way he or she processes sounds, sights, sensations, and movements. It also focuses on how parents, caregivers, therapists, and educators can tailor their interactions/relationships with the child to provide maximal opportunities to achieve the described milestones. **Floortime®** is the technique for implementing this model of intervention for children with ASD. Adults in the child's environment are encouraged to "get down on the floor" and engage in the following set of steps 6 to 10 times per day for 20-minute periods:

a. Pay attention to the child's individual behaviors.

b. Locate an "entry point" into the child's system by imitating/joining in his or her behavior (e.g., jumping, rubbing a spot on the table).

c. Engage the child this way for a few minutes and then introduce variations on the theme for both of you to embrace.

d. Gradually lead the child into mastering the milestones identified above to create the experience of a "shared world" between the child and adult.

Example Profiles

Thomas is a 12-year-old boy who was diagnosed with Asperger's syndrome in second grade (now considered a mild form of ASD according to current DSM-5 guidelines). He is enrolled in a seventh-grade general education program and his academic skills range between average and superior. He tends to answer questions from teachers and others tangentially and in excessive detail. He exhibits difficulty with the rules for initiating conversation and responding appropriately to topics introduced by others. In addition, the teacher and the family report that he consistently interrupts others despite frequent reminders to wait his conversational turn. In general, he does not seem to understand nonverbal cues such as the facial expressions and body language of others. Since childhood, Thomas has had difficulty establishing friendships and has just recently begun to express an awareness of his exclusion from peer groups.

Selection of therapy targets and suggested intervention strategies. Based on Thomas's profile, pragmatic language and executive function are two main areas selected for intervention. Potential pragmatic goals include: (1) adapting the content of his communicative messages to the needs/expectations of different listeners; and (2) improving his ability to recognize and interpret nonverbal communication behaviors. For executive function, a primary goal is to improve Thomas's ability to monitor and inhibit/decrease his persistent conversational interruption behaviors. Although several intervention strategies are applicable in this scenario, social stories and video modeling may be particularly appropriate.

Dominic is 3½-year-old male child old who received a diagnosis of severe ASD at 2 ½ years. He is enrolled in a full-day special education preschool program where he continues to receive services. Dominic displays many classic characteristics of ASD, including:

- Extreme social isolation
- Self-stimulatory behaviors and unprovoked aggression toward others
- Frequent echolalia, which may be a combination of communicative and noncommunicative echoes
- Hypersensitivity to tactile stimuli (e.g., hugging, food textures)
- Severe impairment in receptive and expressive language with moderate intellectual impairment
- Excellent rote memory skills
- Somewhat intact visual/spatial skills

Overall, Dominic does not appear to be interested in communicating with others in his environment.

Selection of therapy targets and suggested intervention strategies. Based on Dominic's profile, the following are suggested as main targets of intervention:

- Increasing the frequency of social interactions
- Decreasing unwanted and aggressive behaviors
- Establishing a larger repertoire of functional communication behaviors

Although several intervention approaches may be appropriate in this case, Functional Communication Therapy (FCT) strategy may be useful in addressing disruptive behaviors. An ABA discrete trial strategy can be utilized to increase on-task attention and compliance in the classroom. In addition, PECS may provide a means of increasing Dominic's ability to initiate communication more effectively with others.

Lilly is an 18-month-old girl who with normal hearing who is at risk for ASD based on the results of a recent evaluation. Lilly was referred for the evaluation by her parents, who are concerned that their daughter's development is very different from that of their other children (Larry, age 4 yrs; Toby, age 6 yrs). Lilly has a positive family history of ASD; her maternal aunt and uncle were diagnosed with autism during childhood. Based on both parental report and clinical evaluation, Lilly shows inconsistent eye contact with parents, siblings, and other familiar persons. She demonstrates a social smile and joint attention but is difficult to engage in social games such as peek-a-boo or in imitative vocal play, both of which require turn-taking. Lilly shows excessive interest in a restricted set of objects and activities, such as her talking monkey and running in and out of a toy house. During the evaluation, some functional play was observed. For example, she kissed a baby doll and when given a toy car, she rolled it on the floor. Her true level of language comprehension was difficult to determine, although below age expectations, as her on-task attention was fleeting and highly distractible. Expressively, Lilly communicated mainly by vocalizations paired with gestures, about half of which the clinician was able to identify as meaningful. Isolated instances of single words (e.g., "no" and "cookie") were noted.

Selection of therapy targets and suggested intervention strategies. Based on Lilly's current profile, she would benefit from family-based language stimulation activities implemented in the home environment. The following are recommended as major areas of focus:

- Turn-taking
- Increasing ability to follow simple directions
- Expanding repertoire of speech sounds and single words relevant to her daily environment

Although several approaches may be appropriate in this case, Reciprocal Imitation Therapy, Floortime, and SCERTS may be particularly useful because these strategies advocate for engaging in child-directed play (imitating what the child does) and shaping that interaction into more functional communication behaviors. Lilly's language development and social communication status should be monitored closely, and a re-evaluation should be scheduled in 6 months unless specific parental concerns arise.

Helpful Hints

1. Include parents and families as full participants on the interdisciplinary team from the beginning of the therapeutic process. Parents, especially keen observers, can provide basic information about their child's preferred and nonpreferred tasks, activities, toys, foods, and so forth. Clinicians also are encouraged to help parents identify and prioritize the behaviors of their child that are most disruptive to the family dynamic at home.

2. Avoid using indirect forms of communication such as indirect requests (e.g., "That cake sure looks good") because individuals with ASD have difficulty reading social cues; direct forms of communication generally are more effective (e.g., "Give me some cake, please").

3. Because individuals with ASD learn in situation-specific ways, we cannot expect them to generalize a skill learned in one situation to another context, or even in the same context at a different time of day. Each context may represent a separate behavioral objective.

4. Older students with high-functioning ASD may benefit from joining networking groups where they can share ideas, voice frustrations, and get suggestions from others who have had similar experiences. Alternatively, local groups can be sought that provide opportunities for social interaction and group social activities.

5. High-functioning individuals with ASD may be misdiagnosed as learning disabled (LD) because they share many of the same presenting behaviors. But, inappropriate diagnosis most often results in inappropriate instruction/intervention strategies, especially programming that does not have a central focus on social communication and interaction.

6. Counsel families, teachers, and others who interact with the child on a regular basis that the communication style of individuals with ASD is frequently "too direct," making others uncomfortable. This directness, however, is a sign that these individuals cannot read the social cues of others or the environment.

7. The clinician and family are encouraged to use visual schedules to build predictability into the daily routines of both children and adolescents.

8. Books are helpful to expose children to emotions and feelings in a nonthreatening way. Titles are available across the age/developmental range. Examples include: *Taking a Bath with the Dog and Other Things That Make Me Happy* (Scott Menchin), *When Sophie Gets Really, Really Angry* (Molly Bang), *I'm Mad* (Elizabeth Cray), and *The Way I Feel* (Janice Cain).

9. Many individuals with high-functioning ASD pursue postsecondary education. Clinicians can provide guidance, resources, and encouragement regarding colleges and universities that serve this population or have programs to support their needs.

10. When working with individuals from culturally and linguistically diverse backgrounds, the perceptions/beliefs of family members regarding appropriate social communication are of critical importance.

11. Often as children's intentional communication improves, a decrease may be noted in unwanted/undesirable behaviors. With the significant growth in technology, clinicians are encouraged to explore the availability of computer programs or "apps" that might be useful for children with ASD, particularly with regard to easy portability into the home environment.

CONCLUSION

This chapter has presented basic information and considerations for ASD issues in intervention at an *introductory* level. This information is intended only as a starting point in the reader's clinical education and training. For in-depth coverage of this area, the following readings are recommended:

Buron, K. D., & Wolfberg, P. (Eds.). (2008). *Learners on the autism spectrum*. Shawnee Mission, KS: APC.

Murray-Slutsky, C., & Paris, B. A. (2013). *Autism interventions: Exploring the spectrum of autism* (2nd ed.). Austin, TX: Hammill Institute.

Prelock, P., & McCauley, R. (Eds.). (2012). *Treatment of autism spectrum disorders: Evidence-based intervention strategies for communication and social interactions (CLI)*. Baltimore, MD: Paul H. Brookes Publishing Co.

Volkmar, F., Rogers, S., Paul, R., & Pelphrey, K. (Eds.). (20014). *Handbook of autism and pervasive developmental disorders* (4th ed.). Hoboken, NJ: Wiley.

ADDITIONAL RESOURCES

Note: There is a wide variety of resources available for addressing autism spectrum disorders. The following list represents a limited number of these resources, with no intended focus on any particular approach to intervention.

American Speech-Language-Hearing Association
2200 Research Blvd.
Rockville, MD 20850
Phone: 301 296-5650
Email: actioncenter@asha.org
Web site: www.asha.org/publications

Social Communication Disorders in Children: Speech-Language Pathologists Can Help
This comprehensive brochure is aimed at parents and families who have concerns about the social communication development of their child. It offers suggestions for promoting social interactions and a list of age-appropriate social communication skill development for infants through adolescents.

Speech-Language Pathologists & Your Child with Autism
Parents are the target audience for this brochure, which describes how SLPs can help children diagnosed with ASD to develop social and communication skills. It also provides a checklist of strategies that parents can use in daily interactions with their child.

LinguiSystems
3100 Fourth Avenue
East Moline, IL 61244
Phone: 800-776-4332
Fax: 800-577-4555
Email: service@linguisystems.com
Web site: http://www.linguisystems.com

Autism and PDD Adolescent Social Skills Lessons

This title refers to a series of workbooks, with each workbook targeting a specific skill. These workbooks can be used with individuals in middle school through adulthood, with topics that include social interaction, behavior management, health and hygiene, and vocational skills. Lessons are supported by pictures to facilitate practice of the targeted skills. These lessons aim to provide individuals with the nonverbal and verbal language skills to navigate social situations encountered in daily life.

Autism and PDD Answering Questions

This set of two workbooks is divided by level/difficulty of questions targeted. These workbooks contain visual supports to help individuals on the autism spectrum to process and use more abstract forms of language. Workbook Level 1 is intended for children ages 3 to 5 years and workbook Level 2 is intended for children ages 5 to 9 years. Various question forms are targeted, including "what" questions, "why" questions, and questions targeting problem-solving skills. For more targeted practice on a specific question type (e.g., "why" questions), the *Autism and PPD More Picture Stories & Language Activities* has a series of workbooks that each target a specific question type.

Autism and PDD Early Intervention

This is a series of workbooks that target prelinguistic skills in children ages 1 to 3 years. Topics covered include joint attention, eating routines, dressing routines, and play skills. The lessons focus on the characters of a boy, a girl, and a bear. The lessons and stories target early vocabulary/concepts and support these skills with colorful visuals and sign language images.

Autism and PDD Picture Stories and Language Activities Social Skills

This is a set of five workbooks that cover social skills in a variety of settings (e.g., home, school, community). The lessons are designed to follow a consistent format to facilitate learning and provide a secure, predictable session. These workbooks use the characters of Matt and Molly to engage children in lessons that depict hypothetical events.

Autism & PDD Things I Can Say and Do

This is a series of workbooks that target social skills that pertain to specific contexts or scenarios. The lessons provide individuals with language skills/phrases to use in context-specific communicative exchanges. Organizational tools/worksheets are provided to individualize lessons to each client. Topics/concepts covered include body parts/clothing, feelings and actions, holidays, weather, seasons, and months.

The Autism Spectrum Disorders IEP Companion

This book provides information on some of the common issues related to communication and behavioral skills that arise in the school setting. It gives advice for treatment planning and considerations during the IEP process, including sensory needs, transitions, and classroom and instructional accommodations. Chapters are divided into skill areas (i.e., social pragmatics, communication) and provide examples of goals and objectives.

The Basic Reading Comprehension Kit for Hyperlexia and Autism

For children ages 5 to 12 years, this kit aims to bridge the gap between a child's ability to decode and comprehend what he or she has read. In particular, it provides strategies for visual imaging skills and sequencing skills in order to support the visual learning style of children with ASD.

Practical Theory of Mind Games

For children 4 to 12 years of age, these lessons target inferencing skills pertaining to social situations. This resource is divided into three sections based on the underlying principles of theory of mind (ToM) deficits, stories and games to teach lessons on inference skills, and discussions of the emotional differences between individuals. This resource includes a CD-ROM to access and print the lessons.

The Source for Intervention in Autism Spectrum Disorders

This resource provides information on issues pertaining to ASD, such as related disorders, theory of mind, and learning styles. This information is then used to develop goals and strategies for intervention as well as activities to use with this population. This book provides advice for working with individuals from the toddler years through adulthood and targets expressive/receptive language, literacy skills, behavioral skills, and functional life skills.

TheraLink Autism & PDD Photo Cards: Asking Questions

This is a set of 270 photographs to engage students in question-asking/answering interactions. The photos depict scenes and have targets to either elicit a question and/or to respond to a question. Picture tasks cover a variety of question types (e.g., "where" questions, "who" questions). Cues and prompts are provided to help with question formulation. This resource can be used on a computer or a tablet with individuals ages 3 to 11 years.

Pro-Ed
8700 Shoal Creek Boulevard
Austin, TX 78757-6897
Phone: 800-897-3202
Fax: 800-397-7633
Web site: http://www.proedinc.com

Educating Students with Autism: A Quick Start Manual

This book is meant for educators as well as related service providers, such as SLPs. It contains chapters on topics such as different treatment approaches, strategies for providing structure to daily life, and communication skills to target. It also provides resources for further information on autism as well as the types of support organizations and programs that are available.

Teaching Perspective-Taking Skills to Children with Autism Spectrum Disorders

This manual provides lessons and activities to use with individuals in preschool through high school. It targets nonverbal communication skills, play skills, and prelinguistic skills. A CD-ROM is included that contains the lesson pages.

Early Start for Young Children with Autism/PDD: Practical Interventions

This is a workbook with information for working with children ages 2 to 5 years. It covers topics such as establishing routines, targeting behavioral issues, implementing visual schedules and calendars, and incorporating play into intervention. The workbook also contains forms that pertain to the lessons and topics covered.

The Speech Bin
School Specialty
P.O. Box 1579
Appleton, WI 54912-1579
Phone: 800-388-3224
Fax: 800-388-6344
Web site: http://store.schoolspecialty.com/

Social Skill Builder: My Community
This CD-ROM program provides social skill lessons pertaining to a variety of social situations and settings. For children ages 5 to 15 years, this program provides children with practice in navigating settings such as a grocery store, restaurant, and a friend's house. Skills targeted include making predictions about what happens in a social context and formulating an appropriate response.

Super Duper Publications
P.O. Box 24997
Greenville, SC 29616
Phone: 800-277-8737
Fax: 800-978-7379
Web site: http://www.superduperinc.com

What Do You Say . . . What Do You Do . . . At School?
This board game can be used for children in grades K–8 and targets social skills that pertain to the school setting. Skills targeted include reasoning, making inferences, and conversational skills. The questions require students to act out situations and verbally problem solve these situations rather than to select an answer from a field of answers. There is a separate game for targeting social skills in the community setting.

Say and Do Social Scenes for Home, School, and Community
This workbook can be used with children in grades K–4. Its lessons present a social scene and then discuss appropriate versus inappropriate responses/actions for these situations. The scenes depict a variety of situations that a child might encounter, including stores, school, and phone conversations.

Simply Social 7 at School
For children in grades 2 through 12, this workbook provides scripted scenarios in order to help children on the autism spectrum to develop social language skills. The workbook targets skills such as conversational skills, turn-taking, using and understanding facial expressions, and understanding figurative language. The workbook also includes a Social Skills Checklist to help identify and target each child's pragmatic language needs.

Positive Pragmatic Game Boards
These game boards consist of a set of five double-sided boards, for a total of 10 board games. Each game targets a specific pragmatic language skill. The skills targeted include

topic maintenance, making requests, identifying and expressing feelings, and giving information on a specified topic.

Social Skills Quick Take Along

This small, laminated booklet contains 600 questions covering 15 areas within the topic of social language skills. Question sections target areas such as formulating apologies in response to a given situation as well as formulating appropriate utterances in response to given social situations. Its smaller format (5" × 3") is designed for on-the-go use.

Social Thinking (Michelle Garcia Winner)

3031 Tisch Way, Suite 800
San Jose, CA 95128
Phone: 408-557-8595
Fax: 408-557-8594
Web site: http://www.socialthinking.com

Social Thinking offers a variety of products and programs for targeting pragmatic language skills. One program, called SuperFlex®, consists of a series of comic books with characters that represent various pragmatic behaviors, such as reacting appropriately to situations and perspective-taking skills. The books, including *You are a Social Detective!,* help students to learn about different characters' traits as well as develop strategies for working on social language skills in relation to these difficulties. Another product is a workbook (*A 5 Could Make Me Lose Control!*) that can be used to develop 5-point rating scales to help individuals identify sources of anxiety or frustration, as well as strategies to mediate these feelings.

CHAPTER 7

The majority of this chapter covers adult aphasia, which is a language-based disorder. In addition, an overview of traumatic brain injury (TBI) is provided. Dementia and right-hemisphere dysfunction are beyond the scope of this chapter. Selected references are provided at the end of this chapter for readers interested in these topics.

APHASIA

Aphasia is a language disorder due to brain damage that results in impairment in the comprehension and/or formulation of language and can affect both the spoken and written modalities. The major cause of aphasia is stroke due to hemorrhage or blockage of blood flow to the brain. Strokes are also referred to as cerebrovascular accidents (CVAs). Other etiologies include tumors, head trauma, and certain disease processes, such as encephalitis. Currently, the incidence of aphasia in the United States is 80,000 individuals, with a prevalence of 1,000,000 individuals; both figures are projected to significantly increase over the next decade as the elderly population increases (National Stroke Association, 2008). Aphasia is associated with damage to the dominant hemisphere for language in the brain, which is the left hemisphere in most individuals. It frequently is accompanied by motor and sensory deficits. As the left hemisphere controls the contralateral (or opposite) side of the body, these motor and sensory impairments are most often right-sided in individuals with aphasia. Common motor impairments are **hemiplegia** or **hemiparesis,** paralysis or weakness on one side of the body, respectively. **Hemianopsia** is a visual field deficit in which an individual cannot see to the right or left of midline in one or both eyes. (Other pertinent medical terms are located in the glossary in Appendix C at the end of the book.)

Classification of Aphasia Syndromes

Historically, there has been an enormous amount of effort devoted to the classification of aphasic types and syndromes. This work has resulted in the development of several different approaches to classification, including site of lesion taxonomies (e.g., Goodglass, Kaplan, & Barresi, 2001; Kertesz, 1979), linguistic structure paradigms (Jakobson, 1964), and modality-oriented systems that address behavioral symptoms of language impairment (e.g., Schuell, Jenkins, & Jimenez-Pabon, 1964). A detailed discussion of the similarities and differences among the various aphasia taxonomies is beyond the scope of this chapter. (See Chapey [2008] for comprehensive reviews of classification issues and approaches.) From a treatment-oriented perspective, we find it clinically useful to adopt the Boston group's (Goodglass et al., 2001) approach to classification, which includes two main categories of aphasia: nonfluent and fluent. This classification system is based on quality of output and involves both oral and written modalities. Within each category, the degree of severity may range from mild to profound.

The profile of **nonfluent aphasias** is one of poor output with relatively spared comprehension. It generally is characterized by reduced vocabulary; agrammatism; and impairments of articulation, rate, and prosody (rhythm, stress, and intonation), resulting in labored and effortful production.

Fluent aphasias consist of impairment in language comprehension with maintenance of normal melodic speech contour. The main characteristics are word-retrieval difficulties, paraphasias (phonemic and semantic), neologisms, perseveration, and the maintenance of normal melodic speech contour.

TABLE 7–1

Terminology Related to Language Deficits in Aphasia

Term	Definition
Agrammatism	Syntactic deficit characterized by omission of function words and grammatical inflections. Semantic aspects of language remain intact. Speech output consists primarily of content words. Example: When asked to describe a picture of a picnic with someone sleeping in a hammock, the client responds, "Food . . . man bed . . . he sleep."
Word-retrieval problems	Difficulty accessing a word from one's mental vocabulary. Severe naming difficulty is termed anomia. Example: When asked to name a hammock in a picture, the client responds, "It's to sleep in . . . under trees . . . you know, with a rope."
Paraphasia	Errors in speech output characterized by the production of unintended sounds, syllables, or words. The two main types are phonemic and semantic. Phonemic paraphasias (also known as literal paraphasias) consist of *extraneous* or *transposed* sounds and syllables or *substitution* of one correctly articulated phoneme for another. Example: When asked to name a hammock in a picture, the client may respond with one of the following: "hammerock," "hackamm," "pammock," respectively. Semantic paraphasias involve unintended substitution of one word for another, usually within the same semantic category. Example: When asked to name a hammock, the client responds, "It's a bed."
Neologism	Invented word that has no true meaning but adheres to the phonological rules of a given language. These errors tend to occur primarily with nouns and verbs rather than function words. Example: When asked to name a hammock in a picture, the client responds, "That's a blick."
Perseveration	Inappropriate continuation of a response after the presentation of a new stimulus. Example: After successfully naming a hammock in a picture, the client continues to respond "hammock" when shown the next three pictures of a chair, key, and glove.

Definitions of key terms related to language deficits in aphasia are presented in Table 7–1. The major categories of fluent and nonfluent aphasia can be further divided into selected subtypes, as shown in Table 7–2. NOTE: Odd language use is not restricted to adults with communication disorders. The following instances are examples from a typical adult that have been observed by or reported to the authors (Roth, 2014, personal communication). Some of the examples are spontaneous comments, while others are portions of conversations.

- In the context of techs working on fixing a website – "They have to create a new aneurysm" (intended meaning = algorithm).
- "Killing two eggs with one stone."
- Speaker A: "I don't like this soup because it is immoral."

  Speaker B: "How can any soup be immoral?"

  Speaker A: "I should have said Swanson. Immoral is a famous chef." (intended meaning of Immoral = Emeril).
- "I've been running around like a chicken without a hat . . . No wait . . . That's not right. I've been running around like a chicken without an egg."
- "Wow, you live close away."
- Speaker A: "He's not the brightest bulb in the . . . What's that saying?"

  Speaker B: "You mean 'drawer'?"

  Speaker A: "No, that's silly."

TABLE 7–2

Classification of Aphasia Syndromes

Syndrome Type	Characteristics
Nonfluent Aphasias	
Broca's	Agrammatism; effortful articulation of phrase-length utterances; impaired prosody and intonation; concomitant apraxia of speech; good comprehension; lesion in the posterior inferior frontal lobe, as well as central and inferior parietal regions
Transcortical motor	Little to no initiation of spontaneous speech; output similar to Broca's but excellent imitation (even of long utterances); relatively intact comprehension; lesion in the medial-frontal cortex, involving the supplementary motor area
Global	Severe deficits in all areas of language comprehension and production; output may be limited to stereotypic utterances; lesion encompasses both pre- and postrolandic speech zones
Fluent Aphasias	
Wernicke's	Fluent but often meaningless speech (jargon); impaired comprehension; good articulation, intonation, and prosody; lesion in the posterior portion of the first temporal gyrus of the left hemisphere
Conduction	Relatively fluent speech; frequent phonemic paraphasias; marked difficulty with imitation; good language comprehension; lesion in the arcuate fasciculus, deep supramarginal gyrus, or superior temporal gyrus
Anomic	Significant word-finding difficulties in the presence of otherwise fluent and grammatical speech; good comprehension; lesion in the angular gyrus region

SOURCE: Adapted from Hedge, M.N. (2001). Introduction to communicative disorders (3rd ed.). Austin, TX: Pro-Ed.

TREATMENT EFFICACY/EVIDENCE-BASED PRACTICE

As part of the natural recovery process, the brain regains some of its speech, language, and motor functions after an injury. The greatest amount of this **spontaneous recovery** occurs during the first 2 to 3 months. However, changes may continue to be noted for a period of up to 1 year after onset. Following the period of spontaneous recovery, individuals may demonstrate varying degrees of gradual improvement, in some cases months or years after the initial brain injury. Several factors influence the degree of spontaneous early recovery and ultimate prognosis. These include the size, location, and etiology of the lesion; type and severity of the initial aphasia (particularly verbal comprehension); age at onset; and overall health of the client (Kertesz, 1979; Kertesz & McCabe, 1977; Pedersen, Vintner, & Olsen, 2004). The most predictive indicator of long-term recovery is initial aphasia severity, along with lesion site and size (Plowman, Hentz, & Ellis, 2011). In general, lesions located in the temporoparietal region are associated with a poorer prognosis. Studies also indicate that hemorrhagic strokes have a more remarkable recovery pattern than those due to blockage of cerebral blood flow (i.e., embolism or thrombosis). As a rule, prognosis is more favorable for younger clients and for those without additional medical problems. During spontaneous recovery, the initial aphasia syndrome may evolve into a different (usually milder) classification type.

Historically, there has been controversy over the efficacy of aphasia therapy. Some studies have suggested that any objective improvement seen in a client's status is attributable to the brain's spontaneous recovery rather than a result of treatment effects (e.g., Sarno, Silverman, & Sands, 1970). Others contend that aphasia treatment results in measurable gains in communicative functioning through both traditional and group treatment models (e.g., Elman & Bernstein-Ellis, 1999; Wertz et al., 1981). Evidence indicates that speech and language treatment is effective in improving functional communication, as well as receptive and expressive language skills, in individuals with stroke-induced aphasia (Brady, Kelly, Godwin, & Enderby, 2012). In part, this controversy is a result of methodological problems associated with obtaining matched subject samples and the ethical dilemma of withholding treatment from individuals assigned to control-group conditions.

To confound the issue further, disagreement also exists regarding the optimal time to initiate therapy. The main source of contention is whether to initiate therapy immediately or wait until the spontaneous recovery process has run its course. The available data do not adequately solve the problem of separating spontaneous recovery changes from treatment effects. Several studies have reported that delaying initiation of treatment had no significant negative impact on client progress (Sarno & Levita, 1971; Sarno et al., 1970; Wertz et al., 1986). However, most clinicians advocate early intervention based on the premise that treatment may serve to accelerate the natural process of spontaneous recovery.

In 1996, Holland, Fromm, De Ruyter, and Stein published a comprehensive summary of available data on treatment efficacy for aphasia. They reviewed large- and small-group studies, single-subject studies, and program evaluation data from several rehabilitation sites throughout the country. Their overall conclusion was that aphasia therapy is efficacious in that treated clients make significantly more improvement than untreated clients. The analysis resulted in several additional conclusions:

- Most of the large-group studies indicated that treatment benefits are greatest for individuals with a single, left-hemisphere stroke.

- Small-group and single-subject studies suggested that treatment is effective for clients with chronic aphasia well beyond the period of spontaneous recovery.

- Client improvement is greatest when therapy is provided on a frequent basis over a period of at least 5 to 6 months.

- Program evaluation data from inpatient rehabilitation settings suggested that the greatest amount of functional improvement occurs in receptive language skills, followed by speech production and expressive language skills.

- The literature is unclear regarding the extent to which severity of aphasia, type of aphasia, or client age influence treatment outcome.

- Further research is needed to determine which treatment techniques are most efficacious for specific types of aphasic impairment.

Robey (1998) conducted a meta-analysis of 55 multiple-subject studies to examine clinical outcomes in the treatment of aphasia. His findings, which confirm and extend those of earlier studies, include the following:

- In all stages of recovery, clients who receive treatment demonstrate outcomes superior to untreated individuals. This is particularly true when treatment is initiated during the acute phase of recovery.

- Clients who receive 2 or more hours per week of intervention during the acute and post-acute stages exhibit greater gains than those receiving services on a less intense schedule.

- Even individuals with severe aphasia benefit substantially from intervention provided by speech-language pathologists (SLPs).

- Outcome information is still needed regarding the effects of different intervention approaches on different types of aphasia.

Pulvermuller and Berthier (2008) and Cherney, Patterson, Raymer, Frymark, & Schooling (2008) also have provided evidence that intensity of treatment has moderate positive effects on language performance in individuals with chronic aphasia. Intervention characterized by massed practice on a frequent basis over a short period of time appears to be beneficial in both early and later stages of aphasia recovery. These authors reported preliminary findings of a modest positive effect for an approach to aphasia treatment, constraint-induced language therapy (CILT). A description of CILT is provided in the next section of this chapter.

Some researchers argue that early intervention targeting linguistic tasks (e.g., semantics, phonology) benefits individuals with aphasia more than deferring treatment (Nouwens, Dippel, De Jong-Hagelstein et al., 2013). Moreover, it is posited that the focus on linguistic tasks rather than functional communication tasks increases blood flow to linguistic regions of the brain, thus supporting communicative gains in these areas early on in the recovery process (Nouwens et al., 2013).

In addition to the question of when to commence treatment, research also has been conducted to investigate the optimal duration for treatment. In a meta-analysis of research studies on treatment gains with chronic aphasia, several studies yielded evidence supporting the continuation of treatment beyond the early intervention phases for gains in communication skills as well as executive function skills (Korner-Bitensky, 2013). Further support for ongoing intervention was found in a 2011 study of individuals with chronic aphasia in Italy. Researchers found evidence that if therapy is intensive enough, gains can be noted even in cases of chronic aphasia (Basso & Macis, 2011). Raymer et al. (2008) also reviewed literature that found greater gains from continued treatment of aphasia versus dismissal from treatment. It was purported that treatment often is discontinued too early and/or is not intensive enough with cases of chronic aphasia (Basso & Macis, 2011). As individuals with chronic aphasia will have long-term deficits, the authors stressed the role of caregivers in providing language stimulation and practice daily for maintenance of therapeutic gains (Basso & Macis, 2011).

In summary, evidence indicates that speech-language treatment is effective in improving communication and receptive/expressive language skills in individuals with stroke-induced aphasia.

TREATMENT FOR APHASIA

The overall goal of aphasia therapy is to improve a client's communication skills to the highest degree possible within the constraints of the neurological damage. The majority of individuals with aphasia will experience at least some residual language deficits throughout their lifetimes. For this reason, clinicians must decide when to shift the focus of treatment from a "cure" to "care" orientation. The goal of treatment changes from recovery of premorbid language skills to establishing compensatory/maintenance strategies for functional language skills (Teasell, Foley, & Salter, 2011). To devise an appropriate and effective intervention program, the clinician must have thorough knowledge of prognostic variables as well as familiarity with the most predictable patterns of recovery that are associated with the different aphasia subtypes. For example, one common recovery pattern is for a global aphasia to evolve into a chronic Broca's aphasia. Few well-designed studies evaluate aphasia therapy in terms of optimal frequency, duration, or the relative value of different methods. This is especially true in the area of fluent aphasia. Therefore, SLPs should design intervention programs in accordance with individual clients' presenting clinical profiles as well as premorbid status factors such as intellectual level, education, and reading ability. In addition, cultural and linguistic differences should be considered across instructional and interpersonal aspects of therapy. Very few individuals with aphasia are completely unable to comprehend auditory information, and conversely, few have perfectly preserved auditory comprehension skills. The goal of the SLP is to recognize both spared areas of function in clients with severe aphasia and subtle areas of weakness in clients with mild aphasia.

Neuroplasticity

Another factor to consider when planning intervention is neuroplasticity, the brain's ability to restructure its neural networks in response to internal and external stimuli. Neuroplasticity is associated with learning in the intact brain and thus relearning in cases of brain damage (Kleim & Jones, 2008). Neural rewiring can manifest itself in several different ways. For example, neural regions adjacent to the lesion may adopt some of the functions attributed to the affected area. In addition, right-hemisphere sites that parallel the affected left-hemisphere areas may start performing functions once attributed to the lesioned area (Torres, Drebing, & Hamilton, 2013). Focusing on brains with damaged tissue, Kleim and Jones (2008) provide a summary of the research on neuroplasticity by outlining 10 principles that can be used to inform treatment plans in relation to speech-language therapy.

One component of neuroplasticity that is currently being debated involves the severity of the brain damage. Although limited, there are some studies that provide evidence for neuroplasticity occurring even in cases of severely damaged tissue. In a study examining brain-stimulation techniques, two patients with substantial lesions corresponding to global aphasia showed behavioral changes from intervention (Barwood et al., 2012). In addition, Johansson's (2011) literature review of melodic intonation therapy (MIT) that shows gains made by patients with severe nonfluent aphasia were a result of MIT intervention.

Neuroplasticity Principle	Relation to Speech-Language Therapy
1. Use it or lose it	Because damage to neural connections has occurred, intervention tasks should target these damaged connections to stimulate that area of the brain to promote the restructuring of these areas as well as to prevent further degradation.
2. Use it to improve it	This principle purports that neuroplasticity can be induced through activities that target damaged neural regions and that this practice can improve a person's ability with the targeted skill.
3. Specificity matters	Specificity refers both to the neural region where change is expected and to the task being trained. Because it is a damaged brain, the process of learning is different from typical learning. Thus, neural changes are often limited and noted strictly in relation to the targeted task rather than being widespread in nature, impacting associated tasks/neural regions.
4. Repetition matters	Repetition of a targeted skill is important to both establishing the behavioral change and neural remodeling as well as to helping to maintain the change.
5. Intensity matters	It is important to note that it is possible for intervention to be too intense and thus negatively impact the client's progress, especially early on in the process. However, this principle provides evidence that the greater the intensity (e.g., the number of trials), the greater the long-term effect of the intervention. Treatment schedules can be altered during the recovery process, starting off slowly in the acute phase and increasing in intensity as the patient enters the chronic phase (Raymer et al., 2008).

(continues)

Neuroplasticity Principle	Relation to Speech-Language Therapy
6. Time matters	Because neural remodeling occurs spontaneously after damage to the brain, consideration must be given for when to commence treatment. Indeed, evidence from animal studies has demonstrated that early intervention can have a negative impact if too intense (Raymer et al., 2008). However, intervention can be viewed as augmenting and directing the neural restructuring already under way. Although not conclusive, early intervention seems to be effective, especially in preventing further loss of skills.
7. Salience matters	The relevance of the activities and targeted skills to the client's daily life is an important factor in promoting therapeutic gains; without motivation, the client is likely to be less engaged in therapy and the neural response will be not be as great.
8. Age matters	Because atrophy naturally occurs in typically aging brains, the age at which a person experiences brain damage may have implications for the level of decline that he or she is already experiencing. However, other factors such as mental and physical status pre-insult are important to consider when setting goals, projecting progress, and identifying treatment outcomes.
9. Transference matters	This principle refers to rewiring that is noted in one neural region as a result of targeted plasticity in a related region. Planning intervention to target more complex stimuli can also result in transference within a given linguistic skill area. For example, targeting complex stimuli (e.g., atypical items in a categorization task, such as penguin and ostrich for the bird category) facilitates learning of less complex stimuli within the same category (e.g., robin, eagle) (Raymer et al., 2008). In addition to changes transferring from one neural region to another, an individual's abilities (e.g., cognitive status) pre-insult can transfer and influence the progression of recovery.
10. Interference matters	There are several ways in which intervention and/or the individual's actions may induce plasticity that does not have a positive effect on the individual's recovery. For example, an individual may develop compensatory strategies that are not as sophisticated or efficient as the original skill. Further, attempts to rewire one skill may interfere with the neural networks underlying a different skill.

SOURCES: Kleim, J.A., & Jones, T.A. (2008). Principles of experience-dependent neural plasticity: Implications for rehabilitation after brain damage. Journal of Speech, Language, and Hearing Research, 51(1), S225–S239. Raymer, A.M., Kendall, D., Maher, L., Martin, N., Murray, L., Rose, M., Thompson, C.K., Turkstra, L., Altmann, L., Boyle, M., Conway, T., Hula, W., Kearns, K., Rapp, B., Simmons-Mackie, N., & Gonzalez Rothi, L.J. (2008). Translational research in aphasia: From neuroscience to neurorehabilitation. Journal of Speech, Language, and Hearing Research, 51, 259–275.

Theoretical Orientations to Aphasia Treatment

There are two main theoretical orientations to aphasia treatment:

1. **Restorative/Linguistic:** This model of intervention is based on the assumption that an aphasic individual's linguistic knowledge has been disrupted and these skills can be strengthened or restored through direct instruction (Murray & Clark, 2006). The main emphasis of this approach is intensive and repeated participation in therapy activities to improve compromised linguistic functions (e.g., syntax, word finding, and phonology). It encompasses both comprehension and production of oral and written language targets. Restorative therapy techniques are frequently referred to using the terms *neuropsychological* or *neurolinguistic* (Chapey, 2008).

2. **Substitutive/Compensatory:** This approach is based on the premise that language function has been lost in individuals with aphasia. However, the focus of therapy is on establishing functional communication. The procedures are designed to encourage use of whatever modalities are available to the individual to convey messages successfully to listeners (Davis, 2007; Davis & Wilcox, 1981; Simmons-Mackie, 2001, 2008). These may include speaking, gesturing, signing, writing, facial expressions, drawing, and so on. The focus of this "consequence-oriented" model is on the tasks and responsibilities of everyday living and resuming a role in society (Holland, 2008). The selection of functional therapy goals can be guided by the communicative behaviors identified in the Functional Assessment of Communication Skills developed by the American Speech-Language-Hearing Association (Frattali, Thompson, Holland, Wohl, & Ferketic, 2003). This framework specifies 43 communicative behaviors that are grouped according to four domains: (a) social communication; (b) basic needs; (c) reading, writing, and number concepts; and (d) daily planning. Therapy goals also can be selected based on the functional endpoints of aphasia treatment suggested by Holland (1995), which are outlined in Table 7–3. The unit of analysis in this treatment paradigm is always the communicative effectiveness within the dyad (speaker + listener) rather than the client as an individual.

In summary, the restorative/linguistic model targets specific impairments in the linguistic system, whereas the substitutive/compensatory model focuses on the successful exchange of communicative messages rather than the form of those messages. Clinicians are encouraged to use whatever combination of these approaches is best suited to individual clients. In addition, a promising new direction in aphasia treatment is the use of pharmacotherapy. This approach uses drug treatment to restore equilibrium to disrupted neurotransmitter systems, which in turn should facilitate linguistic/cognitive recovery (Cahana-Amitay, Albert, & Oveis, 2013; Murray & Clark, 2006; Steele, 2009). This approach is generally used in conjunction with other forms of aphasia intervention.

Guidelines for Programming and Implementing Therapy

Therapy may focus on improving a client's abilities in listening, speaking, reading, and writing. In the restorative/linguistic model, intervention is programmed according to hierarchies of difficulty (refer to Chapter 1 for detailed information on basic therapy programming). The hierarchies are based on neurolinguistic research that has explored how adults

TABLE 7–3
Long-Term Functional Goals for Aphasia Therapy

1. Communicate to obtain assistance in emergency situations.

   Example: Call 911.

2. Express feelings.

   Example: Make attitudes and emotions known.

3. Convey basic needs.

   Example: Communicate hunger, thirst, fatigue.

4. Follow simple directions.

   Example: Set alarm clock.

5. Engage in social relationships or situations.

   Example: Enjoy social interactions to the degree commensurate with pre-aphasia status.

6. Declare autonomy and independence through action, thought, or opinion.

   Example: Indicate disagreement or difference of opinion.

7. Resume activities that were pleasurable prior to onset of aphasia.

   Example: Enjoy hobbies or grandchildren.

8. Take on some routine responsibility.

   Example: Put out trash, water plants.

9. Keep up with news events.

   Example: Read headlines, watch TV news.

10. Function as an individual independent of the aphasic impairment at least for brief time periods.

    Example: Attend a concert or sports event.

SOURCE: Adapted from Holland, A. (1995). Current realities of aphasia rehabilitation: Time constraints, documentation demands, and functional outcomes. Paper presented at Mid-America Rehabilitation Hospital, Overland Park, KS.

with and without aphasia comprehend and produce language (e.g., Berndt, Mitchum, & Wayland, 1997; Goodglass & Wingfield, 1998; Hillis & Newhart, 2008; Mitchum & Berndt, 2008). Following is a sample hierarchy for the selection and sequencing of therapy targets in the area of verbal expression. This general therapeutic progression also can be applied to each of the other language modalities (listening, reading, and writing).

1. Intervention may begin at the nonverbal level by establishing pointing responses.

2. Single-word tasks that target word retrieval can then be introduced in the form of responsive or confrontation naming. In **responsive naming,** a clinician provides a verbal descriptive phrase to elicit a target label (e.g., "The object that we use to sweep the floor is called a ___"). A **confrontation naming** task is more difficult because it requires the client to name a visual stimulus (e.g., picture or object) without any contextual support.

3. Phrase-length responses can then be targeted through sentence completion activities that require the client to fill in a word or phrase that accurately completes a sentence stem.

4. Finally, sentence-level formulation may be required, in which a client might be asked to describe pictures or the function of objects or respond to direct questions posed by the clinician.

This hierarchy of difficulty focuses on utterance length as the critical factor. However, aphasia therapy entails much more than simply increasing the length of a target response. Several factors can be manipulated while maintaining the same response length. For example, a clinician may decrease the amount of support provided in the form of modeling, cues, and prompts to encourage a client to become a more independent communicator. In addition, therapy can be designed to elicit responses at more sophisticated levels of linguistic complexity (e.g., maintaining a phrase-length response while moving from literal language forms to figurative forms such as idioms, metaphors, and humor). At the single-word level, more complex language forms such as antonyms and synonyms can be elicited through the use of word association tasks. Further, the latency between clinician stimulus and client response also can be manipulated. Once the accuracy of a target behavior has been established, task difficulty can be boosted by increasing the speed of the expected response without altering either the length or linguistic complexity of the utterance. In contrast, preliminary data from single-subject research on individuals with agrammatic aphasia suggest that generalization of sentence production is facilitated when the direction of therapy progresses from more complex to less complex syntactic structures (Thompson, Shapiro, Kiran, & Sobecks, 2003).

Another important component of intervention programming for aphasia is the use of **group therapy** as well as individual sessions (Elman, 2007). An ideal model allows a client to learn new communication behaviors in individual sessions and provides group settings for opportunities to practice and expand these skills in an interactional situation. Group settings also provide a milieu in which clients can socialize and identify with peers who have problems similar to their own. In addition to therapy groups, intervention for aphasia often includes group sessions for family training and counseling. Family members can facilitate the aphasic individual's everyday communication performance by learning and implementing the techniques used by the clinician in therapy sessions. Family counseling is an essential aspect of aphasia therapy. Families may require guidance about how to talk to the affected family member. Specific suggestions are provided in Appendix 7-A. Of all communication disorders, aphasia is the one that causes the most severe adjustment problems for families because of its sudden and abrupt onset. Virtually overnight, a family member experiences dramatic changes in health and personality as well as in the ability to communicate.

Finally, one common technique used with clients who present with word-retrieval deficits is **self-cuing.** These are strategies that can be used by a client to trigger the verbal production of a specific word and include the following:

- Automatic sequences (e.g., days of the week)
- Paired verbal associates (e.g., bread and ___ [*butter*])
- Sentence completion (e.g., We use a broom to sweep the ___ [*floor*])
- Idiomatic expressions (e.g., Look before you ___ [*leap*])

- Alternative words (e.g., synonyms and antonyms)

- Rhyming words (e.g., sounds like *fall*)

- Phonemic cues (e.g., initial sound/syllable of target word)

- Writing the initial letter, syllable, or entire word

- Subordinate category cues (e.g., Pizza and hot dogs are types of ___ [*food*])

- Air tracing (i.e., writing a word in the air with one's finger)

- Gesture or pantomime cues (e.g., pretending to drink from a cup)

- Object or action attributes (e.g., asking questions such as "Which one is sharp?" and "Which one is slow?" about two or more pictures)

Consider three approaches when planning intervention for aphasia: therapist-controlled, therapist-led, and patient-focused (Leach, Cornwall, Fleming, & Haines, 2010). The main factor that differentiates these approaches is the amount of contribution from the clinician versus the individual with aphasia and his/her family members. Leach et al. (2010) advocate for a patient-focused approach when possible because this approach has been found to have a positive impact on the client's motivation and achievement of goals. A patient-focused approach also provides insight into the types of skills that are priorities for intervention. Survey results of 50 post-stroke individuals with aphasia revealed a variety of highly desired intervention goals, including the ability to communicate needs and opinions, an increase in autonomy, the ability to return to social and work activities, and the ability to participate in volunteer work and to help others (Worrall et al., 2011). Patient education is stressed as an important component of intervention, especially in terms of setting realistic goals and understanding the rationale for therapeutic activities (Leach et al., 2010).

Specific Intervention Procedures

Numerous procedures have been used in the rehabilitation of individuals with aphasia. This section briefly describes several of the most common programs identified in the clinical research literature.

Constraint-Induced Language Therapy (Pulvermuller, Hauk, Zohsel, Neininger, & Mohr, 2005; Pulvermuller et al., 2001). Constraint-induced language therapy (CILT) is a promising intervention strategy that is currently undergoing substantial clinical study. CILT is specifically beneficial for individuals with stroke-induced aphasia, although results are considered preliminary (Cherney et al., 2010). It is a restorative/linguistic approach and is built on three main principles:

1. Massed practice (intensive therapy over a relatively short period of consecutive days, such as 30 hours of practice over a 2-week period)

2. Shaping by successive approximation (presenting tasks in small steps of gradually increasing linguistic difficulty within natural communication contexts)

3. Constraint (restriction of the client's use of any compensatory/nonverbal communication strategies)

Although CILT requires intensive intervention, there is evidence that its emphasis on verbal communication is of equal importance in attaining communicative gains (Raymer et al., 2008). In addition, studies indicate that family involvement in this therapeutic intervention is especially important for generalization of linguistic gains; thus family and caregivers are encouraged to monitor and to remind individuals to use verbal means for communication throughout daily communicative exchanges (Johansson, 2011).

In contrast, Rose (2013) presented evidence that gestures and other modalities should not be constrained in therapy and daily communication. This opposing view is based on several properties of gestures within the context of language and communication:

- Gestures are not viewed as an arbitrary component of communication; rather, gestures are posited to contribute to language production through means such as helping an individual to retrieve words and thus to maintain fluency.

- Neurological representations of language are not discrete from motor and sensory domains in the brain; thus, the neurological overlap can be targeted to promote gains in each system.

- Studies have found that people with aphasia tend to utilize gestures more frequently in their communicative interactions than people who do not have aphasia.

- Avoidance or targeted non-use of a skill can have a negative impact on this skill; thus, it may be more difficult for an individual with aphasia to utilize gestures or other modalities in the future if they have gone extended periods avoiding these skills.

Stimulation-Facilitation (Schuell et al., 1964). Stimulation-facilitation is not a specific procedure but rather a general approach to aphasia treatment that incorporates the basic principles of competent intervention (Coelho, Sinotte, & Duffy, 2008). Specific characteristics of this approach, as advocated by Schuell et al., are as follows: (1) the focus of therapy is intensive auditory stimulation to elicit language; (2) a client's incorrect responses are met with increased stimulation rather than corrective feedback; (3) the highest possible number of responses should be elicited in each session; (4) target behaviors are elicited through continual repetition of the clinician's stimulus rather than via direct instruction; and (5) therapy tasks are focused mainly on the semantic and syntactic components of the linguistic system.

Melodic Intonation Therapy (Albert, Sparks, & Helm, 1973). Melodic intonation therapy (MIT) is a restorative/linguistic technique that utilizes "intoning" to facilitate verbal expression in clients who demonstrate severely restricted verbal output and relatively good speech comprehension. This approach uses variations in pitch, tempo/rhythm, and stress to recruit participation of the right hemisphere to improve verbal production in clients with damage to the language-dominant left hemisphere. The MIT program consists of a 15-step hierarchy (Helm-Estabrooks & Albert, 2004; Helm-Estabrooks & Holland, 1998; Sparks, 2001; Sparks & Holland, 1976), which is presented in a condensed form as follows:

1. Client taps out rhythm while listening to clinician's hummed and intoned utterance.
2. Client and clinician intone utterance in unison.
3. Clinician fades out of unison production.
4. Client independently imitates clinician's model of intoned utterance.
5. Client's response is no longer intoned but produced in unison with exaggerated inflection and then gradually shaped to approximate more normal speech prosody.

6. Clinician fades out of unison production.

7. Client independently imitates clinician's model of spoken utterance.

8. Client fades imitative response and spontaneously produces the spoken utterance in response to clinician questions.

MIT generally begins with utterances consisting of two- and three-syllable words and short, commonly used phrases. Longer and more complex utterances are gradually introduced at later stages in the program. Each step in the program has specific scoring procedures. At all levels of stimulus difficulty, it is recommended that the utterance should be produced slowly and with continuous voicing.

The most suitable candidates for MIT are aphasic individuals who demonstrate the following characteristics:

- Unilateral stroke in the left frontal lobe (Broca's area), often extending to the parietal region
- Severely limited verbal output with poor speech articulation
- Extremely poor speech imitation skills
- Relatively spared comprehension of verbal input
- Emotionally stable with good attention span

MIT is not the only therapeutic approach based upon shared neurologic pathways for speech and singing. Tomaino (2012) discusses several other therapeutic strategies that can be used along with MIT to help individuals with nonfluent aphasia:.

- Familiar songs: The practice of singing a familiar song can be used to transfer gains made in singing rhythm to speech rhythm. Clinicians also can use familiar lyrics as a cloze task, singing the first part of the lyric and pausing for the patient to fill in the end of the lyric. In addition to familiar lyrics, a familiar melody can be paired with common social phrases (e.g., How are you?) to assist patients with the fluent production of the phrases.
- Breathing exercises: The use of controlled exhalations can help patients to produce speech sounds and simple syllables. This strategy uses any breathing pattern that is intact and accessible to patients, such as yawning or sighing, to facilitate speech productions.
- Oral-motor exercises: The provision of exaggerated models of the oral-motor movements needed to produce lyrics and/or targeted phrases, with the patient imitating the movements while repeating the phrases.

Gestural Program: Amer-Ind (Skelly, Schinsky, Smith, & Fust, 1974). This substitutive/compensatory technique is a gestural system based on American Indian Hand Talk, in which the gestures stand for basic concepts rather than words. Each signal can represent several different English words. Each gesture is very concrete and easily recognizable (i.e., highly transparent; Campbell & Jackson, 1995). This system is telegraphic in nature in that there is no grammar; rather, the signals are sequenced in a logical order. Amer-Ind can be used as an alternative communication system or as a facilitator of other communication modalities (Coelho, 1990; Peach, 2008; Rao, 2001). This therapy approach is generally used with individuals with severely restricted verbal repertoires resulting from aphasia or apraxia. It also is most effective with clients whose gestural skills are better than their verbal skills. It consists of the following main steps:

1. Use extensive imitation to establish comprehension and production of very common and easily recognized (iconic) gestures such as head nods and shoulder shrugs.

2. Gradually fade imitation in favor of more spontaneous and communicatively meaningful use of the signs.

3. Begin to pair the signs with spoken words after client has mastered several signs.

4. Gradually shape the imitative nature of the client's response to spontaneous production of the sign + word combination in response to clinician questions.

Gesture and Naming Therapy (Caute et al., 2013; Marshall et al., 2012). Two modalities are discretely targeted during intervention with this treatment approach: gesture and verbal modalities. If deemed necessary, the written modality can be used in place of the verbal modality based on individual ability. Treatment follows the same hierarchy for both modalities, with equal time given to each during a therapy session:

1. Recognition-level tasks are used in the initial phase of therapy, with individuals associating gestures and/or words with corresponding pictures.

2. Production-level tasks initially require the individual with aphasia to produce gestures/words corresponding to a picture presented by the therapist.

3. Higher-level production tasks require the individual with aphasia to produce targets that are not known by the clinician and that the clinician must then identify from a field of (a) nonrelated targets and then (b) related targets.

Gestural Program: Visual Action Therapy (Helm-Estabrooks & Albert, 2004). Visual Action Therapy (VAT) is a substitutive/compensatory approach to aphasia intervention that enhances an individual's functional communication skills through the use of representational gestures rather than speech. This nonvocal strategy, designed for severely impaired or globally aphasic individuals, focuses on the production of messages at the single-gesture level. VAT is a hierarchically structured three-level program that utilizes objects, realistic line drawings of the objects, and action pictures depicting a figure appropriately manipulating the objects. Ultimately, the client progresses from matching pictures and objects to the spontaneous use of symbolic hand/arm or mouth/face gestures to communicate simple messages. Currently, there are three VAT program variations: (1) **proximal limb** (focuses on gestures composed of gross movements of the shoulder, arms, and fingers, e.g., sawing), (2) **distal limb** (focuses on gestures composed of finer movements of the hand and fingers, e.g., turning a screwdriver), and (3) **bucco-facial** (focuses on gestures composed of movements of the mouth and face, e.g., whistling). All three VAT variations follow the same basic training sequence, summarized as follows:

1. Client matches and then points to objects and pictures in four different seven-way discrimination tasks.

2. Client is taught to demonstrate appropriate use of each object through clinician modeling and shaping until spontaneous performance is achieved.

3. Clinician points to a specific action picture and client is required to pick up the corresponding object from an array of seven and demonstrate its use.

4. Client locates or points to a specific object from an array of seven in response to pantomime gestures produced by the clinician.

5. Client is required to produce an appropriate pantomime gesture when shown each of the seven objects.

6. Client is shown two randomly selected objects, which are then hidden; one object is then returned to view and the client is encouraged to self-initiate the correct gesture for the one that remains hidden.

In subsequent levels of this technique, the use of real objects is discontinued. Pantomime gestures and action pictures are utilized as stimuli. Appropriate candidates for VAT demonstrate the following characteristics:

Limb VAT (Proximal/Distal)	Bucco-Facial VAT
Unilateral damage to left hemisphere, especially anterior language areas	Unilateral damage to left hemisphere, especially primary language zones
Global aphasia, severe impairments, relatively intact verbal comprehension modalities, moderate to severe limb apraxia	Severely impaired verbal output in spoken and written language
Alert and cooperative with good attention span	Alert and cooperative with good attention span

Promoting Aphasics' Communicative Effectiveness (Davis, 1993; Davis & Wilcox, 1981). Promoting Aphasics' Communicative Effectiveness (PACE) is another example of a substitutive/compensatory approach to aphasia intervention. Therapy is conducted in the context of naturalistic conversation between the clinician and client. The goal is to improve a client's ability to convey intended messages using whatever means of communication available to the individual. In 1981, Davis and Wilcox identified four principles that underlie the implementation of PACE:

1. The clinician and client are to be egalitarian communication partners and take an equal number of turns as speaker and listener. The purpose is to create an interaction pattern that adheres to the turn-taking rules of everyday conversation. It also provides a built-in natural mechanism for the clinician to model a range of appropriate communication styles that the client can incorporate into subsequent messages.

2. The messages that are communicated must contain new information rather than information that is already known to both communication partners. This requirement encourages the speaker to reformulate or revise messages that initially meet with listener confusion.

3. Messages can be exchanged using any vocal or nonvocal modality or combinations of modalities.

4. The clinician provides feedback regarding the communicative effectiveness of messages conveyed by the client; errors in linguistic form of messages are not addressed.

Implementation of these four principles is accomplished through a picture description task in which the clinician and client take turns acting as the sender of a message. The designated sender chooses one picture from a facedown pile (being careful to keep it from the listener's view) and describes it using any available communication modalities. Unlike most intervention programming, PACE requires that the clinician be unaware of the specific stimulus items selected by the client from the pile. The aim of this task is for the speaker to successfully transmit the intended information to the listener.

PACE is a flexible treatment technique that has been used with individuals with various types and degrees of aphasia. These include both fluent aphasic and nonfluent aphasic adults. According to Davis and Wilcox (1981), the pragmatic orientation of PACE makes it a suitable component of any aphasia treatment program regardless of the severity of linguistic impairment.

Script Training (Cherney, Halper, Holland, & Cole, 2008; Holland & Ramage, 2004; Youmans, Holland, Muñoz, & Bourgeois, 2005). This approach is based upon the instance theory of automization, which states that automaticity occurs through the retrieval and practice of skills as a complete set rather than through targeted practice of each component within the set (Youmans et al., 2005). Script training merges components of functional therapy and linguistic therapy: it targets functional phrases with an emphasis on massed practice, a condition that is not naturally a part of functional communication. The ultimate goal of script training therapy is to increase the automaticity of speech productions, even if the automaticity is limited to a set of scripts/contexts (i.e., scripted islands of fluent speech; Youmans et al., 2005). Thus, it has implications for individuals with aphasia who have difficulty with word retrieval and/or fluent speech. Therapy typically consists of the following steps:

1. The client selects several contexts for scripts and then identifies the desired concepts/vocabulary of the script for the clinician. Scripts can be conversational in style or monologue-based if the individual desires to practice telling a story.

2. Script training typically commences at the receptive level, with individuals listening to the targeted phrases modeled for them. Training can be conducted face to face in therapy sessions or through the use of computer software, with an SLP monitoring progress at specified time intervals.

3. Script production starts at the phrase level; intensive targeting of each phrase continues until it is mastered, and the individual then moves on to the next phrase, until the entire script is mastered. Cues, such as choral reading, are provided as needed throughout the training process.

4. Once mastered, the entire script is then practiced with communicative partners. These practice conversations can be varied to enable individuals with aphasia to further practice conversational skills. Variations include practicing with different conversational partners and partners using different prosodic inflections during exchanges.

Response Elaboration Training (Kearns, 1985; Wambaugh & Martinez, 2000; Wambaugh, Nessler, & Wright, 2013). The main goal of Response Elaboration Training (RET) is for clients to regain flexible and creative use of language. Some individuals with aphasia may communicate primarily with nouns and/or at the single word or short phrase level. RET utilizes a loosely structured treatment protocol to help patients increase the variety of words and phrases used in communicative exchanges. Client responses are judged in a more flexible manner; the clinician evaluates the amount and type of information being conveyed in a response rather than trying to elicit a specific response or grammatical form. Each stimulus presented during a therapy session is worked on using the following steps:

- The clinician presents the client with a picture and gives the instruction to talk about the picture.

- After the client responds, the clinician gives a response that either expands upon what the client said or provides a verbal model for the client. The model may be a repetition of the client's response or an example of another possible response.

- The clinician asks a wh- question pertaining to the picture and/or the client's response to elicit another comment from the client.

- After the client responds, the clinician models a response that includes information from the client's response as well as previous discussion of the picture.

- The client is asked to repeat the modeled elaboration from the previous step.

- The clinician repeats the model one final time for reinforcement.

Life Participation Approach to Aphasia (Elman & Bernstein-Ellis, 1999; Lyon, 1998; Simmons-Mackie, 2008). This approach broadens the functional/compensatory orientation to aphasia intervention. The overriding philosophy of the Life Participation Approach to Aphasia is to maximize the client's re-engagement in life and base all therapeutic decision-making on the life concerns identified by clients and their families. Therapeutic goals are designed explicitly to help clients translate newly learned skills to everyday life experiences. The main emphases of this intervention model include the following:

- All individuals with aphasia are entitled to receive services as needed at all stages of recovery.

- Both personal/intrinsic and environmental/extrinsic factors should be incorporated into therapeutic programming. These range on a continuum from obstructive to facilitative and should be identified on a case-by-case basis.

- Success is measured by documented changes in life areas defined as important by clients and their families.

Noninvasive Electrical Brain Stimulation Techniques (Barwood & Murdoch, 2013; Chrysikou & Hamilton, 2011; Martin et al., 2009). The use of magnetic impulses to stimulate targeted areas of the brain is being explored for its therapeutic applications to treating damaged areas of the brain, thus with potential implications for speech, language, and swallowing disorders. This approach is considered noninvasive because it involves the application of electrical currents to the brain through an intact skull. Studies using a type of electrical stimulation called rTMS (repetitive transcranial magnetic stimulation) have provided evidence of neuroplasticity through behavioral changes in patients' abilities to complete naming tasks (Martin et al., 2009). For example, Barwood et al. (2012) used rTMS to suppress neural activation in a region of the right hemisphere, promoting more activation to the associated linguistic area in the left hemisphere. This treatment protocol was found to improve both accuracy as well as response times during naming tasks up to 8 months posttreatment (Barwood et al., 2012).

Another noninvasive brain-stimulation technique, transcranial direct-current stimulation, also has been found to have a positive effect on lexical retrieval skills (Torres et al., 2013). Because most of the current research has focused on cases of nonfluent, chronic aphasia and naming tasks, further information is needed about the relationship between brain stimulation and language gains. This includes whether this technique should be viewed as an alternative or an augmentative approach to traditional language therapy, whether certain neural areas or lesion severities are more responsive to stimulation than others, and whether the gains made through brain stimulation are transient or permanent in nature.

Pharmacotherapy (Berthier, Pulvermuller, Davila, Casares, & Gutierrez, 2011). The use of medications to treat language deficits in aphasia is an area currently being explored in the literature. One study examined the use of several different medicines with individuals with mild- to- moderate severities of aphasia. The study found support for two different medicinal agents (i.e., dopaminergic and chlorinergic agents) with regard to gains in expressive language skills, specifically naming skills and overall fluency (Tanaka, Albert, Fujita, Nonaka, & Yokoyama, 2006). Neurotransmitters, such as dopamine, are often targeted in pharmacotherapy for aphasia treatment based upon the theory that increasing neural activity in targeted brain areas via neurotransmitters will increase neural recovery in these regions (Berthier et al., 2011). Berthier et al. (2011) conducted a systematic review of the literature on pharmacotherapy and aphasia. Common findings among the research studies reviewed included:

- Greater gains in language skills were seen when pharmacotherapy was used in conjunction with speech and language therapy.
- Individuals with chronic aphasia still benefited from pharmacotherapy.
- Individuals with mild- to- moderate aphasia were the best candidates, as individuals with severe aphasia typically did not benefit from pharmacotherapy.
- Language gains were reported in a variety of linguistic skill area depending on the drug therapy used, including fluency, comprehension, and functional communication skills.

Example Profiles

Following are three profiles representative of the communication problems exhibited by individuals with different types of aphasia (Wernicke's, Broca's, and global). These examples have been designed to illustrate the selection of intervention targets as well as specific therapy activities and materials. Most of the chosen activities can be implemented in either individual or group therapy settings.

Mr. Chang is a 39-year-old right-handed male who presented with a severe-profound fluent aphasia (Wernicke's) after sustaining a left parietal CVA 9 months ago. His initial status was characterized by intelligible verbal output and frequent semantic and phonemic paraphasias. No evidence of dysarthria or apraxia of speech was observed. It was noted that the content of Mr. Chang's output was often unrelated to the topic at hand. He demonstrated severe word-retrieval difficulties and significant auditory comprehension deficits, including an inability to answer yes/no questions. Mr. Chang did not demonstrate the ability to point to objects, pictures, or body parts named, nor did he follow any single- or multiple-step commands. His automatic writing of the alphabet was incomplete, although Mr. Chang accurately wrote his name and the numbers 1 to 20. Reading comprehension was poor, but he did demonstrate the ability to match written word stimuli to objects and pictures.

Mr. Chang received speech-language intervention services for several months post-stroke. His current communication status is characterized by occasional semantic and phonemic paraphasias and moderate word-finding deficits. His auditory comprehension skills have improved; Mr. Chang correctly answers simple questions, identifies objects named by others, and inconsistently follows simple single-stage commands, such as, "Put the pencil next to the book." Writing is Mr. Chang's strongest communication modality as evidenced by his ability to write paragraph-length passages with minimal difficulty. Reading comprehension skills are also relatively strong in the areas of word recognition and sentence comprehension.

Mr. Chang's verbal description of the "cookie theft" picture from the Boston Diagnostic Aphasia Examination (Goodglass et al., 2001) is as follows:

> All right well there's a rolly dolly, whatever it is. And the dirl and be and the willy it fall and the fell and he fall down into the drom. And well the waver, water it's all out off for the end. And the mon, mother doing the dibs all the way and she's for the wauby be.

Selection of therapy targets. The areas to be targeted are word retrieval and auditory comprehension. These were selected for two main reasons. First, word retrieval and comprehension are Mr. Chang's most impaired language skills and continue to have the greatest negative impact on his ability to communicate effectively in everyday situations. Second, these areas have shown improvement with therapeutic intervention in the past, suggesting the potential for continued growth.

Sample Activities

(All three activities are based on a substitutive/compensatory approach.)

1. Assemble a pile of 20 pictures of common objects and place them face down on a table. Based on the PACE approach, explain that the clinician and client will take turns selecting pictures from the pile and describing them without showing them. Instruct the client to use any means of communication to convey the contents of each selected picture (e.g., oral naming, oral description of physical appearance of the object, pantomime the function of the object, draw the object, write the name of the object). Emphasize that the purpose of this activity is to successfully communicate the intended message rather than to retrieve a specific label. When a strategy is ineffective and results in listener confusion, encourage the client to reformulate the message using another communication mode. The clinician should use his or her turn as speaker to model various communication strategies. The client's communication effectiveness is measured by the clinician's ability to accurately identify the object pictured.

2. Identify a topic that is meaningful or of interest to the client (e.g., favorite hobby, job, family) and collect 25 identical pairs of picture cards that relate to this theme. Based on pretreatment baseline data, select two self-cuing strategies that will be taught to facilitate the client's retrieval of each verbal label (e.g., air tracing and sentence completion). Demonstrate each technique several times and ask the client to imitate these strategies. Shuffle the deck and deal seven cards to each player. Explain that the object of the activity is to make pairs for all the cards in a player's hand by asking the other player(s), "Do you have a ___?" Instruct the client to use one or both of the self-cuing strategies for every request. The clinician continues to model the tracing and sentence completion procedures during his or her turn.

3. Collect five common objects (e.g., pencil, book, cup, spoon, comb). With these objects in mind, develop a list of 20 single-stage commands that contain three linguistic units (e.g., "Put the *spoon* in the *cup*"; *Give me the book* and the *pencil*"). Place the objects on the table and explain that the client will be given short instructions involving the manipulation of the objects. Instruct the client to write down the first letter of each important word in the direction as a strategy to facilitate comprehension of the verbal command. If the client demonstrates significant difficulty, the clinician can implement the following modifications: (a) reduce speech rate during presentation of stimulus commands, (b) increase redundancy by stating each direction twice before the client responds, and (c) increase the acceptable latency period between the clinician's stimulus presentation and the initiation of the client's response. These strategies will provide the client with needed extra processing time and can be faded gradually as performance improves.

Mr. Sanders is a 63-year-old right-handed male who presented with a moderate-to-severe nonfluent aphasia (Broca's) after suffering a left frontal intercranial hemorrhage 2 months ago. Currently, Mr. Sanders's verbal output is characterized by one- and two-word utterances in which the subject noun phrase and verb phrase are often separated by distinctive pauses. His output consists mainly of content words, with the frequent omission of grammatical markers. Significant word-retrieval difficulties are not noted. Ability to imitate verbal utterances is poor even at the single-word level. Mr. Sanders's output is pragmatically appropriate and reflects relatively intact comprehension of verbal material. He demonstrates the ability to identify many objects and pictures when named by the clinician and follows one- and two-step commands with minimal difficulty. Articulation is awkward and labored, with phoneme distortion errors most prevalent. However, it was noted that Mr. Sanders consistently articulated his last name correctly. Minimal use of stress and intonation patterns results in a notable lack of speech melody. Writing skills are consistent with oral output with regard to both vocabulary and syntax; reading comprehension skills are mildly impaired.

Mr. Sanders's verbal description of the "cookie theft" picture from the Boston Diagnostic Aphasia Examination (Goodglass et al., 2001) is as follows:

uh . . . mother . . . uh . . . she talking to the . . . uh . . . the . . . uh . . . I don't know . . . two cup . . . cookie in jar . . . fall down . . . wash . . . and stool . . . uh . . . tipping . . . boy . . . uh . . . get hurt

Selection of therapy targets. The areas to be targeted are utterance length and syntactic complexity as well as speech prosody. Because the content and use components of Mr. Sanders's linguistic system are relatively intact, utterance length and complexity were chosen to improve the form component of his verbal repertoire. Speech prosody was targeted because it is an essential component of intelligibility. Improved function in this area will facilitate listeners' ability to predict the content of Mr. Sanders's messages despite his articulatory deficits.

Sample Activities

(Activities 1, 2, and 4 are restorative techniques; activity 3 is based on the substitutive/compensatory approach.)

1. (For MIT Step 1.) Arrange seating to ensure that the client can readily see the clinician's mouth. Select stimulus items for this step of MIT with the following considerations in mind: (a) the stimuli must be meaningful and useful to the individual client; (b) stimuli in this early stage of the program should include a heavy concentration of sounds that are easy to visualize (i.e., bilabials); (c) short, simple phrases should be used (e.g., imperatives such as "Stand up," "Open the door"); and (d) an extensive list of high-probability items is necessary so that any given stimulus utterance is not presented too often. Following is a sample list of stimulus items for Mr. Sanders at this MIT level:

watch TV	salt and pepper
take a nap	good morning
bowl of soup	peach pie
make the bed	cup of coffee
read the paper	start the car

Graphically, plot the intonation patterns for each stimulus item before the session begins. (See the following example.)

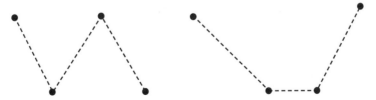

Set criteria for an acceptable response. The clinician takes the client's hand and hums the plotted intonation pattern for a stimulus while tapping the client's hand on the table once for each syllable. Next, the clinician intones (rather than hums) the same prosody pattern using words and continues to tap the client's hand once for each syllable. Avoid a staccato rhythm because continuous voicing facilitates verbal production. After a brief pause, repeat the intoned utterance with client hand tapping. Signal the client to join the clinician in unison repetition of the intoned phrase with assisted hand tapping. If the client's response is acceptable, carry this phrase to Step 3, in which the clinician fades the verbal model partway through the phrase so that the client must finish the utterance alone. The clinician continues to tap the rhythm with the client's hand. If the response is not adequate, pause for several seconds, choose the next item from the stimulus list and repeat the steps outlined previously. (For detailed information regarding the implementation of MIT, refer to Helm-Estabrooks and Albert [2004] and Sparks [2001].)

2. Devise a list of 25 sentence pairs for a cloze task to train production of the regular plural form of nouns. Examples include the following:

> This is one book. These are two (*books*).
>
> He saw one cookie. He saw two (*cookies*).
>
> She washed a dish. She washed all the (*dishes*).
>
> I see the dog. I see lots of (*dogs*).
>
> The plant has one flower. This plant has many (*flowers*).

Gather two pictures that depict common objects for each sentence pair. One should contain a single exemplar of the object and the other multiple exemplars of the same object. Explain to the client that this activity focuses on the production of the plural of nouns. Place the first pair of pictures on the table and demonstrate the activity by pointing to the singleton picture when saying the first sentence and pointing to the multiple picture while producing the second sentence with the correct plural noun form included. For the remaining sentence pairs, the clinician leaves the second sentence unfinished and instructs the client to complete the sentence fragment by supplying the plural noun form.

3. Create a conversational script like the following one, according to the guidelines listed in Appendix 7-B.

a. I can't watch the Orioles anymore.

b. This time they lost to Chicago.

c. And Chicago beat them by 10 runs.

d. They need to get a new coach.

Instruct the client to read the script aloud one sentence at a time. When the client encounters difficulties verbalizing the scripted information, suggest self-cuing strategies to facilitate production of the utterance. Examples include chunking utterances into shorter units, gesturing to convey meaning, and using techniques to trigger word retrieval. Next, video record the client reading the script to a familiar listener who is unacquainted with its content. Coach the listener to concentrate on obtaining the gist of the message rather than focusing on specific words and details. The clinician, client, and familiar listener should evaluate the recording according to the following parameters:

a. How successful was the scripted interaction?

b. What did the speaker/listener find most helpful?

c. What did the speaker/listener find least helpful?

d. What else could have been done by the client, listener, or clinician to facilitate the interaction?

Continue this cycle of coaching and evaluation with increasingly unfamiliar listeners.

4. Develop a list of 20 two-syllable word pairs that have dual intonation patterns. For these pairs, differential stress significantly affects meaning. Stress on the first syllable (indicated in boldface) signals that the word functions as a noun, whereas stress on the second syllable indicates that the word is being used as a verb. Examples include the following:

present/pre**sent**	**con**tract/con**tract**
defect/de**fect**	**re**cord/re**cord**
permit/per**mit**	**con**test/con**test**
convict/con**vict**	**re**fuse/re**fuse**
produce/pro**duce**	**ob**ject/ob**ject**
rebel/re**bel**	**con**vert/con**vert**
contrast/con**trast**	**des**ert/de**sert**
discharge/dis**charge**	**pro**ject/pro**ject**
protest/pro**test**	**sub**ject/sub**ject**
survey/sur**vey**	**ad**dress/ad**dress**

Write each pair on a separate index card and underline or boldface the stressed syllable for each word. Develop a pair of questions or fill-in-the-blank statements for each word that are designed to elicit both noun and verb intonation patterns. For example, queries for the first pair might be: "What do you buy for somebody's birthday?" and "In honor of [insert famous name here]'s great accomplishments, I now ___ him with this award." Instruct the client to choose one index card from the pile and practice both stress patterns in unison with the clinician. The clinician then presents the stimulus question/statement for the noun form and asks the client to look at the index card and spontaneously produce the target word with the appropriate stress pattern. Present the second question/statement to elicit the verb stress pattern indicated on the index card. Repeat this procedure for the remaining word pairs. Task difficulty can be increased by eliciting noun and verb forms in random order.

Mrs. Marshall is a 71-year-old right-handed female who presents with a global aphasia and a right hemiplegia and limb apraxia subsequent to a thrombosis of the middle cerebral artery that resulted in extensive damage to the pre- and postrolandic areas 6 months ago. Her communicative status has not changed substantially since that time.

Currently, Mrs. Marshall demonstrates significant impairment in both language comprehension and language production in all modalities. She exhibits understanding of some simple yes/no questions, such as, "Is your name Polly?" and identifies body parts named by the clinician with approximately 50% accuracy. Mrs. Marshall does not appear to comprehend even simple one-step verbal commands. She relies heavily on nonverbal means to communicate, including facial expressions and head nods to indicate yes/no responses and a gross pointing gesture. Her speech output is limited to stereotypic utterances and neologisms that consist of both real and nonsense words. These are produced with differential stress and intonation and seem to express several communicative intentions. Reading comprehension is extremely poor even at the familiar single-word level. Writing skills are slightly better in that Mrs. Marshall can copy written words with occasional errors but does not exhibit the ability to generate legible written words spontaneously. Overall, she appears alert, attentive, and somewhat frustrated by her inability to communicate.

Mrs. Marshall's verbal description of the "cookie theft" picture from the Boston Diagnostic Aphasia Examination (Goodglass et al., 2001) is as follows:

> I can't. I don't think that . . . What is this? . . . I just don't have that. Oh yeah, right here. That's all.

Selection of therapy targets.   Based on the severity of Mrs. Marshall's deficits, the areas to be targeted are auditory comprehension and functional communication skills. Auditory comprehension was chosen to establish a core receptive vocabulary that is meaningful within the context of her daily activities. Mrs. Marshall's verbal expression appears so limited that even after 6 months she does not represent a good candidate for intervention. Therefore, the substitutive/compensatory approaches of PACE and Amer-Ind will be implemented to facilitate the effectiveness of her relatively stronger nonverbal communication skills. VAT was not considered an appropriate strategy for two reasons. First, the prescribed repertoire of gestural meanings was not deemed to be functional for Mrs. Marshall. Second, this approach requires the ability to perform a seven-way object and picture discrimination task as an initial level of training, which is clearly beyond her auditory comprehension abilities.

Sample Activities

(All three activities are based on a substitutive/compensatory approach.)

1. Consult the client's family members and friends to identify vocabulary items that are most important to Mrs. Marshall. Items may include names of significant others, pets, favorite foods, terms for hobbies and other leisure interests (e.g., knitting, art, TV, and so on), frequently visited locations, and money terms. Select 20 of these items and gather large color pictures of each one (photographs are highly desirable). Complete the following three steps. Step 1: Place each picture card one at a time face up on a table. Name each picture and then point to it to provide a model for the client. Step 2: Present each picture again, name it, and physically assist the client to point to the picture. Step 3: Place two pictures face up on the table, name one, and signal the client to identify the target item by pointing. If the client experiences significant difficulty with the two-way discrimination task in Step 3, reduce the field to a single picture while still requiring a spontaneous pointing response.

2. Gather 25 colored photographs or easily recognizable pictures that depict activities or objects of daily living that are relevant for Mrs. Marshall. These may include brushing teeth, bathing, eating, sleeping, dressing, drinking, church, dentures, toilet, and doctor. Place the stack of pictures facedown on the table. Based on the PACE approach, select one picture from the pile and model several different strategies for communicating the contents of the picture to the client (e.g., oral naming, description of activity/object characteristics, pantomiming action or object function, drawing, rudimentary written cues). Repeat this modeling as necessary. Client

and clinician take turns selecting pictures from the stack. The clinician should use his or her turn as speaker to emphasize that the purpose of this activity is to successfully communicate the intended meaning by whatever means possible rather than to elicit a particular lexical item. Encourage the client to reformulate a message using another communication strategy if the initial attempt is not successful. The client's ability to effectively convey messages is measured by the clinician's success in guessing the identity of the stimulus picture. It is important to recognize that the client's turn as listener requires an identification response. In the event that the client cannot provide an oral label for the picture described by the clinician, an alternative response mode should be made available. This can be accomplished in the following manner: (a) provide a duplicate set of the 25 pictures; (b) display an array of three pictures, including the target and two foils; and (c) instruct the client to indicate the correct stimulus through pointing.

3. Identify three different communication situations that Mrs. Marshall encounters on a daily or weekly basis (e.g., neighbor visits, doctor appointments, and hair-cutting appointments). From the concept illustration section in Skelly (1979), select five concrete and relevant Amer-Ind signals for each situation, such as the following:

Neighbor	Doctor	Hairdresser
hello/goodbye	pain	cut
sit	tired	okay
drink	medicine	comb
eat	nurse	thanks
walk	puzzled	money

(*Note:* Mrs. Marshall's hemiplegia necessitates that the signals chosen can be executed with the left hand.)

Choose one scenario and gather objects and/or pictures that represent the signals to be trained. For the "neighbor" scenario, these might include a chair, a cup, a pretzel, a picture of people entering/leaving a room, and a picture of two women taking a walk. Demonstrate each signal with the corresponding object or picture several times. For example, the concept of "walk" is represented by the following signal: extend left arm in front of body with elbow at shoulder level; palm of hand is down and index/middle fingers are extended pointing down while the hand slowly advances to the right; the extended fingers alternate moving forward, conveying the action of legs walking. Consult Skelly (1979) for explanations and visual illustrations of other Amer-Ind signals.

Place three of the referents on the table, model one of the signals, and encourage the client to identify the appropriate referent. Repeat this procedure until the client reliably recognizes the five target signals.

Place an object/picture on the table, model the corresponding gesture, and require the client to imitate it. If the client demonstrates difficulty with this task, provide physical assistance to shape the response. Once successful and unassisted imitation has been established for a given scenario, gradually fade the clinician's model and elicit more spontaneous and functional productions of the signals through clinician questions or role-playing.

Helpful Hints

1. Keep in mind that there is a basic hierarchy of picture difficulty. One can increase the complexity of a picture description task by progressing from object pictures to action pictures, to pictures denoting location, and then to a series of pictures describing a logical sequence of events.

2. Remember that individuals with aphasia (particularly those of advanced age) often present with concomitant physical or emotional problems that may affect their ability to communicate. Poor performance on therapy tasks may not be attributable to the aphasia per se, but to any of several other factors, including hearing impairment, poor visual acuity or visual field deficits, medication imbalances or side effects, depression, and so on.

3. As a general rule, clients with auditory comprehension deficits benefit from substantial repetition and redundancy of verbal input.

4. Clinicians should consistently use a slower speech rate when interacting with clients with aphasia. Rate of speech may have a significant impact on these individuals' ability to process verbal information.

5. Individuals with global aphasia may benefit from the provision of a *communication book/augmentative device* that contains pictures of familiar objects, people, and events from their daily environment.

6. In the early stages of intervention, clinicians may have to rely heavily on yes/no questions to provide clients with a mechanism for expressing strong feelings of frustration, anxiety, or confusion.

7. Software technology for aphasia intervention is increasingly available from many sources. Clinicians are encouraged to seek out programs with demonstrated efficacy or outcome data.

8. Family participation in therapy should be maximized. Clinicians are encouraged to actively engage family members and caregivers in therapy to promote practice of therapy targets throughout the client's daily activities.

CONCLUSION

This section has presented basic information, protocols, and procedures for aphasia intervention at an introductory level. This material is intended only as a starting point in the reader's clinical education and training. For more in-depth coverage of this area, as well as for information on other cognitive-communication disorders, the following readings are recommended:

Aphasia

Barnes, M., Dobkin, B., & Bogousslavsky, J. (Eds.). (2005). *Recovery after stroke.* New York: Cambridge University Press.

Brookshire, R. H. (2007). *An introduction to neurogenic communication disorders (7th ed.).* St. Louis, MO: C.V. Mosby Co.

Chapey, R. (2008). *Language intervention strategies in aphasia and related neurogenic communication disorders* (5th ed.). Baltimore, MD: Lippincott Williams & Wilkins.

Elman, R. J. (2006). *Group treatment of neurogenic communication disorders: The expert clinician's approach.* San Diego, CA: Plural Publishing.

Helm-Estabrooks, N., & Holland, A. (1998). *Approaches to the treatment of aphasia.* San Diego, CA: Singular Publishing Group.

Tanner, D. C. (2008). *The family guide to surviving stroke and communication disorders. A primer for health care professionals (2nd ed.).* Sudbury, MA: Jones & Bartlett Publishers, LLC.

Right-Hemisphere Dysfunction

Beeman, M. J., & Chiarello, C. (Eds.) (2013). *Right hemisphere language comprehension: Perspectives from cognitive neuroscience.* Mahwah, NJ: Lawrence Erlbaum Associates, Inc.

Myers, P. S. (2008). Communication disorders associated with right hemisphere damage. In R. Chapey (Ed.), *Language intervention strategies in aphasia and related neurogenic communication disorders* (5th ed., pp. 809–828). Baltimore, MD: Lippincott Williams & Wilkins.

Tompkins, C.A. (2012). Rehabilitation for cognitive-communication disorders in right hemisphere brain damage. *Archives of Physical Medicine and Rehabilitation,* 93(1), S61–S69.

Dementia

Bayles, K. A., & Tomoeda, C. K. (2007). *Cognitive-communication disorders of dementia.* San Diego, CA: Plural Publishing.

Bourgeois, M. S., & Hickey, E. M. (2009). *Dementia: From diagnosis to management—a functional approach.* New York, NY: Psychology Press.

Krishnamoorthy, E. S., Prince, M. J., & Cummings, J. L. (Eds.). (2010). *Dementia: A global approach.* New York, NY: Cambridge University Press.

Weiner, M. F., & Lipton, A. M. (2009). *Textbook of Alzheimer disease and other dementias.* Arlington, VA: American Psychiatric Publishing.

ADDITIONAL RESOURCES

Aphasia
AliMed
297 High Street
Dedham, MA 02026
Phone: 800-225-2610
Fax: 800-437-2966
Web site: http://www.alimed.com

Workbook for Cognitive Skills
For adults and adolescents with moderate cognitive impairments or learning disabilities. Target areas include word formation, familiar phrases, definition usage, visual recognition, letter placement, and logical solutions.

Cognitive Reorganization

Includes 4,200+ stimuli plus activities for functional applications help meet the diverse needs of clients who cannot use functional language skills in any organized, sequential, or pragmatic way. Responses may be written, verbal, or graphic.

Building Word Recall from Everyday Situations

This workbook can be used with individuals with mild to severe memory deficits. It targets memory skills by focusing on 12 areas that progress from automatic speech tasks to more volitional language skills (e.g., using yes/no, completing sentences to sequencing events and providing descriptions).

Functional Memory Manual

This workbook provides strategies for increasing memory recall for individuals with mild to severe memory deficits. It contains chapters on topics such as attention, visual recall, and auditory recall.

The Speech Bin
School Specialty
P.O. Box 1579
Appleton, WI 54912-1579
Phone: 800-388-3224
Fax: 800-388-6344
Web site: http://store.schoolspecialty.com

Workbook for Aphasia

For adults with mild-to-moderate language and cognitive deficits. Target areas include word usage, development of syntax, use of factual information, and concrete and abstract reasoning.

Workbook for Language Skills

For adults with mild-to-severe language impairments. Target areas include spelling, sentence completion, sentence construction, sentence comprehension, figurative language, general knowledge, and word recall.

Workbook for Reasoning Skills

For adolescents and adults with mild-to-moderate impairment in problem solving, reasoning, and comprehension skills. Target areas include drawing conclusions, problem solving, following directions, visual/logical sequencing, humor, and numbers/systems.

Pro-Ed
8700 Shoal Creek Boulevard
Austin, TX 78757-6897
Phone: 800-897-3202
Fax: 800-397-7633
Web site: http://www.proedinc.com

Focus on Function: Gaining Essential Communication, 2nd Edition

Targets independent living skills for adolescents and adults by having them practice a variety of daily tasks. Includes reproducible evaluation forms, task cards, picture cards, manipulatives, and practical activities that emphasize everyday verbal, phone, reading, writing, and numerical skills.

Language Activity Resource Kit (LARK), 2nd Edition

A portable kit with objects (two of each), illustrated cards, color photographs, word and phrase cards, and line drawings of the objects in use. Designed especially for the itinerant SLP treating adults with aphasia and/or TBI. Optional LARK workbook with reproducible worksheets can be purchased.

Laureate Software

110 East Spring Street
Winooski, VT 05404-1898
Phone: 800-562-6801
Fax: 802-655-4757
Email: laureate@laureatelearning.com
Web site: http://www.laureatelearning.com

The Words and Concepts Series

Computer software designed to build vocabulary, strengthen language comprehension and word relationships, and develop important concepts. Consists of three instructional programs and three companion game programs, which use a core vocabulary of 40 referential nouns in six related language units: Vocabulary, Categorization, Word Identification by Function, Word Association, and Same and Different Concepts. Most activities contain three levels of difficulty, which can be set to branch among each other, following the progress of the individual.

The Following Directions Series

Computer software that includes eight activities to help clients learn to follow one-level, sequential, and two-level commands using spatial relations concepts and directional terms. Also includes 10 activities to improve clients' ability to follow directions and develop right/left discrimination concepts through activities such as simple left- and right-hand matching, practice crossing midline, and moving objects to left and right using hands in mirrored and nonmirrored positions.

My House, My Town, and My School: The Language Activities of Daily Living Series

These talking instructional computer software programs were designed to help clients understand and express the language they encounter during daily routines. Each program has four different activities designed to increase understanding of object names and their functions or descriptions: Discover Names, Identify Names, Discover Functions, and Identify Functions. In My House, the scenes represent typical rooms in a house: a bedroom, bathroom, dining room, kitchen, living room, and utility room. In My Town, a doctor's office, dentist's office, restaurant, park, city neighborhood, and suburban neighborhood are included.

Apps
Lingraphica
103 Carnegie Center
Suite 204
Princeton, NJ 08540
Phone: 888-274-2742
Fax: 609-275-1311
Web site: www.aphasia.com

Lingraphica is a company devoted to providing resources to individuals with aphasia. Some of the apps focus on facilitating communication, such as SmallTalk Conversational Phrases and SmallTalk Daily Activities. Other apps provide practice for therapy targets for both expressive and receptive language tasks. The TalkPath Speaking app contains naming and speech repetition exercises for memory and word retrieval skills. Receptively, the TalkPath Listening app provides practice answering yes/no and wh-questions as well as identifying associations through matching object pairs.

Tactus Therapy Solutions
Web site: http://tactustherapy.com

Language TherAppy
A collection of four apps that target skills in the following areas: comprehension, naming, writing, and reading. The Comprehension TherAppy App is available in English as well as Spanish and French. Other features include difficulty that adjusts based on performance, exercise scores that can be shared with SLPs, and practice modes that provide supports.

Tactus Therapy Solutions also offers several other apps that target aphasia. The Conversation TherAppy App uses a library of photographs and questions to provide practice using speech at the conversational level. The Category TherAppy App is designed so that it can be used with clients who are verbal and nonverbal. It offers 70 categories ranging from concrete to abstract categories and includes tasks such as picking the one that does not belong or naming additional category items.

TRAUMATIC BRAIN INJURY
(CO-AUTHORED BY EMILY MINEWEASER)

Traumatic brain injury (TBI) results from an external insult to the brain due to numerous causes, including vehicular accidents, gunshot wounds, impact from falls, sports-related injuries, and blasts or explosions. It is estimated that 1.7 million cases of TBI occur annually in the United States. Of these cases, approximately 75 percent are mild in severity, and males are more likely to incur TBIs than females, regardless of age (Centers for Disease Control [CDC], 2013). Resulting damage and deficits vary based on the type and severity of the insult. There are two main classifications of TBI. A **closed head injury (CHI)** results in damage to a widespread area of the brain. The force of the insult or blow is significant and can cause tearing of cell structures. Additionally, the blow or jolt can cause the brain to move back and forth in the skull (contrecoup motion), resulting in multiple points of damage (Coelho et al., 2013). In a **penetrating head injury (PHI)**, damage tends to be concentrated in a specific neurologic region(s) (Coelho et al., 2013). In mild TBI, there are brief changes in or loss of consciousness and memory. In more severe cases, memory loss and periods of unconsciousness are more pronounced. Although not common, aphasia may be a possible result of TBI depending on the extent of damage with CHI or the location of damage with PHI (Coelho et al., 2013; Ylvisaker, Szekeres, & Feeney, 2008). A multitude of symptoms may accompany TBI, including headaches, blurry vision, lethargy, dizziness, sleeping problems, irritability, anxiety, and depression. It can also cause epilepsy and increase the risk for conditions such as Alzheimer's disease, Parkinson's disease, and other brain disorders that become more prevalent with age. From the perspective of the SLP, most cases of TBI involve core deficits in one or more of the following areas: communication, cognition, and behavior. It should be noted that these areas are highly intertwined and many skills represent integration across domain boundaries.

Communication

Communication impairments of clients with TBI typically occur at the discourse level of language (Coelho et al., 2013). Discourse errors can occur at the microstructure or the macrostructure level, with macrostructure typically more impaired (Coelho et al., 2013). The **microstructure (or local structure)** involves lexical/word choice and syntactic organization at the individual sentence level. The **macrostructure (or global structure)** involves higher-level linguistic organization of content across sentences to create a coherent and complete discourse (e.g., cohesion devices for conversation, stories, personal accounts; Coelho et al., 2013; Peach, 2013). In addition to discourse difficulties, other aspects of language may be impaired. Comprehension often becomes difficult, especially with increased linguistic complexity/utterance length, or when abstract topics are discussed (MacDonald & Wiseman-Hakes, 2010). Individuals with TBI often exhibit problems with the social uses of language, or pragmatics. These difficulties include a reduced ability to take the perspective of their listener when formulating messages, recognizing the difference between the intended meanings of their messages and how the listener perceives them, the ability to inhibit socially inappropriate behaviors, or the ability to make inferences about other people's feelings. Individuals with TBI are often judged by society to demonstrate less-than-adequate "social competence" in many areas of daily function. In addition, speech production may be affected due to physical damage to the oral mechanism or due to dysarthria resulting from a neurologic deficit (Cherney et al., 2010).

Cognition

The communication difficulties of individuals with TBI are closely related to accompanying cognitive deficits. Areas of cognition often affected include **executive functioning (EF)**, working memory, problem solving, and attention (Coelho et al., 2013; Ylvisaker et al., 2008). In the area of EF, self-regulation is a frequent problem and may include individuals' difficulty in monitoring, appraising, and inhibiting their own behavior and realistically assessing their strengths and weaknesses. Other EF difficulties include problems in coping with disappointment or anger and reduced ability to regulate and express emotions. Impairments in working memory can cause an individual to struggle with retrieving linguistic information and maintaining thoughts across conversational exchanges. Individuals with TBI often experience difficulties in problem solving such as the effective identifying and sequencing of steps needed to reach logical solutions. Attention difficulties are often characterized by distractibility in noisy environments, lack of sustained concentration, and poor short-term memory.

Behavior

Patients with brain injuries, especially in or near the frontal lobes, often demonstrate deficits in behavioral control (Ylvisaker et al., 2007). These behavioral disorders may manifest themselves externally as aggression, irritability, reduced inhibitions with anger, and inappropriate verbal outputs, or internally as depression, social withdrawal, feelings of awkwardness in social situations, and rigidity (Ylvisaker et al., 2007). Behavioral disturbances also may be related to frustrations that arise from impairments secondary to TBI. Thus, behavioral issues may persist despite improvements in communication or cognitive skills.

Treatment Efficacy/Evidence-Based Practice

By way of introduction, it is important to understand that individuals with TBI constitute a particularly heterogeneous population (MacDonald & Wiseman-Hakes, 2010). Ylvisaker et al. (2007) conducted a systematic review of the literature on therapeutic interventions for individuals with TBI. Each of the 65 studies reviewed reported favorable treatment outcomes from positive behavioral intervention approaches, contingency management principles, or a combination of both elements. More important, 45 of 65 studies reported on various aspects of social validity (the ability to successfully apply intervention procedures to daily life activities). In 2010, MacDonald and Wiseman-Hakes examined systematic reviews across deficit areas (e.g., attention, verbal expression, memory) to determine best practices for treating individuals with brain injury. Evidence supported the use of several metacognitive strategies and/or intervention approaches:

- Incorporation of metacognitive strategies (e.g., self-monitoring skills)
- Individualization of goals based on daily routines (e.g., relevance, social validity)
- Development of self-regulation techniques
- Participation in simulated or real-life scenarios rather than drill-based activities

Cicerone et al. (2011) conducted a literature review on the specific use of cognitive rehabilitation therapy (CRT), a treatment approach that emphasizes utilizing metacognitive strategies and individualizing treatment plans for generalization. They found support for the use of this approach when targeting cognitive skills such as attention, memory, and executive function. In their summary of well-designed research studies for cognitive rehabilitation, Tsaousides and Gordon (2009) indicated that:

1. A neuropsychological assessment is required to develop an appropriate treatment plan.
2. Cognitive therapy can be beneficial regardless of the length of time since the injury and its severity level.
3. Cognitive rehabilitation leads to improvements of psychosocial (e.g., communicating with others in social situations, motivation, mood) as well as cognitive functioning.

Research on military members with **mild TBI (mTBI)** has steadily increased over the past 10 years, as researchers and rehabilitation specialists seek to identify treatment strategies and programs that represent best/preferred practices (Belanger, Kretzmer, Yoash-Gantz, Picket, & Tupler, 2009; Helmick, 2010). Belanger et al. (2009); Lew et al. (2009); Tanielian and Jaycox (2008); and Vanderploeg, Belanger, and Curtiss (2009) identify many challenges, including the following:

- Sparse evidence exists regarding the effectiveness of cognitive rehabilitation for the mTBI population.
- The literature on combat-related mTBI is in the emergent stage.
- The recovery trajectory from combat-related mTBI is complicated by the physically and emotionally traumatic circumstances in which many injuries are sustained.
- Multiple co-morbidities (e.g., concomitant physical injuries to other parts of the body, post-traumatic stress, pain, headaches, acoustic trauma, sensory impairments, depression, substance abuse) are often present.
- The concussions sustained during combat duty can be repetitive and cumulative.
- Difficulty in complying with recommendations for implementation of optimal post-concussion rehabilitation is difficult in deployment and postdeployment settings.

Treatment for Traumatic Brain Injury

SLPs treat individuals with TBI in a variety of settings throughout the rehabilitation process, including intensive care units, acute/subacute rehabilitation hospital settings, and outpatient services (Ylvisaker et al., 2008). The ultimate aim of intervention for TBI is to increase an individual's independence with activities of daily living, including social interactions. Another main goal of TBI rehabilitation is to increase self-awareness and psychosocial skills (coping, anxiety, mood, self-esteem, and self-concept). Treatment approaches may change over the course of the recovery process to match the patient's progress and remaining difficulties. For example, treatment may commence while the individual is still in a coma, with the SLP focusing on providing caregiver education while also monitoring the patient's sensory responses (ASHA, n.d., www.ASHA.org/public/speech/disorders/tbi/). Treatment in the acute care setting also may include reestablishing cognitive skills such as attention which underlie the rehabilitation process.

The selected therapy approach should address the individual's primary presenting deficit(s) in the areas of cognition, communication, and behavior. Individual sessions are beneficial in the initial stages of therapy to establish cognitive and communicative targets (e.g., augmentative communication systems, conversational topic maintenance skills) in a structured setting. Then, group treatment provides opportunities for clients to practice targeted skills within a larger setting and facilitates social support during the rehabilitation process.

Key Elements of Effective Treatments. Various rehabilitation approaches have been reported in the literature. These generally focus on improving executive function skills—for example, Metacognitive Instruction Strategy (O'Neil-Pirozzi, 2011; Solhberg, Ehlardt, & Kennedy, 2005). An additional focus of rehabilitation protocols includes social interaction skills—for example, Social Problem-Solving (Rath, Simon, Langenbahn, Sherr, & Diller, 2003) and Group Interactive Structured Treatment, or GIST (Braden et al., 2010; Hawley &

Newman, 2010). Regardless of the specific approach, there are several key elements that comprise effective programming (Cicerone et al., 2011; Turner-Stokes, Nair, Sedki, Disler, & Wade, 2011):

- Rehabilitation is person-centered and matched to individual needs, strengths, and capacities.
- Treatment addresses cognitive, social, emotional, and functional aspects of communication simultaneously rather than sequentially.
- Intervention encompasses both micro- and macro-level deficits. Although it is important to remediate cognitive deficits, focus is simultaneously placed on the client's real-world circumstances.
- A coordinated interdisciplinary team approach is important for effective treatment, especially for individuals with moderate to severe injuries.
- Intervention for TBI incorporates a strong focus on the role of the family in communicative interactions.
- Programming identifies realistic communication goals for the patient and family. Optimizing/maximizing skills is the primary aim rather than restoring pre-injury levels of function.

Helpful Hints

1. Organizations, such as the Brain Trauma Foundation and the Brain Injury Association of America, were established to provide educational information and other resources for individuals with TBI and their caregivers. In addition to providing information, BrainLine has several resources, such as a question-and-answer page that presents information from the perspective of the individual with TBI.

2. Apps are available, such as TBI resource and mTBI pocket guide that provide education and resources on treatment strategies for TBI.

3. In addition to cognitive-communication deficits, individuals with TBI may also suffer hearing loss. Thus, the recommendations given for patients with hearing loss (e.g., reduce background noise when possible, face the communicative partner) may be beneficial in facilitating communication skills for individuals with TBI.

4. Certain medications for symptoms related to traumatic injury (e.g., pain medications) can have an adverse impact on cognitive-communication skills.

5. External memory aids (e.g., calendars, planners) assist individuals in recalling information as well as in maintaining connections to current events.

6. Telehealth services, such as through video conferencing, promote collaboration among team members throughout the rehabilitation process. SLPs can utilize this technology to assist clients in their transition back into their communities.

7. Augmentative and alternative communication (AAC) devices can be incorporated into therapy to support expressive language skills. In cases of severe impairment, SLPs may identify AAC strategies as a primary mode of communication.

CONCLUSION

This section has presented basic information, protocols, and procedures for TBI at an introductory level. This material is intended only as a starting point in the reader's clinical education and training. For more in-depth coverage of these areas, the following readings are recommended:

Coelho, C., Ylvisaker, M., & Turkstra, L. (2005). Nonstandardized assessment approaches for individuals with traumatic brain injuries. *Seminars in Speech & Language, 26*, 223–241.

Koehler, R., Wilhelm, E., & Shoulson, I. (2011). *Cognitive rehabilitation therapy for traumatic brain injury: Evaluating the evidence.* Washington, DC: The National Academies Press.

Kutzleb, J. A. (2009). *Evidence-based clinical management of traumatic brain injury patients: A collaborative approach.* Ann Arbor, MI: ProQuest, UMI Dissertation Publishing.

McDonald, S., Togher, L., & Code, C. (Eds.). (2013). *Social and communication disorders following traumatic brain injury* (2nd ed.). New York, NY: Psychology Press.

ADDITIONAL RESOURCES

Traumatic Brain Injury
LinguiSystems
3100 Fourth Avenue
East Moline, IL 61244-9700
Phone: 800-776-4332
Fax: 800-577-4555
Web site: http://www.linguisystems.com

CARDS Cognition, Attention, and Recall Drill Set
Set of playing cards with different games and activities that are designed to target specific cognitive skills. There are individual card sets for Memory and for Attention.

Results of Adults Cognition
A workbook with lessons that target the following cognitive skills: memory, problem solving, reasoning, and planning. Designed for individuals 15 years of age and older.

Workbook of Activities for Language and Cognition (WALC)
A series of workbooks that provide lessons to target deficits in language and cognition. Each workbook has its own focus, with activities designed to provide practice in specific language and cognitive skills. Several workbooks will be described in greater detail below.

WALC 2 Cognitive Rehab
This workbook is also available in Spanish. It contains 300 pages of exercises targeting the following cognitive skills: attention (e.g., word search, crossword puzzles), memory (e.g., word retrieval tasks), sequential thought (e.g., ordering steps of activities of daily living), and reasoning (e.g., identifying opposites, completing analogies).

WALC 5 Neurological Rehab

This workbook contains lessons organized by cognitive skill as well as ideas for extending these activities for further practice. Topics include orientation, memory, organization, verbal problem solving, abstract reasoning, and writing. The activities are designed to be functional to promote carryover beyond the therapy setting.

WALC 10 Memory

This workbook helps clients to identify memory strategies that best work for them and then provides practice using these memory strategies in various contexts.

WALC 11 Language for Home Activities

This workbook contains functional lessons to help increase client functioning in their homes and daily lives. The emphasis on home and daily living is meant to increase client participation and motivation to participate in rehabilitation.

APPENDIX 7-A

SUGGESTIONS FOR ENHANCING VERBAL INTERACTION WITH A FAMILY MEMBER WITH APHASIA

- Establish eye contact before you begin speaking.

- Speak slowly and with normal inflection at a natural loudness level.

- Keep messages relatively short and to the point.

- Combine speech with gestures, facial expressions, and other nonverbal communication to clarify the meaning of your messages.

- Pause frequently and check to make sure that you are being understood (e.g., ask yes/no questions such as "Are you following me?"; "Is that clear?").

- Be sure that paper and pencil are readily accessible to communicate your message, if needed.

- Avoid abrupt or rapid changes in topic or speakers.

- Give ample time for the aphasic family member to respond to your message.

- Indicate when you do not understand a message rather than pretending you do.

SOURCE: Adapted from Holland, A. (1995). *Current realities of aphasia rehabilitation: Time constraints, documentation demands, and functional outcomes.* Paper presented at Mid-America Rehabilitation Hospital, Overland Park, KS.

APPENDIX 7-B

GUIDELINES FOR CONVERSATIONAL COACHING

1. SCRIPTWRITING

- Scripts should be brief and written at the upper limits of a client's communicative range.
- Scripts should be written to highlight specific communicative behaviors that the clinician wishes to target. For example, if a client is learning to use synonyms as a compensatory strategy for word-retrieval difficulties, the script should contain words that have many alternate lexical forms (e.g., *car: automobile, SUV, convertible, vehicle, minivan*).
- Scripts should be written in a conversational style.
- Scripts should be written in short utterances to promote successful expression and listener comprehension.

2. LEVELS OF DIFFICULTY

- Communication of shared information with a familiar listener
- Communication of new information with a familiar listener
- Communication of shared information with an unfamiliar listener
- Communication of new information with an unfamiliar listener

3. ADVANTAGES

- Simulates a conversational interaction in a highly structured setting
- Targets both speaker and listener communication behaviors in the same activity
- Permits the modification of both conversational content and communicative strategies
- Permits the observation of client in the role of conversational partner

---

SOURCE: Holland, A. (1995). *Current realities of aphasia rehabilitation: Time constraints, documentation demands, and functional outcomes.* Paper presented at Mid-America Rehabilitation Hospital, Overland Park, KS.

CHAPTER 8

Dysarthria is a speech impairment that involves an impaired ability to execute the motor movements necessary for speech production. Apraxia is also a speech-motor impairment but involves a deficit in the planning and sequencing of movement. The term dysphagia refers to difficulty at any stage of the swallowing process. Discussion of this topic is included in this chapter because it is a frequent co-occurring impairment with speech-motor disorders such as dysarthria and apraxia. These deficits may occur alone or coexist in the same individual. There is a lack of consensus concerning many issues related to each of these disorders, including basic terminology. To minimize confusion, the technical vocabulary used in this chapter was selected for its common usage and clarity.

TREATMENT FOR MOTOR-SPEECH DISORDERS

The optimal goal of therapy for motor-speech disorders is to improve intelligibility within the limits of a client's neurological impairment. Articulation and prosody interact to exert a powerful influence on speech intelligibility. For this reason, therapy designed to improve intelligibility focuses primarily on the modification of these two parameters. Intervention tasks in this paradigm are programmed to progress along a continuum of difficulty from simple automatic responses (e.g., counting from 1 to 10) to more volitional and complex behaviors (e.g., responding to a question such as "What did you do last evening?"). Each client's unique characteristics will determine the most appropriate starting point along this continuum. In general, it is recommended that treatment be initiated as soon as possible to discourage a client's tendency to develop undesirable compensatory speech behaviors (e.g., pharyngeal fricatives).

The concept of drill is fundamental to any therapy program that seeks to directly modify motor-speech behaviors in any of the communication subsystems (respiration, resonance, phonation, articulation, prosody). Because speech is a complex motor skill, intense repetitive practice is more successful in changing this behavior than a therapy approach that relies on cognitive learning (e.g., explanation, modeling). Drill activities are most effective when a single presentation of a stimulus is followed by multiple productions of the target response by the client. Re-presenting the stimulus to elicit each production breaks the cycle of the motor-learning chain (Darley, Aronson, & Brown, 1975; Guadagnoli & Lee, 2004).

In some cases, improved speech intelligibility may not be a realistic goal. Certain neurologic conditions such as Parkinson's disease and multiple sclerosis are progressive and require that the treatment be aimed at slowing down the gradual deterioration of a client's speech. Sometimes, the dysarthria is so severe or the disease process is so rapidly degenerative that speech cannot be the primary mode of communication. With these clients, the main goal of therapy is to provide a functional alternative method of conveying messages. This may include use of gestures, communication boards, or speech synthesizers.

The Dysarthrias

The dysarthrias represent a group of related motor-speech disorders characterized by impaired muscular control over the speech mechanism as a result of central or peripheral nervous system damage. Whereas **apraxia** is a deficit in the planning and sequencing of movement, **dysarthria** represents impaired ability to execute motor movement. Clients with either of these disorders will demonstrate inaccurate and/or labored performance on tasks that require rapid, repetitive movement of the articulators such as **diadochokinesis** (see Appendix 8-A for normative diadochokinetic rates).

The lack of neurological control with dysarthria can affect the motor-speech subsystems of respiration, phonation, resonance, articulation, and prosody. Unlike apraxia, the dysarthrias involve paralysis, weakness, decreased tone, or incoordination of the speech musculature. Muscles can be impaired with respect to range, direction, strength, endurance, speed, or timing. Dysarthria can be manifested as a paucity or an excess of any of these parameters (e.g., reduced range of motion versus involuntary or uninhibited movement). Dysarthria is a consequence of damage to the cortex, cerebellum, brainstem, or peripheral nervous system. Of particular significance are the cranial nerves, which consist of 12 pairs of neuron bundles emerging from the brainstem. See Table 8-1 for a list of the cranial nerves and their function. The major causes of dysarthrias include stroke, brain tumors, head trauma, toxins, and neuromuscular diseases, many of which are degenerative (e.g., Parkinson's, multiple sclerosis, myasthenia gravis). The degree of impairment secondary to dysarthria can range in severity from quite mild to devastatingly profound.

Impairment of the articulators (lips, tongue, mandible, velum) has a greater negative impact on speech intelligibility than do disruptions of the respiratory or laryngeal systems. In dysarthria, the primary contributors to reduced intelligibility are distorted or omitted consonants and vowels, prolonged phonemes, and erratic articulation performance (Rosenbek & LaPointe, 1985).

TABLE 8-1
Cranial Nerves

	Nerve	Function	Type
I	Olfactory	Smell, taste	Sensory
II	Optic	Vision	Sensory
III	Oculomotor	Eye, eyelid, and pupil movement	Motor
IV	Trochlear	Eye movement	Motor
V	Trigeminal	Jaw movement; sensation from jaw, face, and mouth	Mixed
VI	Abducens	Eye movement	Motor
VII	Facial	Facial movement; sensation from anterior tongue	Mixed
VIII	Acoustic (vestibulocochlear)	Balance; hearing	Sensory
IX	Glossopharyngeal	Pharyngeal and palatal movement; sensation from posterior tongue	Mixed
X	Vagus	Movement and sensation from larynx, pharynx, esophagus, and internal organs; branches into inferior and superior laryngeal nerves	Mixed
XI	Spinal accessory	Larynx, chest, shoulder, and neck movement	Motor
XII	Hypoglossal	Tongue movement	Motor

SOURCE: Adapted from Brookshire, R. H. (2007). An introduction to neurogenic communication disorders (7th ed.). St. Louis, MO: C.V. Mosby Co.; Duffy, J. R. (2012). Motor speech disorders: Substrates, differential diagnosis, and management (3rd ed.). St. Louis, MO: Elsevier Mosby.

Classification of the Dysarthrias. The most frequently cited classification system for the dysarthrias is based on the Mayo Clinic research studies conducted by Darley, Aronson, and Brown (1969a, 1969b, 1975). This work has resulted in the identification of the following seven major types of dysarthria, based on differential patterns of neurological impairment and associated speech characteristics: (1) flaccid, (2) spastic, (3) ataxic, (4) hypokinetic, (5) hyperkinetic, (6) mixed, and (7) unilateral upper motor neuron. Table 8-2 presents a comparative outline of the dysarthrias.

TABLE 8–2
Classification of the Dysarthrias

Type	Cause	Site of Lesion	Neuromuscular Status	Speech Characteristics
Flaccid	Bulbar palsy, myasthenia gravis	Lower motor neuron	Weakness, low muscle tone	Indistinct and labored articulation; hypernasality; breathy voice quality
Spastic	Pseudobulbar palsy	Upper motor neuron	Increased muscle tone; reduced range of motion, strength, and speed	Slow, imprecise articulation; hypernasality; strained, strangled, harsh voice quality; monotonous pitch and loudness; short phrasing
Ataxic	Cerebellar disorders	Cerebellum	Inaccurate range, timing, and direction; low muscle tone; reduced speed of movement	Excess and equal stress; irregular articulatory breakdown; slow, inaccurate articulation; rhythm disturbances; phoneme prolongations; some excess loudness
Hypokinetic	Parkinsonism	Extrapyramidal (substantia nigra)	Markedly reduced range and speed of movement; marked muscle rigidity; rest tremors	Monopitch and monoloudness; slow speaking rate with short rushes of speech; long, inappropriate pauses; articulation accuracy fluctuates greatly
Hyperkinetic				
Quick	Chorea, Tourette's syndrome, Huntington's chorea	Extrapyramidal	Rapid, jerky, uncontrolled tic movements	Imprecise articulation; variable rate and loudness; harsh voice; inappropriate pauses; abrupt grunts and barks
Slow	Athetosis, dystonia, dyskinesia	Extrapyramidal	Slow, twisting, writhing movements and postures; variable muscle tone	Irregular articulatory breakdown; monopitch and monoloudness; harsh voice quality

(continues)

TABLE 8–2 *(Continued)*

Type	Cause	Site of Lesion	Neuromuscular Status	Speech Characteristics
Hyperkinetic (continued)				
Tremor	Organic voice tremor, myoclonus	Extrapyramidal	Involuntary, rhythmic movements	Voice tremors with rhythmic phonation breaks; choked, strained voice quality
Mixed	Amyotrophic lateral sclerosis (ALS), multiple sclerosis (MS), Wilson's disease	Multiple motor systems	Muscular weakness; reduced range and speed of motion; some intention tremors	ALS: severely defective articulation; slow rate; noticeable hypernasality; harsh voice quality; marked prosodic disturbances. MS: harsh voice quality; inconsistent rate; inconsistent articulatory precision. Wilson's disease: similar to hypokinetic dysarthria without sudden bursts of speech
Unilateral upper motor neuron	Stroke	Posterior frontal lobe	Lower facial weakness; hemiparesis	Imprecise consonants; irregular articulatory breakdown; harsh voice

SOURCES: Adapted from Darley, F. L., Aronson, A. E., & Brown, J. R. (1975). Motor speech disorders. Philadelphia, PA: Saunders.; Rosenbek, J. C. & LaPointe, L. L. (1985). Treating apraxia of speech. In D. Johns (Ed.), Clinical management of neurogenic communicative disorders (pp. 97–152). Boston, MA: Little, Brown.; Dworkin, J. P. (1991). Motor speech disorders: A treatment guide. St. Louis, MO: Mosby–Year Book.; Freed, D. (2012). Motor speech disorders: Diagnosis and treatment (2nd ed.). Clifton Park, NY: Delmar, Cengage Learning.

No spontaneous recovery is associated with certain dysarthria etiologies, such as amytrophic lateral sclerosis (ALS), Parkinson's disease, and Huntington's chorea. However, some neuromuscular diseases, such as multiple sclerosis, do exhibit periods of remission in which symptoms abate. Prognosis for individuals with dysarthria is affected by many of the same variables that are associated with aphasia and apraxia recovery. In addition, there are two dysarthria-specific factors that significantly influence prognosis: (1) if the underlying neuropathology of the dysarthria involves a degenerative disease process, the prognosis for significant improvement is poor; and (2) the existence of a severe co-occurring aphasia will interfere with a client's ability to benefit from dysarthria therapy.

Treatment Efficacy/Evidence-Based Practice

Experimental and clinical evidence indicates that therapeutic intervention is generally effective for individuals with dysarthria. Yorkston (1996); Kent (2000); Spencer, Yorkton, and Duffy (2003); and Yorkston, Hakel, Beukelman, & Fager, (2007) published summaries of group-treatment studies, single-subject studies, and case profiles that offer the following conclusions regarding treatment efficacy with various types of dysarthria:

- Individuals with Parkinson's disease derive greater benefit from treatment that targets both respiratory (breath support for speech) and phonatory function (loudness) than treatment that focuses on respiratory function alone.

- Speech rate control results in improved sentence intelligibility but not phoneme intelligibility.

- The benefits of therapy for prosody impairment are difficult to determine at this time due to the paucity of information available.

- Various behavioral therapy approaches are effective for individuals with stroke or traumatic brain injury, including feedback of acoustic information, respiratory and speech rate control, and physiological strategies such as biofeedback and reaction times.

- Devices such as palatal lifts result in gains in muscle strength and speech intelligibility for individuals with stroke or traumatic brain injury.

- Further research is needed to determine which intervention approaches are best suited for various types of dysarthria. Treatment studies using randomized clinical trials are required to generate reliable and valid efficacy/outcome information.

- Advanced measurement techniques such as neuroimaging should be increasingly utilized in efficacy studies with larger patient populations.

Treatment for the Dysarthrias

The overall goal of dysarthria therapy is to improve intelligibility and, if possible, speech-motor control. Ultimately, goal setting is influenced by the type and degree of dysarthric impairment. For severely impaired individuals, establishing functional communication through the use of augmentative or alternative systems may be the focus of intervention. In contrast, the aim of therapy for clients with mild dysarthrias is to reestablish speech patterns that closely approximate normal production. Spencer et al. (2003) provide a flowchart to guide clinicians through the assessment and treatment of dysarthria, focusing on the impact of respiratory and phonatory impairments on speech production. The flowchart presents different treatment options and strategies for deficits in respiratory control, phonation, and overall coordination for speech. Even if nonspeech tasks or other supports (e.g., postural changes, prosthetic devices) are incorporated into treatment, the authors emphasize the inclusion of speech tasks for relevance and carryover of skills. If intervention results in progress, therapy may be continued on a follow-up nature, especially in cases of progressive disorders; if sufficient progress has not been made with regard to speech intelligibility and/or communicative effectiveness, the clinician may need to consider exploring augmentative and alternative communication (AAC) options.

Types of Treatment. As outlined in Table 8-2, there are several different types of dysarthria with distinctive speech symptoms. However, the basic issues and approaches to treatment are similar across the dysarthria classifications. In general, there are four basic approaches to dysarthria therapy:

1. *Behavioral:* This is the traditional approach, in which progressively more difficult activities and feedback are used to improve client performance on both nonspeech and speech tasks. This may include use of verbal reinforcement, metronome pacing, biofeedback, delayed auditory feedback, and pacing boards. Biofeedback involves electronic monitoring devices that are used to help a client gain some voluntary control over previously unconscious body functions such as respiration, nasality, and extraneous oral movements. **Delayed auditory feedback (DAF)** is a system in which a client's words are returned to him or her through headphones after an imposed electronic delay of a few milliseconds. **A pacing board**

(Helm, 1979) is a series of divided colored squares used to reduce speech rate by requiring a client to touch one square per syllable or word uttered.

2. *Prosthetic devices:* The use of an artificial device or appliance to replace the function of a missing or impaired part of the speech mechanism. The most common prosthesis used in the treatment of dysarthria is a palatal lift. This is a mechanical device that elevates the soft palate toward the posterior pharyngeal wall to decrease hypernasal resonance in clients with velopharyngeal incompetence (VPI).

3. *Medical and surgical procedures:* The use of drugs and/or surgical procedures to ameliorate deficiencies in the speech production system. A pharyngeal flap and phonosurgery are examples of surgical intervention approaches. **Pharyngeal flap surgery** joins soft tissue from the posterior pharyngeal wall to the soft palate to improve velopharyngeal closure during speech. This procedure is used primarily with hypernasal clients for whom behavioral therapy and prosthetic interventions have been unsuccessful. Three types of **phonosurgery** are associated with treatment for unilateral vocal fold paralysis or paresis: (a) Teflon® or Gelfoam® injection, in which material is injected into the compromised fold to increase its bulk; the additional mass shortens the distance that the healthy fold must travel across midline to make contact with the paralyzed fold; (b) repositioning of the impaired fold toward midline through surgical insertion of a plastic implant; and (c) reinnervation of the thyroarytenoid muscle through implantation of a nerve-muscle pedicle taken from an intact omohyoid muscle. (See Klein and Johns [2009] for a detailed discussion of phonosurgical procedures.)

Intervention for Parkinsonian-like disorders has included neurosurgical techniques such as **pallidotomy**, which involves surgical sectioning of the globus pallidus (a portion of the basal ganglia). This procedure is designed to reduce major movement abnormalities by releasing inhibition in the thalamic and brainstem centers. With respect to speech, this surgical procedure has shown some positive impact on the phonatory and articulatory characteristics of clients with hypokinetic dysarthria (Schulz, Greer, & Friedman, 2000; Schulz, Peterson, Sapienza, Greer, & Friedman, 1999).

Deep brain stimulation (DBS) is a surgical procedure used to treat a variety of disabling neurological symptoms—most commonly Parkinson's disease. DBS uses a surgically implanted, battery-operated device—similar to a heart pacemaker—to electrically stimulate the targeted areas in the brain that control movement. When newer, more promising treatments develop in the future, the DBS procedure can be reversed, allowing individuals to still pursue other treatments as they developed (National Institute of Neurological Disorders and Stroke, 2010).

4. *Augmentative/alternative devices:* Nonvocal modes of communication to supplement or replace speech. These may include communication boards, alphabet boards, gestural systems, computers, and speech synthesizers.

Dysarthria is an impairment that may affect all motor speech subsystems. Treatment of dysarthria is generally based on the hierarchical organization of these subsystems: respiration, phonation, resonance, articulation, and prosody. Following is a brief discussion of basic treatment programming for each of the subsystems.

Respiratory Subsystem. The main respiratory problem of clients with dysarthria is inefficient use of the breath stream for speech, rather than a reduction of vital capacity (total volume of air in the lungs). (*Note:* The normal rate of respiration is 16 breaths per minute.) The goal of intervention for this subsystem is to establish consistent, controlled exhalation of air to support speech production. Following is one basic treatment progression for behavioral training:

1. Establish a stable base for respiratory function through muscle relaxation and adjustments of body posture. For example, (a) progressive relaxation techniques (see Table 9-1 in the next chapter) can be used to decrease muscle stiffness; (b) a supine (lying face-up) position may facilitate loudness. (*Note:* Modifications of posture and seating should always be implemented in consultation with other health care professionals such as physical therapists, occupational therapists, or physicians.)

2. Decrease shallow inhalation and improve control of sustained exhalation by manipulating inspiratory and expiratory cycles in nonspeech breathing. For example, (a) ask the client to take a deep breath and hold it as long as possible while the clinician applies light counterpressure on the abdominal wall; (b) provide visual feedback of the client's expiratory pressure and duration through the use of devices such as manometers or oscilloscopes.

3. Further improve exhalation control by establishing adequate loudness and voice quality while producing speech of increasing length and duration (beginning with isolated phonemes and progressing gradually to longer segments). For example, (a) ask the client to produce and sustain a single phoneme (e.g., /s/) for as long as possible, gradually progress to consonant series (e.g., /s-s-s-s-s-s/) and add vowels and other consonants (e.g., /sa/, /sap/); (b) practice sound sequences with varying patterns of loudness, stress, and intonation, progressing systematically to the level of conversation.

Phonatory Subsystem. Individuals with dysarthria exhibit a wide range of phonatory abnormalities, which vary according to dysarthria type and underlying neurological damage. These problems can be classified into three main patterns of vocal fold movement: hyperadduction, hypoadduction, and incoordination. **Hyperadduction** refers to excessive laryngeal tension and overly forceful closure of the vocal folds, which produces a harsh or strained-strangled voice quality. **Hypoadduction** involves reduced laryngeal muscle tension and inadequate closure of the vocal folds, resulting in a breathy, hoarse voice quality with decreased loudness and pitch control. **Incoordination** can be defined as inconsistent fluctuations of vocal fold vibration cycles that can result in *aphonia* (no voice), asynchronous onset of exhalation and phonation, and inappropriate pitch and loudness breaks. In general, hyperadduction and incoordination of vocal fold movement have less overall impact on speech intelligibility than hypoadduction and are usually not the primary intervention targets for this subsystem.

The aim of intervention for hypoadduction is to achieve efficient vocal fold closure during speech. This goal may be accomplished through phonosurgical procedures or behavioral training. A behavioral training approach can proceed according to the following sequence:

1. Increase control of glottal closure through sustained breath holding. For example, instruct the client to take a deep breath and hold it for as long as possible with a closed-mouth posture.

2. Improve voluntary control of vocal fold abduction-adduction through physical maneuvers that elicit glottal closure (e.g., lifting, pushing, and pulling). For example, (a) instruct the client to assume a seated position, exhale slowly, and at each clinician signal, pull up as hard as possible on the sides of the seat while deliberately attempting to stop the exhalation; (b) introduce phonation by asking the client to produce /a/ at a comfortable loudness level on exhalation and employ the glottal closure maneuver described previously on each clinician signal.

3. Refine the client's control of vocal fold valving through the use of a continuum of speech activities. For example, (a) ask the client to use a physical maneuver to induce reflexive glottal closure (e.g., pull up on the seat) and, on clinician instruction, release glottal closure and produce an isolated vowel with a hard phonatory attack; (b) repeat this procedure with speech stimuli of increasing length and duration (e.g., syllable, word, phrase, sentence, conversation).

One specific technique that addresses both phonatory and respiratory dimensions is the Lee Silverman Voice Technique (LSVT; Fox, Morrison, Ramig, & Sapir, 2002; Fox, Ebersbach, Ramig, & Sapir, 2012; Ramig, Pawlas, & Countryman, 1995; Sapir, Ramig, & Fox, 2008). This intensive approach is designed to improve the perceptual characteristics of voice by targeting loudness. LSVT focuses on increasing phonatory effort, vocal fold adduction, and respiratory support. This 4-week daily program teaches clients to "think loud" in order to produce high-effort, loud phonation. Clients also continuously monitor their vocal loudness and effort. Tasks occur in the context of sustained vowel phonation and progress from reading simple texts to conversation. The overall focus of LSVT is not on the modification of specific speech patterns, but rather on amplifying speech loudness. Studies have found that increased vocal loudness can alter acoustic aspects of speech (e.g., increasing vowel duration, raising fundamental frequency) and these alterations have a positive impact on speech intelligibility (Mahler & Ramig, 2012; Tjaden & Wilding, 2011).

Resonance Subsystem. The two main symptoms of dysarthric impairment in this subsystem are hypernasality and accompanying nasal air emission due to impairment of the velopharyngeal musculature. The overall goal of intervention for resonance problems is to decrease hypernasality through the use of procedures designed to improve a client's ability to generate intraoral air pressure. Behavioral, prosthetic, and surgical approaches can be used to accomplish this goal. A behavioral regimen is most effective with clients who demonstrate mild resonance problems. Following is a basic behavioral treatment sequence:

1. Improve awareness of the degree of nasal resonance through the use of biofeedback devices. For example, instruct the client to produce single sustained vowels alternating between greater and lesser degrees of jaw opening, while using an instrument that measures and visually displays the differential amounts of nasal resonance.

2. Improve ability to generate intraoral air pressure during production of consonant-vowel (CV) syllables that contain initial plosives. For example, instruct the client to alternately produce pairs of CV syllables that differ in the nasality of the initial consonant (e.g., *me/be; no/go; my/pie*).

3. Further refine control of velopharyngeal function during connected speech using biofeedback information. For example, instruct the client to maintain the target range of resonance while producing speech of increasing length and complexity (i.e., isolated words, short phrases, sentences, conversational speech).

For clients with moderate to severe impairments that significantly impact speech intelligibility, a prosthetic or surgical approach may be recommended. A **palatal lift** is considered a reasonable treatment alternative under the following conditions: relatively isolated paresis or paralysis of the velum, lack of excessive spasticity or increased reflex activity in the velopharyngeal area, and adequate dentition to anchor the appliance. **Pharyngeal flap surgery** is generally instituted when behavioral and/or palatal lift approaches have been unsuccessful and when an adequate degree of lateral pharyngeal wall movement is available (see Dworkin [1991]; Freed [2012]; Klein & Johns [2009]; Mason [2013]; and Yorkston, Beukelman, and Bell [1988] for detailed discussions of these procedures). Prosthetic and surgical interventions usually do not result in the restoration of "normal" function. Improvements gained from a palatal lift or pharyngeal flap must be considered in relation to a client's comorbid impairments in other speech subsystems.

Articulatory Subsystem. The overriding aim of articulation therapy for clients with dysarthria is to achieve improved speech sound production within the constraints of the underlying neuromuscular impairment. Intervention for the dysarthrias is similar to traditional articulation therapy with respect to both programming and procedures. However, the neuromuscular involvement associated with dysarthria necessitates an additional emphasis on oral-motor training. The following strategies can be used to facilitate improved function in the articulation subsystem:

1. Oral-motor exercises to normalize muscle tone and increase strength and mobility of articulatory musculature (e.g., lip retraction and pursing, tongue elevation and depression, jaw opening and closing)

2. Phonetic placement through explanation, modeling, and tactile stimulation of correct positioning of the articulators (see Appendix 3-A and Dworkin [1991] for specific training activities)

3. Phonetic shaping that entails the use of intact articulatory movements associated with one phoneme (e.g., /t/ to shape a different phoneme, such as /n/)

4. Overarticulation of speech sounds through exaggeration of some characteristic feature of a specific phoneme (e.g., aspiration, stridency, voicing) or the exaggerated production of a particular consonant in medial or final word position (e.g., *hotel, happen, sock, mud*)

5. Negative practice through the use of minimal pair stimuli (e.g., *mat/pat, mob/mop, cook/took*)

6. Accented speech approaches such as the Accent-based Music Speech Protocol (AMSP; Kim & Jo, 2013) resulted in changes in all of the speech subsystems, including improvements in articulation. This approach requires clients to produce targeted phonemes in a variety of contrasting manners (e.g., while performing stretches, while hand-drumming and producing accented productions). The accented or exaggerated productions were found to increase voicing skills as well as to result in clearer oral motor movements and thus more defined speech productions.

The pattern of articulatory errors, and therefore the specific targets selected for treatment, will vary according to the type of dysarthria. One basic sequence that can be considered in the selection of articulation targets mirrors the order of phoneme acquisition with regard to place of articulation. Therapy may begin with vowels and progress in the following sequence: bilabials → labiodentals → linguadentals → lingua-alveolars → culminating with linguapalatals.

The following task hierarchy can be used to train identified phoneme targets (e.g., /b/; LaPointe & Katz, 2002):

Final position of VC syllables:	/ab/
Final position of CVC syllables:	/tab/
Medial position of VCV syllables:	/aba/
Initial position of CV syllables:	/ba/
Initial position of CVC syllables:	/bag/

Varying positions in multisyllabic words and short phrases

Varying positions in sentences and conversational speech

Some clients with dysarthria may experience extreme difficulty producing particular phonemes (e.g., those that require tongue tip elevation). In such cases, it may be necessary to begin articulation therapy at the isolated phoneme level and/or develop compensatory movements to produce adequate approximations of these speech sounds.

Prosody Subsystem. The speech of clients with dysarthria is often characterized by prosodic and suprasegmental (e.g., stress, pitch) disturbances. Common manifestations include monopitch, monoloudness, excessive and equal stress on each word, inappropriate phrasing and intonation contour patterns, and a tendency to attempt maintenance of premorbid speech rate even when no longer appropriate. (*Note:* The normal speaking rate for adults is 150 to 250 words per minute or 4.4 to 5.9 syllables per second [Goldman-Eisler, 1968]. See Table 8-3 for comparative data regarding normal speech rate.) The ultimate aim of intervention with any symptom in this subsystem is to increase a client's overall speech intelligibility. Following are basic intervention strategies for prosody problems:

1. Improve stress and intonation patterns through contrastive drills. This technique employs identical pairs of stimuli that change in emphasis or meaning as a result of differences solely in stress or intonation. Compound words, sentences, or longer units of connected language can be used. For example, "sun shine" versus "sunshine"; "Bill likes *baseball*" versus "*Bill* likes baseball"; or "Bill likes baseball" versus "Bill likes baseball?"

2. Reduce monopitch and monoloudness through the use of negative practice drills. In this procedure, a client is required to intentionally produce a target behavior using a habitual error pattern, thus highlighting the contrast between the habitual error and the desired response. For example, instruct the client to alternate between habitual and target productions of word pairs with respect to pitch or loudness (e.g., movie versus MOVIE). Stimuli can be systematically programmed to include more complex units of language. Negative practice drills can be used to highlight any aspect of prosody.

TABLE 8–3

Normal Speaking Rates for Adults and Children

Task	Average Speaking Rate	Study
Adults		
Uninterrupted discourse	220–240 words per min (wpm)	Weiner (1984)
Conversational speech	270 wpm 4.4–5.9 syllables per sec (sps)	Calvert & Silverman (1983) Goldman-Eisler (1961)
Oral reading	160–180 wpm 150–190 wpm	Calvert & Silverman (1983) Darley & Spriestersbach (1978)
Responses to questions	115–165 wpm 150–250 wpm	Andrews & Ingham (1971) Goldman-Eisler (1968)
Children		
Responses to questions	Age 3 years: 116–163 syllables per min (spm) 4 years: 117–183 spm 5 years: 109–183 spm	Pindzola, Jenkins, & Lokken (1989)
Conversational speech	1st grade: 125 wpm 5th grade: 142 wpm	Purcell & Runyan (1980)

NOTE: Discrepancies in speaking rates are due to variations in calculation methods (e.g., wpm versus spm) and task differences.

3. Modify speaking rate through manipulation of the number and duration of pauses rather than attempting to alter the articulatory movements required for speech sound production. This can be accomplished through the use of metronomes, pacing boards, DAF, or tapping. In each of these strategies, the client modifies his or her habitual speech rate by producing each syllable or word in unison with the imposed beat or tempo. Speech rate also can be modified by requiring the client to write the initial letter of each word uttered. In theory, modifications to speech rate, such as a reduction in rate, can promote greater speech intelligibility by providing the speaker with more time to focus on articulatory precision and by providing the listener with more time to process the utterance (Lansford, Liss, Caviness, & Utianski, 2011). However, reductions in speech rate can alter the acoustic signal of the utterance in a manner that negatively affects the intelligibility of the message (Tjaden & Wilding, 2011).

Example Profiles

Following are three profiles that characterize the speech disturbances exhibited by individuals with different types of dysarthria (flaccid, hypokinetic, and ataxic). These examples have been designed to illustrate the selection of intervention targets as well as specific therapy activities and materials. Most of the chosen activities can be implemented in either individual or group therapy settings.

Mr. Patel, a 75-year-old male, suffered a brainstem stroke 2 weeks ago. He presents with mild paresis of all limbs, intact receptive and expressive language skills, and a moderate flaccid dysarthria. Assessment of the speech musculature indicates reduced strength and range of motion of the velum, tongue, and lips. Laryngeal movement is judged to be less affected. Respiratory support for speech appears to be within normal limits as measured by his ability to adequately sustain the vowel /a/. Mr. Patel's speech output is characterized by marked hypernasality; breathy voice quality; and slowed, labored articulation. The prosodic features of Mr. Patel's speech are unremarkable. Overall speech intelligibility is rated as 50% to 65% when the context is unknown to the listener.

Selection of therapy targets. The subsystems to be targeted for therapy are resonance and articulation. The first two areas were selected because the degree of Mr. Patel's hypernasality and his slow, imprecise articulation contribute most significantly to a reduction in perceived speech intelligibility.

Sample Activities

Resonance

1. Employ a Nasometer, which is a computerized instrument that calculates and visually displays the ratio of nasal versus nasal + oral acoustic energy. (Consult the *Nasometer Instruction Manual,* Kay Elemetrics Corporation, Pine Brook, New Jersey.) Develop a list of 80 stimuli that include 20 CV, VC, CVC, and VCV syllables containing low or mid vowels and liquid consonants (e.g., CV: *yo* and *ro*; VC: *all* and *air*; CVC: *war, roll*; VCV: *olo* and *airo*). Set the threshold line on the Naso-meter to indicate an acceptable percentage of nasal resonance. Instruct the client to produce each syllable three times while closely watching the computer screen. Explain that the visual display of the client's valving behavior should consistently fall within the targeted range of resonance. The threshold line can be reduced in 5% steps as the client demonstrates increased mastery of velopharyngeal valving. If the client has difficulty achieving success at a particular percentage level, the threshold line can be raised 10%.

Articulatory

2. Instruct the client to elevate the tongue tip to the alveolar ridge and then raise the tongue tip outside the mouth beyond the upper lip. Provide a mirror for visual feedback. Repeat this elevation movement pattern three times and then pause. Continue the activity by gradually increasing the number of repetitions between each pause. To strengthen this lingual movement, use a tongue depressor to push against the tongue tip to provide resistance that the client must overcome during tongue elevation.

Prosody

3. Make a list of 25 sentences, 7 to 10 words in length, and type them on a sheet of paper. Double-space the sentences and leave large spaces between the words in each sentence. Sample sentences include the following:

> I really enjoyed my vacation last month.
>
> I don't know what you mean by that.
>
> The people are walking in the park.
>
> Sometimes I watch TV in the evening.
>
> Do you want spaghetti for dinner tonight?
>
> My family visited the museum in London last year.
>
> I saw your wife at the store yesterday.
>
> What time do you usually get home from work?
>
> I am sad to hear that you are not coming.
>
> I heard there is a big sale at the mall.

Take a piece of paper with the approximate dimensions of a 12-inch ruler and cut a slit in it that is the length and height of the longest word in the sentence set (e.g., *spaghetti* or *yesterday*). The clinician places the slit card over the first sentence and moves it slowly across the paper. Instruct the client to read each word aloud as it is revealed by the slit in the card. After each sentence is completed, remove the card and instruct the client to read the sentence again, maintaining the slowed speech rate of the first production.

Mrs. Fields, a 58-year-old female, presents with a moderate hypokinetic dysarthria that is secondary to Parkinson's disease. Her overall status (including speech musculature) is characterized by muscle rigidity, limited range of movement, and rest tremors (involuntary, rhythmic movements exhibited when muscles are at rest). Voice quality is breathy with monopitch and decreased loudness due to limited capacity and control of the respiratory musculature. Resonance is judged to be unaffected. Mrs. Fields's articulatory precision is mildly to moderately affected and is marked by short bursts of hurried speech separated by grammatically inappropriate and abrupt pauses. She demonstrates reduced prosody of speech. Her speech intelligibility is rated as moderately unintelligible, primarily as a result of vocal abnormalities with a more modest contribution from her articulation errors. Language abilities appear to be within normal limits.

Selection of therapy targets. The areas to be targeted are the respiratory, phonatory, and articulatory subsystems. These were selected according to the subsystem hierarchy. The first two were chosen based on Mrs. Fields's vocal symptoms of breathiness and reduced pitch and loudness. The third was targeted in an effort to increase her intelligibility to its maximum level. Respiration was selected as the initial focus of therapy because it serves as the foundation for all other speech subsystems.

Sample Activities

Respiratory

1. Instruct the client to inhale deeply and hold the breath as the clinician slowly counts to three. Tell the client to exhale slowly while producing rhythmic patterns of a voiceless fricative (e.g., /s/). Sound productions of long and short duration comprise the rhythmic patterns. Following are sample series:
   (_____ = long sound; __ = short sound).

   ___ ___ ___ ___ ___ ___

   ___ ___ ___ ___ ___ ___

   ___ ___ ___ ___ ___ ___ ___

   ___ ___ ___ ___ ___ ___

   ___ ___ ___ ___ ___

   Remind the client that each series must be produced on a single exhalation. This activity can be implemented with any rhythmic pattern and can be extended to gradually introduce additional voiceless fricatives such as /f/, /ʘ/, and /ʃ/.

Phonatory

2. Write the numbers 1 to 10 on 20 index cards. Highlight various combinations of numbers on each card by using bold print or type. Instruct the client to read the digit series on each card with increased loudness on the boldface numbers. Sit within 5 feet of the client and encourage her to project her voice without excessive muscular tension. Use the following series:

1	**2**	3	**4**	5	6	7	**8**	9	10
1	2	**3**	4	5	6	7	8	9	10
1	2	3	4	5	6	7	8	9	10
1	2	3	**4**	**5**	6	7	8	9	10
1	2	3	4	5	6	7	**8**	9	10

   Increase the level of difficulty of this activity by gradually expanding the distance between the client and clinician.

Articulatory

3. Identify the client's articulation errors that result from limited range and strength of the oral musculature. Develop compensatory phonetic placements that effect acceptable approximations of the target sounds. Examples include the following:

Error Sound	Compensatory Placement
/p, b/	Place upper teeth on lower lip and abruptly drop the lower jaw to produce the desired plosive air burst.
/m/	Touch upper teeth to lower lip and produce sound with nasal resonance.
/t, d, l, s, z, n/	Elevate tongue blade to touch alveolar ridge while maintaining tongue tip in lower position.

Mr. Seymour, a 45-year-old male, presents with a mild to moderate ataxic dysarthria as a result of a tumor that caused localized damage to the cerebellum. His current condition is marked by hypotonia, slow and jerky voluntary movements, and inaccurate direction of movement. Mr. Seymour's breath support for speech appears to be adequate. His voice quality, although slightly harsh and monotone, is judged to be within normal limits. Resonance is unremarkable. In spontaneous speech, Mr. Seymour exhibits transient articulatory breakdowns characterized by imprecise consonants and distorted vowels, prolongations of phonemes, and dysprosody of speech due to excessive and equal stress of syllables and words. Overall speech intelligibility is rated at approximately 65% to 75% when the context is unknown to the listener.

Selection of therapy targets. The areas to be targeted are articulation and prosody. These were selected because Mr. Seymour's reduced speech intelligibility is caused primarily by deficits in these two subsystems.

Sample Activities

Articulation

1. Develop three word lists for an intelligibility drill, each of which contains 10 CVC words that are similar except for a single phoneme. Sample word lists follow:

Paul	beer	ban
Ball	dear	pan
Call	fear	can
Mall	near	man
wall	cheer	ran
gall	tear	Dan
Fall	gear	tan
Tall	we're	wan
Hall	hear	Fan
doll	mere	Van

   Print each word on an index card and shuffle the cards so that the words are in random order. Instruct the client to select a card from the deck, keeping it out of the clinician's visual field, and read it aloud. The clinician is unaware of the specific word being produced and must guess the identity of the utterance based solely on the client's intelligibility. The client indicates the accuracy of the clinician's guess. If the clinician's first guess is incorrect, the client repeats the target word once. If the clinician's second guess is erroneous, the clinician reads the index card and models the correct production of the word. The client imitates this model five times, returns the index card to the pile, and draws another card.

Prosody

2. Develop a set of 25 identical sentence pairs that contain at least a subject, verb, and object. Write each pair on a separate index card and underline or boldface a different word in each sentence. Explain that this activity focuses on the ways in which changes in prosody affect sentence meaning. Further explain that the clinician will ask a stimulus question that the client must answer by reading aloud the prosodically appropriate sentence from a corresponding index card. Instruct the client to choose one index card, listen to the stimulus question, and read aloud the correct version, using exaggerated intonation to highlight the boldface word. Examples of pairs of stimulus questions and response sentences include the following:

Question	*Response*
What did you open?	I opened the **door**.
What did you do?	I **opened** the door.
Did she read the email?	She **wrote** the email.
Who wrote the email?	**She** wrote the email.
Whose car is John driving tomorrow?	John is driving **my** car tomorrow.
Is Phil driving your car tomorrow?	**John** is driving my car tomorrow.
What dance is Sadie doing?	Sadie is dancing the **tango** with Mel.
Who is she dancing with?	Sadie is dancing the tango with **Mel**.
Does Tom call Judy often?	Tom **always** calls Judy on her birthday.
When does Tom call Judy?	Tom always calls Judy on her **birthday**.

Prosody

3. Gather several reading passages and highlight the syllables and words that receive primary stress. (*Note:* Stress patterns may vary according to regional dialect.) Instruct the client to read each passage aloud while concentrating on stress, rhythm, and intonation. Explain that this can be achieved by *strongly* emphasizing the boldface portions. Examples of reading materials include the following:

The Little Girl and the Wolf

(From *The Thurber Carnival* by James Thurber, 1945)

One after**noon** a big **wolf** wait**ed** in a **dark for**est for a **li**ttle **girl** to come a**long carry**ing a **bas**ket of **food** to her **grand**mother. **Fin**ally a **li**ttle **girl** **did** come a**long** and **she** was **carry**ing a **bas**ket of **food**. "Are you **carry**ing that **bas**ket to your **grand**mother?" **asked** the **wolf**. The **li**ttle **girl** said **yes**, she **was**. So the **wolf asked** her **where** her **grand**mother **lived** and the **li**ttle **girl told** him and he **dis**appeared into the **wood**.

When the **li**ttle **girl** o**pened** the **door** of her **grand**mother's **house** she **saw** that there was **some**body in **bed** with a **night**cap and **night**gown on. She had a**pproached** no **near**er than **twen**ty-five **feet** from the **bed** when she **saw** that it was **not** her **grand**mother but the **wolf**, for **even** in a **night**cap a **wolf** does **not** look any **more** like your **grand**mother than the **M-G-M li**on looks like Calvin Coolidge. So the little girl took an automatic out of her basket and shot the wolf dead.

Moral: It is not as easy to fool little girls nowadays as it used to be.

Oh When I Was . . .

(From *A Shropshire Lad* by A. E. Housman)

Oh when I was in love with you,

Then I was clean and brave,

And miles around the wonder grew,

How well did I behave.

And now the fancy passes by,

And nothing will remain,

And miles around they'll say that I

Am quite myself again.

Helpful Hints

1. It is important to avoid the tendency to simply instruct a client to slow down, speak up, or try harder. Explicit and intensive drills are required to successfully modify the prosodic features of a client's speech.

2. Verbal instructions for therapy activities may have to be simplified for clients who present with language deficits due to a concomitant aphasia.

3. Mirrors, audiorecordings, and videorecordings are useful adjuncts for developing a client's self-monitoring skills for speech production.

4. When working with adults, it is extremely important to explain why a given task is being implemented rather than merely describing how the task should be performed.

5. Clinicians should be aware that a client's reluctance to perform speech tasks may be related to fears about cosmetic changes (e.g., facial asymmetry, drooling) resulting from oral-facial sensory deficits.

6. Family education is an integral part of therapy programming for clients with dysarthria. For useful handouts about the nature of dysarthria and tips for effective communication strategies, see Yorkston, Miller, and Strand (2004) and Tanner (2008).

7. Given the recent advances in technologically based therapy, clinicians are encouraged to stay abreast of these new approaches.

Apraxia of Speech

Apraxia is an inability to plan and execute volitional motor movements due to central nervous system damage despite intact muscle strength and coordination. This deficit can affect any system that requires purposeful sequences of muscle movement. In a **limb apraxia**, voluntary movements of the extremities are affected in gestures such as waving good-bye or making a fist on command. An **oral apraxia** involves difficulty with nonspeech movements of the oral mechanism such as tongue protrusion and lip pursing on command.

Apraxia of speech (AOS; or verbal apraxia) is a neurologically based articulation disorder characterized by difficulty in positioning speech muscles and sequencing muscle movements for the voluntary production of speech. This disorder is not associated with weakness, slowness, or incoordination of these muscles during automatic and reflexive acts (McNeil, Robin, & Schmidt, 1997). Verbal apraxia is a motor speech disorder; therefore, language comprehension and the grammatical system are not affected. However, it should be noted that apraxia frequently co-occurs with aphasia. It is also important to note that the term apraxia of speech is distinct from the motor speech disorder childhood apraxia of speech (CAS). (For information on CAS, see Chapter 7.) Apraxia results from a lesion in the left frontal lobe near Broca's area. The main causes of apraxia are quite similar to those associated with aphasia and include cerebrovascular accident (CVA), trauma, tumors, and disease processes such as Alzheimer's.

Severity of apraxia ranges along a continuum from very subtle articulatory errors to completely unintelligible speech. At the most extreme level of impairment, an individual may be unable to initiate phonation volitionally. Following are the most significant characteristics of verbal apraxia (Croot, 2002; Duffy, 2012; Wertz, LaPointe, & Rosenbek, 1991):

- Highly unpredictable and inconsistent errors are made, even on repeated attempts at the same word. For example, an individual with apraxia may produce the following sequence in an attempt to produce the word *escalator*: escat, lator, scalator, lescatator, lescator, elescator.

- Substitutions and transpositions are the most frequent types of speech production errors, but omissions and distortions are also common.

- Complex consonant blends are often substituted for simpler phonemes (e.g., "sirondo" for *tornado*).

- There is difficulty initiating speech as evidenced by frequent stops, restarts, long pauses and hesitations, and repetition of initial sounds and syllables.

- Articulatory accuracy deteriorates as word length increases.

- There are visible and audible groping behaviors in which the speaker struggles to achieve appropriate placement of the articulators through trial and error.

- Automatic speech generally contains fewer articulatory errors than purposeful productions. For example, rote recitation of the months of the year may be relatively error-free (i.e., January, February, March . . .), whereas meaningful production of any of these words is likely to include numerous articulation errors (e.g., In response to the clinician question, "When are you going to visit your daughter?" the client says, "Ferry . . . ferrary . . . fruary . . . feboary").

- Client may be aware of the articulation errors but is unable to correct them on subsequent attempts.

- Prosody of speech is atypical with respect to rhythm, word stress, and intonational contour.

- Speech rate is slowed.

As discussed in the previous chapter, a period of spontaneous recovery follows the initial neurological insult. This period may continue for up to 6 months, with the most significant improvement occurring during the first 8 weeks. The prognosis is determined by many of the same factors that affect recovery from aphasia, including size, location, and etiology

TABLE 8–4

Differential Characteristics of Apraxia and Dysarthria

Apraxia	Dysarthria
Articulation is better in involuntary/automatic speech; periods of error-free speech may exist.	Automatic and voluntary speech are similarly impaired; there are no periods of error-free speech.
Errors are unpredictable and highly inconsistent.	Errors are predictable and highly consistent.
Substitution and transposition errors predominate.	Distortion and omission errors predominate.
There is significant difficulty with the initiation of speech, evidenced by hesitations, pauses, restarts, and repetitions.	Initiation of speech is usually not affected.
Visible and audible groping postures of the articulators are evident.	There are no visible or audible groping postures of the articulators.
Deficits occur primarily in articulation and prosody.	All speech processes are involved, including respiration, phonation, articulation, prosody, and resonance.

SOURCE: Adapted from Wertz, R. T., LaPointe, L. L., & Rosenbek, J. C. (1991). Apraxia of speech in adults: The disorder and its management. San Diego, CA: Singular.; LaPointe, L. L., & Katz, R. C. (2002). Neurogenic disorders of speech. In G. H. Shames & N. B. Anderson (Eds.), Human communication disorders (6th ed., pp. 472–509). Boston, MA: Allyn & Bacon.; Duffy, J.R. (2013). Motor speech disorders: Substrates, differential diagnosis, and management. St. Louis, MO: Elseiver Mosby.

of lesion, age at onset, and overall health of the client. However, there are certain apraxia-specific indicators that are associated with a less favorable prognosis. These include (1) presence of an accompanying oral apraxia, particularly lasting more than 2 months, and (2) the severity and duration of an accompanying aphasia.

Although apraxia and dysarthria are both motor-speech disorders, their symptomologies are considerably different. Table 8-4 presents the differentiating characteristics of these disorders.

Treatment Efficacy/Evidence-Based Practice

Few studies have been conducted that directly address either efficacy or outcome issues in apraxia of speech. Van Heugten, Dekker, Deelman, Stehmann-Saris, and Kinebanian, (2000) investigated the effect of a functional treatment program with 33 stroke patients with apraxia and 36 stroke patients without apraxia. Their results suggest that traditional prognostic variables such as cognitive impairment, motor impairment, and advanced age were not related to treatment outcome. McNeil et al. (2010) conducted a study with two individuals with acquired apraxia of speech to determine the effect of augmented feedback on treatment outcomes. Feedback from clinicians as well as visual, biofeedback sources were both found to improve performance on speech tasks. Ballard's (2001) critical review of the existing literature suggests that response generalization effects are slight, especially in the application of trained behaviors to novel situations. Wambaugh, Duffy, McNeil, Robin, and Rogers, (2006) conducted a treatment literature review, with the overall conclusion that individuals with apraxia of speech may show improvement in speech production even when the impairment is chronic. The strongest evidence was found for treatments that focus on the articulatory aspects of speech production. An updated systematic review was conducted by Mauszycki and Wambaugh (2011), citing studies that found evidence for using articulatory-kinematic and rate/rhythm control treatment approaches with AOS.

Treatment for Apraxia of Speech

The ultimate aim of intervention for apraxia of speech (heretofore referred to simply as apraxia) is to increase a client's voluntary control over the articulatory movements necessary for accurate speech production to the limits imposed by the neurological impairment. For clients with severe to profound apraxia, intelligible speech may not be a realistic goal. Therapy for these individuals should focus on developing augmentative or alternative means of communication. The Modified Diadochokinesis Test (MDT) is a psychometrically sound assessment tool for measuring treatment gains, although clinicians are advised implement informal measures, (e.g., conversational level speech) for a more holistic view of patient improvement (Hurkmans, Jonkers, Boonstra, Stewart, & Reinders-Messelink, 2012). Many traditional approaches to intervention for apraxia can be discussed from two basic perspectives: structure (how to teach) and function (what to teach). Information can be found in the following sections.

Structure. Intervention programs for apraxia can be structured in several different ways. The central feature of nearly all approaches is the use of drill; motor learning is dependent on repeated opportunities to practice desired movement patterns.

One well-known paradigm for structuring apraxia therapy is the eight-step task continuum developed by Wertz et al. (1991). This continuum incorporates Milisen's (1954a) concept of "integral stimulation," which emphasizes simultaneous input in multiple modalities, especially auditory and visual. This paradigm utilizes imitation as the primary teaching strategy and attempts to facilitate increased voluntary articulatory control through systematic, gradual fading of clinician cues. Following are the eight steps:

Step 1:	Clinician presents integral stimulation (i.e., "Watch me; listen to me"); clinician and client then produce target utterance in unison.
Step 2:	Clinician presents integral stimulation; and then clinician offers visual cue only (i.e., mouths each utterance without sound) while client simultaneously produces the target utterance aloud.
Step 3:	Clinician presents integral stimulation; and then client imitates target utterance independently.
Step 4:	Repeat Step 3 but require the client to produce target utterance several times in a row without any intervening clinician model.
Step 5:	Clinician presents written stimuli, which client reads aloud.
Step 6:	Clinician presents and then removes written stimuli; client attempts target utterance.
Step 7:	Clinician presents a question designed to elicit target utterance and client responds.
Step 8:	Clinician engages client in role-play situations to elicit target utterance. (This step is most appropriate for target behaviors at the word level and beyond.)

Content. The preceding section on structure presents guidelines for "how to teach," or structure a therapy program. This section focuses on "what to teach," or the content of an intervention program for apraxia. In 1975, Darley et al., recommended a basic treatment progression. This protocol was adapted for discussion in this chapter because of its simplicity and its suitability for almost any degree of apraxic impairment. The point in the progression at which therapy is initiated depends on an individual client's capabilities.

Phase I: Initiate Phonation
Instruct the client to:

- Produce a cough or sigh.
- Prolong exhalation and shift from a cough or sigh to phonation.
- Induce phonation through humming (or singing) in unison with clinician.
- Overlay a variety of mouth opening and tongue configurations to produce vowels and diphthongs.

Phase II: Increase Smoothness and Length of Speech
- Use automatic speech such as TV jingles, the Pledge of Allegiance, rotely memorized poems and songs, and everyday expressions such as "How are you?" or "I feel fine" to experience the feel of easily produced speech.
- Use highly familiar or automatic speech patterns to provide a base for establishing propositional vocabulary, for example, "salt and ___" or "roses are ___."

Phase III: Phonemic Drill
Individuals with apraxia exhibit the least amount of difficulty with vowels, glides, and nasal sounds; more difficulty with plosives; increased difficulty with fricatives and affricates; and the most difficulty with consonant clusters. This hierarchy of difficulty with respect to manner of production can guide the selection of therapy targets for drill work. Once a target phoneme has been identified, voluntary motor control can be increased using Darley et al.'s (1975) suggested 10-step therapy sequence.

Step 1:	Hum the phoneme in isolation: /nnnnn/.
Step 2:	Add a vowel to the consonant target and produce the syllable 20 times (e.g., /na/). Repeat this drill with other vowels.
Step 3:	Produce a series of five or six different CV syllable combinations: nu, na, ny, now, naw.
Step 4:	Produce reduplicative syllables first in isolation (nana, nana, nana; nini, nini, nini) and then in succession (nana, nini, nunu).
Step 5:	Add the target phoneme as the final consonant to form a CVC syllable: nan, nin, nown. As in Step 4, first practice in isolation and then in succession.
Step 6:	Produce the target phoneme in short words with simple phonetic environments: *new, nine, nap, nag, nod, nail, bin, bone, run, loan, dune.*

(continues)

Step 7:	Produce two-word phrases with the target phoneme in the initial position of both monosyllablic words: *not now, no news, near noon, nice night, north nook.*
Step 8:	Repeat Step 7 with target phoneme in the final position of words: *down town, dine in, main man, one gown, lean on.*
Step 9:	Produce two-word utterances in which the target phoneme is in the initial position of the first word and the final position of the second word: *knee pain, need ten, new phone, need loan.*
Step 10:	Produce multiword utterances with some polysyllabic words, gradually expanding them into sentences: *Natalie won the honor; Nan lives near Ned; Napoleon Bonaparte; nutmeg and cinnamon; north of Jefferson County.*

Once a client has mastered the production of several different target phonemes, introduce them in minimal word pairs to facilitate accurate articulatory transition from one target phoneme to another across word boundaries. Examples include *name-game, run-rut, banner-backer.*

Throughout phonemic drill training, encourage the client to anticipate upcoming phonemes in an utterance and plan or mentally rehearse appropriate articulatory postures. As the client's voluntary control over articulatory movements improves, foster more natural-sounding speech by increasing speech rate and highlighting other prosodic features.

Wambaugh et al. (2006) present an alternative perspective on categorization of treatment approaches for apraxia of speech: articulatory/kinematic, rate and/or rhythm, intersystemic/reorganization, and alternative/augmentative.

Articulatory/Kinematic

- Emphasizes regaining adequate points of articulation and sequencing of articulatory gestures
- Often focuses on improving spatial and temporal aspects of speech production
- Includes teaching strategies such as modeling and placement cues

Rate and/or Rhythm

- Focuses on modifying the temporal patterning of speech
- Emphasizes reduced rate of speech to provide additional time for motor planning
- May utilize metronomes, pacing boards, computers, and other devices

Intersystemic/Regorganization

- Utilizes intact modality (e.g., gestures, signing) to facilitate speech production

Alternative/Augmentative

- Utilizes nonspeech communication strategies (e.g., spelling, drawing, gestures, symbols, pictures, writing) to substitute for speech production on a temporary or permanent basis.

Two additional AOS treatment approaches that focus on content at the speech sound and/or phrase level are described next.

Sound Production Treatment (Wambaugh, Kalinyak-Fliszar, West, & Doyle, 1998; Wambaugh & Mauszycki, 2010; Wambaugh & Nessler, 2004)

- Studies have evaluated sound production treatment (SPT) with a range of AOS severities. Treatment targets are individualized based on a client's error patterns; minimal pairs are selected based on the speech sounds produced incorrectly during baseline measures.

- Speech sound errors are addressed according to a hierarchy of support provision.

- Feedback is given after every client production, with further supports provided only if errors persist.

- The SPT hierarchy progresses from minimal prompting to maximal prompting as follows:

  - verbal modeling of targets (say ball . . . tall); client imitation of targets

  - verbal modeling while pointing to letters corresponding to targets; client imitation

  - integral stimulation with error sound or target word (watch me, listen to me, and say it with me; say ball); client imitation

  - verbal modeling of the incorrect word in segments (say b . . . all); client imitation

  - verbal cues as to articulatory placement (start with your lips closed for the /b/) followed by verbal model; client imitation

- If the individual still has difficulty at the highest level of prompting, the next minimal pair is targeted and the cycle is repeated. This approach stresses the motor principles of blocked and random practice of targets through the use of repetitive articulation drills with varying speech targets.

Script Training (Youmans, Youmans, & Hancock, 2011)

- Although developed for people with aphasia, script training has been used with individuals with concomitant apraxia of speech to facilitate greater ease in producing phrase-level speech.

- Training principles remain the same when using script training with AOS.

- Strong emphasis is placed on providing feedback so that the individual does not learn incorrect speech patterns.

- Due to the nature of apraxia, the client's speech will continue to contain errors when using scripted phrases, although the frequency of error productions may be reduced.

- However, gains are expected in speaking confidence, ease, and fluidity.

Example Profiles. Following are two profiles that are representative of the speech characteristics of individuals with apraxia. These examples have been designed to illustrate the selection of intervention targets as well as specific therapy activities and materials. Most of the chosen activities can be implemented in either individual or group therapy settings.

Mrs. Elizondo, a 65-year-old female, exhibits a severe apraxia after surgery to remove a tumor localized in the left frontal lobe. She demonstrates no volitional speech but occasionally produces undifferentiated CV or VC syllables and some automatic utterances (e.g., "Oh my goodness"; "I don't know"). Mild to moderate oral and limb apraxia is present, with no evidence of an accompanying aphasia or hemiparesis. Currently, her sole means of communication is through writing.

Selection of therapy targets. Therapy will focus on ensuring the availability of an alternative mode of communication, the initiation of voluntary phonation, and the facilitation of propositional speech. An alternative system will be implemented to provide Mrs. Elizondo with an immediate means of communicating with others. The severity of her verbal apraxia dictates that treatment begin at the most basic level, which involves elicitation of volitional phonation. Because the only intelligible speech in her repertoire consists of sporadic automatic phrases, this type of utterance will be used to stimulate the production of propositional speech at the single-word level.

Sample Activities

Alternative Means of Communication

1. The prognosis for significant improvement in speech production is difficult to determine so early in the recovery process. Therefore, the clinician should provide Mrs. Elizondo with a functional and reliable way of communicating. Many forms of alternative communication systems are available, including picture boards, alphabet boards, electronic devices, and digitized speech. It is the clinician's responsibility to review the available options and select the method within the client's linguistic and motoric capabilities that is (a) most flexible, allowing for the expression of the broadest possible range of messages, and (b) generates messages that are most easily understood by listeners.

   Given Mrs. Elizondo's current status, writing is judged to be the optimal choice for a nonvocal communication system. This selection was based on the fact that her language skills are essentially unimpaired and that the limb apraxia does not significantly impede her ability to write. At this stage in Mrs. Elizondo's recovery, it is not known whether writing will serve as an interim method of communication or eventually become a true alternative to speech as her permanent, primary mode of communication.

Volitional Phonation

2. (Step 1 of Rosenbek's structural hierarchy and Phase I of the Darley et al. [1975] content hierarchy.) Explain that the clinician will model a vocal behavior (i.e., a cough or sigh) two times. For the first trial, instruct the client to watch and listen carefully. On the second trial, instruct the client to attempt the cough or sigh in unison with the clinician's production. Repeat this sequence until the client can

produce a cough on volition. Progress through the next three tasks in Phase I, using the same "integral stimulation-unison production" training paradigm. These tasks consist of (a) prolonging exhalation to transition from the cough or sigh to phonation, (b) extending phonation through humming, and (c) superimposing mouth opening and different tongue positions over the humming to produce vowels.

Propositional Speech

3. (Adaptation of Step 7 of Rosenbek's structural hierarchy and Phase II of the Darley et al. [1975] content hierarchy.) Develop a set of 25 familiar or high-probability phrases. Examples include the following:

> Salt and ___ (*pepper*)
>
> Cup of ___ (*coffee*)
>
> Knife and ___ (*fork*)
>
> Look before you ___ (*leap*)
>
> Birds of a ___ (*feather*)
>
> Shoes and ___ (*socks*)
>
> Turn over a new ___ (*leaf*)
>
> Paper and ___ (*pencil*)
>
> Peaches and ___ (*cream*)
>
> Bacon and ___ (*eggs*)
>
> Bread and ___ (*butter*)
>
> The early bird catches the ___ (*worm*)

Gather pictures that represent the missing word in each fill-in-the-blank phrase. Explain that the clinician will say a phrase aloud while presenting the corresponding picture. Instruct the client to listen carefully, look at the picture, and produce the target word as quickly as possible. If the client is unsuccessful in the first attempt, the clinician can provide additional cues by demonstrating the appropriate placement of the first phoneme or by modeling the first phoneme aloud.

Mr. Collins, a 58-year-old male, sustained a left frontal lobe CVA 1 year ago, which resulted in a moderate apraxia with an accompanying mild to moderate nonfluent (Broca's) aphasia. He presents with a mild right-sided weakness with no significant oral or limb apraxia. Mr. Collins demonstrates good language comprehension for relatively simple oral and written material. With respect to expression, his utterances are pragmatically appropriate and consist of short, effortful phrases marked by morphological and syntactic errors. Mr. Collins exhibits the ability to imitate verbal utterances; however, his performance deteriorates as utterance length and complexity increase. His speech is characterized by unpredictable articulation errors consisting mainly of sound substitutions and transpositions of plosives, fricatives, and affricates. These errors occur more frequently in multisyllabic utterances. Errors on nasal consonants are noted in connected speech. Speech melody is atypical with respect to stress and intonation; struggle behaviors to achieve accurate articulation placement were clearly visible. Overall, speech is rated as moderately unintelligible, particularly in unknown contexts. Mr. Collins recognizes the inadequacy of his communication skills and is frustrated by them.

Selection of therapy targets. The areas to be targeted are the /m/, /p/, and /s/ phonemes as well as the prosodic feature of stress. These sounds were selected according to the hierarchy of difficulty identified by Darley et al. (1975) based on their experience with apraxic individuals. Stress, particularly at the phrase level, was chosen as a means of increasing Mr. Collins's speech intelligibility.

Sample Activities

1. (Adapted from Steps 5 and 6 of Rosenbek's structural hierarchy and Step 9 of the Darley et al. [1975] phonemic drill sequence.) Develop a list of 25 two-word phrases in which /m/ is in the initial position of the first word and the final position of the second word. Select short words with simple phonetic environments. Write each phrase on an index card and place the pile face-down on the table. Examples include the following:

make time	meet him
my room	miss Tom
mail them	more gum
made ham	meal time
men came	moon beam

   Instruct the client to select the top card and read the phrase aloud. Remove the card and tell the client to repeat the same phrase three times. Following the last production, provide feedback such as "You did a nice job saying /m/ in 'make time'" to expose the client to a clearly articulated indirect model of the target sound. The difficulty of this activity can be increased by gradually incorporating polysyllabic words that contain the target sound into longer phrases and sentences.

2. (Step 4 of Rosenbek's structural hierarchy and Step 3 of the Darley et al. [1975] phonemic drill sequence.) Write the target phoneme in the center of a large index card or sheet of paper and surround it with four vowels or diphthongs (e.g., a, o, ɔ, ə). Arrange the vowels as follows, using traditional spelling rather than phonetic symbols.

$$\begin{array}{ccc} & \text{ah} & \\ & \uparrow & \\ \text{aw} \leftarrow & \text{p} & \rightarrow \text{o} \\ & \downarrow & \\ & \text{uh} & \end{array}$$

Explain to the client that this activity is designed to improve his or her ability to transition quickly from one syllable to another. Instruct the client to watch and listen (integral stimulation) as the clinician models CV syllables at a relatively rapid rate. This is accomplished by pairing the target consonant with each of the four vowels in a clockwise progression from ah to aw. Client imitates the clinician's model of the syllable series 10 times. This activity also can be used to provide intense drill work on all other target phonemes.

3. Create a set of 20 pairs of phrases or short sentences in which manipulations of stress and pause time alter meaning. Examples include the following:

The sky is falling.	This guy is falling.
An ice man.	A nice man.
A man eating shark.	A man-eating shark.
Oranges have a peel.	Oranges have appeal.
He's a gentle man.	He's a gentleman.
What a dark room!	What a darkroom!
I don't like cross words.	I don't like crosswords.

Each phrase/sentence is written on separate index cards, which are then shuffled and placed in a pile face-down on the table. Instruct the client to select one card, keeping it out of the clinician's view, and read it aloud using the appropriate stress pattern. The clinician guesses the utterance based on the client's prosody and coarticulation cues and writes it down on a blank index card. The two cards are then compared to determine whether the client successfully communicated the intended message. If the cards do not match, the clinician models both stress patterns. The client is asked to identify the target pattern and imitate it.

Helpful Hints

1. To avoid or minimize client confusion during the initial stages of phonemic drill training, the clinician should select successive sound targets that are maximally different from one another.

2. A client's success on imitation tasks is sometimes facilitated by the clinician's use of an exaggerated stress or intonation when modeling stimuli.

3. To facilitate the concept of errorless learning, clinicians can provide cuing and/or feedback as promptly as possible in order to promote relearning of correct speech patterns and to prevent acquiring error patterns.

4. A metronome is a particularly effective temporal cue for regulating the pace of a client's speech.

5. For some clients, a productive strategy for promoting speech initiation or output is to encourage them to pair a gesture with a word.

6. Melodic Intonation Therapy (MIT; Helm-Estabrooks & Albert, 2004) can be used successfully to promote speech output; the rhythmic nature of intoning a melody facilitates production for some clients with apraxia.

7. Counseling must frequently address the fact that other individuals may negatively judge a client's intellectual/language comprehension skills based on poor speech intelligibility.

8. Families may require considerable education regarding the nature of apraxia to ensure that the client's inconsistent speech errors are not misperceived as signs of laziness or lack of motivation.

CONCLUSION

This section has presented basic information, protocols, and procedures for dysarthria and AOS intervention at an introductory level. This material is intended only as a starting point in the reader's clinical education and training. For more in-depth coverage of these areas, the following readings are recommended.

Brookshire, R. H. (2007). *An introduction to neurogenic communication disorders* (7th ed.). St. Louis, MO: C.V. Mosby Co.

Duffy, J. R. (2012). *Motor speech disorders: Substrates, differential diagnosis, and management* (3rd ed.). St. Louis, MO: Elsevier Mosby.

Freed, D. (2012). *Motor speech disorders: Diagnosis and treatment* (2nd ed.). Clifton Park, NY: Delmar, Cengage Learning.

Miller, R. M., Strand, E. A., & Britton, D. (2013). *Management of speech and swallowing in degenerative diseases* (3rd ed.). Austin, TX: Pro-Ed.

Webb, W. G., & Adler, R. K. (2007). *Neurology for the speech-language pathologist* (5th ed.). New York, NY: Elsevier Health Science.

ADDITIONAL RESOURCES

Dysarthria and Apraxia of Speech
LinguiSystems
3100 Fourth Avenue
East Moline, IL 61244-9700
Phone: 800-776-4332
Fax: 800-577-4555
Email: linguisys@aol.com
Web site: http://www.linguisystems.com

The Source for Dysarthria
A comprehensive manual that includes information about dysarthria such as the different types, etiologies, evaluation and treatment planning options, and treatment objectives for respiration, phonation, resonance, articulation, and prosody. Also includes examples of documentation and sample reports.

The Source for Apraxia Therapy

A resource that combines a visual-auditory-kinesthetic approach to improve intelligibility in clients with mild, moderate, or severe apraxia. Divided into three sections, which focus on production of words and simple sentences, articulation, fluency, phrasing, and para-linguistic drills.

Pro-Ed
8700 Shoal Creek Boulevard
Austin, TX 78757-6897
Phone: 800-897-3202
Fax: 800-397-7633
Web site: http://www.proedinc.com

The Apraxia of Speech Stimulus Library

Includes a research-based manual, four boxed sets of stimulus cards, and reproducible data collection sheets. Uses high-interest words (depicted graphically or by pictures) and practical phrases to improve production of phonemes and phoneme sequences.

Dysarthria Treatment Manual

Imaginative treatment approach emphasizing self-monitoring and self-reliance. Its practical exercises target oral-motor skills, resonance, relaxation, respiration, prosody, and intelligibility. It offers client and family handouts, a simple communication board, and home practice activities.

Dysarthria Rehabilitation Program, 2nd Edition

For adolescents and adults. Exercises focus on improvement of speech intelligibility through exaggeration of articulatory movements, reduction of speech rate via vowel prolongation, and improvement of speech prosody. Includes 60 pictures, words, and reproducible data-collection and tracking forms for use with multiple clients.

Apps
Lingraphica
103 Carnegie Center
Suite 204
Princeton, NJ 08540
Phone: 888-274-2742
Fax: 609-275-1311
Web site: www.aphasia.com

Lingraphica offers several video apps that provide visual supports of oral motor movements needed to produce speech, from the phoneme level up to words. The Phonemes App and Consonant Blends App focus on individual speech sounds, whereas the Days, Months, Dates App and Letter, Colors, Numbers app provide visuals of the oral motor movements needed to produce words in those categories. There is also a Common Phrases App of functional phrases for individuals to practice connected speech.

SpeakinMotion
Web site: www.speakinmotion.com

VAST Songs 1-Intro
This app is based on the principles of utilizing music to stimulate speech production. It provides supports in multiple modalities, including video visuals, written lyrics, and audio for the user to follow. The tempo can be adjusted as individuals practice songs and conversational phrases and work towards more fluent speech.

Tactus Therapy Solutions
Web site: http://tactustherapy.com

Speech Flip Book
This app enables you to create monosyllabic target words by selecting the speech sounds you want to target in each syllable position. Therapy can be programmed to increase the complexity of syllables from CV or VC up to consonant clusters. It has a recording feature that enables users to practice the targets and then view their performance.

DYSPHAGIA

Dysphagia is a swallowing disorder characterized by difficulty moving food from mouth to stomach, including all the behavioral and physiological aspects of the process (Becker et al., 2011; Clark et al. 2009; Groher & Crary, 2009). Dysphagia occurs in all age groups and may result from a variety of structural or physiological abnormalities. The onset of dysphagia can be acute (e.g., resulting from a stroke) or characterized by gradual deterioration (e.g., resulting from a progressive disease process such as amyotrophic lateral sclerosis). Difficulties can occur in any of the four stages of the normal swallow, which correspond to the approximate location of the food bolus as it moves through the system: (1) preparatory (chewing), (2) oral (back of mouth), (3) pharyngeal (throat), and (4) esophageal (toward stomach). See Edgar (2003) for an extensive review of research on swallowing in normal adults. Intervention designed for preparatory and/or oral stage problems is generally referred to as "feeding" techniques, whereas pharyngeal stage intervention is described as "swallowing" therapy. The role of a speech-language pathologist (SLP) in treatment is generally limited to difficulties in the first three stages of swallowing; problems in the esophageal stage are usually managed medically or surgically.

SLPs have an important role to play in the treatment of swallowing and feeding disorders. Their education and clinical background in the anatomy and physiology of respiration, swallowing, and speech prepare them to perform a variety of functions including:

- Developing and implementing treatment plans for individuals with dysphagia
- Providing education and counseling to patients and their families
- Serving as members of a multidisciplinary/interdisciplinary management team
- Advocating for services for individuals with dysphagia
- Advancing the knowledge base on swallowing and feeding disorders through research activities

Treatment for Dysphagia

The two paramount goals of dysphagia management are: (1) prevention of aspiration, malnutrition, and dehydration; and (2) re-establishment of oral intake of food and liquid. Traditionally, these aims are targeted using approaches such as retraining muscle function, teaching new sequences of muscle activity, or stimulating increased sensory input (Logemann, 1998). A more recent approach, the application of neuromuscular electrical stimulation (NMES) to head and neck muscles, is being currently explored, typically as an adjunct to traditional treatment approaches (Langdon & Blacker, 2010). Clinical decision making is often carried out through a multidisciplinary team, which may include a physician, dietitian, radiologist, or occupational therapist.

Intervention for feeding and swallowing disorders can be categorized into two main approaches: *compensatory strategies* or *therapy strategies*. The goal for compensatory strategies is to eliminate or reduce abnormal symptoms without changing the underlying physiology of the client's swallow. This approach requires minimal cognitive or physical effort from the client and largely involves manipulation of variables such as head postures and bolus presentations.

The goal of therapy strategies is to effect change in the client's swallow pattern. This approach generally focuses on range of motion and coordination/timing of movement. In addition to targeting the mechanical aspects of the swallow, clinicians also consider neurologic principles to determine ways to improve swallowing (e.g., techniques to stimulate nerves or the provision of sensory stimulants; Miller, 2008). Clients must be able to follow instructions and have the capacity to practice exercises independently. Intervention may be implemented indirectly with just saliva or directly with food/liquid. This decision should be made solely on the basis of aspiration findings from radiographic studies (Logemann, 1998).

Logemann (2008) and Leonard and Kendall (2008) provide reviews of the current treatment practices for dysphagia with the caveat that more research is needed on implementation variables such as patient populations for each approach and treatment time durations. A discussion of the treatment approaches follows. Please see Appendix D at the end of the book for a schematic of the vocal tract structures discussed in this section.

Postural Techniques

- Chin down: the downward placement of the chin decreases both the distance between the tongue base and the pharyngeal wall and the airway opening. This postural technique is used with patients who have dysphagia due to a tongue base disorder, a pharyngeal phase delay, or compromised airway protection.

- Chin elevated: this posture uses gravity to move the bolus from an elevated position downward through the oral cavity when sufficient lingual pressure is not present. This posture poses an aspiration risk if the patient has concomitant pharyngeal phase delays. It is typically used with patients whose dysphagia is due to oral tongue factors, such as surgical removal of the tongue or amyotrophic lateral sclerosis (ALS).

- Head turn: in cases of unilateral damage to the pharyngeal wall and/or larynx, turning the head to the weaker side enables the patient to isolate and utilize the stronger side for a safer transportation of the bolus.

- Head tilt: this posture also is used in cases of unilateral damage to the oral cavity or pharyngeal wall. In contrast to the head turn technique, this posture requires tilting the patient's head to the undamaged side to direct the bolus toward the stronger side.

■ Lying down: if damage is bilateral or if laryngeal elevation is reduced, the combination of lying down to swallow with a follow-up swallow will move the bolus and any accompanying residue into the esophagus. The horizontal position of the larynx is intended to reduce the risk of aspiration because gravity will work to accumulate residue that can be controlled and then cleared into the esophagus with the follow-up swallow.

Maneuvers

■ Supraglottic swallow: the patient is instructed to hold his or her breath throughout the entire swallow (before, during, after); holding one's breath causes the vocal folds to close, sealing off the opening of the trachea. Once the swallow is completed, the patient voluntarily coughs and swallows a second time to clear any residue. This maneuver is used with reduced airway protection and/or with patients who have demonstrated aspiration.

■ Super-supraglottic swallow: the "super" part of the maneuver denotes the use of extra effort during the supraglottic swallow approach, typically by pushing down on a hard surface with one's hands. The extra effort may facilitate the use of the false vocal folds via arytenoid movement as additional airway protection.

■ Effortful swallow: extra effort is applied as patients are instructed to squeeze the muscles involved in swallowing hard while completing a swallow. The resulting increase in movement of the tongue base should assist patients with tongue retraction or with clearing residue from the valleculae (two spaces or pockets located in the throat just below the root of the tongue).

■ Mendelsohn maneuver: this maneuver requires self-awareness and the ability to voluntarily segment a swallow into stages. The patient places a hand on his or her throat to feel the laryngeal elevation that occurs in swallowing while taking practice swallows. Once familiar with the concept of laryngeal elevation, the patient is instructed to hold the position of laryngeal elevation for several seconds before completing the swallow and allowing the larynx to drop back to the starting position. The rationale for this maneuver is the increased laryngeal movement and coordination in patients where these abilities are diminished, such as after a brainstem stroke. The Mendelsohn maneuver also may increase duration of upper esophageal sphincter opening, thus facilitating movement of the bolus into the final swallowing phase.

■ Masako maneuver: after firmly holding the tongue tip in place between teeth, the patient then completes a swallow, making sure not to let the tongue release from between the teeth. This maneuver forces the glossopharyngeal muscle to contract with greater effort and is helpful for patients who have reduced pharyngeal contraction.

Exercises

■ Shaker exercises: this series of movements is meant to target both hyolaryngeal movement and upper esophageal opening. While lying down, instruct the patient to raise his or her head while keeping the shoulders on the ground and the mouth closed. The patient holds this position for approximately 1 minute, relaxes the head back down for approximately 1 minute, and then repeats this cycle three more times. This same cycle of holding and relaxing is then repeated 30 times at a faster pace of lift-lower-lift-lower. These exercises can be repeated several times during the day.

- Tongue exercises: in cases of oral phase dysphagia, tongue exercises may be used to target swallow efficiency and strength. Exercises include holding the tongue in a retracted position (horizontal) for several seconds, gargling, and moving the tongue in a horizontal manner anteriorly and posteriorly.

- Transference of treatment effects: Russell, Ciucci, Connor, and Schallert (2010) conducted a systematic review of the literature to see if exercises targeting one function of the cranial sensorimotor system (e.g., swallowing, voice, speech) would result in gains to other functions since there is an overlap of anatomical structures. Several studies indicated positive findings for transference, including one study that found that LSVT voice therapy resulted in improvements in both voice and swallowing abilities in patients with Parkinson's disease.

Sensory Stimuli. With patients who have dysphagia due to decreased sensation in the oral and/or pharyngeal regions (e.g., delayed oral onset of swallow), there are sensory stimuli that can be applied to heighten sensation to these regions. Foods and liquids can be altered for taste (e.g., made more sour), volume (e.g., larger bolus), temperature, or carbonation to increase the sensation of their presentation. In a similar manner, thermal tactile stimulation involves the application of a cold stimulus to increase sensation and to promote a swallow response. Another commonly used sensory technique is the application of increased pressure (e.g., spoon placed on tongue surface) to heighten sensation and facilitate preparation for the presentation of a bolus.

Dietary Changes. Various food textures and consistencies can be implemented on a trial basis to determine which diet reduces aspiration risk and helps with swallow efficiency. Options for altering food textures include pureeing solid foods and adding thickeners to liquids. Publications such as the national dysphagia diet (American Dietetic Association, www.eatright.org) can be consulted for planning therapeutically appropriate dietary choices.

Medical. Three main types of surgical procedures are associated with medical treatment for dysphagia. The first type aims to protect the airway by improving vocal fold function (i.e., injecting the vocal folds with biomaterials to improve their ability to close adequately during a swallow). The second type also targets airway protection, but involves making the tracheal and esophageal segments more distinct (e.g., laryngectomy, stent placement). The third type targets the functioning of the **pharyngeoesophageal segment (pes).** The pes can be dilated to make it larger or can be injected with botulinum toxin to decrease tension.

An additional medical treatment for dysphagia is **neuromuscular electrical stimulation (NMES).** Designed for pharyngeal phase dysphagia, NMES involves electrode placement on the surface of the throat to elicit the muscle contractions needed to swallow (Bulow, Speyer, Baijens, Woisard, & Ekberg, 2008). Furthermore, the purported goal of NMES is to rewire the swallow pattern at the level of the cortex by retraining the muscles at the level of the pharynx (Bulow et al., 2008). One study investigating NMES and neurologic changes found that even though swallow function increased, no changes were noted cortically over a 5-day treatment period (Gallas, Marie, Leroi, & Verin, 2010). A systematic review of literature on NMES found some positive findings. However, the research design of these studies was not robust. One tentative finding from NMES efficacy studies is that patients with mild to moderate dysphagia seem to benefit the most from NMES because there is still some remaining volitional muscle movement (Langdon & Blacker, 2010). However, more information is needed to determine the actual efficacy of this treatment approach (Clark, Lazarus, Arvedson, Schooling, & Frymark, 2009). This treatment approach continues to generate much debate; clinicians are referred to Carter and Humbert (2012) for more information.

Ethical Considerations. Intervention for feeding and swallowing disorders can have life-and-death consequences. Ethical issues in this area are complex and extremely serious (Sharp & Bryant, 2003). At this point, no universal guidelines exist for acceptable amounts of aspiration (i.e., entry of food/liquid into airway below level of the vocal folds). Radiographic evaluation is *absolutely* required to identify the existence, severity, and cause of aspiration. Logemann (1998) suggests oral intake of a given food consistency be prohibited if a client aspirates more than 10 percent of each bolus despite the use of optimal intervention techniques. However, clinicians should be aware that the wishes of clients and/or their families may run contrary to therapeutic recommendations. An instructive example involves a terminally ill client for whom the clinician has determined that oral intake be prohibited due to excessive aspiration under all conditions. Yet the client and family insist on continuing to eat by mouth. The clinician's ethical dilemma is whether to provide information/training on the least harmful way to swallow within a range of life-threatening alternatives. Speech-language pathologists can refer their professional organization (e.g., American Speech-Language-Hearing Association's Code of Ethics) for guidance in dealing with ethical dilemmas. In addition, a survey of speech-language pathologists revealed five elements commonly considered when addressing ethical problems: (1) client well-being and quality of life, (2) professional scope of practice (e.g., roles and responsibilities), (3) establishment of professional relationships with other team members as well as the client and family, (4) economic need to balance resources to provide appropriate services, and (5) acknowledgment that personal and professional value systems may differ (Kenny, Lincoln, & Balandin, 2010).

Helpful Hints

1. If the client's progress plateaus for at least 4 weeks, active therapy can be terminated until/unless status changes.

2. Clinicians must carefully consider the eligibility question: "Will this client benefit from intervention?" Individuals with severe cognitive limitations or advanced motor neuron disease may not be considered good candidates for swallowing treatment.

3. Several factors may complicate the treatment of patients with dysphagia. For example, reduced hearing ability or cognitive decline may make it more difficult for patients to follow directions during treatment and thus additional supports (e.g., text, diagrams) may be beneficial.

4. Patient education through the use of visual supports of the swallowing anatomy and/or biofeedback measures (e.g., ultrasound) may help patients to understand their disorder as well as help them to perform certain treatment exercises.

5. Oral care is extremely important for individuals with dysphagia because there is a risk of aspirating bacteria from the oral cavity. Frequent teeth brushing, gargling, and adequate hydration can help to maintain oral care.

6. The patient's family can learn the various safe swallowing strategies available to help promote independence. These strategies include an upright posture, taking small bites, and alternating bites and sips.

7. Molds are available to make pureed foods more closely resemble the intended food item, which may increase the patient's motivation to eat.

8. Some individuals with dysphagia (e.g., a patient with head/neck cancer who has undergone radiation treatment) have a condition known as xerostomia (excessive dry mouth). Products are available to help patients to replace the saliva and moisture in their mouth.

CONCLUSION

This section presented basic information, protocols, and procedures for intervention with dysphagia at an *introductory* level. This information is intended only as a starting point in the reader's clinical education and training. For more in-depth coverage of this area, the following readings are recommended:

Groher, M., & Crary, M. (2009). Dysphagia: Clinical management in adults and children. St. Louis, MO: Mosby.

Leonard, R., & Kendall, K. (2008). *Dysphagia assessment and treatment planning: A team approach* (2nd ed.). San Diego, CA: Plural Publishing.

Logemann, J. A. (1998). *Evaluation and treatment of swallowing disorders* (2nd ed.). Austin, TX: Pro-Ed.

ADDITIONAL RESOURCES

Dysphagia
LinguiSystems
3100 Fourth Avenue
East Moline, IL 61244-9700
Phone: 800-776-4332
Fax: 800-577-4555
Web site: http://www.linguisystems.com

The Source for Dysphagia, 3rd Edition
This 305-page workbook includes Medicare changes related to swallowing treatment; detailed educational handouts for physicians, patients, and staff; information on fiberoptic endoscopic evaluation of swallowing (FEES); new information on how to perform and interpret a modified barium swallow; and descriptions of new therapy techniques and references to document their efficacy.

The Source for Pediatric Dysphagia
For ages birth to 18, this resource provides information on feeding, swallowing, and treatment goals for young patients. The techniques also can be applied to older children with cerebral palsy, neurological disorders, or any swallowing disorder. From diagnosis through treatment, chapters cover anatomy and physiology, diagnostic procedures, infant feeding techniques, behavioral feeding disorders, goals and treatment objectives, and tools for feeding.

Pro-Ed
8700 Shoal Creek Boulevard
Austin, TX 78757-6897
Phone: 800-897-3202
Fax: 800-397-7633
Web site: http://www.proedinc.com

Pre-Feeding Skills, 2nd Edition

This program for infants to adolescents discusses normal development, limitations, and management of tube feeding, cleft palate, drooling, prematurity, and feeding in autism. It covers evaluation, treatment, oral stimulation, positioning, oral-motor limitations, and nutritional factors. It features reproducibles, mealtime exercises, and Spanish translations of parent questionnaires.

Swallowing Disorders Treatment Manual, 2nd Edition

Hands-on manual covering assessment and treatment with information on how to conduct a patient interview, bedside evaluation, and a videofluoroscopy study. Intervention includes thermal-tactile stimulation, the Mendelsohn maneuver, supraglottic swallow, posture changes in feeding position, diet consistency, oral-motor exercises, and compensatory strategies, as well as reproducible swallowing guidelines. A list of dysphagia products is also included.

AliMed
297 High Street
Dedham, MA 02026
Phone: 800-225-2610
Fax: 800-437-2966
Web site: http://www.alimed.com

Swallow Right, Second Edition

Comprehensive exercise manual for evaluation and treatment of oral myofunctional disorders. Suitable for individual, group, or carryover programming. Program covers theory, treatment, and tracking charts for the three main stages of swallowing.

Practical Applications in Dysphagia

A manual that provides guidelines on how to assess and treat individuals based on the presentation of the dysphagia and/or associated disorders. It also includes resources for recipes and dietary information.

Working with Dysphagia

This workbook is designed to provide information on a variety of disorders associated with dysphagia as well as a variety of settings in which an SLP would work with clients with dysphagia. In addition to assessment and treatment, the text also provides information on related topics such as tracheostomies, ethical issues, and nutritional needs.

Swallow Safely: A Caregiver's Guide to Dysphagia

Provides information in a manner that is beneficial in counseling both the client and the family about dysphagia. It includes information on signs to look for that indicate swallowing difficulties, related problems that may occur, and the treatment options that are available. It also discusses swallowing and how the process can become disordered.

Apps

Lingraphica
103 Carnegie Center
Suite 204
Princeton, NJ 08540
Phone: 888-274-2742
Fax: 609-275-1311
Web site: www.aphasia.com

The SmallTalk Dysphagia App was designed to enable individuals with swallowing disorders to explain their disorder to others, primarily those responsible for their care and/or medical treatment. It utilizes icons as well as spoken phrases so that individuals can communicate the safe swallowing strategies they need implemented while eating and drinking.

Infonet, Inc.
Center for Voice and Swallowing
UCDavis Health System
Web site: http://ucdvoice.org/iswallow.html

iSwallow
This app was designed for supervised use with an SLP. It contains a library of videos of dysphagia exercises that can be selected to create treatment programs. Clients can use the app on their own after instruction from an SLP, with the option to receive alerts for when to complete the exercises.

Northern Speech Services & National Rehabilitation Services Inc.
117 North Elm Street
PO Box 1247
Gaylord, MI 49734
Phone: 888-337-3866
Fax: 888-696-9655
Web site: http://www.northernspeech.com

Dysphagia App
This app is meant for educational purposes. It provides videos of normal swallowing as well as disordered swallowing, with a variety of disorders and swallowing complications to choose from. Videos include "Impairment of Bolus Transport," "Impairment of Pharyngeal Contraction," and "Example of Penetration with Aspiration."

CHAPTER 9

The focus of this chapter is on **stuttering,** the major type of fluency disorder exhibited by children and adults. Cluttering, an associated fluency disorder, is beyond the scope of this chapter. Readers who are interested in this topic are referred to Myers, Bakker, St. Louis, and Raphael (2012); and Ward and Scott (2011).

Stuttering is characterized by an abnormally high frequency and/or duration of stoppages in the forward flow of speech (Andrews & Harris, 1964; Manning, 2010; Wingate, 1964; Yaruss, 1998). Studies indicate that prevalence under age 6 is considerably higher than in later periods in life and that stuttering occurs in approximately 0.72% to 1% of the population (Yairi & Ambrose, 2013), with males outnumbering females by a significant ratio. Many theories have been proposed regarding the cause of stuttering, ranging from genetic and other organic explanations to learned, environmental, or linguistic accounts. Certain theories emphasize differences in cerebral dominance (Travis, 1931), disruptions of speech motor timing (Kent, 1984; Van Riper, 1982), or anticipatory struggle to avoid communicative failure (Bloodstein, 1987; Sheehan, 1958). The covert repair hypothesis proposed by Kolk and colleagues (Howell, 2007; Kolk, 1991; Kolk & Postma, 1997; Postma, 2000; Vasic & Wijnen, 2005) suggests that stutterers may be prone to errors in phonological planning; their attempts to edit these errors prior to producing the utterance are manifested as disfluencies. In addition, several multifactorial theories have emphasized the interaction between stuttering and a variety of intrinsic/extrinsic factors (Metten et al., 2011). One account is the capacities and demands model, which posits that stuttering results from demands for performance that exceed the speaker's capacities in one or more domains (i.e., linguistic, motor, cognitive, or emotional; Starkweather & Gottwald, 2000). The three-factor hypothesis (Wall & Myers, 1995) claims that a combination of psycholinguistic, psychosocial, and physiological factors are involved in the phenomenon of stuttering. The Packman (2012) is multifactorial and includes the following components: (1) underlying deficit in neural processing for spoken language; (2) triggers inherent in spoken language such as variable syllable stress and linguistic complexity; and (3) modulation factors unique to each individual such as emotional reactivity and environmental stressors. In the multifactorial-dynamic model, Smith and colleagues (Smith, 1999; Smith & Kelly, 1997) argue that interaction among these factors occurs on multiple nonlinear levels and that stuttered moments should be viewed as dynamic rather than static events. Similarly, Chang, Horwitz, Ostuni, Reynolds, and Ludlow (2011); De Nil and Kroll (2001); Giraud et al. (2008); and Watkins, Smith, and Howell (2008) interpret the interactionist approach to stuttering by emphasizing that all environmental and intrinsic factors are ultimately filtered through the stutterer's neurophysiological system. Recently, Kang et al. (2010) identified specific gene mutations correlated with stuttering. These mutations involve metabolic deficiencies in the body's ability to process certain enzymes. Epidemiologic studies are being developed to determine the proportion of the world's population that carries these mutations and how many of them are identified as stutterers. In 2012, Jackson, Quesal, and Yaruss discussed the prevailing view of stuttering as a disorder defined by listener-based perceptions of acoustic interruptions. They argued that the disorder is actually more complex than these surface features (e.g., repetitions, prolongations, blocks) and encompasses crucial speaker-based perceptions of "loss of control" along with powerful cognitive and affective variables. Their proposed definition for stuttering includes consideration of a neurobiological lack of integration of the processes of planning and producing language and speech that, upon verbal execution, can lead to interruptions in the acoustic speech signal and physical struggle (e.g., tension). The underlying features may lead to surface behaviors, as well as emotional and cognitive reactions. Individuals may experience severe difficulties in communication, with a highly adverse impact on their quality of life. The specific interactions among linguistic, motor, cognitive, genetic, emotional, and social factors are yet to be determined, as well as their influence on the variable nature and complexity of stuttering. (See Bloodstein and Ratner [2008] for a review of different theoretical positions.)

The onset of stuttering usually occurs between 2 and 5 years of age and may emerge in a sudden or severe manner (Yairi & Ambrose, 1999). Some researchers report that approximately 80% of children who stutter will spontaneously recover before the age of puberty (Andrews & Harris, 1964; Yairi & Ambrose, 1999). Some evidence suggests that spontaneous recovery is a gradual process that may begin within the first year of stuttering and not reach completion until 3 or 4 years post-onset (Yairi & Ambrose, 1999). Differences in terminology, methodology, and interpretation of data make it difficult to compare results (Bothe, Davidow, Bramlett, & Ingham, 2006; Ingham & Bothe, 2001; Onslow & Packman, 1999a, 199b; Prins & Ingham, 2009; Yairi & Ambrose, 1999, 2001, 2013). Many clinicians use a rule of thumb that 50% to 80% of children who stutter will recover with or without treatment (Guitar, 2013). For individuals who continue to stutter, the characteristics of the disorder may gradually change over time. Several viewpoints regarding the development of stuttering have been proposed. Bloodstein (1960) describes a four-phase model that progresses from mild episodic disfluencies to severe, chronic stuttering accompanied by fear and avoidance reactions. Van Riper (1982) suggests a three-stage progression that includes primary, transitional, and secondary phases. A third hypothesis, put forth by Starkweather (1987), indicates that the development of stuttering fluctuates as a result of an individual's changing capacity to accommodate environmental demands for communicative performance. Finally, recent longitudinal data on preschool stutterers suggest that severity of stuttering at onset may remain unchanged up to 3 years post-onset (Sawyer, & Yairi, 2010; Throneburg & Yairi, 2001).

CATEGORIES OF STUTTERING BEHAVIORS

Two main categories of characteristics are associated with stuttering: core behaviors and secondary behaviors.

Core Behaviors

Core behaviors are the basic manifestations that seem beyond the voluntary control of the stutterer and include the following:

- Repetitions of sounds, syllables, or whole words (e.g., c-c-cat; ba-ba-balloon; we-we-we are going)
- Prolongations of single sounds (e.g., sssssoap; fffffishing)
- Blocks of airflow/voicing during speech (inappropriate stoppage of air or voice at any level of the vocal tract)

Secondary Behaviors

Secondary behaviors develop over time as learned reactions to the core behaviors and are categorized as **escape** or **avoidance** behaviors. Escape behaviors occur during a stuttering moment and are attempts to break out of the stutter. Common examples of escape behaviors include head nods, eye blinks, foot taps, and jaw tremors. In the more advanced stages of stuttering, these behaviors may be accompanied by visible struggle and muscular tension. Avoidance behaviors occur in anticipation of a stuttering moment and are attempts to refrain from stuttering at all. Typical avoidance behaviors are circumlocutions (substitutions of less feared vocabulary words), unfilled pauses without accompanying tension and struggle within or between words, and use of "um" or other interjections to postpone speaking.

Developmental Disfluencies Versus Stuttering

Most typically developing children between 2 and 4 years of age display some of the following relatively effortless disfluencies during the normal course of language acquisition (Gregory & Hill, 1993; Pellowski & Conture, 2002; Zebrowski, 1994):

- Hesitations (silent pauses)
- Interjections of sounds, syllables, or words (e.g., "Um, I went to school"; "Did you *you know* find her?")
- Revisions/repetitions of words, phrases, or sentences (e.g., "You have to touch, *no, turn* it"; "I have some . . . *I want you to look at* these baseball cards")
- Normal rhythm and stress patterns
- No tension or tremors noted

It is important to differentiate between these normal disfluencies and the atypical disfluencies in the following list, which are often the early signs of stuttering:

- Three or more *within-word* disfluencies per 100 words (especially fragmentation of syllables)
- Disfluencies on more than 10% of syllables spoken
- Predominant use of prolongations, blocks, and part-word repetitions (as opposed to interjections and whole-word or phrase repetitions)
- Presence of secondary behaviors/increased tension
- Vowel neutralization (schwa) during repetitions (e.g., buh-buh-beat)
- Duration of single instance of disfluency that exceeds two seconds
- Uncontrolled or abrupt changes in pitch or loudness

Ambrose and Yairi's (1999) large-scale study of preschool children provides strong evidence that stuttering can be differentiated from normal disfluency on the basis of three main characteristics: (1) part-word repetition, (2) single-syllable word repetition, and (3) disrhythmic phonation (i.e., prolongations, blocks, and broken words). This differential pattern of disfluency types was significant even at the early stages of stuttering. Pellowski and Conture (2002) also found that the speech of children who stutter (CWS) could be differentiated from the speech of children who do not stutter (CWNS). Specifically, CWS produced approximately two and a half to four times as many total disfluencies as the CWNS. Also, CWS produce an average of 2.0 extra repetition units (per instance of part- or whole-word repetition) than their typically developing counterparts. Zebrowski (1997) suggests that clinical decision-making regarding intervention should be influenced by whether the child demonstrates five important characteristics that are associated with a high probability of recovery:

- 18 months to 3 years of age at onset
- no family history of stuttering or a small number of affected relatives who recovered in childhood
- female
- few to no associated behaviors
- no coexisting phonological or cognitive problems

TREATMENT FOR FLUENCY DISORDERS

Regardless of theoretical orientation, the ultimate aim of most stuttering therapy programs is spontaneous fluency. Fluency can be described as consisting of four primary components: rate, continuity, rhythm, and effort (Andrews et al., 2012; Starkweather, 1985, 1987). Accordingly, spontaneous fluent speech is smooth, relatively rapid, and melodic (as opposed to monotonous), and appears free of conscious physical or mental effort. For people who demonstrate severe stuttering behavior, spontaneous fluency may not be considered a realistic goal. Controlled fluency or acceptable levels of stuttering may be identified as the ultimate goal of treatment for these individuals, depending on the clinician's philosophy of the general nature of stuttering. The client's cultural and linguistic background as well as preferences and priorities also may influence the choice of general approach to intervention. In addition, it is important to recognize that, unlike most other speech and language disorders, relapse is a common phenomenon in stuttering. People who stutter frequently experience periods of increased disfluency after treatment has been terminated. For this reason, periodic follow-up sessions should be an integral part of an effective fluency treatment program. For example, Blood (1995) advocates a cognitive-behavioral relapse management program for adolescents that is instituted following the completion of a traditional course of fluency therapy. This program provides training in five basic areas: problem solving, general communication skills, assertiveness, coping strategies, and establishment of realistic expectations.

Individuals who stutter have been shown to demonstrate performance differences in some language and phonological skills when compared with typical speakers (Anderson & Conture, 2004; Anderson, Wagovich, & Hall, 2006; Cuadrado & Weber-Fox, 2003; Melnick, Conture, & Ohde, 2003). Stuttering also can occur concomitantly with other communication problems such as language or phonology disorders, particularly in preschool and school-age children (Gregory, 2003). Multiple authors (Brent & Yairi, 2012; Smith, Sadagopan, Walsh, & Weber-Fox, 2010) have investigated the association of stuttering with phonology disorders and have come to the conclusion that children with persistent stuttering are at increased risk for phonological and articulation disorders. There are at least four programming alternatives for treating coexisting impairments (Ratner, 1995):

> **Discrete:** A certain amount of therapy time is allotted to treat each disorder in isolation. For example, in a 1-hour therapy session, a clinician may devote 20 minutes to fluency goals and the remaining 40 minutes to articulation goals. Alternatively, a twice-weekly therapy schedule can be divided to spend one session on each disorder area.

Modified cycles: Treatment for one disorder is implemented for a specified block of time (e.g., 6 weeks) and then discontinued. An equivalent time period is then devoted to treatment of the other communicative impairment. This cycle is alternated until long-term goals are achieved for each disorder.

Blended: Therapy goals for one disorder are incorporated into the therapy activities for a second disorder. For example, during articulation activities, the clinician can encourage fluency-enhancing behaviors such as slower speaking rate and increased pause time between conversational turns.

Lagged: This is a modified form of the blended approach that incorporates an initial time delay. Specifically, a period of initial therapy focuses on attaining a predetermined level of mastery in the concomitant disorder area (e.g., phonological or linguistic). Once the child has reached this level of mastery, fluency therapy can begin using the recently mastered phonological/linguistic forms as the basis for practice. Fluency therapy continues to be programmed at comfortable levels of phonological/linguistic demand as the child progressively masters new objectives in the concomitant disorder area.

Treatment Efficacy/Evidence-Based Practice

Efficacy in the area of stuttering therapy is particularly difficult to measure because its definition must incorporate three interrelated factors: (1) objective measures of frequency and duration of stuttered moments, (2) client emotions and attitudes, and (3) the client's amenability to participate in communicative interactions with a variety of partners. The importance of treatment outcomes has been increasingly addressed in the stuttering literature. Prins and Ingham (2009) have attempted to clarify general principles of evidence-based practice as they relate to stuttering from a historical perspective. They present definitional and operational guidelines that can facilitate clinicians' ability to critically evaluate different approaches to stuttering treatment of young children and adults (Blood & Conture, 1998; Cordes & Ingham, 1998; Finn, 2003; Ingham, 2003; Ingham & Riley, 1998; Langevin & Kully, 2003). In 2001, the World Health Organization (WHO) presented a multidimensional classification scheme for describing health status and the experience of disability. This paradigm, the International Classification of Functioning, Disability, and Health (ICF; WHO, 2001), has been adapted by Yaruss (2010) to describe the speaker's experience of the disorder of stuttering. Specifically, this can involve negative affective, behavioral, and cognitive reactions (both from the speaker and the listener), as well as significant limitations in the speaker's ability to participate in daily activities and a negative impact on the speaker's overall quality of life. He advocates for the use of the ICF as a framework for measuring treatment outcomes for persons who stutter. Several authors have conducted systematic reviews of the treatment literature for both children and adults (Bothe et al., 2006; Conture, 1996; Herder, Howard, Nye, & Vanryckeghem, 2006; Prins & Ingham, 2009). The findings from these reports are organized below according to four age groups: preschoolers, school-age children, adolescents, and adults. The overall conclusion is that treatment for fluency disorders is generally effective across age ranges. (For a comprehensive summary of the treatment literature in stuttering, see the appendix in Bloodstein and Ratner [2008].)

- Preschool children benefit from initiation of therapy in the early stages of stuttering.
- Response-contingent intervention is the most well-documented approach for preschoolers who stutter.

- Efficacy information for school-age children and adolescents is scant, although preliminary data are emerging regarding predicting and/or minimizing relapse after treatment.

- Studies of adults indicate that prolonged speech, gentle onsets, self-monitoring, and modeling are among the most effective treatment strategies for remediating stuttering.

- Future efficacy research is needed to address several critical issues, including the relationship between reduced stuttering and naturalness of speech, attitudinal changes, and long-term outcomes (e.g., more than 5 years) of intervention.

An interesting development in the field of treatment efficacy includes the notion of "common factors." First proposed in the field of psychology (Ahn & Wampold, 2001; Kim, Wampold, & Bolt, 2006), this model suggests that efficacy data often shows little difference across treatment regimens, but that variance related to other factors does exist. The alliance between the therapist and the client as well as the quality of clinician expertise seem to have significant influence on treatment effect sizes. This finding was corroborated by a meta-analysis of stuttering treatment conducted by Herder et al. (2006). They came to the conclusion that what is critical for successful treatment outcomes may not be the intervention itself, but rather the knowledge and skill of the clinician.

Intervention Techniques

Various techniques are used in the treatment of stuttering. These include Shames and Florance's (1980) stutter-free speech program, Ryan's (1974) graduated increase in length and complexity model, computer-aided fluency establishment training (Goebel, 1986), Bloodstein's (1975) anticipatory struggle program, and Shine's (1980) systematic fluency training, to name just a few. Frequently, the client's age is a critical factor in determining how intervention will be implemented.

Onslow and colleagues (Arnott et al., 2014; Onslow & Andrews, 1994; Packman et al., 2014) developed the Lidcombe program, a response-contingent approach to stuttering intervention for young children. The central component of this fluency-shaping program is presentation of verbal contingencies for stuttered versus stutter-free speech (i.e., praise versus corrective feedback). It incorporates a strong focus on parental participation as well as a structured maintenance phase.

Philosophically, all the different approaches can be divided into two primary schools of thought: fluency shaping and stuttering modification/management.

Fluency Shaping. Fluency shaping is based on the assumption that stuttering is a learned behavior. The primary goal of fluency shaping is to eliminate disfluencies and gradually change the speaker's habitual speaking pattern to one of fluent speech. This is accomplished through the use of several fluency enhancing techniques:

- **Easy onset/prevoice exhalation:** The speaker is taught to exhale slightly before beginning phonation and reach conversational loudness gradually.

- **Decreased speaking rate (prolonged speech):** The speaker is trained to stretch out the sounds (primarily vowels) in his speech and produce words at a slower-than-normal speaking rate while maintaining normal stress and intonation.

- **Light articulatory contacts:** The speaker is taught to move the articulators in a loose and relaxed manner.

- **Continuous phonation:** The speaker is trained to reduce all breaks between words by maintaining voicing continuously until he naturally needs to take a breath.

The ultimate aim of programs based on a fluency-shaping philosophy is to completely change speech behavior by teaching clients to use these techniques at all times, not just during disfluent moments. These techniques are designed to interfere with the stuttering behaviors, thus reducing them. Overall, most fluency shaping programs can be categorized according to which parameter of communicative interaction is the focus of change: phonation, speech rate, length of utterance, or provision of contingent feedback. Therapy sessions focus solely on acquisition of fluency-enhancing behaviors and generally do not address a client's secondary behaviors or the negative feelings and attitudes that may be associated with the stuttering.

Delayed Auditory Feedback (DAF). This fluency-shaping technique has been widely used in the treatment of stuttering. A speaker's own words are returned through headphones after an imposed electronic delay of a few milliseconds. For normal speakers, the use of DAF disrupts the smooth flow of speech and results in a significant breakdown in fluency. DAF has the opposite effect on the speech of many individuals who stutter; it decreases their speech rate and reduces the number of notable disfluencies. As a general rule, therapy is initiated at a delay time of approximately 250 ms. The time delay is then reduced in 50-ms intervals (i.e., 200 ms, 150 ms, 100 ms, and so on) as the client stabilizes fluency skills at each level. (See Ham [1999]; Huddock and Kalinowski [2014]; and Saltuklaroglu [2011] for detailed information on the implementation of DAF as a clinical procedure.)

Use of DAF in stuttering therapy has been recommended by many authors, including Van Riper (1973); Webster, Schumacher, and Lubker (1970); and Shames and Florance (1980). Proponents of this technique suggest that it tends to generate increased fluency in the early stages of therapy. DAF also is believed to enhance the speaker's ability to monitor oral-sensory feedback cues from his own speech mechanism. Finally, it facilitates a slower speaking rate by increasing a client's syllable duration and phonation time. However, other writers have cautioned about the possible drawbacks of DAF (Sheehan, 1968; Wingate, 1976). Among the most commonly cited disadvantages are difficulty in weaning clients from the DAF equipment and the development of a "DAF voice" (slow, labored, lacking in inflection and stress variation). For a detailed review of the literature on the effects of DAF, see Bloodstein and Ratner (2008).

Recently, numerous **assistive devices** have been developed to treat stuttering from a fluency-shaping perspective. Some devices, such as SpeechEasy, use **frequency-altered feedback** (FAF) as well as DAF to promote fluent speech (Foundas, Mock, Corey, Gol, & Conture, 2013; Stuart, Kalinowski, Rastatter, Saltuklaroglu, & Dayalu, 2004). In FAF, digital technology allows speech signal frequencies to be adjusted without changing a client's speech rate. Other portable devices, such as the Edinborough Masker, permit clients to turn on masking noise in anticipation of a disfluency (Block, Ingham, & Bench, 1996). With the rapid advances in digital technology, other portable devices are likely to become available. The way in which these devices are incorporated into intervention should be determined by the clinician on a case-by-case basis.

Stuttering Modification/Management. Stuttering modification is based on the premise that stuttering may involve a physiological predisposition. The primary goals of stuttering management are to modify each disfluent moment by stuttering more easily and to eliminate struggle and avoidance behaviors (Van Riper, 1973). Gregory (1979) called this the "stutter more fluently" approach. In essence, the strategy is to minimize a client's reaction to loss of speech control rather than to eliminate the disfluencies themselves. These goals are accomplished through the use of a combination of the following techniques:

- **Self-analysis:** Increase the client's awareness of the type, severity, and loci of disfluencies as well as any accompanying secondary behaviors. Attention also may be given to increasing the client's self-awareness of the characteristics of his non-stuttered speech and monitoring his proprioceptive awareness of the oral musculature.
- **Relaxation:** Reduce the client's anxiety and muscle tension through relaxation training (see Table 9-1 for specific steps).
- **Desensitization:** Reduce negative emotions associated with stuttering (e.g., fear, frustration, embarrassment) by decreasing sensitivity to core behaviors and listener reactions through activities such as voluntary stuttering or voluntary exaggeration of a stuttered moment.

In this philosophy, therapy outcomes are not defined strictly by decreases in stuttering frequency counts. Rather, progress is measured along a qualitative continuum as the nature of stuttering shifts from high-struggle speech with syllable fragmentations to less effortful, forward-moving speech.

Clinicians who employ a stuttering modification/management approach work with clients to identify hierarchies of feared speaking situations. These hierarchies are valuable tools for a variety of therapeutic purposes: (1) developing clients' self-awareness and ability to analyze their behavior, (2) recognizing variations in clients' stuttering patterns across different settings, and (3) facilitating development of sequential behavioral objectives and collection of data. (See Figure 9-1 for sample hierarchies.)

TABLE 9–1
Progressive Relaxation Training

Step 1:	Ensure that the client is seated comfortably.
Step 2:	Explain that this procedure involves the deliberate contracting and relaxing of various muscles to help the client recognize and discriminate between muscular tension and relaxation.
Step 3:	Starting at the level of the abdomen, instruct the client to tightly contract his stomach muscles for at least 5 seconds and then relax them. Encourage the client to concentrate on how his muscles feel when they are in a tensed versus relaxed state. Require the client to perform this activity three to five times.
Step 4:	Repeat the contraction-relaxation sequence with other muscle groups moving progressively toward the head (i.e., arms, shoulders, neck, face). The clinician should periodically check the client's level of relaxation during the release phase by placing one hand on the target muscle group and pushing slightly to determine the degree of muscle resistance. Noticeable resistance indicates an insufficient degree of relaxation.
Step 5:	At the level of the face, instruct the client to perform each of the following movement sequences three to five times: clench the mandible against the upper molars and release; pucker and release the lips; push the blade of the tongue strongly against the hard palate and release; tightly close both eyes and then open; frown in an exaggerated manner and relax.

NOTE: The aim of teaching progressive relaxation is to enable the person who stutters to consistently identify instances of excessive muscular tension during speech and to immediately transition into a relaxed state without having to work through the entire stepwise progression.

SOURCE: Adapted from Brutten and Shoemaker (1967), Jacobson (1938), and Ham (1986).

FIGURE 9–1

Climbing the fear hierarchy

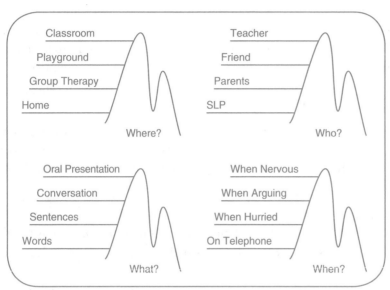

Used by permission of V. Sisskin, University of Maryland

    The following stuttering modification/management techniques are generally intended to be used as a three-part sequence in the following order (Van Riper, 1973):

- **Cancellations:** When experiencing a disfluency, the speaker is encouraged to *complete* the intended word without attempting to break out of the disfluency. After the disfluency has been produced, the speaker is instructed to pause and mentally rehearse a technique for producing the word more fluently (or with an easier stutter) and then repeat the word.

- **Pull-outs:** When experiencing a disfluency, the speaker is taught to stop in the *middle* of the stuttering moment, mentally rehearse the intended word using a fluency-enhancing technique (or easier stuttering pattern), and then reproduce it.

- **Preparatory sets:** The speaker is encouraged to anticipate an imminent disfluency and pause briefly to mentally rehearse fluent (or gentle stuttering) production *before* the word is attempted.

    The ultimate aim of programs based on a stuttering modification/management philosophy is to modify stuttering behaviors to an acceptable level rather than eliminate them entirely. The client's negative attitudes and feelings toward his or her stuttering are typically identified and monitored over time through the administration of attitudinal scales. Therapy sessions also give considerable attention to the reduction of speech fears and secondary behaviors as a means of minimizing the impact of stuttering. Elementary school–age children and adolescents are particularly vulnerable to teasing and negative self-image. Effective therapy programs incorporate activities such as role playing and brainstorming to proactively address these issues. Detailed information on related counseling techniques can be found in Chapter 11.

    Guitar (2013) suggests that long-term fluency goals and clinical methods are two important treatment issues that differentiate fluency-shaping and stuttering modification/

management approaches. With regard to fluency goals, the three possible outcomes of therapy are spontaneous fluency, controlled fluency, and acceptable stuttering. The outcome of choice for both therapy approaches is spontaneous fluency, with a secondary goal of controlled fluency.

Yairi and Seery (2014) suggest that therapists consider three major alternatives when designing long-term treatment for people who stutter: increased fluency, reduced stuttering, and improved cognitive-emotional adjustment. Guitar (20013) and others advocate the integration of fluency shaping and stuttering modification/management techniques in the treatment of stuttering. They believe that stuttering results from an interaction of physiologic factors and learned behaviors. Therefore, facets of each approach are viewed as essential components of an effective treatment paradigm.

Example Profiles

Four profiles representative of fluency problems exhibited by clients of different age ranges (i.e., preschool, school age, and adult) are presented in this section. These examples have been designed to illustrate the selection of intervention targets, specific therapy activities, and materials. Implementation of both fluency shaping and stuttering modification/management approaches is demonstrated for each profile.

Eli is 3 years old and his speech is characterized by hesitations, whole-word or whole-phrase repetitions, and interjections of syllables/words (e.g., "um," "well") with no accompanying struggle behaviors. Analysis of a 200-syllable spontaneous speech sample indicated that 20% of the syllables uttered were disfluent. By parental report, Eli appears to exhibit no awareness of his communication difficulties. Receptive and expressive language abilities, as well as other developmental skills, appear age appropriate.

Selection of therapy targets. The overall communicative profile demonstrated by Eli is consistent with that of a child experiencing normal disfluencies, except for the relatively high frequency of the disfluencies. Based on Eli's disfluency rate and his young chronological age, an indirect approach to treatment is selected. An indirect approach focuses on the modification of the communicative environment rather than on treating the disfluencies themselves. The child's family is taught strategies for adapting their communicative behaviors in ways that create an environment conducive to the production of fluent speech. This is particularly important, because survey evidence indicates that parents may unknowingly exacerbate children's disfluencies by correcting and/or finishing their utterances. Families are encouraged to do the following:

- Listen attentively to the child's message rather than to his speech pattern.
- Avoid speaking for the child; do not fill in or complete the child's message.
- Avoid communicative stresses such as time pressures.
- Decrease demands for verbal performance (e.g., "Tell Aunt Suzie what you did in school today.").
- Avoid interrupting the child or allowing siblings or friends to interrupt (emphasize the rules for turn-taking in conversation).

- Avoid the predominant use of questions that demand lengthy or complex responses in favor of those that require simple one- or two-word answers.
- Avoid using an excessively rapid speech pattern; be sure to model smooth, relaxed speech when talking with the child (Guitar & Marchinkoski, 2001).
- Avoid labeling disfluencies as stuttering.
- Maintain natural eye contact while the child speaks, even during disfluencies.
- Avoid correcting the child's mispronunciations of speech sounds.

An important aspect of the indirect approach is to facilitate parental awareness of the child's fluency status in the home environment. This can be accomplished through use of a fluency observation chart (Form 9–1) in which parents keep a record of each disfluency exhibited by the child at home and the factors that surround it.

It is essential to maintain regular contact with the family to monitor the effectiveness of these strategies in ameliorating the child's disfluencies. A more direct treatment approach should be considered when no significant improvement is reported after a predetermined time period (e.g., 3–4 months), or more immediately if the child's communication performance deteriorates (i.e., demonstrates a higher frequency or longer duration of disfluencies, emergence of struggle behaviors).

Helpful Hints

1. Video recordings of natural family interactions (e.g., birthday party, family vacation, family reunion) can be helpful in identifying the communication patterns used by different family members with the child.

2. The effectiveness of an indirect treatment approach can be enhanced by preparing simple, clear materials that outline the desired communication strategies listed previously. These materials can be given to individuals with whom the child has regular contact (i.e., daycare providers, preschool teachers, babysitters, grandparents, and so on).

3. For families that seem overly sensitive to their child's disfluencies, it may be helpful to have them chart the type and number of disfluencies that occur naturally in everyday conversations among normally fluent speakers.

4. Parents often express feelings of guilt regarding a child's disfluencies. It is important to assure parents that they did not cause the fluency problem and that their consistent use of the recommended communication strategies can be the most powerful, positive facilitator of fluent speech for their child. (Refer to Chapter 11 for additional information on counseling strategies.)

5. Clinicians may need to make parents aware that the severity of their child's stuttering can vary considerably from one day to the next. This inconsistent behavior is typical of stuttering and should not to be interpreted as voluntary in nature or indicative of permanent change in fluency status.

6. In their attempts to minimize disfluent moments, families may inadvertently reduce or alter the amount/variety of verbal exchanges with their children. Clinicians should encourage family members to maintain natural levels of communicative interactions that typically occur in the home environment.

FORM 9–1 HOME FLUENCY OBSERVATION CHART

Child's Name: _____ Informant: _____

INSTRUCTIONS: Over the next week, write down at least five situations in which your child experiences disfluency. Please indicate the circumstances in which the disfluency occurs by recording the information below. It is recommended that a separate recording chart be maintained by each observer.

Date/ Time	Situation/ Topic	Type of Disfluency	Child's Reaction to Disfluency	Listener Name/ Reaction to Disfluency	What Triggered the Disfluency

For each of the remaining profiles, two sets of therapy targets will be presented, one based on a fluency shaping approach and the other on stuttering modification/ management. The sample activities that are included were designed to illustrate how each of these treatment paradigms can be implemented.

Kate is 3 years old and her speech is characterized by hesitations, whole-word/phrase repetitions, and interjections of syllables/words. Unlike Eli in Profile 1, Kate also demonstrates occasional word–initial syllable repetitions, accompanied by the incipient secondary behaviors of eye blinks and head nods. Analysis of a 200-syllable spontaneous speech sample indicated that 23% of the syllables uttered were disfluent. According to her parents, Kate is extremely frustrated by her disfluencies and often states, "I can't say that word." Her receptive and expressive language abilities, as well as other developmental milestones, appear age appropriate.

Selection of therapy targets using a fluency-shaping approach. The behaviors to be targeted are decreased speech rate and easy onset of phonation. These techniques were chosen because they are relatively easy for a young child to conceptualize and generally yield a marked decrease in disfluencies. In addition, the use of easy onset is particularly appropriate because it tends to inhibit the production of word-initial disfluencies.

Sample Activities

Easy Onset of Phonation and Decreased Speaking Rate

1. Fill a large bag or pillowcase with 25 to 30 small toys and objects. Collect pictures of one slow-moving and one fast-moving animal (e.g., whale and rabbit). Point to each picture while modeling the animals' special voices. Demonstrate the whale's voice by producing simple sentences using an exaggerated slow speech rate (approximately three to four syllables per second) and easy onset of phonation. Repeat the same sentences to demonstrate the rabbit's voice with an extremely rapid speech rate and abrupt onset of phonation.

   Select a carrier phrase that begins with a vowel, such as "I have a ___." Tell the child that she should close her eyes and pick one object from the bag. Have the child say the carrier phrase five times, including the name of the chosen object, using the preferred "whale voice" (e.g., "I have a *ball*"). As each utterance is produced, the clinician identifies the child's speech pattern by pointing to one of the animal pictures. Whenever the child's utterance is more like the rabbit's voice, the clinician provides another model of the whale's smooth, easy speaking voice and asks the child to imitate it. The child is then given a brief opportunity to play with the selected toy before repeating the sequence with another toy.

Decreased Speaking Rate and Light Articulatory Contact

2. Obtain an empty coffee can and punch 20 holes (approximately the diameter of a pencil) in the plastic lid. Place a small toy or other prize inside the can. Gather 20 lengths of colored yarn (each approximately 12 inches long) and tie a large knot

at one end of each piece. Put the knotted ends of the strings at the bottom of the can and replace the lid on the can with unknotted ends of each piece protruding slightly through a hole in the lid. Select a book that contains pictures of common objects and activities with which the child is familiar. The clinician shows the child the first picture in the book and models simple three- to five-word sentences (e.g., There's a doggie; I see a baby; The man is running; The house is red) using a very slow, easy speaking voice. The child is required to imitate the sentence using the same speech pattern while pulling one string of yarn through the coffee can lid in a correspondingly slow and gentle manner (until the yarn is stopped by the knot). Model a different sentence for each successive picture until all the yarn pieces are "sprouting" from the can. After the last string has been pulled, the child may remove the lid to find the prize hidden inside.

Selection of therapy targets using a stuttering modification/management approach. Stuttering modification may be of limited usefulness with a child of this age because many of the techniques employed in this approach require relatively advanced cognitive skills beyond the grasp of a 3-year-old child (e.g., self-analysis, cancellations, pull-outs). However, parents can be encouraged to minimize their child's anxiety by using appropriate vocabulary for casual reference to disfluencies (e.g., bumpy speech) and modeling expressions that mirror their child's feelings (e.g., "That one was really tough to say"). One aspect of this approach that can be extremely effective with very young disfluent children is desensitization. Therefore, the goal is to lessen the child's sensitivity to her own disfluencies.

Sample Activities

Desensitization

1. Obtain two Colorform sets (or two simple puzzles) and a deck of 25 cards depicting different agent + action relationships. Give one set (puzzle) to each player and place the card deck face-down on the table. Introduce a "Catch Me if You Can" game by explaining that each person will take a turn picking a card from the deck, placing it face-up on the table, and describing it. The clinician should be prepared to pseudo-stutter (pretend to be disfluent) using the child's habitual pattern on about half of her turns. The child is instructed to listen carefully for any instances of "bumpy" (disfluent) speech during the clinician's or her own turn and to immediately slap the picture as soon as she hears it. The clinician provides feedback regarding the smoothness or bumpiness of every production. The player who correctly slaps the picture first earns a chance to put a piece on the Colorform set. Repeat this sequence until the card deck is depleted.

2. Gather three puppets with movable mouths. One is for the clinician; the others are given to the child. Select a storybook that has a repetitive refrain or story line (e.g., *Green Eggs and Ham*, *The Little Red Hen*, and so on). Explain to the child that her puppets both have "bumpy" voices, but that "Snappy" has more trouble with his words and gets stuck more often than "Max." The clinician uses her puppet to model both voices. The bumpier voice should reflect the child's habitual disfluency pattern in a slightly exaggerated manner and be accompanied by the child's secondary behaviors. The other voice is produced with just a few easy whole-word

repetitions. Tell the child that the clinician's puppet is going to read a story out loud alternately using one or the other of her puppets' voices. The child's puppets will supply the refrain or repetitive line. The child must identify which voice the clinician's puppet is producing by making either Snappy or Max say the refrain in the same voice as the clinician's model. The clinician should gradually increase the frequency with which Max's less bumpy voice is presented as a model for imitation.

Susan is 9 years old and her speech is characterized by part-word repetitions, whole-word repetitions, prolongations of initial sounds (approximately 2 to 3 seconds), and phrase revisions. She was noted to demonstrate several secondary behaviors, of which she did not seem consistently aware. These included excessive leg movements, lip tremors, and eye gaze aversion. Analysis of a 200-syllable spontaneous speech sample indicated that 29% of the syllables uttered were disfluent. According to parental report, Susan is extremely anxious about her speech difficulties. Developmental history is unremarkable and her academic performance is appropriate for her grade level.

Selection of therapy targets using a fluency-shaping approach. The behaviors to be targeted are easy onset of phonation, light articulatory contacts, and decreased speaking rate. An analysis of Susan's disfluency profile indicates that her most severe stuttering characteristics are initial sound prolongations and part-word repetitions. Easy onset and light articulatory contacts were chosen because they are effective in addressing these types of disfluencies, especially when they occur in the word–initial position. Decreased speaking rate is considered a basic intervention technique that generally results in an immediate observable decrease in frequency of stuttering and thus provides the child with success in the very early stages of therapy.

Sample Activities

Easy Onset of Phonation and Light Articulatory Contacts

1. Play a modified version of an "I Spy" game in which the clinician is "it." Before beginning the game, teach the fluency-enhancing techniques of easy onset of phonation and light articulatory contacts. Instruct the child to release a little bit of air before starting her voice and to move her tongue and lips gently during speech. The clinician models each of the target techniques in single words. As soon as the child demonstrates some mastery of these behaviors (e.g., five consecutive correct responses), the I Spy game can be initiated. The clinician thinks of an object in the room and gives the child clues to its identity by describing its attributes one at a time (e.g., "I spy something black"; "I spy something heavy"; and so on), employing a slightly exaggerated rendition of both techniques. After each clue, the child takes one guess at identifying the object (at the single-word level) using both fluency techniques. Continue to present clues until the object is named. In the early phases of therapy, a slight modification of the game is recommended when the child takes his turn to be "it." Following the child's selection of an object, the clinician supplies the carrier phrase, "I spy something . . . ," for the child to complete with a single word clue using the target fluency techniques.

Decreased Speaking Rate

2. Obtain a book/digital list of Mad Libs. Mad Libs are stories or vignettes in which specific parts of speech (e.g., noun, proper noun, adverb, adjective, and so on) have been omitted. When the missing parts are filled in, the result is a semantically absurd and funny text. The clinician selects one of the stories and says, "Give me an example of a ___" for each of the omitted parts of speech. These utterances should be produced with a slightly decreased speaking rate to highlight the target behavior. The child provides a word or phrase, which the clinician inserts into the written story. When all the blanks have been filled in, the child is instructed to read the whole story aloud using a predetermined slow rate of speech. The child then takes a turn choosing a Mad Lib and asks the clinician to supply the missing parts, remembering to use her slow speech rate. Instruct the child to read the completed story aloud to give her maximal opportunities to practice the target behavior. (This task is best used with children who have already demonstrated initial mastery of decreased speaking rate at the level of imitation.)

Selection of therapy targets using a stuttering modification/management approach. Based on Susan's fluency profile, the therapy targets are her secondary behaviors, prolongation of initial sounds, and part-word repetitions. The secondary behaviors were selected because Susan shows little awareness of them and because these behaviors are highly distracting to conversational partners. The prolongations and part-word repetitions were identified as therapy targets because they represent Susan's most severe disfluency types.

Sample Activities

Self-Analysis

1. Obtain a 20- to 30-minute video sample of the child's connected speech that represents her typical pattern and level of disfluencies. Explain to the child that when she stutters, she often exhibits some extra body movements and tends to look away from the listener. Tell her that she and the clinician will review the video to increase her awareness of the occurrence of these accompanying behaviors (i.e., leg movements, lip tremors, and eye gaze aversion). Select one of the secondary characteristics and tell the child that she and the clinician will watch the tape carefully for instances of that behavior. The first person to notice an occurrence of the target should signal by raising her hand. The person who signals correct identifications most frequently is declared the winner. Particularly clear examples of the behaviors may be played again to reinforce the child's understanding of the nature of the secondary characteristic. The initial stages of this activity should entail the use of brief segments of video (about one minute), which can be gradually increased as the child demonstrates greater facility with the task.

Cancellations

2. Compile a list of 25 animal riddles (e.g., Q: Why do chimpanzees like bananas? A: Because they have a-peel). Underline one word in the question part of each riddle, being sure to vary location of the underlined word in the sentence. Tell the child that she is going to read the riddles to the clinician using cancellations.

Before beginning this activity, review this stuttering modification/management technique with the child. Remind the child that whenever she gets stuck on a word, she should complete the stutter without trying to start the word or sentence again. Once the word is finished, the child should pause to think about what went wrong, using the self-analysis skills learned in previous stages of therapy. The child should plan how to correct it by silently rehearsing how it would feel to say the word fluently. Then, have the child repeat the word in a smooth, prolonged manner. Provide the child with several opportunities to practice the technique by modeling some disfluencies and cancellations for her to imitate.

Instruct the child to read the first part of each riddle and to deliberately stutter on the underlined word in the question. Each disfluency should be modified using cancellation. Once the cancellation has been successfully completed, the child can finish reading the whole riddle. Any spontaneous disfluencies that occur on words other than the underlined target should also be cancelled.

Patrick is 29 years old and his speech is characterized by laryngeal blocks and prolongations of initial sounds. Duration of blocks ranges between 2 and 20 seconds, whereas prolongations tend to last 3 to 5 seconds. Patrick was observed to demonstrate numerous secondary behaviors, including head jerks, jaw tremors, eye blinks, and audible inhalation. Analysis of a 200-syllable spontaneous speech sample indicated that 35% of syllables uttered were disfluent. During the case history interview, Patrick stated that stuttering has been a problem since childhood and that he is currently seeking treatment because his disfluencies are interfering with career advancement as well as interpersonal relationships.

Selection of therapy targets using a fluency-shaping approach. The behaviors to be targeted are easy onset of phonation and continuous phonation. These techniques were chosen because they require an open vocal fold posture and therefore inhibit the production of laryngeal blocks, Patrick's most severe type of disfluency.

Sample Activities

Easy Onset of Phonation

1. Draw a graphic representation of two breath curves, like the ones shown in Figure 9-2. Explain that the first drawing represents the usual pattern of speaking, in which voicing (the dotted line) is initiated at the same time as the onset of exhalation (the solid line). Explain to the client that his attempts to use this pattern often result in complete involuntary closure of the vocal folds (i.e., laryngeal blocks). Introduce the second drawing and tell him that it illustrates an alternative phonation pattern that will help prevent these blocks. Explain that the solid line again represents the point at which inhalation ends and exhalation begins and that the

FIGURE 9–2
Breath curves

FIGURE 9–2
Breath curves

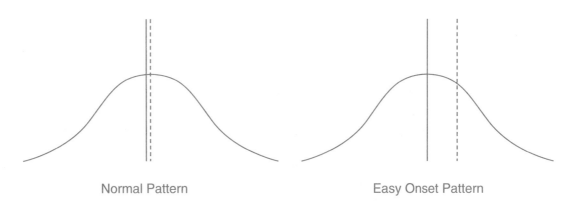

Normal Pattern   Easy Onset Pattern

dotted line has been moved to indicate that his voice should start *after* exhalation has begun. Using the easy onset graph, instruct the client to place his finger at the beginning of the breath curve. Tell him to move his finger slowly along the curve as he inhales. When his finger reaches the solid line, he should begin to exhale slowly and continuously. As his finger reaches the dotted line, the client should *maintain* his open vocal fold posture and smoothly produce an isolated vowel such as /o, a, uh/. Once the client can easily initiate phonation without blocking, the task can progress hierarchically from isolated vowels to h-initial words, and then to more complex units of speech. (See Appendix 9-A for sample phrases, questions, and monologue topics.)

Continuous Phonation

2. Prepare a list of 50 simple three-word phrases (see Appendix 9-A). Introduce the technique of continuous phonation by explaining to the client that he should keep his voice turned on even between words, but without increasing his habitual speech rate. Model use of the technique by first producing an audible yawn, which is characterized by continuous voicing. Produce the yawn a second time, and over-lay a four-word utterance that lasts throughout its duration. Stress the idea that speaking over the yawn results in a smooth, unbroken utterance stream. Instruct the client to produce several audible yawns to heighten his awareness of how it feels to produce smooth, flowing streams of phonation. Read phrases from the prepared list and have the client imitate each stimulus phrase using the yawn technique to emphasize the production of continuous phonation.

Selection of therapy targets using a stuttering modification/management approach. Based on Patrick's fluency profile, the therapy targets are his secondary behaviors, laryngeal blocks, and prolongations of initial sounds. The secondary behaviors were chosen because their bizarre nature tends to invoke severe listener penalty. Patrick's two main disfluency types were selected because both blocks and prolongations interfere significantly with his ability to communicate.

Sample Activities

Desensitization

1. Help the client to generate a list of anxiety-producing speaking situations and arrange them hierarchically from least to most feared. Teach the client a tension reduction procedure such as progressive relaxation (Jacobson, 1938). This technique can be modified specifically for stutterers by using the steps outlined in Table 9-1. Once the client demonstrates the ability to consciously achieve a relaxed state, explain that relaxation will be used to desensitize him to the previously identified feared speaking situations. Beginning with the least feared situation in the hierarchy, instruct the client to use visual imagery to imagine himself in that situation. Tell him to monitor his overall level of muscle tone for any significant increase in tension. Whenever the client identifies an occurrence of excessive tension, he is instructed to employ the relaxation skills learned in progressive relaxation training. Continue to have the client focus on the same speaking situation until he demonstrates the ability to remain relaxed throughout the entire visualization. Once the client can maintain a relaxed state at this level with minimal discernible effort, move to the next situation in the hierarchy. Repeat the visualization-relaxation sequence for each successive entry until the client is effectively desensitized to the thought of all the feared speaking situations in the hierarchy. Once the client can consciously induce a relaxed state, progress to more difficult environments such as including strangers in the therapy session and going outside the clinic setting (e.g., a store or library).

Voluntary Stuttering

2. Introduce the technique of **voluntary stuttering** and the rationale for its use in the treatment process. Explain that this technique requires clients to stutter on purpose and then analyze their own feelings as well as listener reactions. The goal of voluntary stuttering is to reduce/minimize the stutterer's feelings of fear or embarrassment associated with disfluent moments. Model easy repetitions and prolongations for the client during a short conversational interaction. Then instruct the client to produce at least five of these voluntary stutters on nonfeared words during another 3-minute conversation. Provide visual cues (e.g., hand gestures), as necessary, to prompt the client's use of easy repetitions and prolongations. Following the conversation, the client should rank feelings of anxiety on a five-point scale. Once the client is comfortable with this technique in the clinical setting, the task can be implemented gradually in real-world situations with other conversational partners. In addition, the rating scale can be expanded to rank degrees of negative listener reactions.

Freezing

3. Introduce the concept of **freezing,** which involves purposefully extending the moment of stuttering to increase the client's tolerance for and control over core stuttering behaviors. Instruct the client to read aloud lists of short phrases (e.g., those in Appendix 9-A). Explain that when a disfluency occurs, the clinician will signal the client to continue the stutter. The client should maintain the same disfluency pattern (prolongation, repetition, or block) until the clinician signals to release it.

Pull-Outs

4. Obtain a board game suitable for adults that generally requires the production of multiword responses, such as Jeopardy. Explain the rules of the game and inform the client that he will assume the role of contestant. Tell him that each of his responses must contain at least one pseudo or real disfluency, which he will modify using pull-outs. Review this stuttering modification/management technique by reminding the client that whenever he gets stuck on a word, he should (a) stop in the middle of the disfluency; (b) pause to mentally rehearse how it would feel to produce that word fluently; (c) say the word a second time in a smooth, prolonged manner; and (d) complete the rest of the intended utterance without going back to the beginning of the sentence. Provide several opportunities to practice this technique by modeling some disfluencies and pull-outs for him to imitate. Begin the game by instructing the client to choose a topic category and a difficulty level. Read the designated "answer" to which the client must respond in the form of a question that contains a pull-out. Provide the opportunity for the client to produce at least 50 "questions" during the game.

Helpful Hints

1. For each of the activities listed, the difficulty of the task can be manipulated systematically with regard to utterance length using the traditional hierarchy of single words, carrier phrase + word, sentence, two- to four-word sentences, and conversation. Provision of consistent clinician models should be faded gradually until all client responses are spontaneously generated without any model.

2. As therapy progresses, introduce activities that simulate natural speaking situations. For young children, these might include asking for a turn to play with a toy, asking for assistance in completing a puzzle, describing pictures in a book, playing house or tea party, telling stories, and negotiating the rules of a game. For older children and adults, activities may involve talking on the telephone, ordering food at a restaurant, asking for directions, interviewing for a job, and giving presentations in class or at work.

3. Fluency-shaping and stuttering modification/management techniques can be combined within the same therapy session. It is best to begin the session with stuttering modification techniques and then move on to fluency shaping. If implemented in the reverse order, carryover from fluency shaping practice may significantly decrease the number of disfluencies the client produces during the treatment visit. The reduced frequency of stuttering may not provide the client with adequate opportunities to learn and practice stuttering modification/management techniques later in the session.

4. Once the target concepts and techniques have been established in individual sessions, group therapy can be particularly effective for strengthening and refining clients' fluency skills.

5. It is essential for the clinician to monitor her or his reactions to client disfluencies. Even subtle indications of discomfort (e.g., averted eye gaze) may adversely affect the therapeutic relationship between client and clinician.

6. A client's feelings about his stuttering can be monitored over the course of therapy by periodic re-administration of a stuttering attitude checklist (see Form 9-2). Such scales are not intended to be scored quantitatively along a continuum of severity, but rather to provide descriptive information about changes in the client's emotions and attitudes.

7. Families should be encouraged to avoid a conspiracy of silence regarding stuttering. Open acknowledgment and discussion can minimize the feelings of isolation and shame often experienced by individuals who stutter. (Refer to Chapter 11 for additional information on counseling strategies.)

8. Stuttering modification/management therapy frequently results in a noticeable increase in observable disfluencies as the client begins to relinquish habitual avoidance strategies. The focus of counseling at this point is twofold: (a) to help the client understand that this stage of therapy is temporary and (b) to provide consistent and direct support as the client confronts feared speaking situations during this phase.

9. Clinicians should be aware that older students and adolescents (i.e., between approximately 10 and 17 years of age) frequently demonstrate extreme resistance to any type of fluency therapy. Parents may require considerable counseling support to accept the fact that their child may not be emotionally ready to benefit from direct intervention during this period. Clinicians should also reassure parents that willingness to participate in therapy reemerges with increased maturity.

10. Individuals with a long-standing history of severe stuttering often limit their participation in social interactions, resulting in a relative lack of practice with conversational skills in both speaker and listener roles. Clinicians can incorporate pragmatic language goals into the fluency treatment plan in order to facilitate maximal communicative effectiveness.

11. Even if a person who stutters makes no change in the frequency of disfluencies, a significant reduction in the use of postponements and starters (e.g., "uhm," "you know," "well, let me see . . .") can improve the listener's perception of speech.

12. Clinicians should monitor client progress over time and be aware of the difference between a "lapse" (a small slip or mistake) and "relapse" (cessation of newly learned behaviors with a return to previous performance levels).

FORM 9–2 STUTTERING ATTITUDE CHECKLIST

INSTRUCTIONS: Respond to the following by circling "Y" to indicate that "Yes, I agree" or "N" to indicate "No, I do not agree" with each statement. Record your initial reaction rather than analyzing or deliberating over each statement.

1.	Y	N	I often feel that stuttering is my own fault.
2.	Y	N	I find it easy to talk to people in authority such as my teacher or my employer.
3.	Y	N	Sometimes I wonder if I stutter on purpose to get attention.
4.	Y	N	I have more trouble saying some words/sounds than others.
5.	Y	N	Most people think that stutterers are not quite as smart as people who do not stutter.
6.	Y	N	People always seem comfortable when I am talking to them.
7.	Y	N	I think that stuttering is caused by some kind of mental or emotional problem.
8.	Y	N	My stuttering keeps me from doing the kind of work that I would really like to do.
9.	Y	N	I sometimes think that other people are responsible for having caused my stuttering.
10.	Y	N	The way I talk does not embarrass me.
11.	Y	N	Stuttering is my biggest problem.
12.	Y	N	Even when I know the right answer to a question, I often keep silent because of my stuttering.
13.	Y	N	I think speech therapy can help me a great deal.
14.	Y	N	My stuttering would go away if I stopped worrying about it all the time.
15.	Y	N	I feel that I should be able to stop my stuttering without help from anyone else.

SOURCE: Adapted from Andrews, G., & Cutler, J. (1974). Stuttering therapy: The relation between changes in symptom level and attitudes. Journal of Speech and Hearing Disorders, 39(3), 312. ; Cooper, E., & Cooper, C. (2003). Cooper Personalized Fluency Control Therapy for Adolescents and Adults: Clinician's Manual. Austin, TX: Pro-Ed.; and Yaruss, J. S., & Quesal, R. W. (2006). Overall Assessment of the Speaker's Experience of Stuttering (OASES): Documenting multiple outcomes in stuttering treatment. Journal of fluency disorders, 31(2), 90–115.

CONCLUSION

This chapter presented basic information, protocols, and procedures for intervention with fluency disorders at an *introductory* level. This information is intended only as a starting point in the reader's clinical education and training. For more in-depth coverage of this area, the following readings are recommended:

Anderson, J. D., & Conture, E. G. (2004). Sentence-structure priming in young children who do and do not stutter. *Journal of Speech, Language, and Hearing Research, 47*, 552–571.

Bloodstein, O., & Ratner, N. (2008). *A handbook on stuttering* (6th ed.). Clifton Park, NY: Delmar, Cengage Learning.

Guitar, B. (2013). *Stuttering: An integrated approach to its nature and treatment* (3rd ed.). Baltimore, MD: Lippincott Williams & Wilkins.

Manning, W. H. (2010). *Clinical decision making in fluency disorders* (3rd ed.). Clifton Park, NY: Delmar, Cengage Learning.

Yairi, E., & Seery, C. (2014). *Stuttering: Foundations and clinical applications* (2nd ed.). Upper Saddle River, NJ: Pearson Education, Inc.

ADDITIONAL RESOURCES

Pro-Ed
8700 Shoal Creek Boulevard
Austin, TX 78758-9965
Phone: 800-897-3202
Fax: 800-397-7633
Web site: http://www.proedinc.com

50 Great Activities for Children Who Stutter
This practice manual contains 50 activities, most including several possible adaptations. The activities are divided into five categories and include reproducible homework and handouts: Identifying and Exploring Stuttering, Practicing Speech Tools, Learning the Facts, Uncovering Feelings, and Targeting Language and Stuttering Goals.

The Lidcombe Program of Early Stuttering Intervention: A Clinician's Guide
This text is written for clinicians to provide detailed information on the method and implementation of the Lidcombe Program, a parent-conducted, behavioral treatment for stuttering that is designed for children younger than age 6.

Easy Talker: A Fluency Workbook for School-Age Children
For children in grades 3 to 12, this workbook uses a three-step approach for working on and coping with stuttering by focusing on cognition, emotion, and behavior. It incorporates these issues into real-life situations and solutions.

LinguiSystems
3100 Fourth Avenue
P.O. Box 747
East Moline, IL 61244
Phone: 800-776-4332
Fax: 800-577-4555
Web site: www.linguisystems.com

Easy Does It for Fluency: Preschool/Primary and Intermediate Sets
This series provides a manual and a workbook for therapists and students to use during therapy. It provides a direct approach to intervention and addresses the motor, linguistic, and psychosocial aspects of stuttering. The workbook is divided into six levels: getting ready, analyzing, modifying speech production, desensitizing, transferring, and maintaining. The series includes a CD for access to forms, such as parent and teacher letters and home assignments.

The Source for Stuttering and Cluttering
This comprehensive resource for ages 7 to 18 includes all phases of the therapeutic process from assessment through diagnosis and treatment. Tools, tips, activities, and strategies to help develop skills including planning and implementing therapy, providing "real-world" practice, working effectively with parents and teachers, and much more.

Cengage Learning
10650 Toebben Drive
Independence, KY 41051
Phone: 800-354-9706
Fax: 800-487-8488
Web site: http://www.cengage.com

The Child and Adolescent Stuttering Treatment and Activity Resource Guide
This guide provides specific, hands-on activities that can be used in the evaluation of fluency disorders in children. It offers specific decision-making information to help clinicians choose goals to address and gives ideas on activities and strategies that can be used to meet these goals.

Super Duper Publications
P.O. Box 24997
Greenville, SC 29616
Phone: 800-277-8737
Fax: 800-978-7379
Web site: www.superduperinc.com

Working with School-Age Children Who Stutter: Basic Principle Problem Solving
This text is designed to help therapists to problem solve questions and decisions made during stuttering intervention. Case profiles are included to further demonstrate how to apply problem-solving skills to these cases.

Focus on Fluency: A Tool Kit for Creative Therapy and CD-ROM
This kit provides a manual with activities as well as materials for games. Materials include card decks, sentence strips, manipulatives, and game boards. The materials are designed to target the following areas: education, basic communication, desensitization, fluency shaping, and stuttering modification.

Stuttering Foundation of America
1805 Moriah Woods Blvd Suite 3
P.O. Box 11749
Memphis, TN 38111
Phone: 800-992-9392
Fax: 901-761-0484
Web site: www.stutteringhelp.org

Stuttering and Your Child: Help for Parents
Appropriate for viewing in any home, daycare, clinical, or educational setting, this 30-minute video provides parents with up-to-date information about what stuttering is, what is thought to cause and worsen childhood stuttering, and what parents can do to help their child.

Effective Counseling in Stuttering Therapy
This book helps the clinician have a better understanding of the counseling aspect of therapy and suggests ways to use it effectively.

The School-Age Child Who Stutters: Working Effectively with Attitudes and Emotions
This resource focuses on assessing and treating feelings/beliefs in school-age children who stutter. It contains practical, concrete ideas for documentation and strategies to achieve change.

The Power R Game!
This resource uses a game-board format to change attitudes and feelings about stuttering. Contains 94 game cards with 564 statements for directing discussions about stuttering and an additional 50 cards containing diversion scenarios. The second edition provides an updated manual with additional resources and references.

Miscellaneous
Stuttering Home Page – http://www.mnsu.edu/comdis/kuster
This is a comprehensive Web site for individuals who stutter and the professionals who work with them. The site includes information about research and treatment as well as support organizations and conferences.

APPENDIX 9-A

SAMPLE PHRASES, QUESTIONS, AND MONOLOGUES

PHRASES
LIST 1

1.	on his doorstep	9.	cloak and dagger
2.	those turnip greens	10.	be on time
3.	broom and dustpan	11.	in a sand trap
4.	brand new bicycle	12.	that steamy pot
5.	a price tag	13.	in a candy store
6.	an August day	14.	cats and dogs
7.	an afternoon snack	15.	old spark plug
8.	gas station pump	16.	salt and pepper

LIST 2

With "the" in linking position

1.	over the rainbow	9.	melt the butter
2.	behind the tree	10.	in the birdhouse
3.	in the hall	11.	up the hill
4.	over the bridge	12.	close the lid
5.	beside the pool	13.	climb the ladder
6.	in the meadow	14.	dial the phone
7.	ring the doorbell	15.	ride the subway
8.	tour the museum	16.	near the table

(continues)

LIST 3

Two adjacent alveolar phonemes in linking positions

1. in a slump
2. smell an aroma
3. this smeary ink
4. smaller and smaller
5. give a speech
6. stay a while
7. swear under oath
8. all eyes and ears
9. a joyous smile
10. be a small fry
11. spin around
12. sugar and spice
13. clean a stain
14. swam in a race
15. sweltering weather
16. sweep the porch and smoke a cigar

QUESTIONS

What country is shaped like a boot?	(Italy)
What Chinese medical procedure uses needles?	(acupuncture)
Who won the Civil War?	(Union Army)
What are the ditches around castles called?	(moats)
What bird is the emblem of the United States?	(bald eagle)
Who is said to have shot Abraham Lincoln?	(John W. Booth)
In the United States, who takes command if the president dies or leaves office?	(vice president)
What were the last two states admitted to the United States?	(Hawaii and Alaska)
Why did the Pilgrims come to North America?	(freedom of religion)
What book gives synonyms?	(thesaurus)
Who fought in the Gulf War?	(U.S. and Iraq)
What kind of war is fought between people who live in the same country?	(civil war)
Which president was involved in the Watergate scandal?	(Nixon)
Who wrote Hamlet and Macbeth?	(Shakespeare)
What rock star is referred to as "The Boss"?	(Bruce Springsteen)

(continues)

MONOLOGUE TOPICS

Tell me about your summer vacation.

Tell me about the last movie you saw.

What do you like most about your job?

What do you like least about your job?

Tell me about your brothers and sisters.

If you won $10 million in the lottery, what would you do with it?

How would you change things if you had your boss's job?

If you could go anywhere in the world this afternoon, where would it be?

What additional language would you most like to learn and why?

If you could relive any year in your life, which would it be and why?

If you could redesign an automobile, what things would you change?

If you were able to read another person's mind, would you do it?

If you could have three wishes come true, what would they be?

If you were president of the United States, what is the first law you would make?

If you had to choose between being blind or deaf, which would you choose and

why?

CHAPTER 10

This chapter will address impairments in phonation (traditionally referred to as voice disorders) as well as alaryngeal speech resulting from surgical removal of the larynx. To competently diagnose and treat phonatory disorders, clinicians must be well acquainted with the mechanisms involved in normal voice production. The reader is referred to Aronson and Bless (2009); Boone, McFarlane, Von Berg, & Zraick (2013); Seikel, King, and Drumright (2010); and Zemlin (1998) for detailed discussions of laryngeal anatomy and physiology.

VOICE DISORDERS

A voice disorder is a disturbance of pitch, loudness, or quality in relation to an individual's age, gender, and cultural background. Voice disorders are identified on the basis of a listener's judgment rather than by any absolute or standardized criteria for normal voice production. The term **dysphonia** refers to any deviation in phonation, whereas **aphonia** is a term used to indicate the absence of audible phonation.

Appendix D provides a schematic of the vocal tract structures relevant to phonation. In the normal production of voice, the airstream is generated by the lungs. As the air passes through the larynx, the vocal folds are set into vibratory motion, which results in the production of sound (i.e., phonation). The sound continues to travel through the upper vocal tract and is modified by the resonating characteristics of the pharynx and oral and nasal cavities. Loudness and pitch are controlled by different physiologic mechanisms. Loudness is the perceptual counterpart to amplitude (the height of a sound wave). It is determined primarily by the amount and speed of subglottal air pressure. A voice becomes louder when there is an increase in the volume and velocity of the airstream as it passes through the glottis. Pitch is the perceptual correlate of frequency (number of vibratory closing and opening cycles per second). The relative length and thickness of the vocal folds determine voice pitch. The voice becomes higher in pitch when the vocal folds are elongated with a concurrent decrease in mass and an increase in elasticity of the vocal folds. The pitch most frequently used by an individual speaker during spontaneous speech production is known as **fundamental frequency** or **habitual pitch.** The fundamental frequencies used by normal speakers of different ages and genders are shown in Table 10-1.

Normal voices function in at least three pitch ranges or **voice registers.** These are the **pulse** (the lower range of fundamental frequencies), **modal** (the range of fundamental frequencies used in normal speech), and **loft** (the highest range of fundamental frequencies) registers. Each register is characterized by a distinct pattern of vocal fold approximation. The vocal folds vibrate in the same manner throughout a given pitch range; the pattern of vibration changes as the maximum limit for the range is exceeded and a new voice register is entered.

Voice quality is difficult to define but can be described as the aspects of a voice that differentiate it from another voice at identical pitch and loudness levels. It is regulated, at least in part, by the manner and force with which the vocal folds approximate one another. For example, if the folds are loosely approximated during phonation, the resulting voice quality is generally labeled as breathy, whereas overly tense vocal fold approximation is generally associated with a harsh, strained voice quality.

Resonance is another factor that affects voice production. The sound generated at the laryngeal level is amplified or filtered as it passes through the resonating cavities of

TABLE 10–1

Normal Fundamental Frequencies for Males and Females

	Fundamental Frequency (Hz)	
Age in years	Male	Female
1–2	400	400
3	300	300
4	285	285
5–7	265	265
8	250	255
9–13	235	240
14	175	225
15	165	220
16	150	215
17	135	210
18	125	205
20–29	120	227
30–39	112	214
40–49	107	214
50–59	118	214
60–69	112	209
70–79	132	206
80–89	146	197

SOURCE: Adapted from Aronson (1990) Aronson, A. E., & Bless, D. (2009). Clinical voice disorders (4th ed.). New York: Thieme Medical Publishers; Hollien and Shipp (1972) Hollien, H., & Shipp, T. (1972). Speaking fundamental frequency and chronologic age in males. Journal of Speech and Hearing Research, 15, 155–159; Kelley (1977) Kelley, A. (1977). Fundamental frequency measurements of female voices from twenty to ninety years of age. Unpublished manuscript, University of North Carolina at Greensboro; Wilson (1987) Wilson, D. K. (1987). Voice problems of children (3rd ed.). Baltimore, MD: Williams and Wilkins.

the upper vocal tract (i.e., pharynx, oral and nasal cavities). Vocal resonance can be affected by a variety of neurological and structural factors. Information regarding voice symptoms and resonance problems associated with various kinds of dysarthrias was discussed in Chapter 7; resonance problems that accompany cleft palate were described in Chapter 3.

The incidence of voice disorders is not well documented. Some studies suggest that they occur in approximately 3% to 9% of the general population including children and adults (Senturia & Wilson, 1968; Silverman & Zimmer, 1975; Verdolini, 1998, 2000; Yairi, Currin, Bulian, & Yairi, 1974). A recent epidemiologic study investigating voice disorders in adults estimated the prevalence of voice disorders at approximately 7% of this population (Roy et al., 2005). The percentage of adults reporting a past history of voice disorders is higher, around approximately 30%, reflecting the typically transient nature of voice disorders (Roy, Merrill, Gray, & Smith, 2005).

Classification of Voice Disorders

Traditionally, voice disorders have been classified as either organic or functional (Aronson, 1990; Boone, McFarlane, Von Berg, & Zraick, 2013). **Organic** voice disorders result from pathology or disease that affects the anatomy or physiology of the larynx and other regions of the vocal tract. **Functional** voice disorders are dysphonias related to vocal abuse/misuse or psychogenic factors in the absence of an identifiable physical etiology. The distinction between these two diagnostic categories is not always clear. For example, a pattern of long-term vocal abuse may eventually lead to organic pathology of the vocal folds. The most common voice disorders are functional in nature and involve faulty habits of vocal usage (Boone et al., 2013). However, several organic etiologies have a significant impact on voice production.

The speech-language pathologist (SLP) should be familiar with the range of possible organic and functional etiologies and their implications for treatment planning. Table 10-2 lists the most common organic and functional voice problems.

Organic. Many organic factors alter the mass of vocal folds and result in lowered pitch, decreased loudness, and a breathy, hoarse voice quality. These alterations affect the shape, the mobility, and/or the muscular tension of the vocal folds. Lower pitch is a result of the inability of the vocal folds to be lengthened and thinned. Reduced loudness and a breathy, hoarse voice quality will occur if the folds cannot achieve adequate closure (adduction). Examples of these organic factors include the following:

- **Edema** (swelling) related to **laryngitis** (inflammation of the folds and other regions of the larynx, usually caused by bacterial infection)
- Mass lesions such as **tumors,** large **granulomas,** and **papillomas**
- **Neurologic** or **endocrine disorders** (e.g., degenerative diseases such as Parkinsonism and hypothyroidism)
- **Laryngeal webs** (membranes that extend from one vocal fold to the other and partially occlude the airway)
- **Vocal fold paralysis** due to impairment in the recurrent or superior laryngeal nerves that innervate the larynx

TABLE 10–2
Organic and Functional Voice Problems

Organic	Functional
Vocal fold paralysis	Abuse/misuse
Laryngeal webs	Vocal nodules
Papilloma	Contact ulcers
Edema	Ventricular dysphonia
Tumor	Psychogenic
Granuloma	Conversion dysphonia
Neurologic/endocrine disease	Mutational falsetto
Spasmodic dysphonia*	

*Several varieties have been described; etiology is not known.

Functional. Functional voice disorders arise from faulty voice usage or psychogenic factors. Symptoms range from a breathy, whispered voice to a strained, tight voice with inappropriate loudness and pitch.

Vocal abuse/misuse is directly related to excessive muscle tension (i.e., laryngeal hyperfunction). In laryngeal hyperfunction, the pattern of vocal fold closure is abrupt and forceful. The most common types of abuse/misuse include shouting, screaming, and excessive talking as well as excessive coughing or throat clearing. Initiation of phonation is accomplished by **hard glottal attack,** which is characterized by tight glottal closure, increased subglottal air pressure, and explosive abduction (opening) of the folds. Consistent use of faulty patterns can result in pathology (e.g., chronic laryngitis, vocal nodules, or contact ulcers). **Vocal nodules** are benign, whitish protuberances that occur at the junction of the anterior and middle thirds of the vocal folds, the area of maximum impact during vocal fold closure. These callus-like formations prevent complete adduction of the folds and result in a lower pitch and breathy, hoarse voice quality. **Contact ulcers** are benign, bilateral, sore-like lesions on the posterior third of the vocal folds, caused by habitual use of hard glottal attacks and excessively low pitch. Symptoms include hoarseness and laryngeal pain. Another example of vocal misuse is **ventricular dysphonia.** This disorder involves the use of the ventricular folds (false vocal folds) as the primary source of phonation, while the true folds are held in an abducted position.

Psychogenic voice disorders arise from emotional or mental factors such as anxiety, depression, or personality disturbance that interfere with voluntary control over voice production (Aronson, 1990). These disorders may develop subsequent to an occurrence of physiologic changes in the larynx, such as laryngitis, and persist long after the physical symptoms have disappeared. Two primary examples of psychogenic voice disorders are conversion dysphonias and mutational falsetto. **Conversion dysphonias** are the physical manifestations of psychological conflict and range in severity from mild hoarseness to whispering to complete absence of voice (i.e., dysphonia → aphonia → mutism). A **mutational falsetto** is characterized by the continued use of a higher-pitched childhood voice into adolescence and adulthood in the presence of a normal laryngeal system. This condition is seen mainly in males and results in a voice that is high pitched, breathy, hoarse, and gives the overall impression of immaturity.

Spasmodic dysphonia (SD) is a voice disorder that resists easy classification. Several different types of these dysphonias have been described, some of which are considered organic and others functional in origin (Aronson & Bless, 2009; Stemple, Glaze, & Klaben, 2000). However, there is mounting evidence of an underlying neurologic etiology for all types. This growing consensus suggests that SD is a focal dystonia, a condition characterized by involuntary movement in an isolated body part. These abnormal movement patterns occur predominantly during purposeful tasks such as speech and may not affect reflexive functions such as coughing, laughing, or sneezing. This disorder involves severe spasmodic movements of the vocal folds that interrupt the normal adduction-abduction cycle of phonation. The disorder is traditionally divided into two main categories: **adductor spasmodic dysphonia** and **abductor spasmodic dysphonia,** depending on when the vocal fold spasms occur. In the more common adductor type, glottal closure is so tight that the vocal folds cannot vibrate in the usual sustained fashion. This overadduction results in a voice that can be described as hoarse, strained, and staccato. It is accompanied by periodic cessation in phonation (phonation breaks) and sudden, unpredictable changes in pitch (pitch breaks). Abductor spasmodic dysphonia is less common than the adductor type and is characterized by excessive and spasmodic opening of the vocal folds during phonation. This uncontrolled abduction allows a great deal of unphonated air to pass through the larynx, causing a breathy voice quality.

There is a distinct lack of research data regarding prognostic indicators related to voice disorders. The same factors generally associated with improvement of any communication disorder can also be applied to individuals with vocal abnormalities. A favorable outcome is generally associated with structural adequacy of the speech production mechanism with little or no organic impairment, a high degree of client motivation and cooperation, and a client's ability to discriminate and self-monitor target behavior.

Treatment Efficacy/Evidence-Based Practice

Ramig and Verdolini (1998) provided a comprehensive summary of available data on treatment efficacy for voice disorders. They reviewed group and single-subject experimental designs, retrospective analyses, case studies, and program evaluation data. Their overall conclusion was that voice treatment is effective for both functional and organic voice disorders. Their analysis also resulted in several additional conclusions:

- Disorders of vocal misuse and hyperfunction can be effectively treated with a variety of intervention techniques, including biofeedback of laryngeal muscle activity, progressive relaxation, yawn-sigh procedure, and vocal intensity reduction.

- Voice therapy significantly reduces the recurrence of vocal nodules after surgical removal. (See also McCrory [2001], Speyer et al. [2002].)

- Voice therapy is effective in reducing or eliminating contact ulcers for most individuals.

- Lee Silverman Voice Treatment (LSVT) successfully increases vocal fold adduction in individuals with Parkinson's disease. (See also Ramig et al. [2001].)

- A combination of voice therapy and botulinum toxin (Botox®) injection significantly improves laryngeal function for clients with spasmodic dysphonia.

Additional treatment efficacy data have been provided by several investigators and are highlighted below:

- Boutsen, Cannito, Taylor, and Bender (2002) conducted a meta-analysis of efficacy research that showed an overall moderate improvement as a result of Botox® treatment, especially for adductor spasmodic dysphonia. However, they caution that a great deal of variability exists among clients, measurements, and treatment conditions.

- Voice production therapy may be more effective than vocal hygiene education in addressing adults' perceptions of severity levels of their own vocal impairment (Behrman, Rutledge, Hembree, & Sheridan, 2008).

- Vocal amplification has been found to be an effective treatment alternative for voice disorders in adults (Roy et al., 2002, 2003).

- Advances in technological measurement of voice characteristics (e.g., vibratory patterns in young children's vocal folds, videostroboscopic endoscopy, and vocal fold histopathology) are likely to significantly influence future treatment efficacy research (Hooper, 2004).

Additional studies have been conducted to investigate evidence-based practice (EBP) for specific voice disorders and conditions. Misono and Merati (2012) investigated several treatments for unilateral vocal fold paralysis and found evidence supporting the use of laryngeal surgery and/or injections to the larynx over the use of laryngeal electromyography.

A recent systematic review of the literature on EBP and voice assessment was conducted by Roy et al. (2013). Although one of the main findings was that there is a need for further research on EBP for voice assessments, the authors made several recommendations based on the current research:

- Laryngeal-based imaging measures (e.g., endoscopy) are recommended as a primary means of assessment due to the objective nature of these measurements.

- Subjective assessments, such as auditory-perceptual measures, are used more frequently by SLPs and can provide beneficial supplemental information about the nature of a voice disorder as well as recommendations for therapy.

TREATMENT FOR VOICE DISORDERS

The goal of treatment for voice disorders is to help a client produce a voice of the best possible pitch, loudness, and quality in relation to the individual's age and gender within the context of his or her cultural and linguistic background. There are three main approaches to voice treatment: (1) medical, (2) environmental, and (3) behavioral. Medical interventions include surgery, medication, and radiation (e.g., removal of vocal fold polyps). Environmental strategies involve modifying a client's daily surroundings or helping a client adjust to the vocal demands of his or her environment (e.g., suggesting the use of a microphone or visual communication system for a client employed in a noisy workplace). Behavioral strategies (also referred to as symptomatic voice therapy) consist of intervention techniques designed to modify specific vocal symptoms such as hoarseness, breathiness, and monoloudness (Casper & Murry, 2000; Stemple et al., 2000).

The approach to intervention for some organic voice disorders is strictly medical. For example, papillomas (wartlike growths on the inner margin of the vocal folds) are effectively treated only through surgical removal. Other organic disorders are best treated through a combination of medical and behavioral therapies. For instance, treatment for a neurological disorder such as Parkinson's disease generally consists of medications as well as symptomatic voice therapy. Functional voice disorders are usually treated effectively with voice therapy alone.

Numerous intervention techniques for voice disorders have been described in the literature. Certain approaches are applicable to any voice disorder regardless of symptomatology or etiology. These include the following:

- *Listening skills:* These techniques are used to increase the client's awareness of his or her vocal behaviors. The clinician demonstrates and contrasts appropriate and inappropriate vocal behaviors. The client is asked to identify and discriminate between the two in live and recorded samples.

- *Respiratory control:* These strategies are used to optimize respiratory support for voice production. Attention is given to posture, breathing patterns, and expiratory control for phonation. The client may be asked to prolong phonation for as long as possible at a variety of different pitch and intensity levels.

- *Vocal rest:* Reduction or elimination of phonation is sometimes recommended to limit laryngeal irritation and to permit the vocal folds to recover from surgery or misuse. A client may be asked to modify or totally refrain from talking for a specified amount of time (usually 4 days to 2 weeks). Individuals most likely to be placed on vocal rest have (1) fluid-filled lesions that may rupture (e.g., cysts), (2) vascular conditions such as hematoma, or (3) just undergone laryngeal surgery. The strategy of complete voice rest is highly controversial with regard to its value and practicality.

Intervention Techniques

This section is devoted to a discussion of therapy techniques associated with specific voice abnormalities. Although the organic versus functional paradigm was appropriate for a description of voice disorder classification, we find it clinically more useful to organize treatment information according to the following four categories: vocal hyperfunction, vocal hypofunction, psychogenic disorders, and spastic dysphonias.

Vocal Hyperfunction. This category includes any voice disorder characterized by excessive laryngeal tension or overly forceful closure of the vocal folds. It consists primarily of dysphonias related to vocal abuse or misuse. The majority of voice problems encountered by speech-language pathologists are related to vocal hyperfunction caused by vocal abuse or misuse. The following techniques are useful in treating symptoms associated with laryngeal hyperfunction (Boone et al., 2013; Prater, Swift, Deem, & Miller, 1999). The overall aims of these techniques are (1) to reduce muscular tension and (2) to eliminate abusive vocal behaviors.

Relaxing Muscles. Techniques can be directed specifically to the vocal tract musculature or toward relaxation of the whole body. One method of tension reduction for the muscles of the larynx is the adoption of an open-mouth posture during speech, because muscular tension in the jaw area is usually related to tension in the laryngeal musculature. The client visualizes the contrasting mouth postures of a ventriloquist and an opera singer. The client then practices speaking alternately with a closed-mouth and open-mouth posture in front of a mirror. Other vocal relaxation techniques include laryngeal massage and head and neck rolls. (For step-by-step instructions, see Prater, Swift, Deem, and Miller [1999].) One of the most common approaches to tension reduction for the whole body is progressive relaxation, which was described in detail in Chapter 7. Muscle relaxation typically is used in conjunction with one or more of the other therapy techniques in this category.

Reducing Loudness. The client reads short phrases or sentences aloud, using a different intensity level for each one. A lower intensity level that is optimal for the client is identified (described by Boone et al. [2013] as the voice to use when not wanting to waken a sleeping person). This quieter voice is practiced in drills that require reading utterances of increasing length (i.e., single sentences → multiple sentences → short paragraphs).

Softening Glottal Attacks. Several techniques can be used to soften hard glottal attacks:

- *Yawn-sigh:* The client yawns in a natural manner and phonates a gentle sigh on exhalation. Once relaxed phonation is mastered, the client produces words on the exhalation. Begin with single words that begin with /h/ or a vowel and progress to four to five words per exhalation. The eventual goal is for the client to induce easy phonation by imagining the relaxed oral feeling associated with the yawn-sigh approach.

- *Chewing:* The client chews in a natural but exaggerated manner while simultaneously producing phonation (Froeschels, 1952). Start with vowels and gradually increase the length of the utterance on successive exhalations. The client practices variations in pitch and loudness levels while chewing/phonating. Relaxation of laryngeal musculature should be maintained.

- *Easy onset:* The client produces syllable combinations of /h/ + vowel to practice relaxed initiation of phonation. This phoneme sequence establishes airflow through the glottis prior to phonation. Gradually lengthen utterances to polysyllabic words and short sentences. Expand the drills to include other voiceless fricatives and other sound classes.

- *Chant talk:* The client listens to and imitates a recording of chanting, a speaking pattern characterized by the production of words in a continuous unbroken monotone, prolongation of vowels, and lack of syllable stress (e.g., Gregorian chant). Once this speaking style can be reliably produced, the client reads aloud for 20-second periods, alternating between habitual voice and chant talk.

Adjusting Pitch. A habitual pitch that requires the least amount of physical effort and tension results in the most pleasant-sounding voice. The client produces "um-hum" with a closed-mouth posture using a rising inflection. This vocalization should simulate the conversational device that is commonly used to signal agreement with a partner's statement. Once identified, a pitch pipe can be used to provide a model for the client to imitate. Begin with isolated vowels and progress to single words, sentences, and paragraphs. Instrumentation (e.g., Visi-Pitch II from Kay Elemetrics Corporation) can be used to provide visual feedback, which helps the client maintain appropriate pitch use for longer periods of time.

Adjusting Pitch as Related to Transgender Voice. Although speech sound articulation, pragmatic language skills, and nonverbal communication are recognized as potential targets of intervention with transgender/transsexual individuals, the major focus with this client group tends to be vocal behaviors. Several aspects of voice production are generally considered to differ between males and females. Specifically, fundamental frequency range (particularly maximal fundamental frequency), average fundamental frequency, formant frequencies, and average intensity are considered important to listeners' perceptions of gender. Clients who have undergone transgender procedures have several options for altering their voice, if desired. Voice therapy can target alterationof pitch and/or register to more closely approximate the vocal attributes of the new gender. Biofeedback instruments can be beneficial in assisting clients to achieve a targeted pitch and register. Phonosurgical procedures also are available to alter the structural and mechanical components of the vocal tract. See the following sources for more information on vocal behaviors in this population: Oates and Dacakis (1997); Rammage, Morrison, and Nichol (2001); Freidenberg (2002); Pickering and Baker (2012); and Adler, Hirsch, and Mordaunt (2012).

Phonating on Inhalation. The client inhales slowly while attempting to phonate a hum as modeled by the clinician. Once this behavior is reliably established, the client attempts to phonate on exhalation and match the pitch produced during the previous inhalation.

Gradually, phonation is produced only on exhalation and at a wide variety of pitch levels. This technique is often used with cases of ventricular phonation because phonating on inhalation requires the use of the true vocal folds rather than the false folds.

Lessac-Madsen Resonant Voice Therapy (LMRVT). This treatment approach can be used to address both vocal hyperfunction and hypofunction (see the following section on hypofunction). Treatment protocols begin with stretching exercises to position the vocal folds slightly ajar. Clients then perform syllable and sentence level tasks while maintaining this vocal fold position. The aim of LMRVT is to produce a strong voice with the minimal amount of intra-oral pressure needed. LMRVT is also preventative in nature by tailoring vocal hygiene protocols to each client in order to promote the use of treatment exercises and target behaviors in the client's habitual speech pattern. See Seligman (2005) for more information on this technique.

Flow Phonation. This treatment method focuses on airflow management as a means of retraining a natural airflow for speech. Clients that have developed maladaptive breathing and/or muscle contraction patterns during speech benefit from flow phonation techniques. Vocal stretching is one of the main components used to retrain natural phonation. The client works from controlled exhalations to adding in voicing to his or her phonation until airflow for speech sounds can be sustained and produced in a balanced manner. See Gartner-Schmidt (2006) for more information on this technique.

Manual Circumlaryngeal Techniques. In this approach, the speech-language pathologist uses his or her hand to massage and/or to reposture the larynx. Several maneuvers can be used to return the larynx to a more neutral position. The client is directed to phonate when the larynx is in a more neutral position to promote developing awareness of correct vocal positioning and target vocal production behaviors. This approach is used primarily with clients who have muscular tension or organic lesions that have resulted in maladaptive vocal habits. See Gartner-Schmidt (2006) for more information on this technique.

Cough Suppression. In cases of a refractory chronic cough, a speech-language pathologist can provide education as well as treatment to patients to reduce cough frequency. Treatment typically focuses on vocal hygiene and techniques to minimize the cough reflux (e.g., cough suppression swallow and breathing patterns). This approach is non-pharmacological and typically requires only a few sessions of treatment to educate the patient for home practice and implementation of methods. See Ryan, Vertigan, Bone, and Gibson (2010) for more information on this technique.

Vocal Hypofunction. This category refers to voice disorders characterized by incomplete closure of the vocal folds. It involves dysphonias resulting from neurologic disorders such as unilateral vocal fold paralysis, myasthenia gravis, and muscular dystrophy. The techniques described next are useful in treating symptoms associated with laryngeal hypofunction (Boone et. al, 2013). The main purposes of these techniques are to achieve firmer closure of the vocal folds and/or compensatory movements (e.g., one fold moves across the midline to compensate for the other in unilateral paralysis).

Pushing/Pulling. The client engages in forceful muscular activity that elicits reflexive glottal closure (Froeschels, Kastein, & Weiss, 1955). These activities should be used for short periods of time and discontinued as soon as the client demonstrates an awareness of the "feel" of tighter vocal fold closure. Care must be taken to ensure that an overly hyperfunctional behavior does not occur. In one method, the client is seated in a chair, firmly grasps each side of the seat, and pushes downward with both arms while producing a vowel such as /a/. A variation of this activity requires the client to raise both fists to the level of the chest with the elbows extended outward. The client then pushes both fists downward forcefully while producing a vowel sound as loudly as possible. A third method requires the client to link the fingers of both hands together at the level of the chest and to pull in opposite directions while producing a vowel such as /a/. Length of phonation should be gradually increased while maintaining the improved loudness and voice quality.

Increasing Loudness. In some cases, loudness can be improved by establishing a more efficient respiratory pattern (i.e., abdominal-diaphragmatic breathing). The client lies supine and places one hand on the chest and the other on the abdomen. The client inhales through the nose and closely monitors movement of the abdomen (not the chest) while exhaling through the mouth. During subsequent respiratory cycles, the client deliberately relaxes the abdominal muscles during inhalation and tenses the same muscles during exhalation. Once this respiratory pattern has been established, the client begins to produce prolonged vowels on exhalation at an increased level of loudness. Progress occurs from vowels to syllables to words to phrases to sentences. Vocal loudness also can be addressed through the use of the pushing/pulling techniques described in the previous section.

A programmed approach to remediating reduced vocal loudness in clients with Parkinson's disease is the **Lee Silverman Voice Treatment** (Neel, 2009; Ramig, 1998; Ramig, Pawlas, & Countryman, 1995; Ward, Theodoros, Murdoch, & Silburn, 2000). This approach utilizes high-phonatory-effort tasks to increase vocal fold adduction and respiratory support. The goal of this program is to improve functional speech intelligibility to a realistic level. A minimum of 16 intensive individual sessions within a 4-week period is required regardless of a client's severity of impairment. The program also provides specific guidelines for post-treatment maintenance and reevaluation.

Paradoxical Vocal Fold Dysfunction. There are several theories as to the etiology of paradoxical vocal fold dysfunction, a disorder characterized by aberrant adducting movements of the vocal folds during inhalation and/or exhalation. Possible etiologies include psychological disorders, neurologic factors, possible laryngeal dystonia, and irritation of the laryngeal tract (Mathers-Schmidt, 2001). Patients with paradoxical vocal fold dysfunction often present with asthma-like symptoms such as stridor, dyspnea, and feelings of tightness in the chest or larynx. The SLP serves as part of a team along with other domains, such psychologists and otolaryngologists, in order to differentially diagnosis this disorder and to determine contributing factors in order to inform the rehabilitation process.

Respiratory Retraining. These techniques are used with clients with paradoxical vocal fold movement disorders. Gartner-Schmidt (2006) recommends making respiration the main focus of therapy, with breathing rhythm used to help retrain clients with a natural breathing pattern to support phonation and speech. Clients perform breathing exercises that require inhalation of air through the nose, passage through a relaxed oral cavity, and then exhalation through a slightly tense labial posture (e.g., the articulatory placement for /s/).

Psychogenic. This category involves voice disorders that arise from psychological or emotional factors. Symptoms associated with psychogenic voice disorders range from mild dysphonia to complete loss of voice and can involve pitch, loudness, or voice quality. The overall purpose of treatment is to reestablish a client's access to his or her own normal voice. This purpose is generally achieved through three sequential stages of intervention (Aronson, 1990):

1. Client education. The clinician discusses available medical reports with the client and emphasizes that the client's laryngeal anatomy and physiology are intact and, more important, that the client is capable of producing a normal voice.

2. Symptomatic therapy. The clinician attempts to elicit normal phonation through vegetative vocal functions. The client produces a variety of these sounds (i.e., coughing, throat clearing, laughing, gargling, humming). When normal phonation occurs during one of the vegetative behaviors, it should be brought to the client's attention immediately. The client then extends this normal voice into vowels, single words, and sentences. For clients with mutational falsetto, inhalation phonation (as described in the section on hyperfunction) also may be an effective technique for eliciting normal phonation.

3. Referral. The clinician considers the possibility that voice intervention alone is insufficient to resolve a client's underlying emotional problems and may counsel the client to seek psychological or psychiatric services as needed.

Spasmodic Dysphonia. This category encompasses two distinct types of voice disorders characterized by spasms that result in abnormalities of vocal fold approximation. Adductor spasmodic dysphonia has been treated with a variety of surgical and medical interventions. In general, the surgical approach focuses on removal of a small segment (resection) of the recurrent laryngeal nerve to improve vocal fold function (Berke et al., 1999; Dedo & Izdebski, 1983). More recently, injection of **botulinum toxin (Botox®)** into the vocal folds has become the treatment of choice for this type of dysphonia (Blitzer, Brin, Fahn, & Lovelace, 1988; Boutsen et al., 2002; Langeveld et al., 2001; Sulica, 2004; Sulica, Blitzer, Brin, & Stewart, 2003). Botox® injections are also used to treat the abductor type of SD, although with somewhat less effectiveness. According to Blitzer, Brin, and Stewart's (1998) retrospective analysis, adductor SD patients demonstrated approximately 90% normal vocal function over an average of 15 weeks, whereas adductor SD patients had an average benefit of almost 67% normal function over an average of 10.5 weeks.

Spasmodic dysphonias are also treated with symptomatic voice techniques, although voice therapy alone usually does not result in significantly improved voice production. These techniques are similar to those employed for treating laryngeal hyperfunction/hypofunction and are generally used on a trial basis before and after medical intervention. The overall goal of symptomatic voice therapy is to help the client achieve the best possible voice, with the recognition that normal voice quality may never be regained.

Premedical Therapy Techniques. Techniques aimed at reducing laryngeal muscle tension are employed, including chewing, chant talk, yawn-sigh, and easy onset. (See the section on vocal hyperfunction for a description of these techniques.)

Postmedical Therapy Techniques. Techniques aimed at decreasing breathiness, increasing loudness, and establishing a new pitch are employed, including pushing/pulling and abdominal-diaphragmatic breathing. (See the section on vocal hypofunction for a description of these techniques.)

Example Profiles

The following three profiles represent typical dysphonias of children and adults with different types of voice disorders. These examples have been designed to illustrate the selection of intervention targets as well as specific therapy activities and materials. Most of the chosen activities are easily implemented in either individual or group therapy settings.

Brian, an 8-year-old male, presents with a hoarse, low-pitched voice. Otolaryngological findings reveal prominent bilateral vocal nodules approximately 2 mm in size. Both vocal folds are swollen and irritated. Case history information obtained from his parents indicates that Brian is an extremely active child whose play activities are frequently accompanied by shouting and screaming. According to his mom, "Brian talks incessantly, from the moment he wakes up until it's time for bed." She also reported that Brian likes to make "sound effects," including car noises and monster voices. Brian shows no awareness of the dysphonic nature of his voice. Both Brian's parents and his classroom teacher noted that his voice quality deteriorates as the day progresses.

Selection of therapy targets. The overall communicative profile demonstrated by Brian is consistent with a dysphonia caused by vocal abuse/misuse. Based on his age and the pattern of hyperfunctional vocal behaviors, therapy will focus on the following areas: (1) identification of vocally abusive situations, (2) establishment of the target voice, and (3) elimination of the abusive behaviors. Most children with voice disorders do not recognize that a problem exists. Therefore, an important aspect of this approach is to facilitate an awareness in Brian, his parents, and his teacher of what constitutes abusive vocal behaviors, as well as the situations in which these behaviors most frequently occur.

Sample Activities

Identify Situations Associated with Vocal Abuse

1. Observe Brian in home, play, and school settings for specified units of time (e.g., 15 minutes, recess period, and so on) to identify instances of hyperfunctional vocal behavior. Use this information to establish baselines regarding the type, context, and frequency of vocal abuse/misuse. These observations should be conducted on at least three occasions to ensure gathering of a representative sample of Brian's

communicative behavior. Interviews with family members and others also can yield useful information regarding Brian's habitual vocal patterns. Develop a list of his most common types of vocal abuse/misuse and the situations in which they most frequently occur. Review this list with Brian and discuss how these behaviors have bothered his voice.

Establishing the Target Voice

2. Help Brian generate a list of 25 of his "likes" and "dislikes." Likes might include soccer, computer games, ping-pong, and playing with his best friend, Ian. Dislikes might include homework, broccoli, brushing his teeth, going shopping, and cleaning his room. Gather pictures or photographs depicting each item and tack the positive and negative items to separate walls. Model an excessively loud voice and a more desirable quiet voice until Brian can easily imitate each pattern. Explain to Brian that he will talk about the pictured items, alternately using his old loud voice and the new quieter voice. Instruct Brian to select one picture from the negative set and produce it along with the carrier phrase, "I don't like ___ ," using his old voice pattern. Then ask him to choose an item from the positive group and say the carrier phrase, "I do like ___ ," using the target voice. Encourage Brian to pay attention to the differences in how these voices sound and feel. Continue to compare and contrast the desirable and undesirable loudness levels by repeating this alternating sequence until all items have been named.

Elimination of Abusive Vocal Behaviors

3. Provide Brian with a tally card or a simple behavioral response counter. Instruct Brian to record each time he catches himself yelling during a given time period. The clinician should specify time periods in which there will likely be at least 10 instances of the abusive behavior (e.g., recess). Have Brian tally the number of recorded behaviors at the end of each day and plot the number on a simple graph like the one shown in Form 10-1. As Brian's ability to accurately identify instances of vocal abuses improves, the specified time frame for self-monitoring can be progressively increased.

FORM 10–1 VOCAL ABUSE CHART

Client's Name: _____   Setting: _____

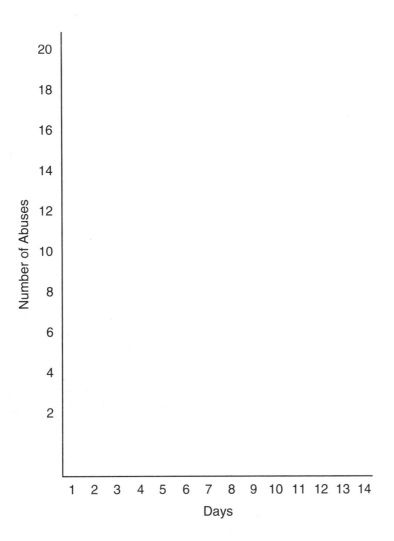

Mr. Abdul, a 48-year-old professor of political science, reports a 2-year history of hoarseness and throat pain associated with teaching. He states that these symptoms are more severe during summer school because lecture periods are substantially longer than during the fall and spring semesters. A video of a typical lecture indicates that Mr. Abdul's speaking style in the classroom can be described as loud, forceful, and low pitched. In addition, Mr. Abdul is a member of a local repertory theater company and frequently performs in plays and musicals. A recent laryngoscopic examination reveals the presence of bilateral contact ulcers.

Selection of therapy targets. The aspects of voice production to be targeted are inappropriately low pitch, abrupt initiation of phonation, and excessive loudness. These features were selected because they constitute the primary symptoms of laryngeal hyperfunction in Mr. Abdul's profile.

Sample Activities

Adjusting Voice Pitch

1. Determine the client's optimal pitch through the procedure described in the section on treatment techniques for vocal hyperfunction. Devise a list 25 sentences for a cloze task. Examples include the following:

    I'm going to the store and I'm going to buy some _____.

    I'm going on a trip and I'm packing _____.

    I'm going on a picnic and I'm taking _____.

    My favorite chili is made with _____.

    On our last vacation, we visited _____.

    If I win the lottery, I would buy _____.

    I'm sending a birthday card to _____.

    My favorite baseball player is _____.

    Last night for dinner I had _____.

    This old car needs new _____.

    Explain that the clinician will read each sentence and present a cue or prompt (e.g., pitch pipe, piano note) representing the client's optimum pitch. Then the client completes the statement with a single word using the targeted pitch level. The difficulty level of this task can be increased by requiring the client to answer with a series of items rather than a single word.

Softening Glottal Attacks

2. The clinician models a soft glottal attack by yawning and producing single words that begin with /h/ or a vowel during the exhalation. Once the client can easily imitate this relaxed initiation of phonation, utterances can be progressively lengthened and may include initial phonemes other than /h/.

Explain to the client that the game of 20 Questions will be used to practice the yawn-sigh approach to phonation at the carrier phrase level. Instruct the client to think of a person, place, or thing. The clinician then asks yes/no questions to determine the correct answer. Emphasize that the client should employ the yawn-sigh approach at the beginning of each response to the clinician's queries. For example:

Clinician: Are you thinking of a person?

Client: Yes, I'm thinking of a person.

Clinician: Is the person a female?

Client: No, the person is not a female.

Clinician: Is the person alive?

Client: Yes, the person is alive.

Task difficulty can be increased by reversing roles and instructing the client to spontaneously formulate the questions.

Reducing Loudness

3. Identify the optimal loudness level for the client as described in the section on vocal hyperfunction. Select list-like reading materials that can be easily divided into segments corresponding to single breath groups (e.g., directions to a destination such as a restaurant or movie theater, a recipe, instructions for assembling or operating a DVD player, and so on). Write each topic on an index card or sheet of paper and clearly delineate the utterance to be produced on each exhalation. Sample formats may include the following:

Directions

Turn left at the second traffic light./Pass the gas station on the right./Go two blocks and make your first left./The restaurant will be on your right.

Recipe

1. Combine flour and sugar in a bowl.
2. Add melted butter and one egg.
3. Mix thoroughly until batter is stiff.
4. Drop by the spoonful onto cookie sheet.
5. Bake at 350 degrees for 20 minutes.

Model reading each utterance aloud on a single exhalation. Instruct the client to imitate each production using the optimal loudness level identified previously.

Mrs. Simon, a 39-year-old female, was diagnosed with right unilateral adductor vocal fold paralysis 2 months ago. She sustained damage to the vagus nerve as a result of intubation during surgery. Mrs. Simon presents with an extremely quiet, weak, and breathy voice.

Also evident are a hoarse vocal quality and low pitch with occasional pitch breaks. Decisions regarding surgical interventions such as phonosurgery are deferred for 6 months to allow for any spontaneous recovery of laryngeal function.

Selection of therapy targets. The vocal symptoms to be targeted are breathy, hoarse voice quality and reduced loudness level. These areas were chosen because they represent the primary characteristics of laryngeal hypofunction in Mrs. Simon's profile.

Sample Activities

Pushing/Pulling

1. Instruct the client to use one of the pushing/pulling techniques described in the section on laryngeal hypofunction to achieve firmer vocal fold approximation during phonation. Once closure has been achieved, emphasize the importance of an easy, relaxed pattern. Begin with prolongation of single vowels and progress hierarchically to the level of connected speech. At the connected speech level, the clinician poses simple questions and the client responds while employing the pushing/pulling technique. Sample questions include the following:

   Where do you live?

   How long have you lived there?

   Do you have any brothers or sisters?

   What are their names?

   When is your birthday?

   Where do you work?

   What was your first job?

   What has been your favorite vacation?

   What did you do last weekend?

   What kind of car do you drive?

   What kind of car would you like to drive?

   What are your hobbies?

   What is your favorite movie?

   What do you like most about your job?

   What is your favorite holiday?

Increasing Loudness

2. Instruct the client to use the abdominal-diaphragmatic breathing pattern with phonation as discussed in the section on vocal hypofunction to achieve increased loudness. Stimuli may begin at the level of isolated vowels and advance systematically to the discourse level. At the discourse level, the clinician creates several written dialogues and provides two copies of each scenario. Assign the client one of the roles. Instruct her to place one hand on her abdomen to monitor the use of the target breathing pattern while reading her lines in the script. Following are sample scripts; additional dialogues can be found in Appendix 10-A.

Calling Information

Operator: Hello. What city please?

Caller: College Park.

O: Yes?

C: I'd like the number for the post office on Route 1.

O: Thank you. That number is 555-2200.

Ordering a Pizza

Operator: Thank you for calling the pizzeria. Can you hold please?

Caller: Yes.

O: Thanks for holding. Can I take your order?

C: Yes, I'd like a large pepperoni pizza with extra cheese.

O: Any sodas with that?

C: I'll take two large sodas.

O: What's your address?

C: 1600 Pennsylvania Avenue.

O: And the phone number?

C: 203-4000.

O: OK. We'll be there in 30 minutes or less.

C: What's the total?

O: $14.50.

C: Thanks.

Helpful Hints

1. Clients with voice disorders that result from psychogenic factors, such as conversion dysphonias, may regain a completely normal voice within a single session.

2. Puppets can be very useful in negative practice activities for children who demonstrate dysphonias related to hyperfunction. For example, large or ugly puppets can adopt the abusive vocal pattern, while small or attractive puppets speak in the target voice.

3. With respect to the treatment of conversion disorders, the clinician must recognize that, although the voice is not actually lost, the loss of voice control is very real to the client.

4. Relatively loud masking or ambient noise can be useful for increasing loudness in some clients with weak, ineffective voices.

5. Irritating substances such as tobacco or alcohol can exacerbate the symptoms of an existing dysphonia.

6. Clinicians should be able to translate anatomical, physiological, and medical terminology used by other professionals (e.g., otolaryngologists) into clear and understandable explanations of a client's voice disorder.

7. Some aspects of voice production are difficult to explain verbally; use of visual imagery such as a Nasometer™ or computer display often helps clients grasp these concepts in a more concrete manner.

8. Despite the effectiveness of Botox® injections, a client with long-standing spasmodic dysphonia may persist in the tendency to "push out" his or her voice. This type of individual may benefit from direct counseling/education to realize that his or her habit of effortful phonation is now unnecessary.

9. Therapy techniques that involve massage or other tactile stimulation may be inappropriate for clients who are hypersensitive or resistant to touch.

ALARYNGEAL SPEECH

Alaryngeal speech refers to voice that emanates from a sound source other than the larynx. The surgical procedure known as **total laryngectomy** involves complete removal of the larynx due to malignant tumor or severe trauma. During total laryngectomy surgery, the larynx and its intrinsic muscles as well as the hyoid bone are removed. The trachea is then surgically attached to an opening (stoma) created in the neck just above the notch of the sternum. As a result, air from the lungs can no longer enter the vocal tract, and the voicing source has been removed, making normal phonation impossible. In addition to surgery, some individuals with laryngeal cancer may receive pre- or postoperative radiation and/or chemotherapy. In fact, a study (Weber et al., 2003) indicates that patients who receive simultaneous chemotherapy and radiation therapy are less likely to require surgical removal of the larynx. Although concurrent chemoradiation is the widely used approach, a similar surgical approach is starting to gain attention. Near-total laryngectomy is a surgical procedure that preserves the voice by removing only certain parts of the laryngeal structures. Because only portions of the larynx are removed, near-total laryngectomy is only appropriate in patients with cancer localized to specific areas (D'Cruz, Sharma, & Pai, 2012).

A preoperative visit by the speech-language pathologist plays an important role. The clinician can clearly explain the consequences of the surgical procedure on voice production and describe various methods of alaryngeal speech production. The visit also provides an ideal opportunity for assessment of the individual's habitual speaking patterns prior to surgery. Prater et al. (1999) suggest that the following factors be noted during the preoperative visit: (1) articulatory proficiency, (2) conversational speech rate, (3) dialectal patterns, and (4) degree of mouth opening used in conversation. Client and family counseling forms a major part of this preoperative visit and continues throughout the therapeutic process. Overall personal adjustment can facilitate successful long-term rehabilitation efforts (Schuster et al., 2003). The goal of therapy for individuals with laryngectomies is to establish an alternative mode of sound production that can be used for communication. Many factors may affect the prognosis for successful intervention:

- Extent of surgery (especially if significant portions of the tongue are also removed)
- Presence of significant hearing impairment (greatly reduces an individual's ability to acquire alaryngeal speech)
- Presence of excessive esophageal muscle tone

- Lengthy course of concurrent radiation treatment (may produce side effects that interfere with easy acquisition of alaryngeal speech)
- Limitations in cognitive, linguistic, or emotional status (may negatively affect an individual's ability to learn alaryngeal speech)

TREATMENT FOR ALARYNGEAL CLIENTS

The search for an alternative method of sound production subsequent to laryngectomy is based on three general sources: external mechanical devices, functional use of the sphincterlike tissue at the junction of the **pharynx and esophagus (PE segment)** to produce esophageal speech, or the use of a prosthetic voice device inserted into a surgically created opening. The clinician should consult with the physician prior to and after surgery regarding the most appropriate form of alaryngeal speech for a given individual.

Mechanical Devices

Pneumatic Aids. These devices consist of a plastic housing that is held over the stoma connected to a small unit with a reed, and a tube that is placed in the mouth. Air exhaled from the lungs through the stoma vibrates the reed, and the sound is carried to the oral cavity through the tubing. The speaker articulates this sound to produce speech.

Electronic Aids. Several types of electronic artificial larynges provide a battery-powered sound source, including the following:

- *Neck devices:* A handheld sound source (e.g., an electrolarynx) is placed against the neck. Sound is transmitted through the skin into the vocal tract. The clinician locates the most supple area on the client's neck and the aid is placed there, with the head of the aid in full contact with the skin. Typically, the best location is approximately 1–2 inches below the mandible near the midline of the neck. The client is instructed to hold the electrolarynx in his nondominant hand and turn it on while simultaneously shaping monosyllabic words containing bilabial consonants as clearly as possible. The client should be cautioned against the instinct to forcefully exhale because this results in stoma noise that distracts the listener. As longer utterances are produced, the client must learn to turn the electrolarynx off during natural speech pauses and coordinate initiation of articulatory movement with finger movement for the "on" switch. The intelligibility of speech produced with an electrolarynx is greatly enhanced by the use of precise articulatory movements and reduced speaking rate. The feasibility of a hands-free electrolarynx is currently being explored. For example, one possible hands-free model utilizes oral movements, such as lingual movements to active denture-based switches (Wan, Wu, Wu, Wang, & Wan, 2012).
- *Oral devices:* These devices are similar to the pneumatic aid described previously, except the sound source is battery driven rather than arising from air exhaled through the stoma. Tubing should be placed in a corner of the mouth and angled up toward the hard palate to ensure that it is not occluded by the tongue or cheek. The client learns to articulate the sound carried to the oral cavity by the tubing. This type of aid is often used immediately after surgery because it does not interfere with sutures or swollen tissues. As with the neck version, training in the use of this device generally begins with monosyllabic words that contain bilabial consonants.

There are some disadvantages to the use of artificial larynges. The quality of the sound source is often judged as "unnatural," and these devices severely restrict the individual's ability to vary the pitch and loudness of his or her speech. However, there are also many positive aspects to the use of an artificial larynx. The device can be demonstrated prior to surgery and can be employed in the immediate postoperative period. The device also provides a means of communication that can be learned rapidly by most clients. Some laryngectomees will continue to use an electrolarynx as the primary method of communication; others will employ it as a temporary alternative until they master other forms of alaryngeal communication.

Esophageal Speech

This method of communication consists of using air passing through a narrow constriction in the esophagus as an alternative source of sound for speech (Graham, 2005). The quality of sound produced is perceived as more natural than that generated by an electrolarynx. The client's ability to rapidly intake and expel air from the esophagus and perform precise articulatory movements is the most critical aspect of effective esophageal speech. According to Casper and Colton (1998), at least one-third of laryngectomees will be unable to produce esophageal speech that is intelligible for daily communication purposes. Esophageal speech production operates on the principle that air of greater pressure in one location (mouth) will flow to a location of lesser pressure (esophagus) if the locations are connected (PE segment). The six main goals of intervention with esophageal speech as originally identified by Aronson in 1980 remain unchanged (Prater et al., 1999):

1. Easily and rapidly phonate on demand.
2. Use a rapid method of air intake.
3. Keep a short latency period between air intake and phonation.
4. Produce four to nine syllables per air charge.
5. Speak at a rate of 85 to 129 words per minute.
6. Speak with adequate intelligibility.

The basic sequence of training for esophageal speech includes the following steps:

Step 1: Establishing esophageal voice

Step 2: Gaining and maintaining control over production

Step 3: Increasing intelligibility of esophageal speech

Step 4: Increasing length of utterance production

Step 5: Mastering conversational nuances of pitch, loudness, and stress patterns

Esophageal speech training should begin as soon as possible after the client's discharge from the hospital. One rule of thumb states that an individual is ready to start learning esophageal speech when he or she can tolerate oral ingestion of food. A moderate pace of therapy is recommended. Although many clients are extremely eager to master this procedure, therapy that proceeds too rapidly may result in unintelligible, forced speech with excessive stoma noise. (See Table 10-3 for basic guidelines for home practice of esophageal speech techniques.)

TABLE 10–3
Homework Guidelines for Esophageal Speakers

1. Have reasonable expectations, especially during the initial period of treatment. It takes time to establish effective patterns of muscle control over esophageal speech production.

2. Practice for short, consistent periods (e.g., 10 minutes per hour) rather than for lengthy periods of time.

3. Exaggerated breathing patterns (either on inhalation or exhalation) do not make esophageal speech clearer or easier to understand.

4. Use of excessive muscular force does not make esophageal speech more intelligible; it only wears you out.

There are four main techniques for obtaining an esophageal air supply. From most to least efficient, they are consonant-injection, glossopharyngeal press, inhalation, and swallowing. Therefore, it is generally recommended that the clinician begin with the consonant-injection method. If the client is unsuccessful, proceed sequentially through the other methods until the client can consistently initiate phonation. At that point, the clinician may want to retry one of the more efficient methods.

Consonant-Injection Method. This method uses the intraoral air pressure that normally builds during production of high-pressure consonants, such as stops and fricatives, to inflate the esophagus. It has been described as the most efficient technique of esophageal air intake because air can be injected *simultaneously* with the production of a consonant rather than only during a pause or phrase interval. This results in minimal or no interruption in communication, unlike the other three methods.

Step 1: Client forces air into the esophagus by producing a whispered plosive bilabial consonant, such as /p/, repetitively four to five times. This repeated compression of air in the oral cavity should force some air into the esophagus.

Step 2: Client expels the air from the esophagus and attempts to phonate /pə/.

Step 3: Gradually introduce other voiceless plosives, fricatives, and affricates paired with /ə/ at the syllable level.

Step 4: Introduce monosyllabic words containing high-pressure consonants such as *pay, tap, toy, skate, stop, scotch.*

Step 5: Extend phonation to phrases that contain a preponderance of both voiced and voiceless high-pressure consonants such as "make it dark," "stop that cab," "cut the cake," and "take that skate."

For some clients, this method may be less effective with stimulus items that consist mainly of vowels and low-pressure consonants. The relatively open-mouth articulatory configurations of these sounds may not allow the buildup of sufficient air pressure to insufflate the esophagus.

Glossopharyngeal Press Method. This method achieves esophageal air intake through tongue movements and is a useful alternative to consonant-injection for utterances loaded with low-pressure phonemes.

Step 1: Client closes lips and anchors the tongue tip against the alveolar ridge.

Step 2: The posterior portion of the tongue is moved backward along the hard and soft palates to pump air into the esophagus.

Step 3: The client expels air from esophagus and attempts to phonate vowels or monosyllables. Extend length of utterance as the client's mastery of voluntary phonation improves.

Remind the client to refrain from actually completing a swallow when employing this technique.

Inhalation Method. In this method, air is supplied to the esophagus through relaxation of the PE segment during pulmonary inhalation. The expansion and contraction of chest muscles are used to direct air into the esophagus.

Step 1: The client inhales rapidly through the nose or covers the stoma midway through a quick inhalation.

Step 2: The client immediately expels the air and attempts production of /a/.

Step 3: Consonant-vowel (CV) syllables that contain stops are gradually introduced and content progresses to monosyllabic words.

Swallow Method. This method utilizes a controlled swallowing pattern to inject air into the esophagus. It is based on the fact that the PE segment tends to open spontaneously during a swallow because air is forced backward by the posterior movement of the tongue. This is the least efficient method of air injection and should be used only as a last resort. Primary disadvantages include (1) the extended latency between initiation of a swallow and the production of phonation; (2) the accumulation of air in the stomach as a result of repeated attempts at rapid swallowing; and (3) the inability to produce rapid, repetitive dry swallows as required for speech.

Step 1: The client swallows in a normal fashion by moving the tongue backward toward the pharynx.

Step 2: The client releases air and attempts to produce a CV syllable with an alveolar stop consonant such as "ta" and "da."

Tracheoesophageal (TE) Speech

This method is an alternative to esophageal speech (Blom, Singer, & Hamaker, 1998). A small device made of silicone is inserted into a surgically created opening between the trachea and esophagus to allow air from the lungs to reach the PE segment. This procedure can be performed during the primary laryngectomy surgery or at a later date. This technique, called **tracheoesophageal puncture (TEP),** may be the quickest way for a client to regain near-normal speech after the larynx has been removed. Compared to users of artificial larynges, TE speakers report more positive long-term outcomes with regard to their communication abilities and their overall sense of well-being (Gress & Singer, 2005; Stajner-Katusic, Horga, Musura, & Globlek, 2006; Ward et al., 2003). Patient selection for this procedure is often made by the surgeon. However, the clinician should be aware of some guidelines that are relevant to the selection of candidates for TEP. First, the client's overall health should be stable in all areas other than the laryngectomy. For example, an individual with poor respiratory function due to emphysema might not be able to generate enough pressure to move pulmonary air through the prosthesis to the PE segment.

Second, the client should possess the manual dexterity and cognitive skills required to use and care for the prosthesis on a daily basis. Ideally, the clinician should be involved in evaluating the suitability of a client for the TEP procedure; sizing the prosthesis; and training the client to insert, remove, and clean the prosthesis.

Once the fistula (punctured area) has healed sufficiently and the prosthesis has been inserted, the clinician may begin intervention according to this basic sequence of steps:

Step 1: Ask the client to inhale and then phonate on exhalation while the clinician uses a finger to occlude the stoma. It is important that the stoma be covered completely but with gentle pressure.

Step 2: The client digitally occludes the stoma during exhalation and attempts to phonate sustained sounds or words. Utterances should become longer and more effortless at a fairly rapid rate. (*Note:* Use of a tracheostoma valve can eliminate the need for manual occlusion of the stoma during speech production.)

For more information regarding this topic, consult the technical report published by the American Speech-Language-Hearing Association in 2004.

Example Profile

The following profile illustrates characteristics typical of individuals who have undergone surgical removal of the larynx. Unlike other profiles throughout the book, the activities presented in this section are designed to illustrate a progression of intervention strategies that would be implemented over time with a single individual.

Mr. Evans, a 62-year-old male, underwent a total laryngectomy 3 months ago as a result of squamous cell carcinoma. Sutures have been removed, and he is currently able to take food by mouth. He received a postsurgical regimen of radiation treatment for 8 weeks. Currently, Mr. Evans communicates with an electrolarynx and by writing.

Selection of therapy targets. The targets selected based on this profile illustrate the typical progression of esophageal speech programming and include (1) establishing phonation, (2) increasing duration of phonation, and (3) refining vocal pitch and intensity. One activity will address each of the target areas.

Sample Activities

Consonant-Injection Method

1. Instruct the client in the consonant-injection method of esophageal sound production as described in the section on esophageal speech. Once Mr. Evans can produce /pə/ rapidly in 10 consecutive trials, introduce CV syllables containing

other voiceless plosives, fricatives, and affricates and then progress to monosyllabic words containing high-pressure consonants. Example stimuli include the following:

CV Syllables	CVC Words
/tə/	cup
/tɔ/	tub
/ti/	pat
/to/	cut
/kæ/	bag
/kɛ/	cheese
/ki/	church
/kʊ/	bit
/sə/	punch
/so/	cash
/sʊ/	bed
/si/	cat
/tʃʌ/	day
/tʃo/	date
/tʃə/	ghost

Increasing Duration of Phonation

2. Once esophageal speech has been reliably established at the level of monosyllabic CVC words, focus on increasing the duration of phonation. Write a list of three- to five-word phrases that are loaded with voiced and voiceless high-pressure consonants. Instruct the client to read these longer stimuli aloud while maintaining a consistent pattern of phonation. Sample stimuli include the following:

   Stop that cab

   Get the cup

   Buy the boot

   Touch the cat

   Pull the tag

   Call the cop

   Go to bed

   The time of day

   Put it in the bank

   A day at the beach

   Teach the kids

   Shut the door

Make it good

Coach the team

Get in the tub

Put on the cap

A lot of cash

Cash in the chips

Cut the tape

As the client progresses, the difficulty of this task can be increased. Write each phrase on separate index cards, shuffle the cards, and place the deck face-down on the table. The client draws the top card from the pile without exposing its contents, reads it aloud, and the clinician attempts to imitate it. Emphasize that the clinician will be relying solely on the intelligibility of the client's esophageal speech to identify the entire phrase.

Refining Pitch and Intensity

3. The next phase of therapy focuses on refining communicative effectiveness by improving the client's ability to manipulate the pitch and loudness characteristics of esophageal speech (to the extent possible). Develop 10 groups of three-sentence sets. Each set should contain declarative, interrogative, and tag question versions of the same sentence (three to five words in length). Write each set on a single index card. Instruct the client to select a card and read each of the three sentences aloud using the appropriate alterations of pitch and increased loudness on the second and third versions. Encourage the client to try a variety of different head postures, which may facilitate increased pitch and loudness (e.g., slight head turning, chin lowering, head and chin extension). Examples include the following:

   They know she's gone.

   They know she's gone?

   They know she's gone, don't they?

   There's no hot water.

   There's no hot water?

   There's no hot water, is there?

   The office opens at 9 A.M.

   The office opens at 9 A.M.?

   The office opens at 9 A.M., doesn't it?

   Mr. Smith is her dentist.

   Mr. Smith is her dentist?

   Mr. Smith is her dentist, isn't he?

   They're going to the mall.

   They're going to the mall?

   They're going to the mall, aren't they?

   The weather has improved.

   The weather has improved?

The weather has improved, hasn't it?

It won't work for me.

It won't work for me?

It won't work for me, will it?

They shoot horses.

They shoot horses?

They shoot horses, don't they?

The budget was vetoed.

The budget was vetoed?

The budget was vetoed, wasn't it?

This is delicious soup.

This is delicious soup?

This is delicious soup, isn't it?

Helpful Hints

1. It is important for the client to avoid the use of excessive muscular tension during the production of esophageal speech. Overly rapid and effortful phonation is often accompanied by undesirable and distracting behaviors such as stoma noise, grimacing, and audible clunking during air injection.

2. A client can learn to self-monitor stoma noise using a microphone, stethoscope, or his or her hand held in front of the stoma.

3. The clinician may want to avoid the use of velar plosives such as /k/ in the early stages of esophageal speech training to prevent inadvertent production of pharyngeal speech (i.e., a Donald Duck voice).

4. The clinician needs to remember that esophageal speakers have much smaller reservoirs of air available for speech (i.e., less than 5 mL) than normal speakers (i.e., greater than 5 L). Therefore, they have a reduced capacity to generate lengthy utterances on a single injection of air.

5. Whenever possible, the clinician should arrange for the client to meet with a successful esophageal speaker either immediately prior to or following surgery. This visit can accomplish several goals at once. It serves as a motivator for the client; it demonstrates the communicative effectiveness of esophageal speech; and it allows the client and family to ask specific questions about the entire rehabilitation process.

6. A nonspeech communication system may need to be provided on an interim basis while the client is learning one of the alternative sound production methods.

7. Clinicians should be aware that clients may experience difficulty focusing on therapy goals due to preoccupation with global issues such as physical survival, economic pressures, and self-identity.

8. WebWhispers (http://webwhispers.org/library/esophagealspeech.asp) is an informational support site for individuals with laryngectomies and laryngeal cancer. The site includes several representative samples of laryngeal speech.

CONCLUSION

This chapter has presented basic information, protocols, and procedures for intervention with voice disorders at an *introductory* level. This information is intended only as a starting point in the reader's clinical education and training. For in-depth coverage of these areas, the following readings are recommended:

Andrews, M., & Summers, A., (2001). *Voice treatment for children and adolescents.* Clifton Park, NY: Cengage Learning.

Aronson, A. E., & Bless, D. (2009). *Clinical voice disorders* (4th ed.). New York: Thieme Medical Publishers.

Boone, D. R., McFarlane, S. C., Von Berg, S., & Zraick, R. (2013). *The voice and voice therapy* (9th ed.). San Francisco, CA: Allyn & Bacon.

Casper, J. K., & Colton, R. H. (1998). *Clinical manual for laryngectomy and head/neck cancer rehabilitation* (2nd ed.). Clifton Park, NY: Cengage Learning.

Prater, R. J., Swift, R., W., Deem, J. F., & Miller, L. (1999). *Manual of voice therapy* (2nd ed.). Austin, TX: Pro-Ed.

Salmon, S. J. (Ed.). (1999). *Alaryngeal speech rehabilitation: For clinicians by clinicians* (2nd ed.). Austin, TX: Pro-Ed.

Sapienza, C., & Ruddy, B. H. (2012). *Voice disorders* (2nd ed.). San Diego, CA: Plural Publishing.

Wilson, D. K. (1987). *Voice problems of children* (3rd ed.). Baltimore, MD: Williams and Wilkins.

ADDITIONAL RESOURCES

The Speech Bin
School Specialty
P.O. Box 1579
Appleton, WI 54912-1579
Phone: 800-388-3224
Fax: 800-388-6344
Web site: http://store.schoolspecialty.com/

The Boone Voice Program for Children
This is a cognitive approach to diagnosing and treating children's voice disorders. The kit includes an assessment manual, a remediation manual, and an audiotape.

Abilitations Speech Bin Special Needs Voice Buddies Playing Cards
These sets of playing cards depict characters that help teach children about vocal abuse by identifying both negative and positive vocal techniques and behaviors.

Using Your Best Voice
These worksheets and activities are designed to teach 3- to 11-year-olds important vocal concepts: how to demonstrate appropriate voice patterns, interpret meanings and feelings in vocal and nonverbal behaviors, and practice effective nonverbal behaviors.

Activities are presented in three sections—finding, practicing, and showing others your best voice—for voice disorders including hyperfunction, hypofunction, resonance, pitch, loudness, and rate/timing.

LinguiSystems
3100 Fourth Avenue
East Moline, IL 61244
Phone: 800-776-4332
Fax: 800-577-4555
Email: service@linguisystems.com
Web site: http://www.linguisystems.com

The Source for Children's Voice Disorders
This book provides information on assessing and treating voice disorders. It addresses vocal hyperfunction and abuse as well as other issues associated with the vocal tract (e.g., resonance). Includes a CD of reproducible forms as well as an informational PowerPoint presentation.

The Source for Voice Disorders: Adolescent and Adult
This book provides clinicians with assessment and treatment procedures. It discusses a variety of pathologies and how to address them through therapy. The book comes with a CD that contains handouts on evaluation procedures, therapy exercises, patient questionnaires, and educational resources.

Pro-Ed
8700 Shoal Creek Boulevard
Austin, TX 78757-6897
Phone: 800-897-3202
Fax: 800-397-7633
Web site: http://www.proedinc.com

Manual of Voice Therapy, 2nd edition
This comprehensive reference includes information for pediatric through adult clients. It includes information about the various conditions that lead to voice disorders, the most recent developments in treatment methods and approaches, instrumentation, related medico-surgical management, counseling, and the challenges in management of voice disorders. This resource also contains a set of reproducible informational handouts for clients and families.

The Voice Diagnostic Protocol
This book serves to provide clinicians with information on how to assess voice disorders with a comprehensive approach. It has chapters that focus on the following topics: pitch, loudness, quality, respiratory control, dysphonias, and case studies. It also includes forms and materials for the evaluation process.

Clinical Management of Voice Disorders, 4th edition
This text addresses voice disorders, starting with anatomy and physiology and continuing to discuss a variety of evaluation procedures and tools, such as endoscopy and

electroglottography. The book also includes information on a variety of voice disorders by category, including neurogenic disorders, psychogenic disorders, and laryngectomies.

Voice Assessment Protocol for Children and Adults (VAP)

This assessment procedure can be used with clients ages 4 to 18. The kit contains an examiner's manual, audiocassette, and protocols. It assesses voice by examining pitch, loudness, quality, and rate.

Amazon.com, Inc.

Web site: www.amazon.com

Easy Does It for Voice

This is a vocal abuse detection and reduction program for children ages 6 to 12. It can be used with individuals or groups and includes reproducible tracking charts, parent and medical letters, and a voice evaluation form.

The Boone Voice Program for Adults, 2nd edition

This program includes stimulus and practice materials, explanations of normal voice and vocal pathologies, and 15 approaches for achieving better voice quality. Kit includes evaluation and remediation manuals, an audiotape, and practice sheets.

Clinical Manual for Laryngectomy and Head/Neck Cancer Rehabilitation

This text addresses the full scope of rehabilitation of the client with head/neck cancer. It includes current approaches to the rehabilitation of clients who have had a laryngectomy, as well as those whose cancer resulted in the removal of structures in the oral and/or pharyngeal cavities.

Working with Voice Disorders

This spiral-bound text is meant to assist clinicians with the assessment and treatment of voice disorders. The text contains sections on anatomy and physiology, disorders, and treatment approaches. It is meant to encompass the entire rehabilitation process, starting with information for gathering a case history and progressing all the way through treatment sessions.

Micro Video Corporation

1935 Pauline Blvd, Suite H
Ann Arbor, MI 48103
Phone: 800-537-2182
Fax: 734-996-3838
Web site: http://www.videovoice.com

Video Voice

For use with clients aged preschool to adult, this computer software covers 15 areas of vocal function, including volume awareness and control, intonation and stress, pitch training, and voice quality. Activities are conducted in a game format in which the model's voice can be replaced with the clinician's or client's voice to facilitate responses across different speakers. Correct/incorrect productions are visually displayed for the client and the program records the data.

Super Duper Publications
P.O. Box 24997
Greenville, SC 29616
Phone: 800-277-8737
Fax: 800-978-7379
Web site: www.superduperinc.com

Martha Mouse and Baby Bear: Preschool Voice Worksheets Book
This book depicts the characters of Baby Bear and Martha Mouse in a variety of scenarios. The purpose of the book is to educate children as to the importance of healthy voice techniques. The book is spiral-bound and contains 64 educational worksheets.

Voice Adventures Card Deck
These cards contain illustrations of the characters Baby Bear and Martha Mouse. Different situations are presented on each card that the client has to identify as depicting positive or negative vocal behaviors. The cards are stored in a tin box and come in pairs for use in games.

Cengage Learning
10650 Toebben Drive
Independence, KY 41051
Phone: 800-354-9706
Fax: 800-487-8488
Web site: http://www.cengage.com

Voice Treatment for Children and Adolescents
This book presents information on the practical assessment and treatment of voice disorders in children through a review of recent research and technological advancements in the area of voice. It also contains problem-solving and team intervention models appropriate for SLPs working in clinical, school, or medical settings.

Singing Voice Rehabilitation: A Guide for the Voice Teacher and Speech-Language Pathologist
Written by a SLP who also is a voice teacher, this book addresses the rehabilitation process by discussing the anatomy of the vocal mechanism in relation to singing. It advocates for voice therapy as an important component of vocal training.

APPENDIX 10-A

ADDITIONAL DIALOGUE SCRIPTS FOR VOICE THERAPY ACTIVITIES

MAKING A DENTAL APPOINTMENT

Secretary: Hello, can I help you?

Customer: Yes, I need to make an appointment with Dr. Brown.

S: Have you ever been here before?

C: No.

S: OK. What are you coming in for?

C: I need my teeth cleaned and checked.

S: OK. What day would you like to come in?

C: Are there any openings next Thursday?

S: Morning or afternoon?

C: I'd prefer the morning, and after 11 o'clock if possible.

S: I have an opening at 1 o'clock. Is that OK?

C: Yes, that's fine.

S: OK. Then we'll see you next Thursday at 1 o'clock.

C: What should I do if I have to cancel?

S: You need to call us and cancel at least 24 hours in advance.

C: And will my insurance cover it? I am insured by the local public school system.

S: Yes. We are a preferred provider for that insurance. Just bring in your card on the day of the appointment.
C: OK. Thank you very much. See you next Thursday.

GOING TO A RESTAURANT

Hostess: Would you like to be seated at the bar or in the formal dining room?

Customer: The dining room, please.

H: Right this way. Your waitress will be right with you.

C: Thank you very much.

Waitress: Can I take your order?

(continues)

C: I'll take a hamburger and a large order of fries.

W: Would you like anything to drink with that?

C: I'd like a large soda.

W: OK. I'll be right back with your drink.

Waitress brings the soda.

C: Excuse me—can I also get a salad?

W: Sure. What type of dressing would you like?

C: The house dressing would be fine.

Waitress comes to clear the table.

W: How was everything?

C: The food was really great.

W: I'm glad to hear that. Would you care for any dessert?

C: I don't think so.

W: What about some coffee?

C: I'll just take the check.

W: OK. I'll be right back.

BUYING A CAR

Salesperson: Good afternoon. Can I help you with something?

Buyer: Yes, I'm interested in buying a used car.

S: Did you have a particular car in mind?

B: Well, I was looking at this sedan yesterday, but I have a few questions about it.

S: OK. What are they?

B: What year car is it?

S: A 2012.

B: And how many miles does it have on it?

S: 35,000.

B: Oh, that's not very many.

S: No, and it's in really good condition.

B: What other features does it have?

S: It has an automatic transmission, GPS, and a sunroof.

B: Would it be possible for me to take it for a test-drive?

S: Sure—let me get the keys.

After the test-drive

S: So, what did you think?

(continues)

B: It drives great. What kind of deal can you give me on it?

S: Well, with your first-time buyer discount I can give it to you for $11,500.

B: Would I be able to pay it off by paying $350 a month?

S: Yes, that's no problem. Should I go draw up the paperwork?

B: Not today—I'll get back to you.

OPENING A BANK ACCOUNT

Teller: Good afternoon. What can I do for you today?

Customer: I'd like to open an account.

T: Checking or savings?

C: Both types of accounts.

T: Do you want a debit card with the account also?

C: Is there a charge when I use the card?

T: Only if you use it at a bank other than this one.

C: I'll take one then. Is there a monthly charge on the account?

T: Will you make more than 25 transactions per month?

C: I usually make fewer than that.

T: We have an account that's free if you post fewer than 25 transactions a month.

C: What if I make more?

T: You'll be charged $1.00 for every electronic transaction beyond the limit.

C: Are there any other free accounts?

T: We have another type of account that requires a minimum monthly balance of $1,000.

C: I'd like to go with the first type of account.

T: How much money will you be initially depositing?

C: I have $300.

T: Here is your account number.

C: OK. Thanks for all your help.

GETTING WORK DONE ON YOUR CAR

Mechanic: Hi, can I help you?

Customer: Yes, I need to have some work done on my car.

M: What's wrong with it?

C: Well, it needs an oil change, the brakes are squealing really badly, and the tires need to be rotated.

(continues)

M: Can you leave it here today?

C: Yes, but I need to have it back by 6 P.M. tonight.

M: That's fine. We'll take a look at it and give you a call within the next two hours to let you know what's wrong.

C: OK—thanks.

MAKING A VETERINARY APPOINTMENT

Vet: Hello, can I help you?

Caller: Yes, I'd like to make an appointment for my dog.

V: What is your last name?

C: (Client states his/her last name.)

V: What's the dog's name?

C: Scruffy.

V: OK. What's he coming in for?

C: He just needs his shots updated.

V: We have a spot open Saturday at noon. How's that?

C: Saturday at noon is fine.

V: OK. We'll see you then.

CHAPTER 11

Counseling can be defined as an interpersonal relationship that is intended to alleviate emotional stress arising from or contributing to the primary communicative disorder. There are several theoretical schools of thought regarding the counseling process. Some of the most common include behavioral (Skinner, 1953), humanistic (Rogers, 1951), cognitive (Ellis, 1977), existential (Yalom, 1980), and interpersonal (Sullivan, 1953) orientations. This chapter takes an eclectic approach to counseling and integrates the following underlying assumptions of several theoretical models (Flasher & Fogle, 2012):

1. Human behavior can change or be changed.
2. Some behaviors (e.g., inadequate, dysfunctional, undesirable) warrant change.
3. Particular counseling techniques/interventions will effect change in client behavior.
4. Clients generally acknowledge the possibility that change will occur.
5. Clinicians expect clients to be actively involved in the therapeutic counseling process.

In speech-language intervention, counseling is an essential aspect of the therapeutic process and fulfills several important functions:

- It allows the clinician to impart basic information to clients and their families.
- It provides opportunities for clients to verbalize feelings, fears, and uncertainties.
- It serves as an emotionally supportive milieu in which clients are comfortable making attitudinal and behavioral changes.

Although counseling is recognized as an integral part of treatment, clinicians often do not receive formal education or training in basic counseling skills. Many clinicians feel uncomfortable with this aspect of their professional role and are uncertain about the differences between psychotherapy and counseling. Psychotherapy involves the identification of unconscious patterns of behavior in a client in order to effect major personality changes. In contrast, counseling focuses on helping a client acknowledge feelings and engage in problem solving to make personal adjustments.

Counseling is the aspect of speech-language therapy that focuses on the person rather than the disorder. An effective therapeutic relationship must be built on mutual confidence, trust, respect, and consideration (Luterman, 2006; Rollin, 2000). Client and family perceptions of positive therapeutic/counseling relationships include the following characteristics:

- Sensitivity to and empathy for their feelings and circumstances
- Respect for them as individuals
- Honest, yet tactful, presentation of potentially unpleasant or emotionally charged information
- Motivation to actively participate in the therapy process
- Careful listening by the clinician that promotes effective communication and allows for the "venting" of feelings

Several variables can influence the counseling process. Both client and clinician bring their own needs, values, feelings, experiences, and expectations to the therapeutic relationship (Flasher & Fogle, 2012). However, it is important for the clinician to practice selfless listening (e.g., to set aside his or her own personal views) in order to identify the client's concerns and to foster feelings of trust and security (Luterman, 2006). Both participants must recognize that the client's welfare is the central concern of the relationship and work together to improve the client's communicative status. It is important to understand that individual clients require varying amounts of time to form a bond of trust with another person. Therefore, clinicians need to be patient with clients who are slower to risk self-disclosure. In addition, clinicians must realize that, in most cases, a communicative disorder is a family problem rather than a problem of a single individual. Thus, counseling must address clients in the context of their overall life situations. Clinicians are encouraged to look beyond the observable aspects of client and family behavior and consider their internal emotional and affective states as well (Geller & Foley, 2009).

Counseling is an ongoing process and should not be viewed as a one-time event. It is incorporated into diagnostic as well as treatment sessions. In some cases, counseling may constitute the treatment process itself. For example, an intervention program for a person who stutters may consist entirely of counseling sessions that focus on reducing anxiety, boosting self-confidence, and modifying the environment to eliminate communicative stress. It's important for clinicians to realize that clients frequently receive services from multiple sources. Thus, collaboration among the professionals is crucial in communicating consistent counseling messages in order to minimize client/family misunderstanding and confusion.

Counseling is a relationship, and for any relationship to be successful, boundaries must be established (Flasher & Fogle, 2012; Stone & Olswang, 1989). This is a necessary first step, because boundaries define the function and role of each participant and clarify what will or will not be part of the therapeutic relationship. Setting specific parameters reduces anxiety for clients whose expectations about therapy may be confused or unclear. In the initial stage of intervention, the clinician is responsible for ensuring that boundaries are established and understood.

Clinicians also need to recognize the limits of their training/experience and realize when referrals need to be made to professionals with specialized counseling expertise (Flasher & Fogle, 2012). Situations that are clearly beyond the scope of practice for a speech-language pathologist (SLP) may involve either the content or the style of the interaction. Content refers to the topic areas discussed within the therapeutic relationship. Topics that are generally considered inappropriate for discussion within the domain of speech-language pathology may include a client's marital problems, chronic depression, or unrelated health problems. Style involves the manner in which the clinician and client interact. Examples of inappropriate style include a client's unhealthy dependency on the clinician, unpredictable and repeated fluctuations of mood and temper, or undue anxiety on the part of the clinician before and after each therapy session.

FIVE KEY TRAITS OF AN EFFECTIVE COUNSELOR*

Many authors have discussed the interpersonal attributes of clinicians as counselors. Five key characteristics are presented here:

1. *Appropriate sharing*: Clinicians are often eager to establish a genuine connection with clients and their families. However, it is important for clinicians to recognize personal boundaries during these professional interactions. The type and amount

---

*Adapted from Shames (2000) and Luterman (2008).

of personal information that a clinician shares with clients should be carefully monitored, ensuring that the focus of counseling remains clearly on the clients and their needs. Clinicians should maintain objectivity regarding their personal relationship with clients (e.g., the difference between "being friendly" and "being a friend"; Shipley & Roseberry-McKibbin, 2006). An example of inappropriate sharing might be the following:

Client: I just can't seem to get members of my family to stop giving me advice about my stuttering.

Clinician: I know what you mean. My boyfriend is like that whenever I try to tell him about a problem I'm having.

2. *Nonjudgmental*: Counseling requires clinicians to provide support and encouragement to clients and families throughout the therapy process. Care should be taken to ensure that this feedback is not presented in terms of "good versus bad" or "right versus wrong." It is also important that clinicians refrain from imposing their own belief system/values onto their clients/families. An example of inappropriately judgmental behavior might be the following:

Client's wife: We really don't go to museums anymore because my husband has to use the wheelchair since his stroke.

Clinician: That shouldn't stop you! All museums these days have handicapped access and I'm sure your husband would enjoy visiting them.

3. *Tolerant of crying and emotional language*: There are points during the therapeutic process when clients may become emotional. These emotions can range from extreme happiness to hostility to self-pity. Beginning clinicians often feel the most uncomfortable with negative emotions such as crying or anger and seek to cut them off quickly. Yet effective counseling requires clinicians to recognize that allowing clients to express negative emotions can have therapeutic value. An example of appropriate tolerance for emotional behavior might be the following:

Client: (*crying and shouting*) It's just too hard—I'll never learn how to read!

Clinician: (*waits until outburst is over*) It's OK to be upset—I know you're really frustrated today.

4. *Client- or family-centered*: The driving forces behind counseling are the needs and priorities of clients and their families. Effective counselors recognize that these needs may be in conflict with their own plan for intervention. The ability to adapt and accommodate clients' views while maintaining appropriate therapeutic focus is critical for successful counseling. An example of accommodating parental input might be the following:

Client's parent: Benjamin isn't cooperating in therapy because he's bored. Can you use songs instead? He really likes singing.

Clinician: Singing won't really help him learn to produce novel two- to three-word utterances. But we can use songs for our therapy goal on production of final consonants.

5. *Refrains from solving client issues*: Counseling is not designed to solve or prescribe solutions to client problems. Clients who discuss problems in therapy often just need someone to listen and are really not looking for specific advice. Effective counseling helps clients work toward identifying their own solutions for themselves and their families.

Another key aspect to being an effective counselor is continued dedication to professional literature and evidence-based practices (Holland & Nelson, 2014). In addition to remaining updated on current practices, certain disorders and conditions will require SLPs to research other fields for a fuller understanding of their client's status. For example, a communication disorder associated with a degenerative disease would lead an SLP to obtain information on the medical characteristics and prognosis of the disease, including the projected timeline and expected trajectory of symptoms so as to inform treatment plans and to manage expectations (Holland & Nelson, 2014).

STAGES OF COUNSELING

Counseling is a dynamic process that continues throughout the course of a treatment program. As therapy progresses, the nature of counseling evolves through three main phases.

Establishing the Therapeutic Relationship

In this first phase, one of the clinician's primary responsibilities is to provide clients and their families with information. This information may pertain to the nature of the communicative disorder, possible treatment options, specific therapy techniques, the prognosis for improvement, and the level of commitment that therapy will require from the client and family. Clinicians must be sensitive to the amount of information that a client or family can handle at a given time. For example, the impact of an initial diagnosis of a communicative disorder may be devastating and preclude the processing of any other information presented at that time. Moreover, cognition becomes limited when emotions are elevated, making it difficult to process additional information (Luterman, 2006). When establishing a therapeutic relationship, the clinician functions in a directive role and assumes primary responsibility for setting the therapeutic agenda. The clinician determines the topics to be discussed, the activities to be performed, and the parameters of the client–clinician interpersonal relationship.

Implementing Counseling Intervention

This is the "work" stage of the client–clinician relationship. The focus of the counseling process shifts from an educational/informative mode to a problem-solving orientation. It is essential for clinicians to use their listening skills carefully in order to recognize the difference between "teaching moments" and "counseling moments." See the Helpful Hints section for books in the popular literature that provide insight into the lives of individuals with communication impairments. Therapy activities begin to focus directly on the client's deficits, and demands for behavioral change become more intense. Individual clients may demonstrate a variety of coping strategies or defense mechanisms such as avoidance, escape, humor, rationalization/intellectualization, and passive-aggression (Fogle & Flasher, 2012; Tanner, 2003). The client may begin to experience feelings of vulnerability, anxiety, and frustration, which may give rise to behaviors that are disruptive to the therapy process. Commonly seen manifestations may include (1) consistently arriving late for sessions, (2) chronically failing to complete homework assignments, (3) resisting therapy activities perceived as "too difficult," or (4) refusing/"forgetting" to attempt new communicative behaviors outside of the therapy setting. The clinician needs to recognize the feelings that motivate these behaviors in the client and focus counseling efforts on resolving these issues. In this phase, the clinician begins to function in a more nondirective mode. The client is encouraged to assume more active responsibility for self-motivation and for determining the therapeutic agenda.

Terminating the Therapeutic Relationship

At this final stage, the clinician lays the groundwork for the closure of the relationship by preparing the client to become his or her own therapist (i.e., shifting the locus of control). Counseling efforts focus on validating accurate client perceptions and encouraging the client to assume full responsibility for maintaining the behavioral changes that have been accomplished in therapy. Counseling also should be directed toward ensuring that the client leaves therapy with a genuine conceptual understanding and healthy perspective regarding the nature of the communicative disorder. Clinicians should encourage clients to actively use self-advocacy skills in order to promote successful communicative outcomes once the therapeutic relationship has ended.

CLIENT AND FAMILY EMOTIONAL REACTIONS TO COMMUNICATIVE DISORDERS

Clients and their families often receive the diagnosis of a communicative impairment with a great sense of loss. This sense of loss can be manifested through a variety of strong emotional responses. Clinicians need to be aware of the range of possible emotions that clients or families may experience at different stages in the therapy process. The most common reactions that clinicians must recognize and be prepared to handle are the following:

- *Grief* is deep sorrow in response to a significant loss. There have been numerous attempts to identify the stages of the grieving process. Kübler-Ross (1969) discussed five stages, which include initial denial that a disorder exists, a bargaining phase in which "deals" are offered to ameliorate the severity or existence of the disorder (e.g., "If Billy stops stuttering, I'll never criticize him again"), and an acceptance stage in which the client and family adjust to the loss as a fact of life and begin focusing efforts toward rehabilitation. Alternatively, Luterman (2008) identified four stages of coping: denial, resistance, affirmation, and integration. See Tanner (2008) for a simple discussion of the acceptance of unwanted change following stroke.

- *Anger* is a strong feeling of displeasure characterized by resentment, hostility, or rage. With respect to a communicative disorder, anger is often an instinctive attempt at self-protection resulting from fear, powerlessness, and frustration. Sometimes, spouses or parents experience feelings of anger toward the family member with the communicative impairment. However, they perceive this reaction as socially unacceptable, and therefore may transfer their angry feelings toward the clinician.

- *Depression* is anger turned inward that results in passivity and feelings of helplessness. The client realizes that previous stages of anger and bargaining were ineffective and that the fact of the communication disorder must be faced. Depression is a relatively common emotion encountered in the counseling process. The clinician should be aware that this emotional state can become self-perpetuating and seriously impede a client's therapy progress.

- *Guilt* refers to self-blame and is frequently demonstrated by a client's immediate family members. These feelings tend to center around two types of issues: "Did I do something to cause (or contribute to) John's communicative disorder?" and "Am I getting the right type and amount of therapy for John?" Parents and family members may not necessarily verbalize these feelings but may act them out in the form of behavioral extremes, such as withdrawal from or over-involvement in the therapeutic process. Clinicians need to be aware that some questions or comments routinely addressed to family members may inadvertently trigger feelings of guilt (e.g., "When did you first seek therapy for John's problem?" or "How do you deal with John's behavior at home?").

- *Shame* is an emotional state characterized by a negative evaluation of one's entire self and is accompanied by feelings of worthlessness and failure. It generates strong avoidance behaviors that may have a significant impact on a client's ability to participate effectively in counseling. Shame can be difficult to detect because there is no easily recognized facial expression or other overt manifestation, as in anger or depression.

- *Anxiety* refers to feelings of apprehension or distress that are generally not directly related to an immediate situation. This reaction may be present throughout the therapeutic process. During the initial stages of intervention, clients and their families are often uncertain about what to expect and also may question whether the clinician can truly help them. As therapy progresses, the focus of client anxiety may shift to the educational, vocational, or social repercussions of the communicative disorder.

- *Inadequacy* encompasses feelings of insufficiency or incompetence. Clients and their families frequently are overwhelmed by the diagnosis and implications of a communicative disorder. As a result, they rely heavily on the information and support provided by the clinician, especially in the initial stages of intervention. If feelings of confidence and self-esteem are not cultivated, this dependent relationship is likely to continue, and the clinician can become cast in the role of "rescuer" rather than a facilitator of change (Luterman, 2008).

- *Isolation* is a sense of personal detachment and remoteness from society. It can be self-imposed or result from others' rejection of the client. Isolation may arise from feelings such as inadequacy and low self-esteem, or from the perception that no one else can truly understand the client's situation. Strong feelings of isolation may exacerbate the intensity or duration of all the emotional reactions just discussed. The client's isolation from social interactions may severely impede the clinician's ability to establish an effective counseling relationship.

Clients rarely verbalize these emotions directly. Therefore, the clinician must be a keen observer of nonverbal and vocal behaviors that may be indicative of client distress. (See Form 11-1 for a behavioral checklist.)

COUNSELING TECHNIQUES FOR COMMUNICATIVE DISORDERS

One of the primary goals of counseling is to help clients and their families cope with the reality of the communicative disorder and foster the perspective that it constitutes only one aspect of the client's overall identity. The clinician's role is to assist clients in assuming responsibility for their own behavior and decisions. This goal is generally achieved through implementation of a variety of counseling techniques. Selection of specific procedures will depend on the personalities of the client and clinician as well as the constraints imposed by the communicative disorder. The following section briefly describes several of the counseling techniques most commonly used by SLPs.

- *Desensitization:* The client is guided through a hierarchy of situations from least to most anxiety provoking within the context of a safe and relaxed counseling environment. For example, a college student with a severe lisp can be gradually exposed to feared speaking situations that range from (1) an informal conversation with the clinician, (2) a formal presentation to the clinician, and (3) the same formal presentation to unfamiliar listeners in a classroom setting.

- *Relaxation:* Tension is reduced in muscle groups to alleviate a client's feelings of anxiety. For example, a client with a hyperfunctional voice disorder can be instructed to (1) alternately contract and release laryngeal muscles, (2) mentally visualize a peaceful setting, and (3) engage in deep diaphragmatic breathing.

- *Counterquestion:* A client may ask questions that appear to be requests for technical information but are actually intended to gain the clinician's confirmation or validation of a decision that has already been made. The clinician can respond to these types of remarks by posing a counterquestion that encourages the client to reveal the true intent of the original query. For example, a clinician may recognize that a mother who repeatedly inquires about the interpretation of her child's cognitive and language test scores may not truly be seeking technical information. The clinician can pose a counterquestion such as "Is there something in particular about these test scores that bothers you?" At this point, the mother may acknowledge that she recently refused to allow an Individualized Education Plan (IEP) team to label her child as "mentally retarded," and she is actually seeking support for this decision from the clinician.

- *Reframing:* A client or family is encouraged to modify views or attitudes toward a negative situation that cannot be changed. For example, a clinician may point out that family members have analyzed and improved their interpersonal relationships as a result of the client's stroke and subsequent aphasia. This technique should be introduced in the later stages of the therapeutic relationship only after the client or family has demonstrated a genuine acceptance of the communicative disorder.

- *Open-ended and indirect questions:* Questions are formulated in a manner that does not restrict the client or family's response to a simple one- or two-word utterance. This technique is used to elicit spontaneous and detailed responses that provide insight into the client's attitudes, knowledge, and feelings. One common example of an open-ended question is: "What are your major concerns about wearing a hearing aid?" A typical indirect question is: "I'd be interested in knowing your opinion of the new hearing aid."

- *Role-playing:* Problematic situations associated with the communicative disorder are identified, and structured opportunities are provided for a client to act out more appropriate behaviors in hypothetical contexts. For example, an adolescent who frequently misunderstands conversational messages may refuse to request clarification because "people will think I am stupid." Scripted scenarios can be developed and used to rehearse specific repair strategies for obtaining needed information without embarrassment.

- *Empathetic listening:* The clinician reflects back the content or emotions expressed by a client's message in a nonjudgmental manner. This is generally accomplished by merely repeating or rephrasing the client's comments in an objective fashion. Effective listening is characterized by consistent eye contact, attentive body language, and behaviors that encourage continued communication such as head nods and "um hmm."

- *Paraphrasing content:* The clinician rephrases a client's message or statement in his or her own words. This "mirroring" allows the client to hear the message from another source and gives him or her the opportunity to amplify, clarify, correct, revise, or confirm the meaning.

- *Summarizing content:* This technique involves succinct, accurate paraphrasing of larger segments of client interaction (e.g., at least 10–15 minutes). The intent is for the clinician to capture the overall gist of the important elements of the preceding discourse.

- *Silence:* The clinician refrains from speaking in order to shift the conversational floor to the client. A purposeful silence can provide the client with a communicative disorder with the time needed to formulate responses. Also, clinicians who meet a client utterance with purposeful silence rather than an immediate rejoinder may encourage the client to share additional information that would not otherwise have been expressed. Beginning clinicians typically are uncomfortable with even brief silences during their interactions with clients. Counseling skills can be greatly enhanced by learning the judicious use of purposeful silences in the clinical setting. (See Form 11-2 for a checklist that clinicians can use to monitor their own verbal and nonverbal behaviors during counseling sessions.)

In addition to overall strategies, Flasher and Fogle (2012) provide counseling guidance with regard to specific communication disorders, including:

- Client age often factors into the counseling approach with individuals who stutter. For example, counseling may not be as direct with a preschool-aged individual as with an adult client.

- Voice disorders and associated changes in vocal characteristics can impact a person's self-identity as well as degree of social interactions. Intervention may need to target improving vocal quality while also addressing issues of vocal use with regards to daily activities.

- Dysphagia and swallowing protocols can cause a client to feel uncomfortable during meals, an activity of daily living that has a strong social component. Ongoing discussions with the client and his or her family are important to managing concerns that arise as the client adjusts to the current situation.

FORM 11–1 CLIENT NONVERBAL AND VOCAL BEHAVIOR CHECKLIST

INSTRUCTIONS: Observe a live or recorded counseling session. Answer each of the following items by circling the letter in each set of three that corresponds to the most appropriate description of the client's nonverbal behaviors.

1. How is the client sitting?

   a. Rigidly   a. Very near the clinician   a. In constant motion

   b. Relaxed   b. At an average distance   b. In typical motion

   c. Slouched   c. Very far from the clinician   c. Motionless

2. How does the client look?

   a. Nervous   a. Happy   a. Well dressed   a. Friendly

   b. At ease   b. Concerned   b. Appropriately dressed   b. Business-like

   c. Passive   c. Upset   c. Disheveled   c. Belligerent

3. How does the client communicate?

   a. Very quickly   a. Loudly   a. High-pitched voice

   b. At a normal rate   b. At normal intensity   b. Average voice

   c. Very slowly   c. Quietly   c. Low-pitched voice

   a. With appropriate affect and intonation   a. With many gestures

   b. With inappropriate affect and intonation   b. With some gestures

   c. With no affect or intonation   c. With no gestures

SOURCE: Adapted from McDonald and Haney (1997) McDonald, P. A., & Haney, M. (1997). Counseling the older adult: A training manual in clinical gerontology. San Francisco, CA: Jossey-Bass.

FORM 11–2 CLINICIAN/COUNSELOR BEHAVIOR CHECKLIST

INSTRUCTIONS: Observe a live or recorded counseling session. Respond to each statement with "Yes," "No," or "Not applicable" to describe the clinician's counseling behaviors.

(Note: Y = Yes; N = No; NA = Not applicable)

Nonverbal

_____	1. The clinician maintained appropriate eye contact with the client.
_____	2. The clinician was alert and responded with an animated facial expression.
_____	3. The clinician refrained from nonverbally reinforcing the client's off-task or irrelevant remarks (i.e., head nods).
_____	4. The clinician demonstrated relaxed body posture.
_____	5. The clinician leaned forward as the client spoke.
_____	6. The clinician used a variety of vocal intonation patterns.
_____	7. The clinician's voice was sufficiently loud to be heard by the client.
_____	8. The clinician used intermittent vocalization (e.g., mm-hmm) during the client's on-task, relevant remarks.

Verbal

_____	1. The clinician's remarks usually addressed the most important aspects of each of the client's utterances.
_____	2. The clinician encouraged the client to express feelings about the communicative disorder.
_____	3. The clinician verbally identified and responded to the client's feelings.
_____	4. Most of the clinician's questions were open-ended in nature and required more than a one- or two-word response from the client.
_____	5. The clinician did not monopolize the available talk time in the session.
_____	6. The clinician used purposeful silences to encourage the client to elaborate on responses.
_____	7. The clinician made verbal responses that supported or reinforced some of the client's statements.
_____	8. The clinician occasionally restated or clarified the client's remarks.
_____	9. The clinician expressed a desire to understand the client's feelings and attitudes about the communication problem.
_____	10. The clinician answered directly when the client asked for information or an opinion.
_____	11. The clinician occasionally used counterquestions to respond to certain client queries.
_____	12. The clinician occasionally offered an alternative and more positive perspective of some situation that the client has identified as distressing.
_____	13. The clinician summarized key points of the session at appropriate junctures.

SOURCE: Adapted from Cormier and Hackney (2008) Cormier, L. S. & Hackney, H. (2008). Counseling strategies and interventions (7th ed.). Princeton, NC: Merrill.

Group Counseling

Some SLPs coordinate sessions that function as emotional support groups for clients and their families. Provision of therapy within a group setting can foster elements important to counseling, thus helping the group members to make progress (Erdman, 2009). Some of these factors include universality (i.e., the knowledge that an individual is not the only one experiencing a particular communication disorder), altruism (i.e., the feeling of self-importance and happiness that arises from providing support to other group members), and imitative behaviors (i.e., the development of compensatory strategies from watching other members) (Erdman, 2009).

Clinicians need to be knowledgeable about group dynamics and be aware of the issues that tend to arise in this setting. Effective counseling skills enable the clinician to do the following:

- Determine appropriate composition and size of a group
- Set the procedures and norms for group interactions
- Promote an atmosphere of trust and unity among the group members
- Assume a less directive leadership role as the group matures
- Encourage a particular group member to risk self-disclosure
- Manage a dominant member who is monopolizing the group's time
- Manage confrontational interactions between or among group members
- Determine the hidden agendas of individual group members
- Extinguish comments and behaviors that detract from therapy goals
- Reinforce group members who make constructive comments to other group members
- Recognize an individual group member's need for more specialized counseling services and broach the topic skillfully
- Determine the appropriate juncture for terminating a group

(See Chapter 1 for a detailed discussion of the advantages and disadvantages of group sessions.)

Family Systems Counseling

Based on family systems theory, this approach acknowledges the central role that the family plays in a client's development and progress. Key concepts of this theory are: (1) change in one family member affects the entire family system, (2) the family unit is greater than the sum of its parts, and (3) families exist within the context of the larger society. In this view, families are dynamic units with specific communication and interaction patterns (Begun, 1996). Effective clinicians incorporate this family-centered perspective into their counseling efforts. It is noteworthy that such consideration is actually required by federal law under the provisions of the Individuals with Disabilities Education Act (2004).

An increasing variety of family structures are represented in clinical caseloads. Several societal factors contribute to this diversity, including differing cultural/ethnic backgrounds, poverty, and single-parent households, among a host of others. Accordingly, clinicians can expect a wide range of family involvement/participation in the intervention process. Therefore, the clinician's counseling efforts should be designed on a case-by-case basis to accommodate the needs of each family.

Helpful Hints

1. The value of counseling is severely compromised if a clinician's personal feelings become a factor in the therapeutic relationship.

2. Important points can be emphasized by reiterating them in different ways at various stages of the counseling relationship.

3. The provision of a brief summary at the end of a counseling session may help the client focus on the most important points that were discussed. A written summary also may help the client to understand and remember terminology related to his or her communication disorder (e.g., dysarthria, anatomical terms).

4. A client's feelings and attitudes generally cannot be changed by the clinician's presentation of rational argument alone.

5. The purpose of counseling is to provide a client with the information needed to manage and to treat the communication disorder; it is not intended to ameliorate problems in the client's personal life.

6. Reluctance, resentment, and opposition are predictable client reactions in the counseling process and should not evoke feelings of defensiveness on the part of the clinician.

7. A clinician's use of phrases such as "It is my impression . . ." or "I hear you saying . . ." are less likely to trigger defensive behaviors from a client than more direct statements such as "You are . . ." or "You can't . . ."

8. It is important for clinicians to realize that the overuse of positive remarks causes such reinforcers to become meaningless.

9. Counseling is more effective if it periodically acknowledges a client's strengths rather than focusing solely on weaknesses or limitations.

10. Clinicians should refrain from pressing a client for self-disclosure too early in the counseling relationship because it may actually increase a client's reluctance to confide in the clinician.

11. Sometimes, conflict within a group can be a sign that the group is working well as a unit. It frequently indicates that group members have developed a sense of trust and feel secure enough to disagree openly with each other.

12. Counseling that loses its focus or purpose becomes mere conversation and accomplishes little.

13. Clinicians can learn to identify "teaching" versus "counseling" moments. For example, some questions may be truly asked to request information (e.g., When did my child acquire this disorder?). However, sometimes the clinician may be able to discern that a question is meant more to address personal concerns (e.g., Did the parent have a role in the development of a communication disorder?).

14. The following books may help clinicians develop their empathetic listening skills and sharpen insights about living with communication disorders:

    - Bauby, J-D. (1997). *The diving bell and the butterfly: A memoir of life in death.* New York: Knopf.

    - Grandin, T. (2011). *The way I see it: A personal look at autism and Asperger's* (2nd ed.). Arlington, TX: Future Horizons.

- Haddon, M. (2003). *The curious incident of the dog in the night-time.* New York: Doubleday.

- Sacks, O. (2000). *Seeing voices: A journey into the world of the deaf.* New York: Knopf.

CONCLUSION

This chapter presented basic information, protocols, and procedures for counseling at an *introductory* level. This information is intended only as a starting point in the reader's clinical education and training. For more in-depth coverage of this area, the following readings are recommended:

Flasher, L. V., & Fogle, P. T. (2012). *Counseling skills for speech-language pathologists and audiologists* (2nd ed.). Clifton Park, NY: Cengage Learning.

Luterman, D. M. (2008). *Counseling persons with communication disorders and their families* (5th ed.). Austin, TX: Pro-Ed.

Shipley, K. G., & Roseberry-McKibben, C. (2006). *Interviewing and counseling in communicative disorders: Principles and procedures* (3rd ed.). Austin, TX: Pro-Ed.

ADDITIONAL RESOURCES

Pro-Ed
8700 Shoal Creek Boulevard
Austin, TX 78757-6897
Phone: 800-897-3202
Fax: 800-397-7633
Web site: http://www.proedinc.com

***Interviewing and Counseling in Communicative Disorders: Principles and Procedures,* 3rd edition**
This resource addresses issues such as various interviewing and counseling activities, stages of interviewing and counseling, and skills and techniques for effective interviewing and counseling. It also discusses areas such as multicultural factors, professional and ethical matters, and dealing with difficult situations.

***Lifespan Perspectives on the Family and Disability,* 2nd edition**
This resource examines how families cope, adapt, and grow through the challenge of living with a child with a disability. A family-centered focus is presented within a life-span framework: infancy/early childhood, school years, transition from school to adult life, adult years.

***Rehabilitation Counseling: Basics and Beyond,* 5th edition**
This text provides clinicians with theoretical, research-based approaches to counseling as well as experience-driven practices. The authors frame counseling from the viewpoint of federal laws (e.g., Americans with Disabilities Amendment Act) as well as the issues that arise at different developmental stages (e.g., vocations/careers, sexual development).

Counseling Persons with Communication Disorders and Their Families
This resource helps professionals incorporate some of the knowledge and skills of trained counselors into their work with clients and families. Includes a free Instructor's Manual upon request.

Cengage Learning
10650 Toebben Drive
Independence, KY 41051
Phone: 800-354-9706
Web site: http://www.cengagebrain.com

Counseling Skills for Speech-Language Pathologists and Audiologists
Written by a clinical psychologist and an SLP, this text presents basic and advanced counseling skills as they are used by students and professionals in the communication sciences working with individuals with communication disorders. It places the theories of counseling and the therapeutic process in real-life contexts that are applicable to SLPs and audiologists.

CHAPTER 12

This topic is an evolving area of discussion that include many important constructs, such as language, culture, ethnicity/race, geography, degree of acculturation, background, family type, values, and belief systems. The term *culture* can also encompass individuals with disabilities, such as the Deaf culture (Battle, 2012). For the sake of simplicity and clarity, this chapter will use the term **cultural and linguistic diversity (CLD)** to represent this broad range of variables. In addition, there are a variety of terms used to describe individuals who are acquiring a second language. The most common include *dual language learners*, *English learners*, and **English language learners (ELLs).** Again, for the sake of simplicity and clarity, this chapter will use the term *ELL* to represent these individuals. Similarly, the term *bilingual*, as used in this chapter, refers to individuals who speak two or more languages. L1 refers to an individual's native language, whereas L2 represents the second language.

In a related vein, dialects are variations within a single language and may encompass phonological, syntactic, semantic, and pragmatic components. Dialects may be associated with geographic, socioeconomic, or cultural/ethnic factors. Examples of dialects in English include African American English (AAE), Appalachian English, and Cajun English. Competent users of multiple languages or dialects often engage in **code-switching,** alternating use of each language/dialect depending on the context or listener needs.

The changing demographics of the United States have important implications for speech-language pathologists (SLPs) to consider. Currently, the CLD population represents approximately 25% of the U.S. population and 14% of students enrolled in public schools. This number is projected to increase to over 30–50% between 2000 and 2015 (U.S. Bureau of the Census, 2000). If communication disorders occur at the same prevalence rate as in the general U.S. population, then approximately 6.2 million CLD Americans currently have a communication disorder (Battle, 2012). The number of ELL students receiving speech-language services doubled between 1990 and 2000 and continues to rise. The majority of these students tend to be classified as demonstrating a learning disability (U.S. Department of Education, 2009). In the adult population, there is a steady increase in the number of CLD individuals receiving intervention for neurogenic communication disorders (Centeno, 2009).

At least 13% of individuals living in the United States speak a primary language other than English. An estimated 11 million children in the United States are bilingual (National Center for Education Statistics, 2009). When individuals in this group demonstrate communication disorders, they may not be able to effectively participate in or derive maximal benefit from intervention. Unfortunately, about 5% of certified SLPs across the country can deliver clinical services in a language other than English, with slightly more than half of bilingual SLPs listing Spanish as the other language (ASHA, 2002b, 2012; Roseberry-McKibbin, Brice, & O'Hanlon, 2005).

Each year, thousands of children from other countries are adopted by American families. However, international adoption numbers have been on the decline within the past decade, decreasing from 22,734 children adopted in 2005 to 8,668 children adopted in 2012 (U.S. Department of State, 2014). These **international adoptees,** increasingly from China and Eastern Europe, sometimes spend their earliest years in settings characterized by inadequate nutrition, lack of stimulation, and lack of interpersonal/social interaction (Hwa-Froelich, 2009). As a result, they show evidence of a fundamental attachment disorder and demonstrate significant developmental impairments, especially in cognitive, linguistic, and behavioral skills. Due to the increasing rate of referral for assessment and treatment for this population, SLPs need to be aware that the age of adoption appears to be the most critical factor in eventual language outcome. Longitudinal studies indicate that children who are adopted after 2 to 3 years of age tend to show significant delays in acquisition of English (Glennen & Masters, 2002; Roberts et al., 2005). Still, some internationally adopted children will demonstrate language acquisition skills in the normal range, but generally below their native English-speaking peers. A study comparing language acquisition in individuals adopted from China and Canadian-born children acquiring French found that certain aspects of language may be more difficult for children to acquire as they learn their second "first" language. Among their difficulties were receptive syntax and morphology and expressive vocabulary (Gauthier & Genesee, 2011).

There are several broad categories of CLD variables to consider in delivery of intervention services. The following sections illustrate them with three examples.

SOCIOECONOMIC STATUS (SES)

Socioeconomic status (SES) is a way of ranking relative position in a society based on class, status, and power. It is frequently represented by financial resources/wealth, level of education, and occupation.

Clients of lower SES may be primarily concerned with practical issues of daily living that revolve around making ends meet, both financially and personally. Their priority in therapy may be to seek immediate solutions and concrete, observable behavioral changes. An intervention approach that focuses on increasing self-awareness and insight into the personal dynamics associated with a communication disorder may not be highly valued. Recommendations and referrals that may arise from the intervention process should be made with full consideration of each client's financial and personal situation. Qualls and Muñoz (2005) suggest that SES may be a better predictor of cognitive-communicative behaviors than other factors such as racial-ethnic background. In addition, maternal education level has been found to positively correlate with children's vocabulary knowledge (Hammer et al., 2012).

CULTURAL/ETHNIC BACKGROUND

Prior to initiating the intervention process, clinicians should engage in self-reflection to identify core aspects of their own values and belief systems. Roseberry-McKibbin (2007) identified several assumptions that are common to clinicians reared in mainstream American culture. Examples include:

- Punctuality is an indicator of mutual respect in a therapeutic relationship.
- In meetings, value is placed on "getting to the point" quickly and directly.
- The age and gender of the clinician relative to the client are much less important than the clinician's level of competence.
- Written documentation is an integral component of all interactions with clients/families.
- Treatment is warranted even for individuals with no observable physical disability.
- The ultimate goal of intervention is independent functioning.

These beliefs may be in substantial contrast to those held by individuals from CLD backgrounds. Some examples of these differences are discussed here in an attempt to illustrate the scope of knowledge required to develop multicultural competence.

Cultural competence has been defined as the "ability to think, feel, and act in ways that acknowledge, respect and build upon ethnic, cultural, and linguistic diversity" (Lynch & Hanson, 2011). In its 2011 position statement, the American Speech-Language Hearing Association (ASHA) described cultural competence as a clinician's ability to adjust his or her views and behavior in relation to another culture's norms. Culturally competent clinicians demonstrate understanding of the impact of cultural differences on individual behavior. Within the clinical setting, flexibility is important in adapting and reacting to CLD variables. However, it is important for clinicians to recognize that individual differences exist even within specific cultural groups. To avoid stereotyping, clinicians should view clients as individuals first and members of particular ethnicities or cultures second (ASHA, 2011; Battle, 2012; Kuo & Hu, 2002; Pedersen, Draguns, Lonner, & Trimble, 2002; Roseberry-McKibbin, 2007).

Members of various cultures have widely differing views regarding the nature and appropriate treatment of communication disorders. Use of professional terminology varies widely from country to country and may affect clinician–client communication during the intervention process. For example, the term *dyslexia* in Russia is confined to those with reading problems only. However, in Italy, the same term refers to writing difficulties as well (Smythe & Everatt, 2002). Even issues as fundamental as whether a disability exists or should be treated are subject to cultural interpretation (Adler, n.d.). Battle (1997) highlights this point by contrasting the belief systems of Native American and Chinese cultures. Native Americans embrace a philosophy that life should be in harmony with nature. Thus, a communication disorder may be considered a part of life that should be accepted rather than changed. In contrast, Chinese cultural tradition regards a disability as an irreversible punishment for the transgressions of ancestors. Members of either culture, therefore, may be reluctant to engage in the therapeutic process. Other consequences of cultural differences may become obvious when parental expectations of a child differ from school expectations. Thus, the child receives "mixed messages" and has to find a way to resolve the conflict between the two sets of expectations.

Numerous other culture-specific factors may have an influence on the clinician's approach to clients with communication disorders and their families. Battle (2012) provides the following illustrations:

- Islamic tradition does not permit a female client to receive therapy services from a male clinician. Extended family members may expect to participate in therapy sessions and might be offended if they are excluded.

- Hinduism allows no photographs or videotapes of female clients.

- Japanese mothers tend to use less verbal (and more nonverbal) communication behaviors than middle-class American mothers when interacting with their young children.

- Hispanic families may experience difficulty acknowledging disabilities that have no visible physical manifestations (e.g., language or articulation disorder, dyslexia, and so on).

- Asian cultures often view social skills as a critical component of intelligence, whereas Western European cultures' model of intelligence involves innate cognitive skills.

LINGUISTIC DIFFERENCES

In addition to SES and cultural/ethnic factors, the intervention process may be affected by language differences with clients from diverse backgrounds. These differences involve nonverbal, paralinguistic, and verbal aspects of communication. With respect to nonverbal behaviors, beginning clinicians may assume that certain communication behaviors have universal meanings. In fact, tremendous variation exists in the interpretation of paralinguistic expressions. Three examples that are particularly relevant to therapy provided by SLPs are eye contact, smiling, and seating arrangement. Caucasian Americans exhibit a much greater degree of eye contact as listeners than as speakers, while African Americans tend to demonstrate the opposite pattern (i.e., greater eye contact when speaking than listening). Moreover, Asians/Pacific Islanders often perceive eye contact as an expression of hostility, whereas Native Americans tend to interpret direct eye contact as a sign of disrespect. Similar variation exists with respect to smiling: Western cultures assign positive meaning to this facial expression; the Japanese culture associates smiling with shyness or embarrassment; and other Asian cultures may interpret smiling as a sign of weakness or superficiality. Finally, Westerners seem to prefer a seating arrangement in which the client and clinician face each other across a table. On the other hand, Native Americans may be most comfortable with a side-by-side arrangement (Sue & Sue, 1999).

In the United States, native language speakers of tonal languages have increased from 1.2 million in 1990 to more than 2 million in 2000, when Chinese became the third most widely spoken language in the country (Wong, Perrachione, Gunasekera, & Chandrasekaran, 2009). Chinese is considered a tonal language, in which pitch is used to discriminate between the meanings of individual words (e.g., /ma/ can have at least three meanings depending on the lexical tone used by the speaker). These lexical tones vary within a speaker's pitch range and change over time. The ability to perceive lexical tones is correlated with activity in the language-dominant left hemisphere of the brain for native speakers of tonal languages. In contrast, lexical tones presented to native speakers of nontonal languages tend to activate the right hemisphere of the brain, because the tones carry no linguistic relevance for them.

Clearly, verbal language differences are culturally determined and may influence semantic, phonologic, syntactic, and morphologic behaviors. Moreover, pragmatic language issues such as appropriate topics of conversation, turn-taking rules, and the effects of social status between communication partners are culturally bound. For specific information regarding nonverbal and verbal characteristics of three main cultural groups—African American, Hispanic, and Asian—refer to Tables 12-1 through 12-9.

CLINICAL CONSIDERATIONS FOR CHILDREN

Provision of effective intervention for children from CLD backgrounds requires basic knowledge of second-language acquisition in childhood. This knowledge base includes important terminology, patterns of L2 acquisition, and models of bilingual education.

TABLE 12–1

Consonant Sound Production Characteristics of African American English (AAE)

Phoneme	Description
/n/	Replaced by nasalized vowel in the final position (e.g., bin → /bɪ̃/)
/w, d/	Omitted in initial position for specific words (e.g., was → /əz/; don't → /ont/)
/ŋ/	Replaced by /n/ especially in final position (e.g., going → /goɪn/)
/l, r/	Omitted in medial and final positions (e.g., poor → /po/) Replaced occasionally by /ə/ in final position (e.g., pill → /pɪə/; here /hiə/)
/θ/	Replaced by /t/ or /f/ in initial, medial, and final positions (e.g., author → /ɔfə/; math → /mæf/)
/ð/	Replaced by /d/ in initial position and /d/ or /v/ in medial and final positions (e.g., this → /dɪs/; mother → /mʌvɚ/)
/z/	Omitted or replaced by /d/ before nasal sounds (e.g., isn't /ɪdnt/)

Blends

/str/	Replaced by /skr/ (e.g., street → /skrit/)
/ʃr/	Replaced by /str/ (e.g., shrill → /strɪl/)
/θr/	Replaced by /θ/ (e.g., throw → /θo/)
/pr, br, gr, kr/	Omission of /r/ (e.g., apron → /epən/; agriculture → /æglkəltʃɚ/)

Consonant Clusters

/sk, nd, sp, ft, ld, dʒd, st, sd, nt/	Deletion of second consonant in final word position (e.g., left → /lɛf/; cold → /kol/; desk → /dɛs/)

SOURCE: Bailey, G., & Thomas, E. (1998). Some aspects of African-American vernacular English phonology. In S. Mufwene, J. Rickford, G. Bailey, & J. Baugh (Eds.), African-American English: History and use (pp. 85–109). London: Routledge. Adapted from Bailey and Thomas (1998), Goldstein (2000) Goldstein, B. (2000). Cultural and linguistic diversity resource guide for speech-language pathologists. Clifton Park, NY: Cengage Learning., Owens (2001) Owens, R. E. (2011). Language development: An introduction (8th ed.). Needham Heights, MA: Allyn & Bacon. , Fasold and Wolfram (1970) Fasold, R., & Wolfram, W. (1970). Some linguistic features of Negro dialect. In R. Fasold & R. Shuy (Eds.), Teaching standard English in the inner city (pp. 41–86). Washington, DC: Center for Applied Linguistics. , and -Williams and Wolfram (1977) Williams, R., & Wolfram, W. (1977). Social dialects: Differences vs. disorders. Washington, DC: -American Speech-Language-Hearing -Association.

Terminology

There are three main types of bilingualism:

- **Ambilingual:** Speaks both languages with the proficiency of a native speaker
- **Equilingual:** Communicates effectively in both languages
- **Semilingual:** Demonstrates poor mastery of both L1 and L2

Mastery of a language can be described in two major ways:

- **Proficiency:** Competence in or mastery of a given language; may change over time
- **Dominance:** Preference for or comfort with a specific language in a particular context

Acquisition of L2 can be described according to two major functions (Butler, 2013; Cummins, 1984):

- **Basic Interpersonal Communication Skills (BICS):** Use of language for social purposes (e.g., conversation, play, requesting, greetings). It is often supported by contextual cues, gestures, or facial expressions and takes 2 to 3 years to develop fully.

TABLE 12–2
Morphologic and Syntactic Characteristics of African American English (AAE)

Structure	Description
Verbs	
Regular past –ed	Not obligatory and frequently omitted (e.g., I **talk** to him last week)
Irregular past	May remain uninflected or regularized with "–ed" (e.g., He **begin** work yesterday; She **knowed** all about it)
Regular present third-person singular	Not obligatory and frequently omitted (e.g., John **sleep** too much)
Irregular present third-person singular	Not obligatory and frequently omitted (e.g., He always **do** silly things)
Future tense	"Will" is replaced by "gonna"; "will" is omitted preceding the verb "be" (e.g., The dog **gonna** bite you; I **be** back tomorrow)
Copula and auxiliary	Not obligatory and may be omitted if contractible (e.g., He **ready;** They **eating**)
Perfect tense	"Been" is used to signify action in the distant past (e.g., He died long ago → He **been** dead)
Habitual state	Ongoing or general states are marked by uninflected "be" (e.g., She **be** funny)
Modals	Double modals are permissible with forms such as *might, could,* and *should* (e.g., They **might could** come)
Noun Phrases	
Regular plural –s	Not obligatory and frequently omitted when quantifiers are present (e.g., I see three **book** over there)
Irregular plural	May be doubly inflected (e.g., Help me find the **childrens**)
Possessive –'s	Not obligatory and frequently omitted when word order indicates possession (e.g., **Debbie** bike got wet)
Pronouns	
Apposition	Pronoun immediately follows the referent noun (e.g., My brother **he** bigger than you)
Relative pronouns	Not obligatory and frequently omitted (e.g., There's the **dog bit** me)
Reflexive pronouns	Reflexive -*self* form can be extended to possessive pronouns (e.g., **hisself; theirself**)
Demonstratives	Certain demonstrative/pronominal phrases are permissible (e.g., **These here** apples; **Them there** toys)
Adverbs and Adjectives	
Comparatives and superlatives	The forms –*er* and –*est* can be extended to many adjectives (e.g., **worser, horriblest**)
	The modifiers *more* and *most* can be added to comparative and superlative forms (e.g., **more taller; most oldest**)

(continues)

TABLE 12–2 *(Continued)*

Structure	Description
Adverbs and Adjectives (Continued)	
Intensifiers	Certain modifiers can be added to adverbs or adjectives for emphasis (e.g., **right** quick; **plumb** crazy)
Negation	
Ain't	"Ain't" is a permissible negative form (e.g., I **ain't** got any money)
Multiple negation	Double and triple negative markers are permissible (e.g., **Nobody don't** like me; **Nobody don't never** talk to him)
Interrogatives	
Indirect questions	The inverted form may be used for indirect questions (e.g., I wonder what **was he** singing)
	The uninverted form may be used for direct questions (e.g., What **he was** eating?)
	The conditional conjunction *if* is replaced by *do* (e.g., I wonder **do** you hear me?)

SOURCES: Adapted from Fasold and Wolfram (1970) Fasold, R., & Wolfram, W. (1970). Some linguistic features of Negro dialect. In R. Fasold & R. Shuy (Eds.), Teaching standard English in the inner city (pp. 41–86). Washington, DC: Center for Applied Linguistics. , Goldstein (2000) Goldstein, B. (2000). Cultural and linguistic diversity resource guide for speech-language pathologists. Clifton Park, NY: Delmar Cengage Learning. , Owens (2001) Owens, R. E. (2011). Language development: An introduction (8th ed.). Needham Heights, MA: Allyn & Bacon. , Roseberry-McKibbin (1995) Roseberry-McKibbin, C. (2008). Multicultural students with special language needs (3rd ed.). Oceanside, CA: Academic Communication Associates. , Washington and Craig (1994) Washington, J., & Craig, H. (1994). Dialect forms during discourse of poor, urban African-American preschoolers. Journal of Speech and Hearing Research, 37, 816–823. , and Williams, R., & Wolfram, W. (1977). Social dialects: Differences vs. disorders. Washington, DC: American Speech-Language-Hearing -Association. Williams and Wolfram (1977).

- **Cognitive-Academic Language Proficiency Skills (CALPS):** Use of language effectively for academic learning purposes (e.g., make inferences, compare and contrast, synthesize). Contextual cues and other supports are usually not available, so the individual must primarily rely on the linguistic code itself to derive meaning. This set of language skills generally takes about 5 to 7 years to develop fully.

L1 and L2 can influence one another in the following reciprocal ways:

- **Language Interference/Transfer:** The grammar, vocabulary, phonology, or pragmatics of L1 may have an impact on the production of utterances in L2. These effects are frequently perceived as errors.
- **Language Loss:** Previously mastered skills in L1 can be negatively affected by the introduction of L2. If usage of L1 decreases significantly, the child will likely lose some degree of proficiency in that language.

Patterns of Second Language Acquisition

There are two major patterns of L2 acquisition:

- **Simultaneous** (Patterson & Pearson, 2012): Child is exposed to and acquires L1 and L2 from birth. In this ideal although rare scenario, the child develops BICS in both languages with relatively equivalent levels of proficiency.

TABLE 12–3
Pragmatic Characteristics of African American English (AAE)

- Direct eye contact is used in the speaker role, whereas indirect eye contact is associated with the listener role. Speakers of other dialects may interpret this indirect eye contact as inattentiveness or disrespect.

- Interruptions during conversation are permissible and the role of speaker is yielded to the most assertive conversational partner. This interaction pattern may be interpreted by non-AAE speakers as impolite or rude.

- Silence is used as a communication strategy in unfamiliar situations or to refute a speaker's statement. In other dialects, this silence may be interpreted as lack of knowledge or acceptance of the speaker's statement.

- Questions about personal matters such as family, health, and education are considered rude and discourteous when addressed to a new acquaintance.

- Humor and sarcasm are highly valued aspects of communicative interactions and are often expressed in ritualized exchanges of insults and comebacks. These interactions may be misinterpreted by non-AAE speakers as instances of negative and hostile behavior.

- Conversations are considered to be private; verbal contributions from individuals outside the immediate conversational group are perceived as impolite eavesdropping behavior (even if the comments were intended to be helpful).

- Intense and demonstrative speech behavior is permissible in public conversational interactions. Speakers of other dialects may interpret this emotional display as irresponsible or in bad taste.

SOURCE: Adapted from Kamhi, Pollack, and Harris (1996) Kamhi, A., Pollock, K., & Harris, J. (1996). Communication development and disorders in African-American children. Baltimore, MD: Brookes. ; Paul, R. (2006). Language disorders from infancy to adolescence: Assessment and intervention. Boston, MA: Mosby. Paul (2007).

- **Sequential/Successive** (Kayser, 2012): L2 is introduced later in childhood, usually after 3 years of age, when a significant portion of BICS in L1 is already in place.

The age or stage at which L2 is introduced strongly influences the degree of bilingualism that a child will demonstrate. For example, if L2 is introduced in the early primary grades, then the child will tend to present as *equilingual* (i.e., able to communicate effectively in either language). Children who are exposed to L2 at later ages or grade levels will generally present in a manner that more closely resembles *semilingual* (i.e., does not demonstrate native proficiency in either language). In addition to the age of exposure, the relative amounts that each language is used as well as the contexts in which each are used also affect the degree of bilingualism (Hammer et al., 2012).

Educational Models

Various educational approaches exist for children from CLD backgrounds:

- **Immersion:** L1 is de-emphasized and all instruction is conducted in L2.

- **Transitional:** L1 is used to teach L2 until students can acquire the classroom curriculum effectively in L2 (at which point L1 is faded out).

- **Maintenance:** Both L1 and L2 continue to be used in instructional settings to varying degrees, with the goal of maintaining some level of proficiency in the child's native language.

TABLE 12–4

Speech Sound Production Characteristics of Spanish-Influenced English (SIE)

Phoneme	Description
/ɪ, æ/	Do not exist in Spanish and are replaced by other vowels (e.g., mister → /mistɚ/)
/d/	Dentalized in medial position
/ŋ/	Replaced by /n/ in the final position (e.g., song → /sɔn/)
/j/	Replaced by /dʒ/ in initial position (e.g., you → / dʒu/)
/ʃ/	Replaced by /tʃ/ in all positions (e.g., sheet → /tʃit/; washer → /wɔtʃɚ/)
/tʃ/	Replaced by /ʃ/ in all positions (e.g., chain → /ʃen/; teacher → /tiʃɚ/)
/dʒ/	Replaced by /j/ in initial and medial positions (e.g., major → /mejɚ/)
/θ/	Replaced by /t/ in initial and final positions and omitted in medial position (e.g., think → /tɪnk/; baths → /bæs/)
/v/	Replaced by /b/ in all positions (e.g., vowel → /baʊl/; oven → /ʌbɛn/)
/z/	Replaced by /s/ in all positions (e.g., zero → /siro/; blizzard → /blɪsɚd/)
/ð/	Replaced by /d/ in initial and final positions; replaced by /d/, /v/, or /θ/ in medial position (e.g., they → /de/; brother → /brʌθɚ/)
	Consonants in the final position are usually devoiced (e.g., cab → /kæp/; bug → /bʌk/)
	A schwa or /ɛ/ is often added before consonant blends beginning with /s/ (e.g., speech → /əspitʃ/; slow → /ɛslo/)

SOURCE: Adapted from Battle (2002) Battle, D. E. (2012). Communication disorders in multicultural and international populations (4th Ed.). St. Louis, MO: Mosby., Goldstein (2000) Goldstein, B. (2000). Cultural and linguistic diversity resource guide for speech-language pathologists. Clifton Park, NY: Delmar Cengage Learning., Owens (2001) Owens, R. E. (2011). Language development: An introduction (8th ed.). Needham Heights, MA: Allyn & Bacon., and Paul (2007) Paul, R. (2006). Language disorders from infancy to adolescence: Assessment and intervention. Boston, MA: Mosby.

CLINICAL CONSIDERATIONS FOR ADULT POPULATIONS

Very little information is available to guide clinicians in the treatment of adults from CLD backgrounds. Following is a compilation of clinically relevant information that SLPs can incorporate into the development and delivery of intervention (Adler, n.d.; Centeno, 2009; Faroqi-Shah, Frymark, Mullen, & Wang, 2010; Kohnert, 2009; Wong et al., 2009):

- Language disorders often exist in both languages. Thus, assessments in each language are necessary to determine the types of linguistic difficulties in each language.

- For bilingual speakers, the same type and severity of aphasia may be present in both languages, or severity may be greater in one language (even after adjusting for premorbid proficiency levels).

- An effective approach for enhancing recovery from aphasia in bilingual speakers includes an emphasis on cross-linguistic generalization from a treated to an untreated language.

TABLE 12–5

Morphologic and Syntactic Characteristics of Spanish-Influenced English (SIE)

Structure	Description
Verbs	
Regular past –ed	Not obligatory and frequently omitted (e.g., I **talk** to him last week)
Regular present third-person singular	Not obligatory and frequently omitted (e.g., John **sleep** too much)
Future	Use of *go* + *to* with omission of the verb *to be* as well as the progressive marker *–ing* (e.g., I **go to** store)
Copula	Occasional use of *have* instead of *be* in certain instances (e.g., I **have** fourteen years)
Noun Phrases	
Regular plural –s	Not obligatory and frequently omitted (e.g., I see three **book** over there)
Possessive –'s	Replaced by prepositional phrase following the noun (e.g., This is the shirt **of my brother**)
Articles	Not obligatory and frequently omitted (e.g., They went **to movie**)
Pronouns	
Possessive pronouns	Replaced with article in reference to body parts (e.g., I broke **the** leg)
Subject pronouns	May be omitted when subject is specified in the preceding utterance (e.g., Maria is pretty. **Got** a new dress)
Adjectives	
Comparative –er	Replaced by modifier *more* (e.g., That table is **more** long)
Negation	
No	*No* replaces "auxiliary + *not*" before a verb (e.g., He **no** drink milk)
	No replaces *don't* in imperative forms (e.g., **No** touch that)
Interrogatives	
Inversion	Not obligatory and replaced by rising intonation (e.g., **Mama is** gone?)
Do insertion	Not obligatory and frequently omitted (e.g., **You want** more soup?)

Source: Adapted from Battle (2002) Battle, D. E. (2012). Communication disorders in multicultural and international populations (4th Ed.). St. Louis, MO: Mosby., Goldstein, B. (2000). Cultural and linguistic diversity resource guide for speech-language pathologists. Clifton Park, NY: Delmar Cengage Learning., Owens, R. E. (2011). Language development: An introduction (8th ed.). Needham Heights, MA: Allyn & Bacon., and Paul, R. (2006). Language disorders from infancy to adolescence: Assessment and intervention. Boston, MA: Mosby. , Goldstein (2000), Owens (2001), and Paul (2001).

TABLE 12–6
Pragmatic Characteristics of Spanish-Influenced English (SIE)

■ Indirect eye contact is used in conversation to convey attentiveness or respect. Speakers of other dialects may interpret this behavior in the opposite manner.

■ Distance between speakers during conversation is relatively close.

■ Touching one's communication partner is common during conversations. This contact may be perceived as offensive by speakers of other cultural orientations.

■ Interruptions during conversation are permissible. This pattern of interaction may be interpreted by non-SIE speakers as impolite or rude.

■ Formal or business conversations are opened with personal questions and remarks, which can be extensive. Speakers of other dialects may interpret this style of conversational initiation as intrusive, a sign of procrastination, or as "a waste of time."

SOURCE: Adapted from Kayser (1998) Kayser, H. (1998). Assessment and inter-vention resource for Hispanic children. San Diego, CA: Singular. and Paul, R. (2006). Language disorders from infancy to adolescence: Assessment and intervention. Boston, MA: Mosby. Paul (2001).

TABLE 12–7
Speech Sound Production Characteristics of Asian-Influenced English (AIE)

■ Speakers of AIE may shorten, lengthen, or otherwise distort English vowels. For example native speakers of Mandarin may produce *bead* as /bɪd/ or *fit* as /fit/.

■ AIE speakers tend to omit or distort final consonants because the rule systems of many Asian languages highly restrict or eliminate consonant sounds in the final position (e.g., *did* → /dɪ/).

■ In many Asian languages, /r/ and /l/ are not categorized as distinctly separate phonemes. As a result, these sounds may be used interchangeably in English (e.g., *rice* → /laɪs/).

■ Consonant blends are uncommon in many Asian languages. AIE speakers tend to simplify clusters either by inserting a /ə/ into the blend (e.g., speakers of Chinese and Japanese) or by omitting the entire cluster (e.g., speakers of Vietnamese).

■ Several Asian languages are predominantly monosyllabic in nature. AIE speakers may shorten or misplace stress on multisyllabic words (e.g., sepa'rately).

■ Asian languages such as Chinese, Vietnamese, or Laotian use changes in "tone" (prosody) to signify changes in word meaning. In contrast tonal changes in English are used to differentiate declarative from interrogative utterances and to convey communicative intent (e.g., sarcasm, humor, protest). AIE speakers may experience difficulty acquiring English intonation patterns and their messages may frequently be misinterpreted.

SOURCE: Adapted from Cheng (1987a, 1987b) andCheng, L. L. (1987a). As-sessing Asian language performance: Guidelines for assessing limited-English-proficient students. Gaithersburg, MD: Aspen., Cheng, L. L. (1987b). Cross-cultural and linguistic considerations in working with Asian populations. ASHA, 29, 33–38., and Owens, R. E. (2011). Language development: An introduction (8th ed.). Needham Heights, MA: Allyn & Bacon. Owens (2001).

■ Word retrieval can be improved in bilingual aphasia by selecting training stimuli that are similar in both meaning and phonetic form across L1 and L2 (e.g., *plate/plato* rather than *apple/manzana*). This clinical concept also applies to emphasizing the underlying processes that are common to both languages (e.g., attention, categorization, problem-solving strategies).

■ Repeated presentation of therapy stimuli may improve ability to gain or regain cognitive skills in L1 or L2.

TABLE 12–8

Morphologic and Syntactic Characteristics of Asian-Influenced English (AIE)

Structure	Description
Verbs	
Regular past –ed	Not obligatory and frequently omitted (e.g., He **walk** home yesterday)
Irregular past	May be regularized with –ed or doubly inflected, even in the perfect tense (e.g., He **sleeped** in the bed; He **didn't ran** home; He **had wented**)
Singular present	Not obligatory and frequently omitted in third person; overly inflected in second person (e.g., He usually **walk** to school; You **talks** too loud)
Auxiliary	*Be* and *do* may be omitted or remain uninflected (e.g., He **eating** dinner now; He **do** not know her)
Perfect tense	Marker –en is not obligatory and frequently omitted (e.g., I **have speak** to her)
Noun Phrases	
Regular plural –s	Not obligatory and frequently omitted when quantifiers are present (e.g., I have **three shirt**)
Irregular plural	May be doubly inflected and overregularized (e.g., She brushed her **teeths**)
Possessive –'s	Not obligatory and frequently omitted (e.g., That my **mom** hat)
Pronouns	
Possessive	Pronoun usage may be confused (e.g., I see **she** car)
Case	Subject and object pronouns may be confused (e.g., **Him** coming soon)
Gender	Male and female pronouns may be confused (e.g., I meet **her** wife)
Demonstratives	Singular and plural pronouns may be confused (e.g., He own **that** cars)
Adjectives	
Comparatives	The form –er may be extended to many adjectives (e.g., **gooder, honester**)
	The modifier *more* may be added to comparative forms (e.g., She is **more shorter** than me)
Negation	
Multiple negation	Double negative markers are permissible (e.g., He **didn't** have **none**)
No	*No* replaces "auxiliary + *not*" (e.g., He **no** live here)
Interrogatives	
Inversion	Not obligatory and replaced by rising intonation (e.g., **You are** coming home?)
Do insertion	Not obligatory and frequently omitted (e.g., **You see** her today?)

(continues)

TABLE 12–8 *(Continued)*

Structure	Description
Prepositions	May be omitted or confused (e.g., I put **it drawer;** I am at kitchen)
Conjunctions	Not obligatory and frequently omitted (e.g., **Brother sister** went home)
Articles	May be omitted or overused (e.g., I saw **boy;** I go to **the school**)
Word Order	Changes in word order frequently occur (e.g., I have **car new;** **Book mine** got lost; He put **down it**)

SOURCE: Adapted from Cheng (1987b) Cheng, L. L. (1987b). Cross-cultural and linguistic considera-tions in working with Asian populations. ASHA, 29, 33–38. and Owens (2001) Owens, R. E. (2011). Language development: An introduction (8th ed.). Needham Heights, MA: Allyn & Bacon.

TABLE 12–9

Pragmatic Characteristics of Asian-Influenced English (AIE)

- Direct eye contact is avoided; indirect eye contact is used in conversation to convey respect. Speakers of other dialects may interpret this behavior unfavorably.

- Interruptions during conversations are considered impolite. Children who ask questions or interrupt teachers during classroom lectures are considered disobedient. Western cultures may perceive this behavior (i.e., not asking questions during lecture) as passive and nonparticipatory.

- Third-party introductions are preferred to informal self-introductions, especially when interacting with individuals of high status. Non-AIE speakers may regard this preference for formal introductions as unfriendly or aloof behavior.

- Questions about age, marital status, or employment are considered appropriate even of new acquaintances in order to establish proper social distance between or among the speakers. Western cultures may regard such queries as inappropriate or nosy, especially in initial conversations.

- Professionals are automatically treated with respect and are regarded as authorities.

- Kinship terms may be used with elders who are not family members as an indication of respect.

- Embarrassment is a common reaction to praise; humility is emphasized and highly valued.

- Feelings are not openly exhibited; public affection is not displayed. The facial expressions of AIE speakers may remain impassive even when being provoked or reprimanded. Western speakers may perceive this affect as indifference or insensitivity.

- Giggling may reflect shyness or embarrassment rather than amusement.

- Direct and open disagreement is infrequent, particularly with individuals regarded as high-status professionals or authorities. Speakers in Western cultures may misinterpret this behavior as an indication of agreement.

SOURCE: Adapted from Cheng (1987a, 1987b) Cheng, L. L. (1987a). Assessing Asian language performance: Guidelines for assessing limited-English-proficient students. Gaithersburg, MD: Aspen., Cheng, L. L. (1987b). Cross-cultural and linguistic considerations in working with Asian populations. ASHA, 29, 33–38., and Langdon, H. W., & Cheng, L. R. (2002). Collaborating with interpreters and translators. Eau Claire, WI: Thinking Publications. Langdon and Cheng (2002).

- Therapy provided only in L2 results in positive outcomes even with bilingual speakers with chronic aphasia. Direct treatment in L2 alone does not harm L1 unless it is accompanied by a recommendation to avoid use of L1 outside the clinic setting. However, complete inattention to one language in the clinical setting, combined with a recommendation to avoid using it outside the clinic, may result in a persistent and greater impairment in that language.

- Speech-language intervention most often is conducted in the language that is common to both the clinician and the client. For this reason, programming should incorporate stimulation/facilitation strategies for the non-treated language in environments outside of the clinical setting.

For dysarthric speakers of tonal languages (i.e., when single-word meanings are conveyed by tones), therapy that targets pitch variation at the single-word level may be the most effective approach for improving a client's ability to accurately produce the tones. Therapy can be structured to emphasize functional communication that involves longer utterances accompanied by more contextual cues for the listener. This strategy will decrease dependence on single-word production, which is highly reliant on tone variation to signal meaning.

CLINICAL CONSIDERATIONS FOR MULTILINGUAL POPULATIONS WITH LANGUAGE DISORDERS

As in typically developing individuals, there are many factors that influence the effects of multilingualism on individuals with developmental disorders. Goral and Conner's (2013) literature review provides guidance for treating multilingual individuals with language disorders. Although the literature is currently limited in this area, there are several findings that can inform intervention as well as provide information for multilingual and multicultural families:

- When possible, a bilingual approach to therapy with individuals with specific language impairment (SLI) can result in benefits to both languages. Furthermore, L2 gains from bilingual treatment were comparable to L2 treatment alone.

- For SLI, treatment in L1 has been found to benefit L2 abilities, although the opposite scenario of treatment in L2 has not been found to provide much benefit to L1.

- No evidence supports the notion that exposing individuals with autism spectrum disorders to multiple languages will negatively impact their abilities to learn and use multiple languages.

- Although individuals with Down syndrome can learn to effectively communicate in multiple languages, strategies such as repetition and highly structured language interventions may be necessary to facilitate multiple language learning.

In addition to cultural and linguistic diversity, SLPs also face a diverse variety of disorders within their scope of practice. Factors and strategies to consider with regard to specific disorders and conditions among CLD populations include:

- Individuals with brain injury (e.g., traumatic brain injury [TBI], aphasia) may feel socially isolated depending on cultural views on neurogenic disorders. Participation in rehabilitation also may differ based upon a culture's view of possible treatments and outcomes (Qualls, 2012).

■ Dysphagia intervention in CLD populations requires consideration of factors such as the role of food and meals within the culture, nutrition and health issues related to dietary preferences of a culture, and culture-specific dietary restrictions (Qualls, 2012).

■ The linguistic properties of a language can impact the manner in which motor speech disorders manifest. For example, intervention for an individual with dysarthria who speaks a tonal language may require a greater emphasis on targeting suprasegmental aspects than intervention for an individual who speaks a non-tonal language (Qualls, 2012).

■ Some cultures may have theories as to the cause of certain disorders, such as stuttering, that are not based in scientific evidence (Robinson, 2012). Patient and caregiver counseling can help promote greater understanding of communication disorders and the role of intervention.

■ Voice and the vocal characteristics that are considered normal vary from culture to culture. Thus, an individual may not perceive his or her voice as disordered in a new cultural context (e.g., nasality). Conversely, an SLP may not perceive certain vocal qualities as disordered (e.g., vocal volume). Pretreatment interviews and assessments can help an SLP to ascertain the client's motives for seeking intervention (Behlau & Murray, 2012).

Helpful Hints

1. Children from Spanish-speaking and African American backgrounds tend to learn vocabulary words more effectively in tasks that involve descriptions and functions of target words rather than in tasks that emphasize labeling.

2. Some vocabulary words are differentially harder for specific CLD groups of children because of reduced exposure to certain words and/or prior experiences. In the selection of vocabulary targets, clinicians need to consider a child's prior knowledge and experiences rather than using curriculum as the sole source of material.

3. Use formal titles and full names when addressing adult clients. First names or nicknames may be considered condescending or offensive.

4. Clinicians should make every effort to learn the correct pronunciation of clients' and family members' names.

5. There may be cultural inhibitions about sharing personal information. Clinicians should carefully explain the meaning and parameters of confidentiality in the clinical process.

6. When intervention requires information gathering about family members or personal issues, the clinician should review standardized questionnaires and omit or modify items as appropriate given a client's specific background.

7. Clients from CLD backgrounds may require additional support in developing mainstream cultural knowledge (e.g., history, arts, news events) to facilitate their acquisition of reading and writing skills.

8. Use of dialects such as AAE should not be assumed to be a given for any particular individual. Use of AAE may be influenced by factors such as age, SES, and geographic region.

9. A speaker's use of code-switching should not be interpreted as an indicator of poor linguistic mastery. In fact, a speaker of multiple languages or dialects should be encouraged to code-switch strategically to maximize communication success in different environments with different listeners.

10. The role of the family varies in different cultures. This aspect may impact factors such as the point of contact for a family as well as the family's view on completing homework assignments in the home environment.

11. Although it is important to be aware of CLD factors when planning intervention, it is also important to note that individual variation occurs within cultures. Thus, a client's cultural and linguistic preferences are best identified through interactions that will either confirm or alter expected CLD norms.

12. Interpreters may be needed to discuss intervention progress with family members. In addition, ASHA provides resources (e.g., informational brochures) that are written in other languages to help provide information to linguistically diverse clients.

13. In-service trainings on CLD, especially the aspects specific to the cultures and languages present in one's work environment, can provide beneficial information for staff members (e.g., teachers, other therapists) to use when interacting with clients from diverse backgrounds.

CONCLUSION

This chapter has presented basic information and considerations for multicultural issues in intervention at an *introductory* level. This information is intended only as a starting point in the reader's clinical education and training. For in-depth coverage of this area, the following readings are recommended:

Battle, D. E. (2012). *Communication disorders in multicultural and international populations* (4th ed.).St. Louis, MO: Mosby.

Bhatia, T. K., & Ritchie, W. C. (Eds.). (2013). *The handbook of bilingualism and multilingualism.* Malden, MA: Wiley-Blackwell.

Centeno, J. G. (2009). Issues and principles in service delivery to communicatively impaired-minority bilingual adults in neurorehabilitation. *Seminars in Speech and Language, 30*(3), 139–152.

Cummins, J. (1984). *Bilingualism and special education: Issues in assessment and pedagogy.* Clevedon, England: Multilingual Matters.

Faroqi-Shah, Y., Frymark, T., Mullen, R., & Wang, B. (2010). Effect of treatment for bilingual individuals with aphasia: A systematic review of the evidence. *Journal of Neurolinguistics, 23,* 319–341.

Glennen, S., & Masters, M. G. (2002). Typical and atypical language development in infants and toddlers adopted from Eastern Europe. *American Journal of Speech and Language Therapy, 11,* 417–433.

Goldstein, B. (2000). *Cultural and linguistic diversity resource guide for speech-language pathologists.* Clifton Park, NY: Cengage Learning.

Grech, H., & McLeod, S. (2012). *Multilingual speech and language development and disorders.* In D. E. Battle (Ed.), *Communication disorders in multicultural and international populations* (pp. 205–232). St. Louis, MO: Mosby.

Hwa-Froelich, D. A. (2009). Communication development in infants and toddlers adopted from abroad. *Topics in Language Disorders, 29*(1), 27–44.

Kohnert, K. (2009). Cross-language generalization following treatment in bilingual speakers with aphasia: A review. *Seminars in Speech and Language,* 30, 174–186.

Lynch, E., & Hanson, M. (Eds.). (2011). *Developing cross cultural competence: A guide for working with children and their families* (4th ed.). Baltimore: Paul H. Brookes.

Patterson, J. L., & Pearson, B. Z. (2012). Bilingual lexical development, assessment, and intervention. In B. Goldstein (Ed.), *Bilingual language development and disorders in Spanish-English speakers* (2nd ed., pp. 113–130). Baltimore, MD: Paul H. Brookes.

Paul, R. (2006). *Language disorders from infancy to adolescence: Assessment and intervention* (3rd ed.). Boston: C. V. Mosby.

Pearson, C. (2001, October 23). *Internationally adopted children: Issues and challenges. The ASHA Leader, 6*(19). Publication of the American Speech-Language-Hearing Association.

Qualls, C. D., & Muñoz, M. L. (2005). Race-ethnicity, socioeconomic status, and cognitive-communicative functioning in individuals with neurogenic communication disorders: Clinical implications and research directions. *ECHO: E-Journal for Black and Other Ethnic Group Research and Practices in Communication Sciences and Disorders,* 1, 30–39.

Roberts, J., Pollock, K., Krakow, R., Price, J., Fulmer, K., & Wang, P. (2005). Language development in preschool-aged children adopted from China. *Journal of Speech-Language-Hearing Research,* 48, 93–107.

Roseberry-McKibbin, C. (2007). *Language disorders in children: A multicultural and case perspective.* Boston: Allyn & Bacon.

Roseberry-McKibbin, C., Brice, A., & O'Hanlon, L. (2005). Serving English language learners in public school settings: A national survey. *Language, Speech, and Hearing Services in Schools, 36*(I), 48–61.

U.S. Department of Education. (2009). Retrieved from http://www.ed.gov/

Wong, P. C. M., Perrachione, T. K., Gunasekera, G., & Chandrasekaran, B. (2009). Communication disorders in speakers of tone languages: Etiological bases and clinical considerations. *Seminars in Speech and Language, 30*(3), 162–173.

APPENDIX A

Preamble

The preservation of the highest standards of integrity and ethical principles is vital to the responsible discharge of obligations by speech-language pathologists, audiologists, and speech, language, and hearing scientists. This Code of Ethics sets forth the fundamental principles and rules considered essential to this purpose.

Every individual who is (a) a member of the American Speech-Language-Hearing Association, whether certified or not, (b) a nonmember holding the Certificate of Clinical Competence from the Association, (c) an applicant for membership or certification, or (d) a Clinical Fellow seeking to fulfill standards for certification shall abide by this Code of Ethics.

Any violation of the spirit and purpose of this Code shall be considered unethical. Failure to specify any particular responsibility or practice in this Code of Ethics shall not be construed as denial of the existence of such responsibilities or practices.

The fundamentals of ethical conduct are described by Principles of Ethics and by Rules of Ethics as they relate to the responsibility to persons served, the public, speech-language pathologists, audiologists, and speech, language, and hearing scientists, and to the conduct of research and scholarly activities.

Principles of Ethics, aspirational and inspirational in nature, form the underlying moral basis for the Code of Ethics. Individuals shall observe these principles as affirmative obligations under all conditions of professional activity.

Rules of Ethics are specific statements of minimally acceptable professional conduct or of prohibitions and are applicable to all individuals.

Principle of Ethics I

Individuals shall honor their responsibility to hold paramount the welfare of persons they serve professionally or who are participants in research and scholarly activities, and they shall treat animals involved in research in a humane manner.

Rules of Ethics

A. Individuals shall provide all services competently.

B. Individuals shall use every resource, including referral when appropriate, to ensure that high-quality service is provided.

C. Individuals shall not discriminate in the delivery of professional services or the conduct of research and scholarly activities on the basis of race or ethnicity, gender, gender identity/gender expression, age, religion, national origin, sexual orientation, or disability.

D. Individuals shall not misrepresent the credentials of assistants, technicians, support personnel, students, Clinical Fellows, or any others under their supervision, and they shall inform those they serve professionally of the name and professional credentials of persons providing services.

E. Individuals who hold the Certificate of Clinical Competence shall not delegate tasks that require the unique skills, knowledge, and judgment that are within the scope of their profession to assistants, technicians, support personnel, or any nonprofessionals over whom they have supervisory responsibility.

F. Individuals who hold the Certificate of Clinical Competence may delegate tasks related to provision of clinical services to assistants, technicians, support personnel, or any other persons only if those services are appropriately supervised, realizing that the responsibility for client welfare remains with the certified individual.

G. Individuals who hold the Certificate of Clinical Competence may delegate tasks related to provision of clinical services that require the unique skills, knowledge, and judgment that are within the scope of practice of their profession to students only if those services are appropriately supervised. The responsibility for client welfare remains with the certified individual.

H. Individuals shall fully inform the persons they serve of the nature and possible effects of services rendered and products dispensed, and they shall inform participants in research about the possible effects of their participation in research conducted.

I. Individuals shall evaluate the effectiveness of services rendered and of products dispensed, and they shall provide services or dispense products only when benefit can reasonably be expected.

J. Individuals shall not guarantee the results of any treatment or procedure, directly or by implication; however, they may make a reasonable statement of prognosis.

K. Individuals shall not provide clinical services solely by correspondence.

L. Individuals may practice by telecommunication (e.g., telehealth/e-health), where not prohibited by law.

M. Individuals shall adequately maintain and appropriately secure records of professional services rendered, research and scholarly activities conducted, and products dispensed, and they shall allow access to these records only when authorized or when required by law.

N. Individuals shall not reveal, without authorization, any professional or personal information about identified persons served professionally or identified participants involved in research and scholarly activities unless doing so is necessary to protect the welfare of the person or of the community or is otherwise required by law.

O. Individuals shall not charge for services not rendered, nor shall they misrepresent services rendered, products dispensed, or research and scholarly activities conducted.

P. Individuals shall enroll and include persons as participants in research or teaching demonstrations only if their participation is voluntary, without coercion, and with their informed consent.

Q. Individuals whose professional services are adversely affected by substance abuse or other health-related conditions shall seek professional assistance and, where appropriate, withdraw from the affected areas of practice.

R. Individuals shall not discontinue service to those they are serving without providing reasonable notice.

Principle of Ethics II

Individuals shall honor their responsibility to achieve and maintain the highest level of professional competence and performance.

Rules of Ethics

A. Individuals shall engage in the provision of clinical services only when they hold the appropriate Certificate of Clinical Competence or when they are in the certification process and are supervised by an individual who holds the appropriate Certificate of Clinical Competence.

B. Individuals shall engage in only those aspects of the professions that are within the scope of their professional practice and competence, considering their level of education, training, and experience.

C. Individuals shall engage in lifelong learning to maintain and enhance professional competence and performance.

D. Individuals shall not require or permit their professional staff to provide services or conduct research activities that exceed the staff member's competence, level of education, training, and experience.

E. Individuals shall ensure that all equipment used to provide services or to conduct research and scholarly activities is in proper working order and is properly calibrated.

Principle of Ethics III

Individuals shall honor their responsibility to the public by promoting public understanding of the professions, by supporting the development of services designed to fulfill the unmet needs of the public, and by providing accurate information in all communications involving any aspect of the professions, including the dissemination of research findings and scholarly activities, and the promotion, marketing, and advertising of products and services.

Rules of Ethics

A. Individuals shall not misrepresent their credentials, competence, education, training, experience, or scholarly or research contributions.

B. Individuals shall not participate in professional activities that constitute a conflict of interest.

C. Individuals shall refer those served professionally solely on the basis of the interest of those being referred and not on any personal interest, financial or otherwise.

D. Individuals shall not misrepresent research, diagnostic information, services rendered, results of services rendered, products dispensed, or the effects of products dispensed.

E. Individuals shall not defraud or engage in any scheme to defraud in connection with obtaining payment, reimbursement, or grants for services rendered, research conducted, or products dispensed.

F. Individuals' statements to the public shall provide accurate information about the nature and management of communication disorders, about the professions, about professional services, about products for sale, and about research and scholarly activities.

G. Individuals' statements to the public when advertising, announcing, and marketing their professional services; reporting research results; and promoting products shall adhere to professional standards and shall not contain misrepresentations.

Principle of Ethics IV

Individuals shall honor their responsibilities to the professions and their relationships with colleagues, students, and members of other professions and disciplines.

Rules of Ethics

A. Individuals shall uphold the dignity and autonomy of the professions, maintain harmonious interprofessional and intraprofessional relationships, and accept the professions' self-imposed standards.

B. Individuals shall prohibit anyone under their supervision from engaging in any practice that violates the Code of Ethics.

C. Individuals shall not engage in dishonesty, fraud, deceit, or misrepresentation.

D. Individuals shall not engage in any form of unlawful harassment, including sexual harassment or power abuse.

E. Individuals shall not engage in any other form of conduct that adversely reflects on the professions or on the individual's fitness to serve persons professionally.

F. Individuals shall not engage in sexual activities with clients, students, or research participants over whom they exercise professional authority or power.

G. Individuals shall assign credit only to those who have contributed to a publication, presentation, or product. Credit shall be assigned in proportion to the contribution and only with the contributor's consent.

H. Individuals shall reference the source when using other persons' ideas, research, presentations, or products in written, oral, or any other media presentation or summary.

I. Individuals' statements to colleagues about professional services, research results, and products shall adhere to prevailing professional standards and shall contain no misrepresentations.

J. Individuals shall not provide professional services without exercising independent professional judgment, regardless of referral source or prescription.

K. Individuals shall not discriminate in their relationships with colleagues, students, and members of other professions and disciplines on the basis of race or ethnicity, gender, gender identity/gender expression, age, religion, national origin, sexual orientation, or disability.

L. Individuals shall not file or encourage others to file complaints that disregard or ignore facts that would disprove the allegation, nor should the Code of Ethics be used for personal reprisal, as a means of addressing personal animosity, or as a vehicle for retaliation.

M. Individuals who have reason to believe that the Code of Ethics has been violated shall inform the Board of Ethics.

N. Individuals shall comply fully with the policies of the Board of Ethics in its consideration and adjudication of complaints of violations of the Code of Ethics.

APPENDIX B

TABLE B–1

International Phonetic Alphabet Symbols for English Vowels

Phonetic Symbol	Example	Phonetic Transcription
i	*wheel*	[wil]
ɪ	*this*	[ðɪs]
e	*plane*	[pleɪn], [plen]
ɛ	*bed*	[bɛd]
æ	*matches*	[mætʃɪz]
a	*hot*	[hat]
ɔ	*clause*	[klɔz]
o	*stove*	[stov]
ʊ	*put*	[pʊt]
u	*blue*	[blu]
ʌ	*cup*	[kʌp] (stressed)
ə	*umbrella*	[ʌmbrɛlə] (unstressed)
aɪ	*knife*	[naɪf]
aʊ	*shout*	[ʃaʊt]
ɔɪ	*boy*	[bɔɪ]
ɝ	*squirrel*	[skwɝl] (stressed)
ɚ	*zipper*	[zɪpɚ] (unstressed)

TABLE B–2

International Phonetic Alphabet Symbols for English Consonants

Phonetic Symbol	Example	Phonetic Transcription
p	*plane*	[plen]
b	*bed*	[bɛd]
t	*toy*	[tɔɪ]
d	*dot*	[dat]
k	*cup*	[kʌp] (stressed)
g	*glue*	[glu]
h	*hot*	[hat]
ʔ	*mitten*	[mɪʔn]
m	*matches*	[mætʃɪz]
n	*knife*	[naɪf]

(continues)

TABLE B–2 (*Continued*)

Phonetic Symbol	Example	Phonetic Transcription
ŋ	*swing*	[swIŋ]
f	*fast*	[fæst]
v	*voice*	[vɔIs]
θ	*thick*	[θIk]
ð	*this*	[ðIs]
s	*squirrel*	[skwɝl] (stressed)
z	*zipper*	[zIpɚ] (unstressed)
ʃ	*shovel*	[ʃʌvəl]
ʒ	*measure*	[mɛʒɝ]
tʃ	*chicken*	[tʃIkIn]
l	*lamp*	[læmp]
r	*rabbit*	[ræbIt]
j	*yellow*	[jɛlo]
w	*wagon*	[wægən]
dʒ	*jumping*	[dʒʌmpIŋ]

APPENDIX C

ACUTE CARE: Intense medical intervention to stabilize physical condition and ensure survival.

ALZHEIMER'S DISEASE: Progressive dementia caused by cerebral atrophy, resulting in memory loss, confusion, and speech disturbances, beginning in late middle age, with death occurring in 5 to 10 years.

AMYOTROPHIC LATERAL SCLEROSIS (ALS): Progressive disease of the spinal cord, resulting in degenerative muscular atrophy with accompanying mixed dysarthria.

ANGULAR GYRUS: Prominent rounded elevation (convolution) in the posterior portion of the parietal lobe.

ANOXIA: Lack of oxygen in the blood supply to the brain.

ARCUATE FASCICULUS: Nerve fiber bundle in the brain that transmits impulses from Wernicke's area to Broca's area.

ATAXIA: Impairment in movement and balance resulting from cerebellar damage; a type of dysarthria characterized by articulation, rhythm, loudness, and stress disturbances.

BIOFEEDBACK MECHANISMS: Equipment, such as ultrasound imaging, that provides real-time feedback on a client's performance on specified speech and/or swallowing tasks.

BOLUS: Rounded mass of food prepared by the mouth for swallowing.

BRAINSTEM: Lower section of the brain that connects the spinal cord to the cerebrum; regulates functions such as breathing and blood pressure.

BROCA'S AREA: Motor speech area in the frontal lobe dominant for speech and language (usually left).

BULBAR PALSY: Impairment and atrophy of the oral mechanism (lips, tongue, pharynx, and so on) due to lesions in the medulla oblongata region of the brainstem.

CAROTID ARTERY: A major pathway of blood supply from the heart to the brain.

CATASTROPHIC REACTION: Sudden and extreme emotional/physical response to ordinary events or situations often exhibited by individuals with brain injury.

CENTRAL NERVOUS SYSTEM: The brain, brainstem, and spinal cord.

CHOREA: Irregular, spasmodic, involuntary movements of the face and extremities.

CORTEX: Convoluted outer layer of the brain responsible for higher-level sensory and motor functions.

COMPUTED TOMOGRAPHY (CT SCAN): Sophisticated X-ray technique that provides cross-sectional images of the body.

DEMENTIA: General deterioration of mental faculties characterized by disorientation as well as impaired judgment, memory, and intellect.

DYSKINESIA: Impairment in the ability to perform voluntary movements.

DYSPHAGIA: Impairment in the ability to swallow normally.

DYSTONIA: A state of abnormal muscle tone (increased or decreased) associated with involuntary rhythmic twisting of the trunk or extremities.

EDEMA: Swelling resulting from an excessive amount of fluid retention in cells or tissues.

EXTRAPYRAMIDAL: Nerve fibers involved in regulation of automatic, subconscious aspects of motor coordination and posture.

FLACCID: Inability of a muscle to contract volitionally; relaxed, flabby, without tone; hypotonicity.

FMRI: The use of magnetic resonance imaging (MRI) to learn which regions of the brain are active in a specific function, as in speech.

Frontal Lobe: Largest lobe of the brain located at the anterior portion of the cerebrum; responsible for primary motor control for all parts of the body.

Hematoma: A pooling of blood in an organ, tissue, or other area.

Hemorrhage: Escape of blood through ruptured blood vessels.

Huntington's Chorea: Progressive neuromuscular disorder, usually beginning between the ages of 30 and 50 years, characterized by irregular and involuntary movements in the face and limbs; accompanied by gradual deterioration of mental status, resulting in dementia.

Hyperkinesia: Excessive, uncontrolled movement of any part of the body.

Infarct: An area of dead tissue resulting from an interruption of blood supply.

Ischemia: Decrease in blood supply due to mechanical obstruction (mainly narrowing of arteries). Cerebral ischemia involves a deficiency in the supply of the blood to the brain. Transient ischemic attacks (TIAs) generally last less than 24 hours.

Laryngectomy: Surgical procedure in which the larynx is removed, typically due to cancer.

Magnetic Resonance Imaging (MRI): Computerized scan that utilizes nuclear magnetic resonance to produce cross-sectional images of the body.

Multiple Sclerosis (MS): Progressive neuromuscular disorder resulting in paralysis, tremors, and speech disturbances; begins in early adulthood and is marked by periods of exacerbations and remissions.

Myasthenia Gravis: Progressive muscular disorder resulting from impaired conduction of neural impulses to the muscles, beginning in the face and throat.

Myoclonus: Spasms in a muscle or group of muscles.

Neuromuscular Electrical Stimulation (NMES): The application of electrical impulses transcutaneously to muscles with diminished functioning in order to retrain muscle movements.

Neuroplasticity: The brain's ability to restructure its neural networks in response to internal and external stimuli.

Non-Invasive Electrical Brain Stimulation: The use of magnetic impulses to stimulate targeted areas of the brain through an intact skull to effect behavioral changes. Two forms are currently being investigated for application to communication disorders: repetitive transcranial magnetic stimulation (rTMS) and transcranial direct-current stimulation (tDCS).

Nystagmus: Involuntary movement of the eyes often exhibited by individuals with brain injury.

Parietal Lobe: The medial and upper lateral areas of the cerebrum responsible for reception and analysis of tactile and kinesthetic sensory impulses (touch and muscle movement awareness).

Parkinson's Disease: Degenerative neurological syndrome characterized by rhythmic tremors, muscle rigidity, masklike face, general muscular weakness, and limp posture; often accompanied by a hypokinetic dysarthria.

Peripheral Nervous System: Nerve bundles outside of the brain and spinal cord.

PET Scan: Positron emission tomography; a highly specialized imaging technique that uses short-lived radioactive substances to produce three-dimensional colored images of those substances functioning within the body.

Pharyngoesophageal Segment (PE Segment): Anatomical region that separates the pharynx from the esophagus.

PHARYNX: Anatomical region posterior to the oral cavity, below the nasal cavity, and above the esophagus.

PREMORBID: Preceding the occurrence of the disease or lesion.

PSEUDOBULBAR PALSY: Impairments in swallowing, chewing, and articulation due to bilateral upper motor neuron damage.

PYRAMIDAL: Two nerve bundles originating in the sensorimotor area of the cortex inserting into the spinal cord; responsible for refined, spatially oriented, voluntary movements.

ROLANDIC FISSURE: A prominent groove on the lateral portion of each hemisphere, forming the boundary between the frontal and parietal lobes.

SEIZURE: Episode of excessive electrical activity in the brain.

SPASTIC: Muscle contraction that is involuntary and jerky; hypertonicity.

SUBACUTE CARE: Rehabilitation program for individuals with stable medical conditions that provides daily nursing care and a range of other treatment services such as physical therapy, occupational therapy, and so on.

SUPRAMARGINAL GYRUS: Prominent rounded elevation (convolution) in the inferior half of the parietal lobe, surrounding the posterior part of the Sylvian fissure.

TEMPORAL GYRUS: Prominent rounded elevation (convolution) in the lateral surface of the temporal lobe.

TEMPORAL LOBE: Lower lateral portion of the cerebrum, responsible for sensation and interpretation of auditory impulses.

TONGUE BASE: Posterior portion of the tongue that extends downward into the pharynx (throat).

TOURETTE'S SYNDROME: Neurological disorder characterized by verbal and facial tics, coprolalia (cursing), and motor incoordination; usually beginning in childhood.

TRAUMATIC BRAIN INJURY (TBI): Open or closed head injury resulting from impact or penetrating force.

TREMOR: Repetitive and involuntary shaking or vibration of a body part or muscle group.

VALLECULAE: Two spaces or pockets located in the throat just below the root of the tongue.

WERNICKE'S AREA: Large region of the temporal lobe responsible for auditory language comprehension.

WILSON'S DISEASE: Metabolic disorder associated with damage to the basal ganglia due to inadequate processing of the dietary intake of copper; often accompanied by mixed dysarthria.

XEROSTOMIA: An excessively dry mouth due to diminished saliva production following radiation treatments to the head/neck regions.

APPENDIX D

Appendix D–1
Lateral View of Pharyngeal Cavity Divisions

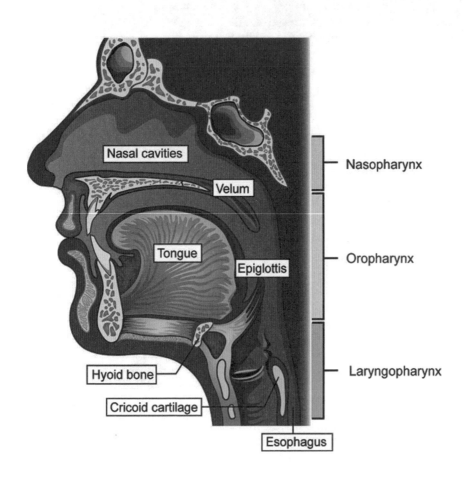

References

Adams, M. J., Foorman, B. R., Lundberg, I., & Beeler, T. (1998). *Phonemic awareness in young children.* Baltimore, MD: Brookes.

Adler, R. (n. d.). *Multicultural issues.* Retrieved from http://www.speechpathology.com/ask-the-experts/multicultural-issues-932

Adler, R., Hirsch, S., & Mordaunt, M. (2012). *Voice and communication therapy for the transgender/transsexual client: A comprehensive clinical guide* (6th ed.). San Diego, CA: Plural Publishing.

Ahn, H. N., & Wampold, B. E. (2001). Where oh where are the specific ingredients? A meta-analysis of component studies in counseling and psychotherapy. *Journal of Counseling Psychology, 48*(3), 251.

Albert, M., Sparks, R., & Helm, N., (1973). Melodic intonation therapy for aphasia. *Archives of Neurology, 29*, 130–131.

Alexander, R., Boehme, R., & Cupps, B. (1993). *Normal development of functional motor skills: The first year of life.* Tucson, AZ: Therapy Skill Builders.

Ambrose, N. G., & Yairi, E. (1999). Normative disfluency data for early childhood stuttering. *Journal of Speech, Language, and Hearing Research, 42*, 895–909.

American Psychiatric Association. (2013). *Diagnostic and statistical manual of mental disorders-5.* Washington, DC: American Psychiatric Publishing.

American Speech-Language-Hearing Association. (2000b). *Roles and responsibilities of speech-language pathologists with respect to reading and writing in children and adolescents: Position statement, technical report, and guidelines.* Rockville, MD: ASHA.

American Speech-Language-Hearing Association. (2002b). *Communication development and disorders in multicultural populations: Readings and related materials.* Rockville, MD: ASHA.

American Speech-Language-Hearing Association. (2004). Evaluation and treatment for -tracheoesophageal puncture and prosthesis: Technical report. *ASHA Supplement, 24.* Rockville, MD: ASHA.

American Speech-Language-Hearing Association. (2007a). *Childhood apraxia of speech: Position statement.* Rockville, MD: ASHA.

American Speech-Language Hearing Association. (2007b). *Scope of practice in speech-language pathology.* Retrieved from http://www.asha.org/policy

American Speech-Language-Hearing Association. (2008). *Roles and responsibilities of speech- language pathologists in early intervention: Position statement, technical report, and guidelines.* Rockville, MD: ASHA.

American Speech-Language-Hearing Association. (2010). *Code of ethics.* Retrieved from http://www.asha.org/policy/

American Speech-Language-Hearing Association. (2011). *Cultural competence.* Retrieved from http://www.asha.org/Practice-Portal/Professional-Issues/Cultural-Competence/

American Speech-Language-Hearing Association. (2012). *Demographic profile of ASHA members providing bilingual services.* Retrieved from http://www.asha.org/uploadedFiles/Demographic-Profile-Bilingual-Spanish-Service-Members.pdf

Americans with Disabilities Act of 1990, 42 U.S.C.A. § 12101 *et seq.* (West 1993).

Anderson, J. D., & Conture, E. G. (2004). Sentence-structure priming in young children who do and do not stutter. *Journal of Speech, Language, and Hearing Research, 47*, 552–571.

Anderson, J., Wagovich, S., & Hall, N. (2006). Nonword repetition skills in young children who do and do not stutter. *Journal of Fluency Disorders, 31*, 177–199.

Anderson, K. L., & Goldstein, H. (2004). Speech perception benefits of FM and infrared devices to children with hearing aids in a typical classroom. *Language, Speech, and Hearing Services in Schools, 35*, 169–184.

Andrews, C., O'Brian, S., Onslow, M., Harrison, E., Packman, A., & Menzies, R. (2012). Syllable-timed speech treatment for school age children who stutter: A Phase I trial. *Language, Speech, and Hearing Services in Schools, 43*, 359–369.

Andrews, G., & Harris, M. (1964). *The syndrome of stuttering.* Clinics in Developmental Medicine, no. 17. London: Spastics Society Medical Education and Information Unit in Association with Heinemann Medical Books.

Andrews, J., Leigh, I., & Weiner, M. (2004). *Deaf people: Evolving perspectives from psychology, education, and sociology.* San Francisco, CA: Allyn & Bacon.

Arciuli, J., Stevens, K., Trembath, D., & Simpson, I. (2013). The relationship between parent report of adaptive behavior and direct assessment of reading ability in children with autism spectrum disorders. *Journal of Speech, Language, and Hearing Research, 56*(6), 1837–1844. doi: 10.1044/1092-4388(2013/12-0034)

Arnott, S., Onslow, M., O'Brian, S., Packman, A., Jones, M., & Block, S. (2014). Group Lidcombe Program treatment for early stuttering: A randomized controlled trial. *Journal of Speech, Language, and Hearing Research.*

Asperger, H. (1944). Die "Autistischen Psychopathen" im Kindesalter. *European Archives of Psychiatry and Clinical Neuroscience, 117*(1), 76–136.

Association on Higher Education and Disability (AHEAD). (2008). Retrieved from https://www.ahead.org/

Baddeley, A. D. (2007). *Working memory, thought, and action.* New York: Oxford University Press.

Badian, N. A. (1999). Reading disability defined as a discrepancy between listening and reading comprehension. *Journal of Learning Disabilities, 32,* 138–148.

Baker, E., & McLeod, S. (2011). Evidence-based practice for children with speech sound disorders: Part 1 narrative review. *Language, Speech, and Hearing Services in Schools, 42*(2), 102–139.

Baker, S. K., Simmons, D. C., & Kameenui, E. J. (1998). Vocabulary acquisition: Reading bases. In D. C. Simmons & E. J. Kameenui (Eds.), *What reading research tells us about children with diverse learning needs: Bases and basics* (pp. 183–217). Mahwah, NJ: Lawrence Erlbaum.

Ballard, K. J. (2001). Response generalization in apraxia of speech treatments: Taking another look. *Journal of Communication Disorders, 34,* 3–20.

Ballard, K. J., Robin, D. A., McCabe, P., & McDonald, J. (2010). A treatment for dysprosody in childhood apraxia of speech. *Journal of Speech, Language, and Hearing Research, 53*(5), 1227–1245.

Barkley, R. A. (1996). Linkages between attention and executive functions. In G. R. Lyon & N. A. Krasnegor (Eds.), *Attention, memory, and executive function* (pp. 307–325). Baltimore, MD: Brookes.

Barkley, R. A. (1997). *ADHD and the nature of self-control.* New York: Guilford Press.

Barlow, J. A., & Gierut, J. A. (2002). Minimal pair approaches to phonological remediation. *Seminars in Speech and Language, 23,* 57–67.

Barnes, M., Dobkin, B., & Bogousslavsky, J. (Eds.). (2005). *Recovery after stroke.* New York: Cambridge University Press.

Baron-Cohen S., Leslie, A. M. & Frith, U. (1985). Does the autistic child have a "theory of mind"? *Cognition, 21,* 37–46.

Barwood, C. H. S., & Murdoch, B. E. (2013). rTMS as a treatment for neurogenic communication and swallowing disorders. *Acta Neurologica Scandinavica 127*(2), 77–91.

Barwood, C. H. S., Murdoch, B. E. Whelan, B. M., Lloyd, D., Riek, S., O'Sullivan , J. D., . . . & Wong, A. (2012). Improved receptive and expressive language abilities in nonfluent aphasic stroke patients after application of rTMS: An open protocol case series. *Brain Stimulation, 5,* 274–286.

Basso, A., & Macis, M. (2011). Therapy efficacy in chronic aphasia. *Behavioral Neurology, 24,* 317–325. doi: 10.3233/BEN-2011-0342

Bates, E., & MacWhinney, B. (1987). Competition, variation, and language learning. In B. MacWhinney (Ed.), *Mechanisms of language learning* (pp. 157–194). Hillsdale, NJ: Lawrence Erlbaum.

Battle, D. E. (1997). Multicultural considerations in counseling communicatively disordered persons and their families. In T. A. Crowe (Ed.), *Applications of counseling in speech-language pathology and audiology* (pp. 118–141). Baltimore, MD: Williams & Wilkins.

Battle, D. E. (2012). *Communication disorders in multicultural and international populations* (4th ed.). St. Louis, MO: Mosby.

Bauman-Waengler, J. (2007). *Articulatory and phonological impairments: A clinical focus* (3rd ed.). Boston, MA: Allyn & Bacon.

Beck, A. R., & Dennis, M. (1997). Speech-language pathologists' and teachers' perceptions of classroom-based interventions. *Language, Speech, and Hearing Services in Schools, 28,* 146–153.

Beck, I. L., McKeown, M. G., & Kucan, L. (2013). *Bringing words to life: Robust vocabulary instruction.* New York: Guilford Press.

Becker, R., Nieczaj, R., Egge, K., Moll, A., Meinhardt, M., & Schulz, R. J. (2011). Functional dysphagia therapy and PEG treatment in a clinical geriatric setting. *Dysphagia, 26*(2), 108–116.

Begun, A. L. (1996). Family systems and family-centered care. In P. Rosin, A. D. Whitehead, L. I. Tuchman, G. S. Jesien, A. L. Begun, & L. Irwin (Eds.), *Partnerships in family-centered care: A guide to collaborative early intervention* (pp. 33–63). Baltimore, MD: Brookes.

Behlau, M., & Murray, T. (2012). Internationa and intercultural aspects of voice and voice disorders. In D. E. Battle (Ed.), *Communication disorders in multicultural and international populations* (4th ed., pp. 174–207). St. Louis, MO: Mosby.

Behrman, A., Rutledge, J., Hembree, A., & Sheridan, S. (2008). Vocal hygiene education, voice production therapy, and the role of patient adherence: A treatment effectiveness study in women with phonotrauma. *Journal of Speech, Language, and Hearing Research, 51,* 350–366.

Belanger, H. G., Kretzmer, T., Yoash-Gantz, R., Picket, T., & Tupler, L. A. (2009). Cognitive sequelae of blast-related versus other mechanisms of brain trauma. *Journal of the International Neuropsychological Society, 15,* 1–8.

Bellini, S., & Akullian, J. (2007). A meta-analysis of video modeling and video self-modeling interventions for children and adolescents with autism spectrum disorders. *Exceptional Children 73*(3), 264–287.

Bellon-Harn, M. L. (2012). Dose frequency: Comparison of language outcomes in preschool children with language impairment. *Child Language Teaching and Therapy, 28*(2), 225–240.

Bennett, T. A., Szatmari, P., Bryson, S., Duku, E., Vaccarella, L., & Tuff, L. (2013). Theory of mind, language and adaptive functioning in ASD: A neuroconstructivist perspective. *Journal of the Canadian Academy of Child and Adolescent Psychiatry, 22*, 13–19.

Berke, G. S., Blackwell, K. E., Gerratt, B. R., Verneil, A., Jackson, K. S., & Sercarz, J. A. (1999). Selective laryngeal adductor denervation-reinervation: A new surgical treatment for adductor spasmodic dysphonia. *Annals of Otology, Rhinology, and Laryngology, 108*, 227–231.

Berndt, R. S., Mitchum, C. C., & Wayland, S. (1997). Patterns of sentence comprehension in aphasia: A consideration of three hypotheses. *Brain and Language, 60*, 197–221.

Bernthal, J. E., & Bankson, N. W. (2013). *Articulation and phonological disorders* (7th ed.). Boston, MA: Pearson.

Berthier, M. L., Pulvermuller, F., Davila, G., Casares, N. G., & Gutierrez, A. (2011). Drug therapy of post-stroke aphasia: A review of current evidence. *Neuropsychology Review 21*, 302–317.

Blache, S. (1989). A distinctive feature approach. In N. Creaghead, P. Newman, W. Secord (Eds.), *Assessment and remediation of articulatory and phonological disorders* (pp. 361–382). Columbus, OH: Charles E. Merrill.

Blitzer, A., Brin, M. F., Fahn, S., & Lovelace, R. E. (1988). Localized injections of botulinum toxin for the treatment of focal laryngeal dystonia (spastic dysphonia). *Laryngoscope, 98*, 193–197.

Blitzer, A., Brin, M. F., & Stewart, C. (1998). Botulinum toxin management of spasmodic dysphonia (laryngeal dystonia): A 12-year experience in more than 900 patients. *Laryngoscope, 108*, 1435–1441.

Block, S., Ingham, R., & Bench, R. (1996). The effects of the Edinburgh Masker on stuttering. *Australian Journal of Human Communication Disorders, 24*, 11–18.

Blom, E. D, Singer, M. I., & Hamaker, R. C. (1998). *Tracheoesophageal voice restoration following total laryngectomy.* San Diego, CA: Singular.

Blood, G. W. (1995). POWER2: Relapse management with adolescents who stutter. *Language, Speech, and Hearing Services in Schools, 26*, 169–179.

Blood, G. W., & Conture, E. G. (1998). Outcomes measurement issues in fluency disorders. In C. M. Frattali (Ed.), *Measuring outcomes in speech-language pathology* (pp. 387–405). New York: Thieme.

Bloodstein, O. (1960). The development of stuttering: II. Development phases. *Journal of Speech and Hearing Disorders, 25*, 366–376.

Bloodstein, O. (1975). Stuttering as tension and fragmentation. In J. Eisenson (Ed.), *Stuttering: A second symposium* (pp. 1–96). New York: Harper & Row.

Bloodstein, O. (1987). *A handbook on stuttering.* Chicago, IL: National Easter Seals Society.

Bloodstein, O., & Ratner, N. (2008). *A handbook on stuttering* (6th ed.). Clifton Park, NY: Delmar Cengage Learning.

Bloom, L. (1973). *One word at a time: The use of single-word utterances before syntax.* New York: The Hague Mouton.

Bloom, P. (2000). *How children learn the meanings of words.* Cambridge, MA: MIT Press.

Blosser, J., & Neidecker, E. A. (2002). *School programs in speech-language pathology: Organization and service delivery* (4th ed.). Boston, MA: Allyn & Bacon.

Bondy, A. S., & Frost, L. A. (1994). The picture exchange communication system. *Focus on Autism and Other Developmental Disabilities, 9*(3), 1–19.

Boone, D. R., McFarlane, S. C., Von Berg, S., & Zraick, R. (2013). *The voice and voice therapy* (9th ed.). San Francisco, CA: Allyn & Bacon.

Bothe, A. K., Davidow, J. H., Bramlett, R. E., & Ingham, R. J. (2006). Stuttering treatment research 1970–2005: I. Systematic review incorporating trial quality assessment of behavioral, cognitive, and related approaches. *American Journal of Speech-Language Pathology, 15*, 321–341.

Boutsen, F. R., Cannito, M. P., Taylor, M., & Bender, B. K. (2002). Botox treatment in adductor spasmodic dysphonia: A meta-analysis. *Journal of Speech, Language, and Hearing Research, 45*, 469–481.

Boyd, B. A., Odom, S. L., Humphreys, B. P., & Sam, A. M. (2010). Infants and toddlers with ASD: Early identification and early intervention. *Journal of Early Intervention, 32*, 75–98.

Braden, C., Hawley, L., Newman, J., Morey, C., Gerber, D., & Harrison-Felix, C. (2010). Social communication skills group treatment: A feasibility study for persons with traumatic brain injury and comorbid conditions. *Brain Injury, 24*(11), 1298–1310.

Brady, M. C., Kelly, H., Godwin, J., & Enderby, P. (2012). Speech and language therapy for aphasia following stroke. *Cochrane Database of Systematic Reviews, 5*, CD000425.

Brady, N. C., Marquis, J., Fleming, K., & McLean, L. (2004). Prelinguistic predictors of language growth in children with developmental disabilities. *Journal of Speech, Language & Hearing Research, 47*, 663–677.

Breit-Smith, A., Justice, L. M., McGinty, A. S., & Kaderavek, J. (2009). How often and how much? Intensity of print referencing intervention. *Topics in Language Disorders, 29*, 360–369.

Brennan-Jones, C. G., White, J., Rush, R. W., & Law, J. (2014). Auditory-verbal frtherapy for promoting spoken language development in children with permanent hearing impairments. *Cochrane Database of Systematic Reviews, 3*.

Brent, G., & Yairi, E. (2012). Disfluency patterns and phonological skills near stuttering onset. *Journal of Communication Disorders, 45*, 426–438.

Brown, R. (1968). *Words and things.* New York: The Free Press.

Bruner, J. (1974). The organization of early skilled action. In M. P. M. Richards (Ed.), *The integration of a child into a social world* (pp. 167–184). London: Cambridge University Press.

Bruner, J. (1977). Early social interaction and language acquisition. In H. R. Schaffer (Ed.), *Studies in mother-infant interaction* (pp. 271–289). New York: Academic Press.

Bruner, J. (1983). *Child's talk: Learning to use language.* (pp. 67–88). New York: W.W. Norton & Co.

Bruner, J. S. (1960). *The process of education: A searching discussion of school education opening new paths to learning and teaching.* Vintage Books.

Brutten, E., & Shoemaker, D. (1967). *The modification of stuttering.* Englewood Cliffs, NJ: Prentice Hall.

Bulow, M., Speyer, R., Baijens, L., Woisard, V., & Ekberg, O. (2008). Neuromuscular electrical stimulation (NMES) in stroke patients with oral and pharyngeal dysfunction. *Dysphagia, 23*(3), 302–309.

Bunton, K. (2008). Speech vs. nonspeech: Different tasks, different neural organizations. *Seminars in Speech and Language, 29,* 267–275.

Burns, S. M., Griffin, P., & Snow, C. E. (1999). *Starting out right: A guide to promoting children's reading success.* Washington, DC: National Academy Press.

Butler, Y. G. (2013). Bilingualism/multilingualism and second-language acquisition. In T. K. Bhatia & W. C. Ritchie (Eds.), *The handbook of bilingualism and multilingualism* (pp. 109–136). Malden, MA: Wiley-Blackwell.

Caesar, L. G. (2013). Providing early intervention services to diverse populations: Are speech-language pathologists prepared? *Infants & Young Children, 26*(2), 126–146.

Cahana-Amitay, D., Albert, M. L., Oveis, A. (2013). Psycholinguistics of aphasia pharmacotherapy: Asking the right questions. *Aphasiology 27,* 1–22.

Calandrella, A. M., & Wilcox, M. J. (2000). Predicting language outcomes for pre-linguistic children with developmental delay. *Journal of Speech, Language, and Hearing, 43,* 1061–1071.

Campbell, C. R., & Jackson, S. T. (1995). Transparency of one-handed Amer-Ind hand signals to nonfamiliar viewers. *Journal of Speech and Hearing Research, 38,* 1284–1289.

Carlisle, J. F., Goodwin, A. P. (2014). Morphemes matter: How morphological knowledge contributes to reading and writing. In C. A. Stone, E. R. Silliman, B. J. Ehren, & G. P. Wallach (Eds.), *Handbook of language and literacy: Development and disorders* (pp. 265–282). New York: Guilford Press.

Carter, J., & Humbert, I. A. (2012). E-stim for dysphagia: Yes or no. *The ASHA Leader, 4.*

Carter, A. S., Messinger, D. S., Stone, W. L., Celimli, S., Nahmias, A. S., & Yoder, P. (2011). A randomized controlled trial of Hanen's 'More Than Words' in toddlers with early autism symptoms. *Journal of Child Psychology and Psychiatry, 52*(7), 741–752.

Casper, J. K., & Colton, R. H. (1998). *Clinical manual for laryngectomy and head/neck cancer rehabilitation* (2nd ed.). San Diego, CA: Delmar, Cengage Learning.

Casper, J. K., & Murry, T. (2000). Voice therapy methods in dysphonia. *Otolaryngologic Clinics of North America, 33,* 983–1002.

Catts, H. W., Hogan, T. P., & Adlof, S. M. (2005). Developing changes in reading and reading disabilities. In H. W. Catts & A. G. Kamhi (Eds.), *The connections between language and reading disabilities* (pp. 50–71). Mahwah, NJ: Lawrence Erlbaum.

Caute, A., Pring, T., Cocks, N., Cruice, M., Best, W., & Marshall, J. (2013). Enhancing communication through gesture and naming therapy. *Journal of Speech, Language, and Hearing Research, 56*(1), 337–351.

Centeno, J. G. (2009). Issues and principles in service delivery to communicatively impaired-minority bilingual adults in neurorehabilitation. *Seminars in Speech and Language, 30*(3), 139–152.

Centers for Disease Control and Prevention (CDC). (2013). *Traumatic brain injury in the United States: Fact sheet.* Retrieved from http://www.cdc.gov/traumaticbrain injury/get_the_facts.html

Centers for Disease Control and Prevention (CDC). (2014). Prevalence of autism spectrum disorder among children aged 8 Years. *Autism and Developmental Disabilities Monitoring Network. 63,* 1–21.

Chang, S. E., Horwitz, B., Ostuni, J., Reynolds, R., & Ludlow, C. (2011). Evidence of left frontal inferior-premotor structural and functional connectivity deficits in adults who stutter. *Cerebral Cortex, 21,* 2507–2518.

Chapey, R. (2008). *Language intervention strategies in aphasia and related neurogenic communication disorders* (5th ed.). Baltimore, MD: Lippincott Williams & Wilkins.

Charlop, M. H., & Milstein, J. P. (1989). Teaching autistic children conversational speech using video modeling. *Journal of Applied Behavior Analysis, 22*(3), 275–285.

Cherney, L. R., Halper, A. S., Holland, A. L., & Cole, R. (2008). Computerized script training for aphasia: Preliminary results. *American Journal of Speech-Language Pathology, 17*(1), 19–34.

Cherney, L. R., Gardner, P., Logemann, J. A., Newman, L. A., O'Neil-Pirozzi, T., Roth, C. R., & Solomon, N. P. (2010). The role of speech-language pathology and audiology in the optimal management of the service member returning from Iraq or Afghanistan with a blast-related head injury: Position of the Communication Sciences and Disorders Clinical Trials Research Group. *Journal of Head Trauma Rehabilitation, 25*(3), 219–224.

Cherney, L. R., Patterson, J. P., Raymer, A., Frymark, T., & Schooling, T. (2008). Evidence-based systematic review: Effects of intensity of treatment and constraint-induced language therapy for individuals with stroke-induced aphasia. *Journal of Speech, Language & Hearing Research, 51,* 1282–1299.

Chin, S. B., Tsai, P. L., & Gao, S. (2003). Connected speech intelligibility of children with cochlear implants and children with normal hearing. *American Journal of Speech-Language Pathology, 12,* 440–451.

Chomsky, N. (1965). *Aspects of a theory of syntax.* Cambridge, MA: MIT Press.

Chomsky, N., & Halle, M. (1968). *The sound pattern of English.* New York: Harper & Row.

Chrysikou, E. G., & Hamilton, R. H. (2011). Noninvasive brain stimulation in the treatment of aphasia: Exploring interhemispheric relationships and their implications for neurorehabilitation. *Restorative Neurology & Neuroscience 29*(6), 375–394.

Chumpelik, D. (1984). The PROMPT system of therapy: Theoretical framework and applications for developmental apraxia of speech. *Seminars in Speech and Language, 5,* 139–155.

Cicerone, K. D., Langenbahn, D. M., Braden, C., Malec, J. F., Kalmar, K., Fraas, M., et al. (2011). Evidence-based cognitive rehabilitation: Updated review of the literature from 2003 through 2008. *Archives of Physical Medicine and Rehabilitation, 92,* 519–530.

Cirrin, F. M., & Gillam, R. B. (2008). Language intervention practices for school-age children with spoken language disorders: A systematic review. *Language, Speech, and Hearing Services in Schools, 39,* S110–S137.

Cirrin, F. M., Schooling, T. L., Nelson, N. W., Diehl, S. F., Flynn, P. F., Staskowski, M., . . . & Adamczyk, D. F. (2010). Evidence-based systematic review: Effects of different service delivery models on communication outcomes for elementary school-age children. *Language, Speech, and Hearing Services in Schools, 41*(3), 233–264.

Clark, H. (2003). Neuromuscular treatments for speech and swallowing: A tutorial. *American Journal of Speech-Language Pathology, 12,* 400–415.

Clark, H., Lazarus, C., Arvedson, J., Schooling, T., & Frymark, T. (2009). Evidence-based systematic review: Effects of neuromuscular electrical stimulation on swallowing and neural activation. *American Journal of Speech-Language Pathology, 18,* 361–375.

Clark, J. G. (1981). Uses and abuses of hearing loss classification. *Asha, 23,* 493–500.

Coelho, C., Lê, K., Mozeiko, J., Hamilton, M., Tyler, E., Krueger, F., & Grafman, J. (2013). Characterizing discourse deficits following penetrating head injury: A preliminary model. *American Journal of Speech-Language Pathology, 22*(2), S438–S448.

Coelho, C. A. (1990). Acquisition and generalization of simple manual sign grammars by aphasic subjects. *Journal of Communication Disorders, 23,* 383–400.

Coelho, C. A., Sinotte, M. P., & Duffy, J. R. (2008). Schuell's stimulation approach to rehabilitation. In R. Chapey (Ed.), *Language intervention strategies in aphasia and related neurogenic communication disorders* (pp. 403–449). Baltimore, MD: Lippincott Williams & Wilkins.

Coggins, T. E., & Carpenter, R. L. (1981). The Communicative Intention Inventory: A system for coding children's early intentional communication. *Applied Psycholinguistics, 2,* 235–252.

Cohn, E. R., & Waltzlaf, V. J. (2011). Privacy and internet-based telepractice. *SIG 18 Perspectives on Telepractice, 1*(1), 26–37.

Coleman, M. R., Roth, F. P., & West, T. (2009). *RoadMap to PreK RTI: Applying response to intervention in preschool settings.* New York: National Center for Learning Disabilities.

Conture, E. G. (1996). Treatment efficacy: Stuttering. *Journal of Speech and Hearing Research, 39,* S18–S26.

Cooper, E., & Cooper, C. (2003). *Cooper Personalized Fluency Control Therapy for Adolescents and Adults: Clinician's Manual.* Austin, TX: Pro-Ed.

Cordes, A. K., & Ingham, R. J. (1998). *Treatment efficacy for stuttering: A search for empirical bases.* San Diego, CA: Singular.

Cornett, R. O. (1967). Cued speech. *American Annals of the Deaf, 112,* 3–13.

Croot, K. (2002). Diagnosis of AOS: Definition and criteria. *Seminars in Speech and Language, 23,* 267–279.

Cuadrado, E. M., & Weber-Fox, C. M. (2003). Atypical syntactic processing in individuals who -stutter: Evidence from event-related brain potentials and behavioral measures. *Journal of Speech, Language, and Hearing Research, 46,* 960–976.

Cummins, J. (1984). *Bilingualism and special education: Issues in assessment and pedagogy.* Clevedon, England: Multilingual Matters.

D'Cruz, A. K., Sharma, S., & Pai, P. S. (2012). Current status of near-total laryngectomy: review. *The Journal of Laryngology & Otology, 126,* 556–562.

Dalton, B., Pisha, B., Eagleton, M., Coyne, P., & Deysher, S. (2002). *Engaging in the text: Final report to the U.S. Department of Education.* Peabody, MA: CAST.

Darley, F. L., Aronson, A. E., & Brown, J. R. (1969a). Clusters of deviant speech dimensions in the dysarthrias. *Journal of Speech and Hearing Research, 12,* 462–496.

Darley, F. L., Aronson, A. E., & Brown, J. R. (1969b). Differential diagnostic patterns of dysarthria. *Journal of Speech and Hearing Research, 12,* 246–269.

Darley, F. L., Aronson, A. E., & Brown, J. R. (1975). *Motor speech disorders.* Philadelphia, PA: Saunders.

Davis, G. A. (1993). *A survey of adult aphasia and related language disorders.* Boston, MA: Allyn & Bacon.

Davis, G. A. (2007). Cognitive pragmatics of language disorders in adults. *Seminars in Speech & Language, 28,* 111–121.

Davis, G. A., & Wilcox, M. J. (1981). Incorporating parameters of natural conversation in aphasia treatment. In R. Chapey (Ed.), *Language intervention strategies in adult aphasia* (pp. 169–193). Baltimore, MD: Williams & Wilkins.

Dawson, G., & Bernier, R. (2013). A quarter century of progress on the early detection and treatment of autism spectrum disorder. *Development and Psychopathology, 25,* 1455–1472.

Dedo, H. H., & Izdebski, K. (1983). Intermediate results of 306 laryngeal nerve sections for spastic dysphonia. *Laryngoscope, 93,* 9–15.

De Nil, L. F., & Kroll, R. M. (2001). Searching for the neural basis of stuttering treatment outcome: Recent neuroimaging studies. *Clinical Linguistics & Phonetics, 15*(1–2), 163–168.

Denton, C. A., Cirino, P. T., Barth, A. E., Romain, M., Vaughn, S., Wexler, J., . . . & Fletcher, J. M. (2011). An experimental study of scheduling and duration of "Tier 2" first-grade reading intervention. *Journal of Research on Educational Effectiveness, 4*(3), 208–230.

Diamond, K. E., Justice, L. M., Siegler, R. S., & Snyder, P. A. (2013). *Synthesis of IES research on early intervention and early childhood education.* Washington, DC: National Center for Special Education Research, Institute of Education Sciences, U. S. Department of Education.

Dockrell, J. J. (2014). Developmental variations in the production of written text: Challenges for students who struggle with writing. In C.A. Stone, E. R. Silliman, B. J. Heren & G. P. Wallach (Eds.), *Handbook of language and literacy: Development and disorders.* (2nd ed., pp. 505–523). New York: The Guilford Press.

Dodd, B., & Bradford, A. (2000). A comparison of the three therapy methods for children with different types of developmental phonological disorder. *International Journal of Language & Communication Disorders, 35,* 189–209.

Dodd, B., Holm, A., Crosbie, S., & McIntosh, B. (2010). Core vocabulary intervention for inconsistent speech disorder. In L. Williams, S. McLeod, & R. McCauley (Eds.), *Interventions for speech sound disorders in children* (pp. 117–136). Baltimore, MD: Brookes.

Duffy, J. R. (2012). *Motor speech disorders: Substrates, differential diagnosis, and management* (3rd ed.). St. Louis, MO: Elsevier Mosby.

Duhon, G. J., Mesmer, E. M., Atkins, M. E., Greguson, L. A., & Olinger, E. S. (2009). Quantifying intervention intensity: A systematic approach to evaluating student responses to increasing intervention frequency. *Journal of Behavioral Education, 18,* 101–118.

Durand, M. (1990). *Severe behavior problems: A functional communication training approach.* New York: Guilford.

Dworkin, J. P. (1991). *Motor speech disorders: A treatment guide.* St. Louis, MO: Mosby–Year Book.

Dykens, E. M., & Lense, M. (2011). Intellectual disabilities and autism spectrum disorder: a cautionary note. *Autism Spectrum Disorders,* 261–269.

Ebbers, S. M., & Denton, C. A. (2008). A root awakening: Vocabulary instruction for older students with reading difficulties. *Learning Disabilities Research & Practice, 23*(2), 90–102.

Edeal, D., & Gildersleeve-Neumann, C. (2011). The importance of production frequency in therapy for childhood apraxia of speech. *American Journal of Speech-Language Pathology, 20,* 95–110.

Edgar, J. D. (2003). Respiration and swallowing in healthy adults and infants. *Perspectives on Swallowing and Swallowing Disorders, 12,* 2–6.

Ellis, A. (1977). The basic clinical theory of rational-emotive therapy. In A. Ellis & R. Grieger (Eds.), *Handbook of rational-emotive therapy* (pp. 3–34). New York: Springer.

Elman, R. J. (2007). The importance of aphasia group treatment for rebuilding community and health. *Topics in Language Disorders, 27,* 300–308.

Elman, R. J., & Bernstein-Ellis, E. (1999). The efficacy of group communication treatment in adults with chronic aphasia. *Journal of Speech, Language, and Hearing Research, 42,* 411–419.

Elsabbagh, M., & Johnson, M. H. (2010). Getting answers from babies about autism. *Trends in Cognitive Sciences, 14*(2), 81–87.

Erdman, S. A. (2009). Therapeutic factors in group counseling: Implications for audiologic rehabilitation. *SIG 7 Perspectives on Aural Rehabilitation and Its Instrumentation, 16*(1), 15–28.

Erikson, E. H. (1968). *Identity: Youth and crisis.* New York: W. W. Norton.

Ertmer, D., & Goffman, L. (2011). Speech production accuracy and variability in young cochlear implant recipients: Comparisons with typically developing age-peers. *Journal of Speech, Language, and Hearing Research February, 54,* 177–189.

Ertmer, D. J. (2005). *The source for children with cochlear implants.* East Moline, IL: LinguiSystems, Inc.

Ertmer, D. J., Young, N. M., & Nathani, S. (2007). Profiles of vocal development in young cochlear implant recipients. *Journal of Speech, Language & Hearing Research, 50,* 393–407.

Faroqi-Shah, Y., Frymark, T., Mullen, R., & Wang, B. (2010). Effect of treatment for bilingual individuals with aphasia: a systematic review of the evidence. *Journal of Neurolinguistics, 23,* 319–341.

Ferrier, L. J. (1978). Some observations of errors in context. In N. Waterson & C. Snow (Eds.), *The development of communication* (pp. 301–309). New York: Wiley.

Fey, M. (1985). *Language intervention with young children.* Baltimore, MD: Allyn & Bacon.

Fey, M. E. (1986). *Language intervention with young children.* San Diego, CA: College Hill Press.

Fey, M. E., Richard, G. J., Geffner, D., Kamhi, A. G., Medwetsky, L., Paul, D., . . . & Schooling, T. (2011). Auditory processing disorder and auditory/language interventions: An evidence-based systematic review. *Language, Speech, and Hearing Services in Schools, 42*(3), 246–264.

Fey, M. E., Yoder, P. J., Warren, S. F., & Bredin-Oja, S. L. (2013). Is more better? Milieu communication teaching in toddlers with intellectual disabilities. *Journal of Speech, Language, and Hearing Research, 56*(2), 679–693.

Finn, P. (2003). Evidence-based treatment of stuttering: II. Clinical significance of behavioral stuttering treatments. *Journal of Fluency Disorders, 28,* 209–218.

Flasher, L. V., & Fogle, P. T. (2012). *Counseling skills for speech-language pathologists and audiologists* (2nd ed.). Clifton Park, NY: Delmar Cengage Learning.

Fodor, J. A. (1975). *The language of thought* (Vol. 5). Harvard University Press.

Forrest, K. (2002). Are oral-motor exercises useful in the treatment of phonological/articulatory disorders? *Seminars in Speech and Language, 23,* 15–26.

Foundas, A. L., Mock, J. R., Corey, D. M., Golob, E. J., & Conture, E. G. (2013). The SpeechEasy device in stuttering and nonstuttering adults: Fluency effects while speaking and reading. *Brain and Language, 126*(2), 141–150.

Fox, C., Ebersbach, G., Ramig, L., & Sapir, S. (2012). LSVT LOUD and LSVT BIG: Behavioral treatment programs for speech and body movement in Parkinson Disease. *Parkinsons Disease, 2012,* 1–12. doi: 10.1155/2012/391946

Fox, C., Morrison, C., Ramig, L., & Sapir, S. (2002). Current perspectives on the Lee Silverman Voice Treatment (LSVT) for individuals with idiopathic Parkinson disease (IPD). *American Journal of Speech Language Pathology, 11,* 111–123.

Franzone, E. (2009). *Steps for implementation: Functional communication training*. Madison, WI: The National Professional Development Center on Autism Spectrum Disorders. Waisman Center, Univeristy of Wisconsin.

Frattali, C. M., Thompson, C. K., Holland, A. I., Wohl, C. B., & Ferketic, M. M. (2003). *Functional Assessment of Communication Skills for Adults (FACS)*. Rockville, MD: ASHA.

Freed, D. (2012). *Motor speech disorders: Diagnosis and treatment* (2nd ed.). Clifton Park, NY: Delmar, Cengage Learning.

Freidenberg, C. B. (2002). Working with male-to-female transgendered clients: Clinical considerations. *Contemporary Issues in Communication Sciences and Disorders, 29,* 43–58.

Froeschels, E. (1952). Chewing method as therapy. *Archives of Otolaryngology, 56,* 427–434.

Froeschels, E., Kastein, S., & Weiss, D. A. (1955). A method of therapy for paralytic conditions of the mechanisms of phonation, respiration and glutination. *Journal of Speech and Hearing Disorders, 20,* 365–370.

Fuchs, D., & Fuchs, L. S. (2006). Introduction to Response to Intervention: What, why, and how valid is it? *Reading Research Quarterly, 41,* 92–99.

Fuchs, L. S. (2002). Best practices in defining student goals and outcomes. In A. Thomas & J. Grimes (Eds.), *Best practices in school psychology IV* (pp. 553–563). Bethesda, MD: National Association of School Psychologists.

Fuchs, L. S. (2003). Assessing intervention responsiveness: Conceptual and technical issues. *Learning Disabilities Research & Practice, 18,* 172–186.

Gallas, S., Marie, J. P., Leroi, A. M., & Verin, E. (2010). Sensory transcutaneous electrical stimulation improves post-stroke dysphagic patients. *Dysphagia, 25,* 291–297.

Gartner-Schmidt, J. (2006). Voice therapy for the treatment of voice disorders. In B. J. Bailey, J. T. Johnson, & S. D. Newlands (Eds.), *Head and neck surgery: Otolaryngology,* (4th ed., pp. 883–894). Philadelphia, PA: Lippincott Williams & Wilkins.

Gauthier, K., & Genesee, F. (2011). Language development in internationally adopted children: A special case of early second language learning. *Child Development, 82*(3), 887–901.

Gebers, J. L. (2003). *Books are for talking too!* (3rd ed.). Austin, TX: Pro-Ed.

Geers, A. E. (2002). Factors affecting the development of speech, language, and literacy in children with early cochlear implantation. *Language, Speech, and Hearing Services in Schools, 33,* 172–183.

Geller, E., & Foley, G. M. (2009). Expanding the "ports of entry" for speech-language pathologists: A relational and reflective model for clinical practice. *American Journal of Speech-Language Pathology, 18,* 4–21.

Gierut, J. A. (1998). Treatment efficacy: Functional phonological disorders in children. *Journal of Speech, Language, and Hearing Research, 41,* 85–100.

Gierut, J. A. (2001). Complexity in phonological treatment: Clinical factors. *Language, Speech, and Hearing Services in Schools, 32,* 229–241.

Gierut, J. A. (2007). Phonological complexity and language learnability. *American Journal of Speech-Language Pathology, 16,* 1–12.

Gierut, J. A., Elbert, M., & Dinnsen, D. A. (1987). A functional analysis of phonological knowledge and generalization learning in misarticulating children. *Journal of Speech and Hearing Research, 30,* 462–479.

Giraud, A. L., Neumann, K., Bachoud-Levi, A. C., von Gudenberg, A. W., Euler, H. A., Lanfermann, H., & Preibisch, C. (2008). Severity of dysfluency correlates with basal ganglia activity in persistent developmental stuttering. *Brain and Language, 104*(2), 190–199.

Glennen, S., & Masters, M.G. (2002). Typical and atypical language development in infants and toddlers adopted from Eastern Europe. *American Journal of Speech and Language Therapy, 11,* 417–433.

Goebel, M. (1986). *A computer-aided fluency establishment trainer.* Annandale, VA: Annandale Fluency Clinic.

Golding-Kushner, K. (2000). *Therapy techniques for cleft palate speech and related disorders.* San Diego, CA: Singular.

Goldman-Eisler, F. (1968). *Psycholinguistics: Experiments in spontaneous speech.* New York: Academic Press.

Goodglass, H., Kaplan, E., & Barresi, B. (2001). *The assessment of aphasia and related disorders* (3rd ed.). Philadelphia, PA: Lippincott Williams & Wilkins.

Goodglass, H., & Wingfield, A. (1998). The changing relationship between anatomic and cognitive explanation in the neuropsychology of language. *Journal of Psycholinguistic Research, 27,* 147–165.

Goral, M., & Conner, P. S. (2013). Language disorders in multilingual and multicultural populations. *Annual Review of Applied Linguistics, 33,* 128–161.

Gotham, K., Pickles, A., & Lord, C.(2012). Trajectories of autism severity in children using standardized ADOS scores. *Pediatrics, 130,* 1278–1284.

Graham, M. S. (2005). Taking it to the limits: Achieving proficient esophageal speech. In P. C. Doyle and R. L. Keith (Eds.), *Contemporary considerations in the treatment and rehabilitation of head and neck cancer.* Austin, TX: Pro-Ed.

Graham, S., & Harris, K. R. (1989). Improving learning disabled students' skills at composing essays: Self-instructional strategy training. *Exceptional Children, 56,* 201–214.

Graham, S., Olinghouse, N. G., & Harris, K. R. (2009). Teaching composing to students with learning disabilities: Scientifically-supported recommendations. In G. Troia (Ed.), *Writing instruction and assessment for struggling writers* (pp. 165–186). New York: Guilford Press.

Graham, S., & Perin, D. (2007). *Writing next: Effective strategies to improve writing of adolescents in middle and high schools. A Report to Carnegie Coporation of New York.* New York: Carnegie Corporation.

Grandin, T. (2010). Thinking in Pictures: My Life with Autism. New York: Random House, Inc.

Graves, M. F. (1986). Vocabulary learning and instruction. In E. Z. Rothkopk & L. C. Ehri (Eds.), *Review of research in education* (pp. 49–89). Washington, DC: American Educational Research Association.

Gray, C. (1994). *Comic strip conversations.* Jenison, MI: Jenison Public Schools.

Gray, C. A. (1995). *Social stories: Improving responses of students with autism with accurate social information.* Rockville, MD: Aspen.

Gray, C. A. (1998). Social stories and comic strip conversations with students with Asperger syndrome and high-functioning autism. In E. Schopler, G. B. Mesibov, & L. J. Kunce (Eds.), *Asperger syndrome or high-functioning autism?* (pp. 167–198). New York: Plenum.

Green, J., Charman, T., McConachie, H., Aldred, C., Slonims, V., Howlin, P., . . . & Pickles, A. (2010). Parent-mediated communication-focused treatment in children with autism (PACT): A randomised controlled trial. *The Lancet, 375*(9732), 2152–2160.

Greenspan, S. (1990). How emotional development relates to learning. [Video program guide]. In S. Greenspan (Ed.), *Floor Time: Tuning in to each child (supplement).* New York: Scholastic.

Greenspan, S. I. (1998). Commentary: Guidance for constructing clinical practice guidelines for developmental and learning disorders: Knowledge vs. evidence-based approaches. *The Journal of Developmental and Learning Disorders, 2,* 171–192.

Gregory, H., & Hill, D. (1993). Differential evaluation and differential therapy for stuttering children. In R. Curlee (Ed.), *Stuttering and related disorders of fluency* (pp. 23–44). New York: Thieme-Stratton.

Gregory, H. H. (1979). Controversial issues: Statement and review of the literature. In H. H. Gregory (Ed.), *Controversies about stuttering therapy* (pp. 1–62). Baltimore, MD: University Park Press.

Gregory, H. H. (2003). *Stuttering therapy: Rationale and procedures.* Boston, MA: Allyn & Bacon.

Gress, C., & Singer, M. (2005). Tracheoesophageal voice restoration. In P. Doyle & R. L. Keith (Eds.), *Contemporary consideration in the treatment and rehabilitation of head and neck cancer: Voice, speech, and swallowing* (pp. 431–452). Austin, TX: Pro-Ed.

Grigos, M., Hayden, D., & Eigen, J. (2010). Perceptual and articulatory changes in speech production following PROMPT treatment. *Journal of Medical Speech-Language Pathology, 18*(4), 46–53.

Groher, M., & Crary, M. (2009). *Dysphagia: Clinical management in adults and children.* St. Louis, MO: Mosby.

Grossman, R. B., Bemis, R. H., Skwerer, D. P., & Tager-Flusberg, H. (2013). Lexical and affective prosody in children with high-functioning autism. *Journal of Speech, Language and Hearing Research, 53*(3), 778–793.

Guadagnoli, M. A., & Lee, T.D. (2004). Challenge point: a framework for conceptualizing the effects of various practice conditions in motor learning. *Journal of Motor Behavior 36,* 212–224.

Guitar, B. (2013). *Stuttering: An integrated approach to its nature and treatment* (2nd ed.). Baltimore, MD: Lippincott Williams & Wilkins.

Guitar, B., & Marchinkoski, L. (2001). Influence of mothers' slower speech on their children's speech rate. *Journal of Speech, Language, and Hearing Research, 44,* 853–861.

Guralnick, M. J. (Ed.) (1997). *The effectiveness of early intervention.* Baltimore, MD: Brookes.

Guralnick, M. J. (2011). Why early intervention works: A systems perspective. *Infants and Young Children, 24,* 6–28.

Guralnick, M. J. (2012). Preventative interventions for preterm children: Effectiveness and developmental mechanisms. *Journal of Developmental and Behavioral Pediatrics, 33,* 352–364.

Guralnick, M. J. (2013). Developmental science and preventative interventions for children at environmental risk. *Infants & Young Children, 26,* 270–285.

Hall, P. K. (2000a). A letter to the parent(s) of a child with developmental apraxia of speech. Part I: Speech characteristics of the disorder. *Language, Speech, and Hearing Services in Schools, 31,* 169–172.

Hall, P. K. (2000b). A letter to the parent(s) of a child with developmental apraxia of speech. Part II: The nature and causes of DAS. *Language, Speech, and Hearing Services in Schools, 31,* 173–175.

Hall, P. K. (2000c). A letter to the parent(s) of a child with developmental apraxia of speech. Part III: Other problems often associated with the disorders. *Language, Speech, and Hearing Services in Schools, 31,* 176–178.

Hall, P. K. (2000d). A letter to the parent(s) of a child with developmental apraxia of speech. Part IV: Treatment of DAS. *Language, Speech, and Hearing Services in Schools, 31,* 179–181.

Hall, T. E., Meyer, A., & Rose, D. H. (Eds.). (2012). *Universal design for learning in the classroom: Practical applications.* New York: Guilford.

Halle, J. W., Marshall, A. M., & Spradlin, J. E. (1979). Time delay: A technique to increase language use and generalization in retarded children. *Journal of Applied Behavior Analysis, 12,* 431–439.

Halliday, M. A. K., & Hasan, R. (1975). *Cohesion in English.* London: Longman.

Ham, R. (1986). *Techniques of stuttering therapy.* Englewood Cliffs, NJ: Prentice-Hall.

Ham, R. E. (1999). *Clinical management of stuttering in older children and adults.* Austin, TX: Pro-Ed.

Hammer, C. S., Komaroff, E., Rodriguez, B. L., Lopez, L. M., Scarpino, S. E., & Goldstein, B. (2012). Predicting Spanish-English bilingual children's language abilities. *Journal of Speech, Language, and Hearing Research, 55*(5), 1251–1264.

Harris, K. R., & Graham, S. (1996). *Making the writing process work: Strategies for composition and self-regulation.* Cambridge, MA: Brookline Books.

Hart, B. M., & Risley, T. R. (1974). Using preschool materials to modify the language of disadvantaged children. *Journal of Applied Behavior Analysis, 7,* 243–256.

Hart, B. M., & Rogers-Warren, A. (1978). A milieu approach to teaching language. In R. Schiefelbusch (Ed.), *Language intervention strategies* (pp. 193–235). Baltimore, MD: University Park Press.

Hassink, J., & Wendt, O. (2010). Remediation of phonological disorders in preschool children: Evidence for the cycles approach. *EBP Briefs, 5*(2), 1–6.

Hawley, L., & Newman, J. (2010). Group interactive structured treatment (GIST): A social competence intervention for individuals with brain injury. *Brain Injury, 24*(11), 1292–1397.

Hayden, D., Eigen, J., Walker, A., & Olsen, L. (2010). PROMPT: A tactually grounded model. In L. Williams, S. McLeod, & R. McCauley (Eds.), *Interventions for speech sound disorders in children* (pp. 453-474). Baltimore, MD: Brookes Publishing.

Hayes, J., & Flower, L. (1987). On the structure of the writing process. *Topics in Language Disorders, 7*, 19–30.

Hegde, M. N., & Davis, D. (2010). *Clinical methods and practicum in speech-language pathology* (5th ed.). Clifton Park, NY: Delmar Cengage Learning.

Helm, N. A. (1979). Management of palilalia with a pacing board. *Journal of Speech and Hearing Disorders, 44*, 350–353.

Helm-Estabrooks, N., & Albert, M. L. (2004). *Manual of aphasia and aphasia therapy*. Austin, TX: Pro-Ed.

Helm-Estabrooks, N., & Holland, A. (1998). *Approaches to the treatment of aphasia*. San Diego, CA: Singular.

Helmick, K. (2010). Cognitive rehabilitation for military personnel with mild traumatic brain injury and chronic post-concussional disorder: Results of April 2009 consensus conference. *NeuroRehabilitation, 26*(3), 239–255.

Herder, C., Howards, C., Nye, C., & Vanryckeghem, M. (2006). Effectiveness of behavioral stuttering treatment: A systematic review and meta-analysis. *Contemporary Issues in Communication Science and Disorders, 33*, 61–73.

Highman, C., Hennessy, N., & Leitão, S. (2013). Early development in infants at risk of childhood apraxia of speech: A longitudinal investigation. *Developmental Neuropsychology, 38*(3), 197–210.

Hillis, A. E., & Newhart, M. (2008). Cognitive neuropsychological approaches to treatment of language disorders: Introduction. In R. Chapey (Ed.), *Language intervention strategies in aphasia and related neurogenic communication disorders* (pp. 595–604). Baltimore, MD: Lippincott Williams & Wilkins.

Hodson, B. (2007). *Evaluating and enhancing children's phonological systems: Theory to practice*. Witchita, KS: Phonocomp.

Hodson, B. W. (2004). *Hodson Assessment of Phonological Patterns* (3rd ed.). Austin, TX: Pro-Ed.

Hodson, B. W., & Paden, E. P. (1981). Phonological processes which characterize unintelligible and intelligible speech in early childhood. *Journal of Speech and Hearing Disorders, 46*, 369–373.

Hodson, B. W., & Paden, E. P. (1983). *Targeting intelligible speech: A phonological approach to remediation*. Austin, TX: Pro-Ed.

Hoffman, L., Ireland, M., Hall-Mills, S., & Flynn, P. (2013). Evidence-based speech-language pathology practices in schools: Findings from a national survey. *Language, Speech, and Hearing Services in Schools, 44*, 266–280.

Holland, A. (1995). Current realities of aphasia rehabilitation: Time constraints, documentation demands, and functional outcomes. Paper presented at Mid-America Rehabilitation Hospital, Overland Park, KS.

Holland, A. L. (2008). Semantic memory and language processing in aphasia and dementia. *Seminars in Speech & Language, 29*, 1–1.

Holland, A. L., Fromm, D. S., De Ruyter, F., & Stein, M. (1996). Treatment efficacy: Aphasia. *Journal of Speech and Hearing Research, 39*, 27–39.

Holland, A. L., & Nelson, R. L. (2014). *Counseling in communication disorders: A wellness perspective* (2nd ed.). San Diego, CA: Plural Publishing, Inc.

Holland, A. L., & Ramage, A. E. (2004). Learning from Roger Ross: A clinical journey. In J. F. Duchan & S. Byng (Eds.), *Challenging aphasia therapies: Broadening the discourse and extending the boundaries* (pp. 118–129). New York: Psychology Press.

Hooper, C. R. (2004). Treatment of voice disorders in children. *Language, Speech, and Hearing Services in Schools, 35*, 320–326.

Hoover, J. J., Baca, L., Wexler-Love, E., & Saenz, L. (2008). *National implementation of response to intervention (RTI): Research summary*. Alexandria, VA: National Association of State Directors of Education.

Hoover, J. J., & Patton, J. R. (2009). Role of special educators in multi-tiered instruction. *Intervention in School and Clinic, 43*, 195–202.

Howell, J., & Dean, E. (1994). *Treating phonological disorders in children* (2nd ed.). London, England: Whurr Publishers Ltd.

Howell, P. (2007). Signs of developmental stuttering up to age eight and at 12 plus. *Clinical psychology review, 27*(3), 287–306.

Hsu, A. S., Chater, N., & Vitányi, P. (2011). The probabilistic analysis of language acquisition: Theoretical, computational, and experimental analysis. *Cognition, 120*(3), 380–390.

Hudgins, C. V., & Numbers, F. C. (1942). An investigation of the intelligibility of speech of the deaf. *Genetic Psychology Monographs, 25*, 289–392.

Hudock, D., & Kalinowski, J. (2014). Stuttering inhibition via altered auditory feedback during scripted telephone conversations. *International Journal of Language & Communication Disorders, 49*(1), 139–147.

Hughes, C. A., & Dexter, D. D. (2011). Response to intervention: A research-based summary. *Theory into Practice, 50*(1), 4–11.

Hull, R. (2009). *Introduction to aural rehabilitation*. San Diego, CA: Plural Publishing, Inc.

Hurkmans, J., Jonkers, R., Boonstra, A. M., Stewart, R. W., & Reinders-Messelink, H. A. (2012). Assessing the treatment effects in apraxia of speech: introduction and evaluation of the Modified Diadochokinesis Test. *International Journal of Language and Communication Disorders, 47*(4), 427–436.

Hwa-Froelich, D. A. (2009). Communication development in infants and toddlers adopted from abroad. *Topics in Language Disorders, 29*(1), 27–44.

Individuals with Disabilities Education Act (IDEA). (2011). Retrieved from http://idea.ed.gov

Ingber, S., & Dromi, E. (2010). Actual versus desired family-centered practice in early intervention for children with hearing loss. *Journal of Deaf Studies and Deaf Education, 15*(1), 59–71.

Ingersoll, B., & Lalonde, K. (2010). The impact of object and gesture imitation training on language use in children with autism spectrum disorder. *Journal of Speech, Language, and Hearing Research, 53*(4), 1040–1051.

Ingham, J. C. (2003). Evidence-based treatment of stuttering: I. Definition and application. *Journal of Fluency Disorders, 28*, 197–207.

Ingham, J. C., & Riley, G. (1998). Guidelines for documentation of treatment efficacy for young children who stutter. *Journal of Speech, Language, and Hearing Research, 41*, 753–770.

Ingham, R. J., & Bothe, A. K. (2001). Recovery from early stuttering: Additional issues within the Onslow & Packman-Yairi & Ambrose (1999) exchange. *Journal of Speech, Language, and Hearing Research 44*, 862–867.

Jackson, C., & Schatschneider, C. (2014). Rate of language growth in children with hearing loss in an auditory-verbal early intervention program. *American Annals of the Deaf, 158*(5), 539–554.

Jackson, E., Quesal, R., & Yaruss, J. S. (2012). What is stuttering (revisited). Presentation in International Stuttering Awareness Day Online Conference.

Jacobson, E. (1938). *Progressive relaxation.* Chicago, IL: University of Chicago Press.

Jakobson, R. (1964). Toward a linguistic typology of aphasic impairments. In A. DeReuck & M. O'Connor (Eds.), *Disorders of language* (pp. 21–46). London: Churchill.

Jakobson, R. (1968). *Child language: Aphasia and phonological universals.* The Hague: Mouton.

Jick, H., & Kaye, J. A. (2012). Epidemiology and possible causes of autism. *Pharmacotherapy, 23*, 1524–1530.

Johansson, B. B. (2011). Current trends in stroke rehabilitation. A review with focus on brain plasticity. *Acta Neurologica Scandinavica, 123*(3), 147–159.

Johnson, J., Christie, J., & Yawkey, T. (1987). *Play and early childhood development.* Glenville, IL: Scott, Foresman.

Jones, J. H., Gliga, T., Bedford, R., Charman, T., & Johnson, M. K. (2013). Developmental pathways to autism: A review of prospective studies of infants at risk. *Neuroscience Bio-behavioral Review, 39*, 1–33.

Justice, L. M. (2006). Evidence-based practice, response to intervention, and the prevention of reading difficulties. *Language, Speech, and Hearing Services in Schools, 37*, 284–297.

Justice, L. M., McGinty, A. S., Piasta, S. B., Kaderavek, J. N., & Fan, X. (2010). Print-focused read-alouds in preschool classrooms: Intervention effectiveness and moderators of child outcomes. *Language, Speech, and Hearing Services in Schools, 41*(4), 504–520.

Justice, L. M., Skibbe, L. E., McGinty, A. S., Piasta, S. B., & Petrill, S. (2011). Feasibility, efficacy, and social validity of home-based storybook reading intervention for children with language impairment. *Journal of Speech, Language, and Hearing Research, 54*(2), 523–538.

Kaiser, A. P., & Warren, S. F. (1986). Incidental language teaching: A critical review. *Journal of Speech and Hearing Disorders, 51*, 291–299.

Kalk, L. G., Law, J. K., Landa, R., & Law, P. A. (2010). Onset patterns prior to 36 months in autism spectrum disorders. *Journal of Autism and Developmental Disorders, 40*, 1389–1402.

Kamhi, A. G. (2014). Improving clinical practice for children with language and learning disorders. *Language, Speech, and Hearing Services in Schools, 45*, 92–103.

Kang, C., Riazuddin, S., Mundorff, J., Krasnewich, D., Friedman, P., Mullikin, J. C., & Drayna, D. (2010). Mutations in the lysosomal enzyme targeting pathway and persistent stuttering. *New England Journal of Medicine, 362*(8), 677–685.

Kanner, L. (1943). Autistic disturbances of affective contact. *Nervous Child, 2*, 217–250.

Katz, J. R. (2001). Playing at home: The talk of pretend play. In D. K. Dickinson & P. O. Tabors (Eds.), *Beginning literacy with language* (pp. 53–73). Baltimore, MD: Brookes.

Kavale, K. A., Holdnack, J. A., Mostert, M. P., & Schmied, C. M. (2003). The feasibility of a responsiveness to intervention approach for the identification of specific learning disability: A psychometric alternative. Paper presented at the National Research Center on Learning Disabilities Responsiveness to Intervention Symposium, Kansas City, MO.

Kayser, H. (1998). *Assessment and intervention resource for Hispanic children.* San Diego, CA: Singular.

Kayser, H. (2012). Bilingual language development and language disorders. In D. E. Battle (Ed.), *Communication disorders in multicultural and international populations* (pp. 102–119). St. Louis, MO: Mosby.

Kearns, K. P. (1985). Response elaboration training for patient initiated utterances. In R. H. Brookshire (Ed.), *Clinical aphasiology* (pp. 196–204). Minneapolis, MN: BRK.

Kenny, B., Lincoln, M., & Balandin, S. (2010). Experienced speech-language pathologists' response to ethical dilemmas: An integrated approach to ethical reasoning. *American Journal of Speech-Language Pathology, 19*, 121–134.

Kent, R. D. (1984). Stuttering as a temporal programming disorder. In R. F. Curlee & W. H. Perkins (Eds.), *Nature and treatment of stuttering: New directions* (pp. 283–301). San Diego, CA: College-Hill Press.

Kent, R. D. (2000). Research on speech motor control and its disorders: A review and prospective. *Journal of Communication Disorders, 33*, 391–427.

Kertesz, A. (1979). *Aphasia and associated disorders: Taxonomy, localization and recovery.* New York: Grune & Stratton.

Kertesz, A., & McCabe, P. (1977). Recovery patterns and prognosis in aphasia. *Brain, 100*, 1–18.

Khan, L., & Lewis, N. (2002). *Khan-Lewis phonological analysis.* Circle Pines, MN: American Guidance Service.

Kim, D. M., Wampold, B. E., & Bolt, D. M. (2006). Therapist effects in psychotherapy: A random-effects modeling of the National Institute of Mental Health Treatment of Depression Collaborative Research Program data. *Psychotherapy Research, 16*(2), 161–172.

Kim, S., & Jo, U. (2013). Study of accent-based music speech protocol development for improving voice problems in stroke patients with mixed dysarthria. *NeuroRehabilitation, 32*(1), 185–190.

Kirk, K. I., Ying, E., Miyamoto, R. T., O'Neill, T., Lento, C. L., & Fears, B. (2002). Effects of age at implantation in young children. *Annals of Otology, Rhinology & Laryngology, 111,* 69–73.

Kleim, J. A., & Jones, T. A. (2008). Principles of experience-dependent neural plasticity: Implications for rehabilitation after brain damage. *Journal of Speech, Language, and Hearing Research, 51*(1), S225–S239.

Klein, A., & Johns, M. (2009). *Laryngeal dissection and phonosurgical atlas.* San Diego, CA: Plural.

Kohnert, K. (2009). Cross-language generalization following treatment in bilingual speakers with aphasia: A review. *Seminars in Speech and Language, 30,* 174–86.

Kolk, H. H. J. (1991). Is stuttering a symptom of adaption or of impairment? In H. F. M. Peters, W. Hulstijn, & C. W. Starkweather (Eds.), *Speech motor control and stuttering* (pp. 189–204). Amsterdam, Netherlands: Elsevier Science.

Kolk, H. H. J., & Postma, A. (1997). Stuttering as a covert repair phenomenon. In R. F. Curlee & G. M. Siegel (Eds.), *Nature and treatment of stuttering* (pp. 182–203). Needham Heights, MA: Allyn & Bacon.

Korner-Bitensky, N. (2013). When does stroke rehabilitation end? *International Journal of Stroke 8*(1), 8–10.

Kübler-Ross, E. (1969). *On death and dying.* New York: Macmillan.

Kuehn, D., & Moller, K. (2000). State of the art: Speech and language issues in the cleft palate population. *Cleft Palate Craniofacial Journal, 37,* 348.

Kummer, A. W. (2008). *Cleft palate and craniofacial anomalies: Effects on speech and resonance* (2nd ed.). Clifton Park, NY: Delmar Cengage Learning.

Kuo, J., & Hu, X. (2002). Counseling Asian American adults with speech, language, and swallowing disorders. *Contemporary Issues in Communication Sciences and Disorders, 29,* 35–42.

Lammers, M. J. W., van der Heijden, G. J. M. G., Pourier, V. E. C., & Grolman, W. (2014). Bilateral cochlear implantation in children: A systematic review and best-evidence synthesis. *The Laryngoscope 124*(7), 1694–1699. doi: 10.1002/lary.24582

Langdon, C., & Blacker, D. (2010). Dysphagia in stroke: A new solution. *Stroke research and treatment, 2010,* 1–6. doi: 570403

Langeveld, T. P., van Rossum, M., Houtman, E. H., Zwinderman, A. H., Briaire, J. J., & Baatenburg de Jong, R. J. (2001). Evaluation of voice -quality in adductor spasmodic dysphonia before and after botulinum toxin treatment. *Annals of Otology, Rhinology, and Laryngology, 110,* 627–634.

Langevin, M., & Kully, D. (2003). Evidence-based treatment of stuttering: III. Evidence-based practice in a clinical setting. *Journal of Fluency Disorders, 28,* 219–236.

Lansford, K. L., Liss, J. M., Caviness, J. N., & Utianski, R. L. (2011). A cognitive-perceptual approach to conceptualizing speech intelligibility deficits and remediation practice in hypokinetic dysarthria. *Parkinson's Disease.* doi: 10.4061/2011/150962

Lanter, E., Watson, L. R., Erickson, K. A., & Freeman, D. (2012). Emergent literacy in children with autism: An exploration of developmental and contextual dynamic processes. *Language, Speech and Hearing in Schools, 43*(3), 308–324.

LaPointe, L. L., & Katz, R. C. (2002). Neurogenic disorders of speech. In G. H. Shames & N. B. Anderson (Eds.), *Human communication disorders* (6th ed., pp. 472–509). Boston, MA: Allyn & Bacon.

Lass, N. J., & Pannbacker, M. (2008). The application of evidence-based practice to nonspeech oral motor treatments. *Language, Speech, and Hearing Services in Schools, 39,* 408–421.

Law, J., Garrett, Z., & Nye, C. (2004). The efficacy of treatment for children with developmental speech and language delay/disorder: A meta-analysis. *Journal of Speech, Language & Hearing Research, 47,* 924–943.

Leach, E., Cornwall, P., Fleming, J., & Haines, T. (2010). Patient centered goal-setting in a subacute rehabilitation setting. *Disability and Rehabilitation, 32*(2), 159–172.

Leach, J. M., Scarborough, H., & Rescorla, L. (2003). Late-emerging reading disabilities. *Journal of Educational Psychology, 95,* 211–224.

Lederberg, A. R., Schick, B., & Spencer, P. E. (2013). Language and literacy development of deaf and hard-of-hearing children: Successes and challenges. *Developmental Psychology, 49*(1), 15–30.

Leinonen-Davis, E. (1988). Assessing the functional adequacy of children's phonological systems. *Clinical Linguistics and Phonetics, 2,* 257–270.

Leonard, R., & Kendall, K. (2008). *Dysphagia assessment and treatment planning: A team approach* (2nd ed.). San Diego, CA: Plural.

Lew, H. L., Garvert, D. W., Pogoda, T. K., Hsu, P. T., Devine, J. M., White, D. K., . . . & Goodrich, G. L. (2009). Auditory and visual impairments in patients with blast-related traumatic brain injury: Effect of dual sensory impairment on Functional Independence Measure. *Journal of Rehabilitation, Research, and Development, 46*(6), 819–826.

Lewis, B. A., Freebairn, L. A., Hansen, A., Gerry Taylor, H., Iyengar, S., & Shriberg, L. D. (2004). Family pedigrees of children with suspected childhood apraxia of speech. *Journal of Communication Disorders, 37*(2), 157–175.

Lindgren, K. A., Folstein, S. E., Tomblin, J. B., & Tager-Flusberg, H. (2009). Language and reading abilities of children with autism spectrum disorders and specific language impairment and their first-degree relatives. *Autism Research, 2*(1), 22–38.

Lloyd, C. A., & Masur, E. F. (2014). Infant behaviors influence mothers' provision of responsive and directive behaviors. *Infant Behavior and Development, 37*(3), 276–285.

Logemann, J. A. (1998). *Evaluation and treatment of swallowing disorders* (2nd ed.). Austin, TX: Pro-Ed.

Logemann, J. A. (2008). Treatment of oral and pharyngeal dysphagia. *Physical Medicine and Rehabilitation Clinics of North America, 19,* 803–816.

Lord, C., Petkova, E., Hus, V., Gan, W., Lu, F., Martin, D. M., . . . & Risi, S. (2012). A multisite study of the clinical diagnosis of different autism spectrum disorders. *Archives of general psychiatry, 69*(3), 306–313.

Lovaas, O. I., Koegel, R., Simmons, J. Q., & Long, S. J. (1973). Some generalization and follow-up measures on autistic children in behavior therapy. *Journal of Applied Behavior Analysis, 6*(1), 161–165.

Love, R. (2000). *Childhood motor speech disability* (2nd ed.). Boston, MA: Allyn & Bacon.

Lundberg, I., Olofsson, A., & Wall, S. (1980). Reading and spelling skills in the first school years predicted from phonemic awareness skills in kindergarten. *Scandinavian Journal of Psychology, 21*, 159–173.

Luterman, D. (2006). The counseling relationship. *The ASHA Leader, 11*(4), 8–9.

Luterman, D. M. (2008). *Counseling persons with communication disorders and their families* (5th ed.). Austin, TX: Pro-Ed.

Lynch, E., & Hanson, M. (Eds.). (2011). *Developing cross cultural competence: A guide for working with children and their families* (4th ed.). Baltimore: Paul H. Brookes.

Lyon, J. G. (1998). Treating real-life functionality in a couple coping with severe aphasia. In N. Helm-Estabrooks & A. Holland (Eds.), *Approaches to the treatment of aphasia* (pp. 203–239). San Diego, CA: Singular.

Maas, E., & Farinella, K. (2012). Random versus blocked practice in treatment for childhood apraxia of speech. *Journal of Speech, Language, and Hearing Research, 55*(2), 561–578.

MacArthur, C. A. (2000). New tools for writing: Assistive technology for students with writing difficulties. *Topics in Language Disorders, 20*, 85–100.

MacArthur, C. A. (2009). Reflections on research on writing and technology for struggling writers. *Learning Disabilites Research & Practice, 24*, 93–103.

MacDonald, S., & Wiseman-Hakes, C. (2010). Knowledge translation in ABI rehabilitation: A model for consolidating and applying the evidence for cognitive-communication interventions. *Brain Injury, 24*(3), 486–508.

Mackie, E. (1996). *Oral-motor activities for young children.* East Moline, IL: Lingui Systems.

MacWhinney, B. (2001). The competition model: The input, the context, and the brain. In P. Robinson (Ed.), *Cognition and second language instruction.* New York: Cambridge University Press.

MacWhinney, B. (2002). Rethinking the logical problem of language acquisition. *Journal of Child Language, 29.*

Magill, R. A. (1998). *Motor learning: Concepts and applications.* Boston, MA: McGraw-Hill.

Mahler, L. A., & Ramig, L. O. (2012). Intensive treatment of dysarthria secondary to stroke. *Clinical Linguistics & Phonetics, 26*(8), 681–694.

Malani, M. D., Barina, A., Kludjian, K., & Perkowski, J. (2011). Improving phonemic awareness in children with learning disabilities. *EBP Briefs, 5*, 51–59.

Manning, W. H. (2010). *Clinical decision making in fluency disorders* (3rd ed.). Clifton Park, NY: Cengage.

Manolson, A. (1985). *It takes two to talk: A parent's guide to helping children communicate.* Ontario, Canada: The Hanen Centre.

Marshall, J., Best, W., Cocks, N., Cruice, M., Pring, T., Bulcock, G., . . . & Caute, A. (2012). Gesture and naming therapy for people with severe aphasia: A group study. *Journal of Speech, Language, and Hearing Research, 55*(3), 726–738.

Marshalla, P. R. (1985). The role of reflexes in oral-motor learning: Techniques for improved articulation. *Seminars in Speech and Language, 6*, 317–335.

Martin, F. N., & Clark, J. G. (1996). *Hearing care for children.* Boston: Allyn & Bacon.

Martin, J. (2013). Quality standards for (re)habilitation. *Cochlear Implants International, 14*(S2), S34–S38.

Martin, P. I., Naeser, M. A., Ho, M., Doron, K. W., Kurland, J., Kaplan, J., . . . & Pascual-Leone, A. (2009). Overt naming fMRI pre- and post-TMS: Two nonfluent aphasia patients, with and without improved naming post-TMS. *Brain and Language, 111*(1), 20–35.

Mason, K. N. (2013). Relationship between pre-operative nasalance scores, velopharyngeal, closure patterns, and pharyngeal flap revision rate in patients with velopharyngeal insufficiency. (Unpublished doctoral dissertation). SUNY College, Fredonia, NY.

Mathers-Schmidt, B. A. (2001). Paradoxical vocal fold motion: A tutorial on a complex disorder and the speech-language pathologist's role. *American Journal of Speech-Language Pathology, 10*, 111–125.

Mauszycki, S. C., & Wambaugh, J. (2011, April 26). Acquired apraxia of speech: A treatment overview. *The ASHA Leader.*

McCathren, R. B., Yoder, P. J., & Warren, S. F. (1999). The relationship between prelinguistic vocalization and later expressive vocabulary in young children with developmental delay. *Journal of Speech, Language & Hearing Research, 42*, 915–924.

McCauley, R. J., & Strand, E. A. (2008). Treatment of childhood apraxia of speech: Clinical decision making in the use of nonspeech oral motor exercises. *Seminars in Speech & Language, 29*, 284–293.

McCauley, R. J., Strand, E., Lof, G. L., Schooling, T., & Frymark, T. (2009). Evidence-based systematic review: Effects of nonspeech oral motor exercises on speech. *American Journal of Speech-Language Pathology, 18*, 343–360.

McCrory, E. (2001). Voice therapy outcomes in vocal fold nodules: A retrospective audit. *International Journal of Communication Disorders, 36*, 19–24.

McDonald, E. T. (1964). *Articulation testing and treatment: A sensory motor approach.* Pittsburgh, PA: Stanwix House.

McGinty, A. S., Breit-Smith, A., Fan, X., Justice, L. M., & Kaderavek, J. N. (2011). Does intensity matter? Preschoolers' print knowledge development with a classroom-based intervention. *Early Childhood Research Quarterly, 26*(3), 255–267.

McNeil, M. R., Katz, W. F., Fossett, T. R. D., Garst, D. M., Szuminsky, N. J., Carter, G., & Lim, K. Y. (2010). Effects of online augmented kinematic and perceptual feedback on treatment of speech movements in Apraxia of Speech. *Folia Phoniatrica et Logopaedica, 63*(3), 127–133.

McNeil, M. R., Robin, D. A., & Schmidt, R. A. (1997). Apraxia of speech: Definition, differentiation, and treatment. In M. R. McNeil (Ed.), *Clinical management of sensorimotor speech disorders* (pp. 311–344). New York: Thieme.

McReynolds, L., & Bennett, S. (1972). Distinctive feature generalization in articulation training. *Journal of Speech and Hearing Disorders, 37*, 462–470.

Mehegan, C. C., & Dreifuss, F. E. (1972). Hyperlexia: Exceptional reading ability in brain damaged children. *Neurology, 22*, 1105–1111.

Melnick, K. S., Conture, E. G., & Ohde, R. N. (2003). Phonological priming in picture naming in young children who stutter. *Journal of Speech, Language, and Hearing Research, 46*, 1428–1443.

Mesibov, G. B., & Shea, V. (2010). The TEACCH program in the era of evidence-based practice. *Journal of Autism and Developmental Disorders, 40*(5), 570–579.

Metten, C., Bosshardt, H. G., Jones, M., Eisenhuth, J., Block, S., Carey, B., . . . & Menzies, R. (2011). Dual tasking and stuttering: From the laboratory to the clinic. *Disability and Rehabilitation, 33*(11), 933–944.

Milisen, R. (1954a). A rationale for articulation disorders. *Journal of Speech and Hearing Disorders, 4*, 5–17.

Milisen, R. (1954b). The disorder of articulation: A systematic clinical and experimental approach. *Journal of Speech and Hearing Disorders, Monograph Supplement, 4.*

Miller, A. J. (2008). Neuroscience of swallowing: Strategies for rehabilitation. *Perspectives on Swallowing and Swallowing Disorders, 17*, 121–127. doi: 10.1044/sasd17.4.121

Misono, S., & Merati, A. L. (2012). Evidence-based practice: Evaluation and management of unilateral vocal fold paralysis. *Otolaryngologic Clinics of North America, 45*(5), 1083–1108.

Mitchum, C. C., & Berndt, R. S. (2008). Testing the interplay of structure and meaning in aphasic sentence production. *Aphasiology, 22*, 853–865.

Moore, C. A., & Ruark, J. L. (1996). Does speech emerge from earlier appearing motor behaviors? *Journal of Speech and Hearing Research, 39*, 1034–1047.

Morgan, A. T., & Vogel, A. P. (2008). Intervention for childhood apraxia of speech. *Cochrane Database of Systematic Reviews, 3.*

Morris, S. E., & Klein, M. D. (2000). *Pre-feeding skills: A comprehensive resource for feeding development.* San Antonio, TX: Psychological Corp.

Mowrer, D. E. (1988). *Methods of modifying speech behaviors* (2nd ed.). Long Grove, IL: Waveland Press.

Murray, C. S., Woodruff, A. L., & Vaughn, S. (2010). First-grade student retention within a 3-tier reading framework. *Reading and Writing Quarterly, 26*, 26–50.

Murray, E., McCabe, P., & Ballard, K. (2012). A comparison of two treatments for childhood apraxia of speech: Methods and treatment protocol for a parallel group randomised control trial. *BMC Pediatrics, 12*, 112.

Murray, E., McCabe, P., & Ballard, K. (2014). A systematic review of treatment outcomes for children with childhood apraxia of speech. *American Journal of Speech-Language Pathology.* doi:10.1044/2014_AJSLP-13-0035

Murray, L., & Clark, H. (2006). *Neurogenic disorders of language.* Clifton Park, NY: Delmar Cengage Learning.

Myers, F., Bakker, K., St. Louis, K., & Raphael, L. (2012). Disfluencies in cluttered speech. *Journal of Fluency Disorders, 37*, 9–19.

Nation, K. (2005). Picture naming and developmental reading disorders. *Journal of Research in Reading, 28*, 28–38.

National Autism Center (NAC). (2009b). *Evidence-based practice and autism in the schools: A guide to providing appropriate intervention to students with autism spectrum disorders.* Randolph, MA: NAC.

National Center for Education Statistics. (2009). Retrieved from http://nces.ed.gov/

National Institute of Neurological Disorders & Stroke. (2011). *Deep brain stimulation for Parkinson's disease fact sheet.* Retrieved from http://www.ninds.nih.gov/disorders/deep_brain_stimulation/detail_deep_brain_stimulation.htm

National Stroke Association. (2008). Retrieved from http://www.stroke.org/site/PageNavigator/HOME

Nelson, K. (1973). Structure and strategy in learning to talk. *Society for Research in Child Development Monographs, 38*(1–2 Serial No. 149). (Reprinted in part in Mussen, Conger, & Kagan, *Readings in child development and personality* [3rd. ed.]. Harper & Row, 1975.)

Nelson, N. W. (2014). Classroom-based writing assessment. In C. A. Stone, E. R. Silliman, B. J. Heren, & G. P. Wallach (Eds.), *Handbook of language and literacy: Development and disorders.* (2nd ed., pp. 524–544). New York: The Guilford Press.

Newson, J. (1979). The growth of shared understanding between infant and care-giver. In M. Bullowa (Ed.), *Before speech* (pp. 207–243). New York: Cambridge University Press.

Ninio, A., & Bruner, J. (1978). The achievement and antecedents of labeling. *Journal of Child Language, 5*, 1–14.

Niparko, J. K. (2009). *Cochlear implants: Principles and practices* (2nd ed.). Baltimore, MD: Lippincott Williams & Wilkins.

Nippold, M. (1998). *Later language development: The school age and adolescent years* (2nd ed.). Austin, TX: Pro-Ed.

Nippold, M. A., Hesketh, L. J., Duthie, J. K., & Mansfield, T. C. (2005). Conversational versus expository discourse: A study of syntactic development in children, adolescents and adults. *American Journal of Speech-Language Pathology, 10*, 169–179.

Nippold, M. A., Leonard, L. B., & Kail, R. (1984). Syntactic and conceptual factors in children's understanding of metaphors. *Journal of Speech and Hearing Research, 27*, 197–205.

Nittrouer, S. (1993). The emergence of mature gestural patterns is not uniform: Evidence from an acoustic study. *Journal of Speech and Hearing Research, 36*, 959–972.

Nober, E. H. (1967). Articulation of the deaf. *Exceptional Child, 33*, 611–621.

Norris, J. A., & Hoffman, P. R. (1990). Language intervention within naturalistic environments. *Language, Speech, and Hearing Services in Schools, 21*, 72–84.

Northern, J., & Downs, M. (2002). *Hearing in children.* Baltimore, MD: Lippincott, Williams & Wilkins.

Nouwens, F., Dippel, D. W., de Jong-Hagelstein, M., Visch-Brink, E. G., Koudstaal, P. J., & de Lau, L. M. (2013). Rotterdam-Aphasia Therapy Study (RATS)-3: The efficacy of intensive cognitive-linguistic therapy in the acute stage of aphasia; design of a randomised controlled trial. *Trials, 14*(1), 24.

O'Neil-Pirozzi, T. M. (2011). Evidence supports metacognitive strategy instruction for particular executive functions in young to middle-aged adults with chronic traumatic brain injury. *Evidence-Based Communication Assessment and Intervention, 5,* 85–88.

Oates J., & Dacakis G. (1997). Voice change in transsexuals. *Venereology, 10*(3), 178–187.

Odom, S. L., Boyd, B. A., Hall, L. J., & Hume, K. A. (2010). Evaluation of comprehensive treatment models for individuals with autism spectrum disorders. *Journal of Autism and Developmental Disorders, 40,* 425–437.

Odom, S. L., Collet-Klingenberg, L., Rogers, S. J., & Hatton, D. D. (2010). Evidence-based practices in interventions for children and youth with autism spectrum disorders. *Preventing school failure: Alternative education for children and youth. 54*(4), 275–282.

Ogle, D. (1986). K-W-L: A teaching model that develops active reading of expository text. *The Reading Teacher, 39,* 564–571.

Oller, D. K. (1975). Simplification as the goal of phonological processes in child speech. *Language Learning, 24,* 299–303.

Oller, D. K., & Kelly, C. A. (1974). Phonological substitution processes of a hard-of-hearing child. *Journal of Speech and Hearing Disorders, 39,* 65–74.

Onslow, M., & Andrews, C. (1994). A control/experimental trial of an operant treatment for early stuttering. *Journal of Speech and Hearing Research, 37,* 1244–1260.

Onslow, M., & Packman, A. (1999a). The Lidcombe program of early stuttering intervention. In N. B. Ratner & E. C. Healy (Eds.), *Stuttering research and practice: Bridging the gap* (pp. 193–210). Mahwah, NJ: Lawrence Erlbaum.

Onslow, M., & Packman, A. (1999b). Treatment recovery and spontaneous recovery from early stuttering: The need for consistent methods in collecting and interpreting data. *Journal of Speech, Language, and Hearing Research, 42,* 398–401.

Orosco, M. J., & Klingnen, J. (2010). One school's implementation of RTI with English language learners. *Journal of Learning Disabilities, 43,* 269–288.

Owens, R. E. (2013). *Language disorders: A functional approach to assessment and intervention* (6th ed.). Needham Heights, MA: Allyn & Bacon.

Packman, A. (2012). Theory and therapy in stuttering: A complex relationship. *Journal of Fluency Disorders, 37*(4), 225–233.

Packman, A., Onslow, M., Webber, M., Harrison, E., Arnott, S., Bridgman, K., . . . & Lloyd, W. (2014). *The Lidcombe Program Treatment Guide.* Retrieved from http://sydney.edu.au/health-sciences/asrc/docs/lp_treatment_guide_0314.pdf

Pamplona, M. C., Ysunza, A., & Ramirez, P. (2004). Naturalistic intervention in cleft palate children. *International Journal of Pediatric Otorhinolaryngology, 68,* 75–81.

Patterson, J. L., & Pearson, B. Z. (2012). Bilingual lexical development, assessment, and intervention. In B. Goldstein (Ed.), *Bilingual language development and disorders in Spanish-English speakers* (2nd ed., pp. 113–130). Baltimore, MD: Paul H. Brookes.

Paul, D. R., Blosser, J., & Jakubowitz, M. D. (2006). Principles and challenges for forming successful literacy partnerships. *Topics in Language Disorders, 26,* 5–22.

Paul, R. (2007). *Language disorders from infancy to adolescence: Assessment and intervention.* Boston, MA: Mosby.

Paul, R. (2008). Intervention to improve communication in autism. *Child and Adolescent Psychiatric Clinics of North America, 17,* 835–856.

Paul, R., Augustyn, A., Klin, A., & Volkmar, F. R. (2005). Perception and production of prosody by speakers with autism spectrum disorders. *Journal of Autism and Developmental Disorders, 35*(2), 205–220.

Paul, R., & Roth, F. P. (2011). Characterizing and predicting outcomes of communication delays in infants and toddlers: Implications for clinical practice. *Language, Speech, and Hearing Services in Schools, 42*(3), 331–340.

Peach, R. K. (2008). Global aphasia: Identification and management. In R. Chapey (Ed.), *Language intervention strategies in aphasia and related neurogenic communication disorders* (pp. 565–594). Baltimore, MD: Lippincott Williams & Wilkins.

Peach, R. K. (2013). The cognitive basis for sentence planning difficulties in discourse after traumatic brain injury. *American Journal of Speech-Language Pathology, 22*(2), S285–S297.

Pedersen, P., Draguns, J., Lonner, W., & Trimble, J. (2002). *Counseling across cultures.* Thousand Oaks, CA: Sage.

Pedersen, P. M., Vintner, K., & Olsen, T. S. (2004). Aphasia after stroke: Type, severity, and prognosis. *Cerebrovascular diseases, 17,* 35–43.

Pelatti, C. Y., Justice, L. M., Pentimonti, J. M., & Schmitt, M. B. (2013). Fostering children's emergent literacy development: The role of family practices. In C. A. Stone, E. R. Silliman, B. J. Ehren, & G. P. Wallach (Eds.), *Handbook of language and literacy: Developmental disorders* (pp. 190–203). New York: Guilford Press.

Pellicano, E. (2012). Do autistic symptoms persist across time? Evidence of substantial change in symptomatology over a 3-year period in cognitively able children with autism. *American Journal on Intellectual and Developmental Disabilities, 117*(2), 156–166.

Pellicano, E. (2013). Testing the predictive power of cognitive atypicalities in autistic children: Evidence from a 3-year follow-up study. *Pediatrics, 130,* 1278–1284.

Pellowski, M. W., & Conture, E. G. (2002). Characteristics of speech disfluency and stuttering behaviors in 3- and 4-year-old children. *Journal of Speech, Language, and Hearing Research, 45,* 20–34.

Peterson-Falzone, S., Trost-Cardamone, J., Karnell, M., and Hardin-Jones, M. (2006). *The clinician's guide to treating cleft palate speech.* St. Louis, MO: Mosby Elsevier.

Peterson-Falzone, S. J., Hardin-Jones, M. S., & Karnell, M. (2001). *Cleft palate speech.* St. Louis, MO: Mosby.

Piaget, J. (1951). *Plays, dreams and imitation in childhood.* London: Heinemann.

Piaget, J. (1954). *Origins of intelligence.* New York: Basic Books.

Piaget, J. (1973). *The child and reality: Problems of genetic psychology. (Trans. Arnold Rosin).* New York: Grossman Publishers.

Pickering, J., & Baker, L. (2012). Voice and communication intervention for individuals in the transgender community: An historical perspective and review of the literature. In R. K. Adler, S. Hirsch, & M. Mordaunt (Eds.), *Voice and communication therapy for the transgender/transsexual client: A comprehensive clinical guide* (2nd ed.). San Diego, CA: Plural Publishing.

Pinker, S. (1989). *Learnability and cognition: The acquisition of argument structure.* Cambridge, MA: MIT Press.

Pinker, S. (1996). *Language learnability and language development.* Cambridge, MA: Harvard University Press.

Plotkin, S., Gerber, J. S., & Offit, P. A. (2009). Vaccines and autism: A tale of shifting hypotheses. *Clinical and Infectious Diseases, 48,* 456–461.

Plowman, E. K., Hentz, B., & Ellis, C. (2011). Post-stroke aphasia prognosis: A review of patient-related and stroke-related factors. *Journal of Evaluation in Clinical Practice, 18*(3), 689–694.

Poole, E. (1934). Genetic development of articulation of consonant sounds in speech. *Elementary English Review, 11,* 159–161.

Postma, A. (2000). Detection of errors during speech production: A review of speech monitoring models. *Cognition, 77*(2), 97–132.

Prater, R. J., Swift, R. W., Deem, J. F., & Miller, L. (1999). *Manual of voice therapy* (2nd ed.). Austin, TX: Pro-Ed.

Prather, E., Hedrick, D., & Kern, C. (1975). Articulation development in children aged two to four years. *Journal of Speech and Hearing Disorders, 40,* 179–191.

Prins, D., & Ingham, R. J. (2009). Evidence-based treatment and stuttering: Historical perspective. *Journal of Speech, Language, and Hearing Research, 52(1),* 254–263.

Prizant, B. M. (1983). Language acquisition and communicative behavior in autism toward an understanding of the whole of it. *Journal of Speech and Hearing Disorders, 48*(3), 296–307.

Prizant, B. M., & Duchan, J. F. (1981). The functions of immediate echolalia in autistic children. *Journal of Speech and Hearing Disorders, 46*(3), 241–249.

Prizant, B. M., Wetherby, A. M., Rubin, E., & Laurent, A. C. (2003). The SCERTS Model: A transactional, family-centered approach to enhancing communication and socioemotional abilities of children with autism spectrum disorder. *Infants & Young Children, 16*(4), 296–316.

Pulvermuller, F., & Berthier, M. L. (2008). Aphasia therapy on a neuroscience basis. *Aphasiology, 22,* 563–599.

Pulvermuller, F., Hauk, O., Zohsel, K., Neininger, B., & Mohr, B. (2005). Therapy-related reorganization of language in both hemispheres of patients with chronic aphasia. *NeuroImage, 28,* 481–489.

Pulvermuller, F., Kujala, T., Shtyrov, Y., Simola, J., Tiitinen, H., Alku, P., et al. (2001). Memory traces for words as revealed by the mismatch negativity. *Neuroimage, 14,* 607–616.

Qualls, C. D. (2012). Neurogenic disorders of speech, language, cognition-communication, and swallowing. In D. E. Battle (Ed.), *Communication disorders in multicultural and international populations* (4th ed., pp. 148–163). St. Louis, MO: Mosby.

Qualls, C. D., & Muñoz, M. L. (2005). Race-ethnicity, socioeconomic status, and cognitive-communicative functioning in individuals with neurogenic communication disorders: Clinical implications and research directions. *ECHO: E-Journal for Black and Other Ethnic Group Research and Practices in Communication Sciences and Disorders, 1,* 30–39.

Radziewicz, C., & Antonellis, C. S. (2008). Children with hearing loss: Considerations and implications. In D. K. Bernstein and E. Tiegerman-Farber (Eds.), *Language and communication disorders in children* (pp. 370–402). Boston, MA: Allyn & Bacon.

Ralabate, P. K. (2011). Universal design for learning: Meeting the needs of all students. *The ASHA Leader, 16*(10), 14–17.

Ramig, L. O. (1998). Speech and voice disorders in Parkinson disease and their treatment. In L. Chernery (Ed.), *Topics in geriatric rehabilitation* (pp. 28–43). Gaithersburg, MD: Aspen.

Ramig, L. O., Pawlas, A., & Countryman, S. (1995). *The Lee Silverman Voice Treatment.* Iowa City, IA: National Center for Voice and Speech.

Ramig, L. O., Sapir, S., Countryman, S., Pawlas, A. A., O'Brien, C., Hoehn, M., & Thompson, L. L. (2001). Intensive voice treatment (LSVT) for patients with Parkinson's disease: A 2 year follow up. *Journal of Neurology, Neurosurgery, and Psychiatry, 71,* 493–498.

Ramig, L. O., & Verdolini, K. (1998). Treatment efficacy: Voice disorders. *Journal of Speech, Language, and Hearing Research, 41,* 101–116.

Rammage, L., Morrison, M., & Nichol, H. (2001). *Management of the voice and its disorders.* San Diego, CA: Singular.

Rao, P. R. (2001). Use of Amer-Ind code by persons with severe aphasia. In R. Chapey (Ed.), *Language intervention strategies in aphasia and related neurogenic communication disorders* (pp. 688–702). Baltimore, MD: Lippincott Williams & Wilkins.

Rapin, I., & Dunn, M. (1997). Language disorders in children with autism. *Seminars in Pediatric Neurology, 4*(2), 86–92.

Rath, J. F., Simon, D., Langenbahn, D. M., Sherr, R. L., & Diller, L. (2003). Group treatment of problem-solving deficits in outpatients with traumatic brain injury: A randomised outcome study. *Neuropsychological Rehabilitation, 13*(4), 461–488.

Ratner, N. (1995). Treating the stuttering child with concomitant grammatical or phonological disorders. *Language, Speech, and Hearing Services in Schools, 26,* 180–186.

Ratner, N., & Bruner, J. (1978). Games, social exchange and the acquisition of language. *Journal of Child Language, 5,* 391–402.

Raymer, A. M., Kendall, D., Maher, L., Martin, N., Murray, L., Rose, M., et al. (2008). Translational research in aphasia: From neuroscience to neurorehabilitation.

Journal of Speech, Language, and Hearing Research, 51, 259–275.

Richard, G. J. (2011). Prologue: The role of the speech-language pathologist in identifying and treating children with auditory processing disorders. *Language, Speech, and Hearing Services in Schools, 42,* 241–245.

Rivkin, M. (1986). The teacher's place in children's play. In G. Fein & M. Rivkin (Eds.), *The young child at play* (pp. 213–217). Washington, DC: National Association for the Education of Young Children.

Roberts, J., Pollock, K., Krakow, R., Price, J., Fulmer, K., & Wang, P. (2005). Language development in preschool-aged children adopted from China. *Journal of Speech-Language-Hearing Research, 48,* 93–107.

Robey, R. R. (1998). A meta-analysis of clinical outcomes in the treatment of aphasia. *Journal of Speech, Language, and Hearing Research, 41,* 172–187.

Robin, D. A., Somodi, L. B., & Luschei, E. S. (1991). Measurement of tongue strength and endurance in normal and articulation disordered subjects. In C. A. Moore, K. M. Yorkston, & D. R. Beukelman (Eds.), *Dysarthria and apraxia of speech: Perspectives on management* (pp. 173–184). Baltimore, MD: Brookes.

Robinson, Jr., T. L. (2012). Cultural diversity and fluency disorders. In D. E. Battle (Ed.), *Communication disorders in multicultural and international populations* (4th ed., pp. 164–173). St. Louis, MO: Mosby.

Rogers, C., & Sawyers, J. (1988). *Play in the lives of children.* Washington, DC: National Association for the Education of Young Children.

Rogers, C. R. (1951). *Client-centered therapy.* Boston, MA: Houghton Mifflin.

Rogers, S. J. (2009). What are infant siblings teaching us about autism in infancy? *Autism Research, 2*(3), 125–137.

Rogers, S. J., Hall, T., Osaki, D., Reaven, J., & Herbison, J. (2000). The Denver Model: A comprehensive integrated educational approach to young children with autism and their families. In J. S. Handleman & S. L. Harris (Eds.), *Preschool education programs for children with autism* (pp. 95–133). Austin, TX: PRO-ED.

Rollin, W. (2000). *Counseling individuals with communication disorders: Pyschodynamic and family aspects.* Boston, MA: Butterworth-Heinemann.

Rose, D. H., & Meyer, A. (2000). Universal design for individual differences. *Educational Leadership, 58,* 39–43.

Rose, M. L. (2013). Releasing the constraints on aphasia therapy: The positive impact of gesture and multimodality treatments. *Amercian Journal of Speech-Language Pathology, 22*(2), S227–S239.

Roseberry-McKibbin, C. (2007). *Language disorders in children: A multicultural and case perspective.* Boston: Allyn & Bacon.

Roseberry-McKibbin, C., Brice, A., & O'Hanlon, L. (2005). Serving English language learners in public school settings: A national survey. *Language, Speech, and Hearing Services in Schools, 36*(I), 48–61.

Rosenbek, J. C., & LaPointe, L. L. (1985). Treating apraxia of speech. In D. Johns (Ed.), *Clinical management of neurogenic communicative disorders* (pp. 97–152). Boston, MA: Little, Brown.

Rossetti, L. M. (2001). *Communication intervention: Birth to three.* Clifton Park, NY: Delmar Cengage Learning.

Roth, F. P. (1999). Communicative intervention for children with psychiatric and communication disorders. *Child and adolescent psychiatric clinics of North America, 8*(1), 137–152.

Roth, F. P., & Baden, B. (2001). Investing in emergent literacy intervention: A key role for speech-language pathologists. *Seminars in Speech and Language, 22,* 163–174.

Roth, F. P., Dougherty, D. P., Paul, D. R., & Adamczyk, D. (2010). *RTI in action: Oral language activities for K–2 classrooms.* Rockville, MD: American Speech-Language-Hearing Association.

Roth, F. P., & Spekman, N. J. (1984). Intervention strategies for learning disabled children with oral communication disorders. *Learning Disability Quarterly, 2,* 7–18.

Roth, F. P., & Troia, G. A. (2006). Collaborative efforts to promote emergent literacy and efficient word recognition skills. *Topics in Language Disorders, 26,* 24–41.

Roth, F. P., & Troia, G. A. (2009). Applications of responsiveness to intervention and the speech-language pathologist in elementary school settings. *Seminars in Speech & Language, 30,* 75–89.

Roth, F. P., Troia, G. A., Worthington, C. K., & Dow, K. A. (2002). Promoting the awareness of sounds in speech: An initial report of an early intervention for children with speech and language impairments. *Applied Psycholinguistics, 23,* 535–565.

Roth, F. P., Troia, G. A., Worthington, C. K., & Handy, D. (2006). Promoting awareness of sounds in speech (PASS): The effects of intervention and stimulus characteristics on the blending performance of preschool children with communication impairments. *Learning Disability Quarterly, 29,* 67–88.

Roth, F. P., Worthington, C. K., & Troia, G. A. (2009). PASS: A phonological awareness interventional program for at-risk preschool children. ASHA Convention Presentation.

Roth, F. P., Worthington, C. K., & Troia, G. A. (2012). *Promoting Awareness of Speech Sounds (PASS): A phonological awareness intervention program.* Verona, WI: Attainment, Inc.

Roy, N., Barkmeier-Kramer, J., Sivasankar, M., Eadie, T., Mehta, D., Paul, D., & Hillman, R. E. (2013). Evidence-based clinical voice assessment: A systematic review. *American Journal of Speech-Language Pathology, 22,* 212–226.

Roy, N., Merrill, R. M., Gray, S.D., & Smith, E. M. (2005). Voice disorders in the general population: Prevalence, risk factors, and occupational impact. *The Laryngoscope, 115*(11), 1988–1995.

Roy, N., Weinrich, B., Gray, S., Tanner, K., Stemple, J., & Sapienza, C. (2003). Three treatments for teachers with voice disorders: A randomized clinical trial. *Journal of Speech, Language, and Hearing Research, 46,* 670–688.

Roy, N., Weinrich, B., Gray, S. D., Tanner, K., Toledo, S. W., Dove, H., Corbin-Lewis, K., & Stemple, C. (2002). Voice amplification versus vocal hygiene instruction for teachers with voice disorders: A treatment outcome study. *Journal of Speech, Language, and Hearing Research, 45,* 625–638.

Ruark, J. L., & Moore, C. A. (1997). Coordination of lip muscle activity by 2-year-old children during speech and nonspeech tasks. *Journal of Speech and Hearing Research, 40*, 1373–1385.

Russell, J. A., Ciucci, M. R., Connor, N. P., & Schallert, T. (2010). Targeted exercise therapy for voice and swallow in person with Parkinson's disease. *Brain Research, 1341*, 3–11.

Rvachew, S. (2005). Stimulability and treatment success. *Topics in Language Disorders, 25*, 207–219.

Rvachew, S., Nowak, M., & Cloutier, G. (2004). Effect of phonemic perception training on the speech production and phonological awareness skills of children with expressive phonological delay. *American Journal of Speech-Language Pathology, 13*, 250–263.

Rvachew, S., Rafaat, S., & Martin, M. (1999). Stimulability, speech perception skills, and the treatment of phonological disorders. *American Journal of Speech-Language Pathology, 8*, 33–43.

Ryan, B. P. (1974). *Programmed therapy of stuttering in children and adults*. Springfield, IL: Charles C. Thomas.

Ryan, N. M., Vertigan, A. E., Bone, S., & Gibson, P. G. (2010). Cough reflex sensitivity improves with speech language pathology management of refractory chronic cough. *Cough, 6*(5), 1–8.

Rydell, P., & Prizant, B. (1995). Assessment and intervention strategies for children who use echolalia. In K. Quill (Ed.), *Teaching children with autism: Methods to increase communication and socialization* (pp. 105–129). Albany, NY: Delmar Publishers.

Saltuklaroglu, T. (2012). Assessment and treatment of stuttering using altered auditory feedback. In *The Science and Practice of Stuttering Treatment: A symposium* (pp. 29). New York: John Wiley & Sons.

Sapir, S., Ramig, L., & Fox, C. (2008). Voice, speech, and swallowing disorders. In S. Factor and F. Weiner (Eds.), *Parkinson disease: Diagnosis and clinical management* (pp. 77–97). New York: Demos.

Sarno, M. T., & Levita, E. (1971). Natural course of recovery in severe aphasia. *Archives of Physical Medicine and Rehabilitation, 52*, 175–178.

Sarno, M. T., Silverman, M., & Sands, E. (1970). Speech therapy and language recovery in severe aphasia. *Journal of Speech and Hearing Research, 13*, 607–623.

Sawyer, J., & Yairi, E. (2010). Characteristics of disfluency clusters over time in preschool children who stutter. *Journal of Speech, Language, and Hearing Research, 53*(5), 1191–1205.

Scarborough, H., & Dobrich, W. (1990). Development of children with early language delay. *Journal of Speech and Hearing Research, 33*, 70–83.

Scarborough, H. S. (1998). Early identification of children at risk for reading disabilities. In B. K. Shapiro, P. J. Accardo, & A. J. Capute (Eds.), *Specific reading disabilities: A view of the spectrum* (pp. 75–119). Timonium, MD: York Press.

Schafer, E. C., Amlani, A. M., Seibold, A., Shattuck, P. L. (2007). A meta-analytic comparison of binaural benefits between bilateral cochlear implants and bimodal stimulation. *Journal of the American Academy of Audiology, 18*, 760–776.

Schopler, E., & Reichler, R. J. (1971). Parents as cotherapists in the treatment of psychotic children. *Journal of Autism and Childhood Schizophrenia, 1*, 87–102.

Schuell, H., Jenkins, J. H., & Jimenez-Pabon, E. (1964). *Aphasia in adults: Diagnosis, prognosis and treatment*. New York: Hober-Harper.

Schulz, G. M., Greer, M., & Friedman, W. (2000). Changes in vocal intensity in Parkinson's disease following pallidotomy surgery. *Journal of Voice, 14*, 589–606.

Schulz, G. M., Peterson, T., Sapienza, C., Greer, M., & Friedman, W. (1999). Voice and speech characteristics of persons with Parkinson's disease pre- and post-pallidotomy surgery: Preliminary findings. *Journal of Speech, Language, and Hearing Research, 42*, 1176–1195.

Schumaker, J., Deshler, D., Alley, G., Warner, M., Clark, F., & Nolan, S. (1982). Error monitoring: A learning strategy for improving adolescent performance. In W. Cruickshank & J. Lerner (Eds.), *Best of ACLD* (pp. 179–183). Syracuse, NY: Syracuse University Press.

Schuster, M., Lohscheller, J., Kummer, P., Hoppe, U., Eysholdt, U., & Rosanowski, F. (2003). Quality of life in laryngectomees after prosthetic voice restoration. *Folia Phoniatrica et Logopaedica, 55*, 211–219.

Schweigert, W. A. (1986). The comprehension of familiar and less familiar idioms. *Journal of Psychological Research, 15*, 33–45.

Seikel, J. A., King, D. W., & Drumright, D. G. (2010). *Anatomy and physiology for speech, language, and hearing* (4th ed). Clifton Park, NY: Delmar Cengage Learning.

Self, T. L., Hale, L. S., & Crumrine, D. (2010). Pharmacotherapy and children with autism spectrum disorder: A tutorial for speech-language pathologists. *Language, Speech and Hearing in Schools, 41*(3), 367–375.

Seligmann, E. R. (2005). Lessac-Madsen Resonant Voice Therapy (LMRVT): A brief description and review. Presented at the Summer Vocology Institute, Denver, CO.

Senturia, B. H., & Wilson, F. B. (1968). Otorhinolaryngologic findings in children with voice deviations. *Annals of Otology, Rhinology, and Laryngology, 77*, 1027–1042.

Shames, G. H. (2000). *Counseling the communicatively disabled and their families: A manual for clinicians*. Needham Heights, MA: Allyn & Bacon.

Shames, G. H., & Florance, C. L. (1980). *Stutter-free speech: A goal for therapy*. Columbus, OH: Charles E. Merrill.

Sharp, H. M., & Bryant, K. M. (2003). Ethical issues in dysphagia: When patients refuse assessment or treatment. *Seminars in Speech and Language, 24*, 285–299.

Sheehan, J. G. (1958). Conflict theory of stuttering. In J. Eisenson (Ed.), *Stuttering: A Symposium* (pp. 121–166). New York: Harper and Row.

Sheehan, J. G. (1968). Stuttering as a self-role conflict. In H. H. Gregory (Ed.), *Learning theory and stuttering therapy* (pp. 72–83). Evanston, IL: Northwestern University Press.

Shine, R. E. (1980). Direct management of the beginning stutterer. *Seminars in Speech, Language and Hearing, 1*, 339–350.

Shipley, K. G., & Roseberry-McKibbin, C. (2006). *Interviewing and counseling in communicative disorders: Principles and procedures* (3rd ed.). Austin, TX: Pro-Ed.

Shprintzen, R. J., & Bardach, J. (1995). *Cleft palate speech management: A multidisciplinary approach.* St. Louis, MO: Mosby.

Shriberg, L., Aram, D., & Kwiatkowski, J. (1997a). Developmental apraxia of speech: I. Descriptive and theoretical perspectives. *Journal of Speech, Language, and Hearing Research, 40,* 273–285.

Shriberg, L., Aram, D., & Kwiatkowski, J. (1997b). Developmental apraxia of speech: II. Toward a diagnostic marker. *Journal of Speech, Language, and Hearing Research, 40,* 286–312.

Shriberg, L., Aram, D., & Kwiatkowski, J. (1997c). Developmental apraxia of speech: III. A subtype marked by inappropriate stress. *Journal of Speech, Language, and Hearing Research, 40,* 313–337.

Shriberg, L. D., & Kwiatkowski, J. (1980). *Natural process analysis.* New York: Wiley.

Shumway, S., & Wetherby, A. (2009). Communicative acts by children with ASD in the second year of life. *Journal of Speech, Language, and Hearing Research, 52,* 1139–1156.

Silberberg, N. E., & Silberberg, M. C. (1967). Hyperlexia: Specific word recognition skills in young children. *Exceptional Child, 34,* 41–42.

Silverman, E. M., & Zimmer, C. H. (1975). Incidence of chronic hoarseness among school-age children. *Journal of Speech and Hearing Disorders, 40,* 211–215.

Simmons-Mackie, N. (2001). Social approaches to aphasia intervention. In R. Chapey (Ed.), *Language intervention strategies in aphasia and related neurogenic communication disorders* (pp. 246–268). Baltimore, MD: Lippincott Williams & Wilkins.

Simmons-Mackie, N. (2008). Social approaches to aphasia intervention. In R. Chapey (Ed.), *Language intervention strategies in aphasia and related neurogenic communication disorders* (pp. 290–317). Baltimore, MD: Lippincott Williams & Wilkins.

Sisskin, V. (2002). Therapy planning for school-age children who stutter. *Seminars in Speech and Language, 23,* 173–180.

Skelly, M. (1979). *Amer-Ind gestural code based on universal American Indian hand talk.* New York: Elsevier Science.

Skelly, M., Schinsky, L., Smith, R. W., & Fust, R. S. (1974). American Indian sign (Amerind) as a facilitator of verbalization for oral verbal apraxia. *Journal of Speech and Hearing Disorders, 39,* 445–456.

Skinner, B. F. (1957). *Verbal behavior.* New York: Appleton-Century-Crofts.

Smit, A. B., Hand, L., Freilinger, J., Bernthal, J., & Bird, A. (1990). The Iowa Articulation Norms Project and its Nebraska replication. *Journal of Speech and Hearing Disorders, 55,* 779–798.

Smith, A. (1999). Stuttering: A unified approach to a mulitfactorial, dynamic disorder. In N. B. Ratner & E. C. Healey (Eds.), *Stuttering research and practice: Bridging the gap* (pp. 27–44). Mahwah, NJ: Erlbaum.

Smith, A., & Kelly, E. (1997). Stuttering: A dynamic, multifactorial model. In R. F. Curlee & G. M. Siegel (Eds.), *Nature and treatment of stuttering: New directions* (pp. 204–217). Needham Heights, MA: Allyn & Bacon.

Smith, A., Sadagopan, N., Walsh, B., & Weber-Fox, C. (2010). Increasing phonological complexity reveals heightened instability in inter-articulatory coordination in adults who stutter. *Journal of Fluency Disorders, 35,* 1–18.

Smythe, I., & Everatt, J. (2002). Dyslexia and the multicultural child: Policy into practice. *Topics in Language Disorders, 22,* 71–80.

Sohlberg, M. M., Ehlardt, L., & Kennedy, M. (2005). Instructional techniques in cognitive rehabilitation: A preliminary report. *Seminars in Speech and Language, 26,* 268–279.

Sparks, R. W. (2001). Melodic intonation therapy. In R. Chapey (Ed.), *Language intervention strategies in aphasia and related communication disorders* (pp. 703–717). Baltimore, MD: Lippincott Williams & Wilkins.

Sparks, R. W., Helm, N., & Albert, M. (1974). Aphasia rehabilitation resulting from melodic intonation therapy. *Cortex, 10,* 303.

Sparks, R. W., & Holland, A. L. (1976). Method: Melodic intonation therapy for aphasia. *Journal of Speech and Hearing Disorders, 41,* 287–297.

Speece, D. L., & Hines, S. J. (2008). Identifying children who require different instruction in a response to instruction framework. *Perspectives on Language Learning and Education, 15,* 34–40.

Spekman, N. J., & Roth, F. P. (1984). Intervention strategies for learning disabled children with oral communication disorders. *Learning Disability Quarterly, 7,* 7–18.

Spencer, K. A., Yorkston, K. M., & Duffy, J. R. (2003). Behavioral management of respiratory/phonatory dysfunction from dysarthria: A flowchart for guidance in clinical decision making. *Journal of Medical Speech Language Pathology, 11*(2), xxxix–lxi.

Speyer, R., Weineke, G., Hosseini, E. G., Kempen, P. A., Kersing, W., & Dejonckere, P. H. (2002). Effects of voice therapy as objectively evaluated by digitized laryngeal stroboscopic imaging. *Annals of Otology, Rhinology, and Laryngology, 111,* 902–908.

Stajner-Katusic, S., Horga, D., Musura, M., & Globlek, D. (2006). Voice and speech after laryngectomy. *Clinical Linguistics & Phonetics, 20,* 195–203.

Stanovich, K. E. (1986). Matthew effects in reading: Some consequences of individual differences in the acquisition of literacy. *Reading Research Quarterly, 21,* 360–406.

Starkweather, C. W. (1985). The development of fluency in normal children. In H. H. Gregory (Ed.), *Stuttering therapy: Prevention and intervention with children* (pp. 67–100). Memphis, TN: Speech Foundation of America.

Starkweather, C. W. (1987). *Fluency and stuttering.* Englewood Cliffs, NJ: Prentice Hall.

Starkweather, C. W., & Gottwald, S. R. (2000). The demands and capacities model II: Clinical implications. *Journal of Fluency Disorders, 15,* 143–157.

Steele, R. (2009). On aphasia pharmacotherapy. In *Lingraphica's "Topics in Aphasia" series.* Retrieved from http://www.speechpathology.com/articles/on-aphasia-pharmacotherapy-1187

Stein, N. L., & Glenn, C. G. (1979). An analysis of story comprehension in elementary school children. In R. O. Freedle (Ed.), *New directions in discourse processing* (Vol. 2, pp. 53–120). Norwood, NJ: Ablex.

Stemple, J. C., Glaze, L. E., & Klaben, B. G. (2000). *Clinical voice pathology: Theory and management.* Clifton Park, NY: Delmar Cengage Learning.

Stevens, K., & Hanson, H. (2013). Articulatory-acoustic relations as the basis of distinctive contrasts. In W. J. Hardcastle, J. Laver, & F. E. Gibbon (Eds). *The handbook of phonetic sciences* (pp. 424–444). Hoboken, NJ: Blackwell.

Stinchfield-Hawk, S., & Young, E. (1938). *Children with delayed and defective speech: Motor-kinesthetic factors and their training.* Palo Alto, CA: Stanford University Press.

Stoel-Gammon, C., Stone-Goldman, J., & Glaspey, A. (2002). Pattern-based approaches to phonological therapy. *Seminars in Speech and Language, 23,* 3–13.

Stone, C. A., Silliman, E. R., Ehren, B. J., & Wallach, G. P. (Eds.). (2014). *Handbook of language and literacy: Development and disorders.* New York: Guilford Press.

Stone, J. R., & Olswang, L. B. (1989). The hidden challenge in counseling. *ASHA, 31,* 27–31.

Strand, E., Stoeckel, C., Baas, B. (2006). Treatment of severe childhood apraxia of speech: A treatment efficacy study. *Journal of Medical Speech-Language Pathology, 14*(4), 297–307.

Strangman, N. (2003). Strategy instruction goes digital: Two teachers' perspectives on digital texts with embedded learning supports. *Reading Online, 6,* 9.

Strain, P. S., & Hoyson, M. (2000). The need for longitudinal, intensive social skill intervention LEAP follow-up outcomes for children with autism. *Topics in Early Childhood Special Education, 20*(2), 116–122.

Strode, R., & Chamberlain, C. (2006). *The source for childhood apraxia of speech.* East Moline, IL: Linguisystems.

Stuart, A., Kalinowski, J., Rastatter, M. P., Saltuklaroglu, T., & Dayalu, V. (2004). Investigations of the impact of altered auditory feedback in-the-ear devices on the speech of people who stutter: Initial fitting and 4-month follow-up. *International Journal of Language and Communication Disorders, 39,* 93–113.

Sue, D. W., & Sue, D. (1999). *Counseling the culturally different: Theory and practice.* New York: Wiley.

Sulica, L. (2004). Contemporary management of spasmodic dysphonia. *Current Opinion in Otolaryngology/Head Neck Surgery, 12,* 543–548.

Sulica, L., Blitzer, A., Brin, M., & Stewart, C. (2003). Botulinum toxin management of adductor spasmodic dysphonia after failed recurrent laryngeal nerve section. *Annals of Otology, Rhinology, and Laryngology, 112,* 499–505.

Sullivan, H. (1953). *The interpersonal theory of psychiatry.* New York: Norton.

Svirsky, M. A., Teoh, S., & Neuburger, H. (2004). Development of language and speech perception in congenitally, profoundly deaf children as a function of age at cochlear implantation. *Audiology & Neuro-Otology, 9,* 224–233.

Tager-Flusberg, H., Paul, R., & Lord, C. (2005). Language and communication in autism. *Handbook of Autism and Pervasive Developmental Disorders, 1,* 335–364.

Tager-Flusberg, H., Rogers, S., Cooper, J., Landa, R., Lord, C., Paul, R., . . . & Yoder, P. (2009). Defining spoken language benchmarks and selecting measures of expressive language development for young children with autism spectrum disorders. *Journal of Speech, Language, and Hearing Research, 52*(3), 643–652.

Tanaka, Y., Albert, M. L., Fujita, K., Nonaka, C., & Yokoyama, E. (2006). Treating perseveration improves naming in aphasia. *Brain and Language, 99,* 57–58.

Tanielian, T. L., & Jaycox, L. (Eds.). (2008). *Invisible wounds of war: Psychological and cognitive injuries, their consequences, and services to assist recovery* (Vol. 1). Santa Monica, CA: Rand Corporation.

Tanner, D. C. (2008). *The family guide to surviving stroke and communication disorders* (2nd ed.). Needham HeightsSudbury, MA: Jones & Bartlett Publishers, LLC. Allyn & Bacon.

Tanner, D. C. (2003). *The psychology of neurogenic communication disorders: A primer for health care professionals.* Boston, MA: Allyn & Bacon.

Teasell, R. W., Foley, N. C., & Salter, K. (2011). *Evidence-based review of stroke rehabilitation* (14th ed.). Retrieved from http://www.ebrsr.com

Templin, M. C. (1957). *Certain language skills in children.* Minneapolis, MN: University of Minnesota Press.

Thelen, E., & Smith, L. B. (1994). *A dynamic systems approach to the development of cognition and action.* Cambridge, MA: MIT Press.

Thompson, C. K., Shapiro, L. P., Kiran, S., & Sobecks, J. (2003). The role of syntactic complexity in treatment of sentence deficits in agrammatic aphasia: The complexity account of treatment efficacy (CATE). *Journal of Speech, Language, and Hearing Research, 46,* 591–608.

Throneburg, R. N., & Yairi, E. (2001). Durational, proportionate, and absolute frequency characteristics of disfluencies: A longitudinal study regarding persistence and recovery. *Journal of Speech, Language, and Hearing Research, 44,* 38–52.

Thurber, J. (1945). *The Thurber carnival.* New York: Samuel French, Inc.

Tjaden, K., & Wilding, G. (2011). Effects of speaking task on intelligibility in Parkinson's disease. *Clinical Linguistics & Phonetics, 25*(2), 155–168.

Tobey, E. A., Geers, A. E., Brenner, C., Altuna, D., & Gabbert, G. (2003). Factors associated with development of speech production skills in children implanted by age five. *Ear & Hearing, 24,* 36S–45S.

Tomaino, C. M. (2012). Effective music therapy techniques in the treatment of nonfluent aphasia. *Annals of the New York Academy of Sciences, 1252*(1), 312–317.

Tomasello, M. (2003). *Constructing a language: A usage-based theory of language acquisition.* Cambridge, MA: Harvard University Press.

Torgesen, J. K., & Davis, C. (1996). Individual difference variables that predict response to training in phonological awareness. *Journal of Experimental Child Psychology, 63,* 1–21.

Torgesen, J. K., Wagner, R. K., & Rashotte, C. A. (1994). Longitudinal studies of phonological processing and reading. *Journal of Learning Disabilities, 27,* 276–286.

Torres, J., Drebing, D., & Hamilton, R. (2013). TMS and tDCS in post-stroke aphasia: Integrating novel treatment approaches with mechanisms of plasticity. *Restorative Neurology and Neurosciences, 31*(4), 501–515.

Travis, L. E. (1931). *Speech pathology.* New York: Appleton-Century.

Tsaousides, T., & Gordon, W. A. (2009). Cognitive rehabilitation following traumatic brain injury: Assessment to treatment. *Mount Sinai Journal of Medicine, 76,* 173–181.

Turner-Stokes, L., Nair, A., Sedki, I., Disler, P. B., & Wade, D. T. (2011). Multi-disciplinary rehabilitation for brain injury in working-age adults. *The Cochrane Library,* 1.

Tyler, A. A. (2005). Planning and monitoring intervention programs. In A. G. Kamhi & K. E. Pollock (Eds.), *Phonological disorders in -children: Clinical decision making in assessment and intervention* (pp. 123–137). Baltimore, MD: Brookes.

U.S. Bureau of the Census. (2000). *Statistical abstract of the United States* (119th ed.). Washington, DC: U.S. Department of Commerce.

U.S. Department of Education. (2009). Retrieved from http://www.ed.gov/

U.S. Department of State. (2014). *Intercountry adoption.* Retrieved from http://travel.state.gov/content/adoptionsabroad/en.htmlValian, V. (1992). Categories of first syntax: *be, be+ing,* and nothingness. In J. M. Meisel (Ed.), *The acquisition of verb placement: Functional categories and V2 phenomena in language development* (pp. 401–422). Dordrecht, Netherlands: Kluwer.

Van Heugten, C. M., Dekker, J., Deelman, B. G., Stehmann-Saris, J. C., & Kinebanian, A. (2000). Rehabilitation of stroke patients with apraxia: The role of additional cognitive and motor impairments. *Disability and Rehabilitation, 22,* 547–554.

Van Riper, C. (1973). *The treatment of stuttering.* Englewood Cliffs, NJ: Prentice Hall.

Van Riper, C. (1978). *Speech correction: Principles and methods* (6th ed.). Englewood Cliffs, NJ: Prentice Hall.

Van Riper, C. (1982). *The nature of stuttering* (2nd ed.). Englewood Cliffs, NJ: Prentice Hall.

Vanderploeg, R. D., Belanger, H. G., & Curtiss, G. (2009). Mild traumatic brain injury and posttraumatic stress disorder and their associations with health symptoms. *Archives of Physical Medicine and Rehabilitation, 90*(7), 1084–1093.

Vasic, N., & Wijnen, F. (2005). Stuttering as a monitoring deficit. In R. J. Hartsuiker, R. Bastiaanse, A. Postma, & F. Wijnen (Eds.), *Phonological encoding and monitoring in normal and pathological speech* (p. 226). Hove (East Sussex): Psychology Press.

Vaughn, G. R., & Clark, R. M. (1979). *Speech facilitation: Extraoral and intraoral stimulation techniques for improvement of articulation skills.* Springfield, IL: Charles C. Thomas.

Verdolini, K. (1998). *NCVS guide to vocology.* Iowa City, IA: National Center for Voice and Speech, University of Iowa.

Verdolini, K. (2000). Voice disorders. In J. B. Tomblin, H. L. Morris, & D. C. Spriestersbach (Eds.), *Diagnosis in speech-language pathology* (pp. 233–280). San Diego, CA: Delmar Cengage Learning.

Vygotsky, L. (1978). Interaction between learning and development. In *Mind and society* (pp. 79–91). Cambridge, MA: Harvard University Press.

Vygotsky, L. S. (1962). *Thought and language.* Cambridge, MA: MIT Press.

Wagner, R. K., & Torgesen, J. K. (1987). The nature of phonological processing and its causal role in the acquisition of reading skills. *Psychological Bulletin, 101,* 192–212.

Wagner, R. K., Torgesen, J. K., & Rashotte, C. A. (1994). Development of reading-related phonological processing abilities: New evidence of bidirectional causality from a latent variable longitudinal study. *Developmental Psychology, 30,* 73–87.

Wall, M., & Myers, F. (1995). *Clinical management of childhood stuttering.* Austin, TX: Pro-Ed.

Wambaugh, J. L., Duffy, J. R., McNeil, M. R., Robin, D. A., & Rogers, M. A. (2006). Treatment guidelines for acquired apraxia of speech: Treatment descriptions and recommendations. *Journal of Medical Speech-Language Pathology, 14,* xxxv–lxvii.

Wambaugh, J. L., Kalinyak-Fliszar, M. M., West, J. E., & Doyle, P. J. (1998). Effects of treatment for sound errors in apraxia of speech and aphasia, *Journal of Speech, Language, Hearing Research, 41,* 725–743.

Wambuagh, J. L., & Martinez, A. L. (2000). Effects of modified response elaboration training with apraxic and aphasic speakers. *Aphasiology, 14*(5–6), 603–617.

Wambaugh, J. L., & Mauszycki, S. C. (2010). Sound production treatment: Application with severe apraxia of speech. *Aphasiology, 24*(6–8), 814–825.

Wambaugh, J. L., & Nessler, C. (2004). Modification of sound production treatment for aphasia: Generalization effects. *Aphasiology, 18*(5–7), 407–427.

Wambaugh, J. L., Nessler, C., & Wright, S. (2013). Modified response elaboration training: Application to procedural discourse. *American Journal of Speech-Language Pathology, 22,* S409–S425.

Wan, C., Wu, L., Wu, H., Wang, S., & Wan, M. (2012). Assessment of a method for the automatic on/off control of an electrolarynx via lip deformation. *Journal of Voice, 26*(5), 674e21-30.

Ward, D., & Scott, K. (Eds.). (2011). *Cluttering: A handbook of research, intervention, and education.* New York: Psychology Press.

Ward, E. C., Theodoros, D. G., Murdoch, B. E., & Silburn, P. (2000). Changes in maximum capacity tongue function following the Lee Silverman Voice Treatment Program. *Journal of Medical Speech-Language Pathology, 8*, 331–335.

Warren, S. F., Fey, M. E., & Yoder, P. J. (2007). Differential treatment intensity research: A missing link to creating optimally effective communication interventions. *Special Issue: Language and Communication, 13*, 70–77.

Warren, Z., McPheeters, M. L., Sathe, N., Foss-Feig, J. H., Glasser, M. A., & VanderWeele, J. (2011). A systematic review of early intervention for ASD. *Pediatrics, 127*, 1303–1311.

Watkins, K. E., Smith, S. M., Davis, S., & Howell, P. (2008). Structural and functional abnormalities of the motor system in developmental stuttering. *Brain, 131*, 50–59.

Watt, N., Wetherby, A., & Shumway, S. (2006). Prelinguistic predictors of language outcome at 3 years of age. *Journal of Speech, Language & Hearing Research, 49*, 1224–1237.

Weber, R. S., Berkey, B. A., Forastiere, A., Cooper, J., Maor, M., Goepfert, H., et al. (2003). Outcome of salvage total laryngectomy following organ preservation therapy: The radiation therapy oncology group trial 91-11. *Archives of Otolaryngology, Head & Neck Surgery, 129*, 44–49.

Webster, R., Schumacher, S., & Lubker, B. (1970). Changes in stuttering frequency as a function of various intervals of DAF. *Journal of Abnormal Psychology, 75*, 45–49.

Weiner, F. F. (1981). Treatment of phonological disability using the method of meaningful minimal contrast: Two case studies. *Journal of Speech and Hearing Disorders, 46*, 97–100.

Weiss, C. E., Gordon, M. E., & Lillywhite, H. S. (1987). *Clinical management of articulatory and phonological disorders* (2nd ed.). Baltimore, MD: Williams & Wilkins.

Wertz, R. T., Collins, M. J., Weiss, D. G., Kurtzke, J. F., Friden, T., Brookshire, R. H., et al. (1981). Veteran's Administration cooperative study on aphasia: A comparison of individual and group treatment. *Journal of Speech and Hearing Research, 24*, 580–594.

Wertz, R. T., LaPointe, L. L., & Rosenbek, J. C. (1991). *Apraxia of speech in adults: The disorder and its management.* San Diego, CA: Singular.

Wertz, R. T., Weiss, D. G., Aten, J. L., Brookshire, R. H., Garcia-Bunuel, L., Holland, A. L., et al. (1986). Comparison of clinic, home, and deferred language treatment for aphasia: A Veteran's Administration cooperative study. *Archives of Neurology, 43*, 653–658.

Weston, A., & Bain, B. (2003, November). Current vs. evidence-based practice in phonological intervention: A dilemma. Poster session presented at the Annual Convention of the American Speech-Language-Hearing Association, Chicago, IL.

Wetherby, A. M., & Prizant, B. M. (2000). *Autism spectrum disorders: A transactional developmental perspective.* Baltimore, MD: Brookes.

Whitehurst, G., Fischel, J., Lonigan, C., Valdez-Menchaca, M., Arnold, D., & Smith, M. (1991). Treatment of early expressive language delay: If, when, and how. *Topics in Language Disorders, 11*, 55–68.

Whitehurst, G. J. (2002). *Evidence-based education. Presented to the Institute of Education Sciences.* Washington, DC: U.S. Department of Education.

Whitehurst, G. J., Arnold, D. S., Epstein, J. N., & Angell, A. L. (1994). A picture book reading intervention in day care and home for children from low-income families. *Developmental Psychology, 30*(5), 679–689.

Whitehurst, G. J., & Lonigan, C. J. (1998). Child development and emergent literacy. *Child Development, 69*, 848–872.

Wilcox, M. J., & Woods, J. (2011). Participation as a basis for developing early intervention outcomes. *Language, Speech, and Hearing Services in Schools, 42*(3), 365–378.

Williams, A. L. (2002). Epilogue: Perspectives in the assessment of children's speech. *American Journal of Speech-Language Pathology, 11*, 259–263.

Williams, A. L., McLeod, S., & McCauley, R. J. (Eds.). (2010). *Interventions for speech sound disorders in children.* Baltimore, MD: Brookes.

Wingate, M. E. (1964). Recovery from stuttering. *Journal of Speech and Hearing Disorders, 29*, 312–321.

Wingate, M. E. (1976). *Stuttering: Theory and treatment.* New York: Irvington.

Witwer, A.N., & Lecavalier, L. (2008). Examining the validity of autism spectrum disorder subtypes. *Journal of Autism Developmental Disorders, 38*, 1611–1164.

Wolf, M. (1984). Naming, reading, and the dyslexias: A longitudinal overview. *Annals of Dyslexia, 34*, 87–136.

Wolf, M. (1991). Naming speed and reading: The contribution of the cognitive neurosciences. *Reading Research Quarterly, 26*, 123–141.

Wong, B. Y. L. (2000). Writing strategies instruction for expository essay writing for adolescents with and without learning disabilities. *Topics in Language Disorders, 20*, 29–44.

Wong, C., Odom, S. L., Hume, K., Cox, A. W., Fetting, A., Kucharczyk, S., & Schultz, T. R. (2013). *Evidence-based practices for children, youth, and young adults with autism spectrum disorder.* Chapel Hill, NC: The University of North Carolina, Frank Porter Graham Child Development Institute, Autism Evidence-Based Practice Review Group.

Wong, P. C. M., Perrachione, T. K., Gunasekera, G., & Chandrasekaran, B. (2009). Communication disorders in speakers of tone languages: Etiological bases and clinical considerations. *Seminars in Speech and Language, 30*(3), 162–173.

Woods, J. J., & Brown, J. A. (2011). Family capacity-building and child outcomes to support social development in young children with ASD. *Topics in Language Disorders, 31*, 235–246.

World Health Organization (WHO). (2001). *ICF: International classification of functioning, disability, and health-report.* Geneva, Switzerland: Author. Retrieved from http://www.who.int/classifications/icf/en/

Worrall, L., Sherratt, S., Rogers, P., Howe, T., Hersh, D., Ferguson, A., & Davidson, B. (2011). What people with aphasia want: Their goals according to the ICF. *Aphasiology, 25*(3), 309–322.

Woynaroski, T., Yoder, P. J., Fey, M. E., & Warren, S. F. (2014). A transactional model of spoken vocabulary variation in toddlers with intellectual disabilities. *Journal of Speech, Language, and Hearing Research.* doi:10.1044/2014_JSLHR-L-13-0252

Yairi, E., & Ambrose, N. G. (1999). Early childhood stuttering I: Persistency and recovery rates. *Journal of Speech, Language, and Hearing Research, 42,* 1097–1112.

Yairi, E., & Ambrose, N. G. (2001). Longitudinal studies of childhood stuttering: Evaluation of critiques. *Journal of Speech, Language, and Hearing Research, 44,* 867–872.

Yairi, E., & Ambrose, N. (2013). Epidemiology of stuttering: 21st century advances. *Journal of Fluency Disorders, 38,* 66–87.

Yairi, E., Currin, L. H., Bulian, N., & Yairi, J. (1974). Incidence of hoarseness in school children over a 1 year period. *Journal of Communication Disorders, 7,* 321–328.

Yairi, E., & Seery, C. (2014). *Stuttering: Foundations and clinical applications* (2nd ed.). Upper Saddle River, NJ: Pearson Education, Inc.

Yalom, I. (1980). *Existential psychotherapy.* New York: Basic Books.

Yaruss, J. S. (1998). Describing the consequences of disorders: Stuttering and the International Classification of Impairments, Disabilities, and Handicaps. *Journal of Speech, Language, and Hearing Research, 49,* 249–257.

Yaruss, S. (2010). Assessing quality of life in stuttering treatment outcomes research. *Journal of Fluency Disorders, 35,* 190–202.

Yavas, M., & Lamprecht, R. (1988). Processes and intelligibility in disordered phonology. *Clinical Linguistics and Phonetics, 2,* 329–345.

Yirmiya, N., & Charman, T. (2010). The prodome of autism: early behavioral and biological signs, regression, peri- and post-natal development and genetics. *Journal of Child Psychology and Psychiatry, 51*(4), 432–458.

Ylvisaker, M., Szekeres, S. F., & Feeney, T. J. (2008). Communication disorders associated with traumatic brain injury. In R. Chapey (Ed.), *Language intervention strategies in adult aphasia* (5th ed., pp. 879–962). Baltimore, MD: Lippincott, Williams, & Wilkins.

Ylvisaker, M., Turkstra, L., Coelho, C., Yorkston, K., Kennedy, M., Sohlberg, M., & Avery, J. (2007). Behavioural interventions for children and adults with behaviour disorders after TBI: A systematic review of the evidence. *Brain Injury, 21*(8), 769–805.

Yoder, P., Fey, M. E., & Warren, S. F. (2012). Studying the impact of intensity is important but complicated. *International Journal of Speech-Language Pathology, 14*(5), 410–413.

Yorkston, K. M. (1996). Treatment efficacy: Dysarthria. *Journal of Speech and Hearing Research, 39,* S46–S57.

Yorkston, K. M., Beukelman, D. R., & Bell, K. R. (1988). *Clinical management of dysarthric speakers.* Boston, MA: Little, Brown.

Yorkston, K. M., Hakel, M., Beukelman, D. R., & Fager, S. (2007). Evidence for effectiveness of treatment of loudness, rate, or prosody in dysarthria: A systematic review. *Journal of Medical Speech & Language Pathology, 15,* xi–xxxvi.

Yorkston, K. M., Miller, R. M., & Strand, E. A. (2004). *Management of speech and swallowing in degenerative diseases.* Austin, TX: Pro-Ed.

Youmans, G., Holland, A., Muñoz, M., & Bourgeois, M. (2005). Script training and automaticity in two individuals with aphasia. *Ahasiology, 19*(3–5), 435–450.

Youmans, G., Youmans, S. R., & Hancock, A. B. (2011). Script training treatment for adults with apraxia of speech. *American Journal of Speech-Language Pathology, 20*(1), 23–37.

Zebrowski, P. M. (1994). Stuttering. In J. B. Tomblin, H. L. Morris, & D. C. Spriestersbach (Eds.), *Diagnosis in speech-language pathology* (pp. 215–245). San Diego, CA: Singular.

Zebrowski, P. M. (1997). Assisting young children who stutter and their families: Defining the role of the speech-language pathologist. *American Journal of Speech-Language Pathology, 6*(2), 19–28.

Zemlin, W. R. (1998). *Speech and hearing science.* Needham Heights, MA: Allyn & Bacon.

Zero to Three. (2012). *National center for infants, toddlers, and families.* Retrieved from http://www.zerotothree.org

Index

Pages numbers followed by "t" or "f" indicate that the entry is included in a table or figure.